Core Concepts in Acute Kidney Injury

Sushrut S. Waikar • Patrick T. Murray
Ajay K. Singh
Editors

Core Concepts in Acute Kidney Injury

Springer

Editors
Sushrut S. Waikar
Renal Division
Brigham and Women's Hospital
Harvard Medical School
Boston, MA
USA

Ajay K. Singh
Renal Division
Brigham and Women's Hospital
Harvard Medical School
Boston, MA
USA

Patrick T. Murray
University College Dublin
Dublin
Ireland

ISBN 978-1-4939-8626-2   ISBN 978-1-4939-8628-6 (eBook)
https://doi.org/10.1007/978-1-4939-8628-6

Library of Congress Control Number: 2018950405

Printed on acid-free paper

This Springer imprint is published by the registered company Springer Science+Business Media, LLC part of Springer Nature
The registered company address is: 233 Spring Street, New York, NY 10013, U.S.A.

Preface

Acute kidney injury or AKI refers to an extremely heterogeneous group of clinical conditions that share common diagnostic features: a rise in the serum creatinine concentration and/or a decrease in urine output. These two elements that comprise the diagnostic criteria for AKI reflect major life-sustaining functions of the kidneys, which are to clear the blood of waste products and to regulate circulating plasma volume. A wide array of conditions can acutely injure or impair kidney function and result in a diagnosis of AKI, including tubular injury, tubulointerstitial nephritis, glomerulonephritis, and pre-renal azotemia (functional AKI).

AKI has a multitude of causes. Worldwide, the most common cause of AKI is pre-renal azotemia from diarrheal illnesses. Environmental exposures, toxins, and injuries are among the many environmental factors that can lead to AKI. Over the past 30 years, the advent of new technologies to diagnose and treat human disease has resulted in a whole new set of causes of AKI, such as cardiac surgery, immune checkpoint inhibitors, iodinated contrast media, and various nephrotoxic injuries.

Notions about the natural history of AKI date back to a seminal report by Swann and Merrill in 1953 that espoused sequential phases: initiation, maintenance, extension, and recovery. This description was based on cases of severe oligoanuric AKI in hospitalized individuals at the Peter Bent Brigham Hospital who had conditions barely recognizable in today's modern hospitals, such as transfusion reactions (25%), distilled water irrigation or infusion (9%), and carbon tetrachloride toxicity (8%)—in addition to more recognizable entities such as postoperative hemorrhage (21%). AKI today frequently does not adhere to the idealized phases outlined by Swann and Merrill.

The importance of AKI as a public health issue in both the developed and developing world is indisputable. AKI is a major risk factor for prolonged length of stay, mortality, and subsequent cardiovascular disease and chronic kidney disease. AKI continues to evolve as our population ages, new environmental threats arise, and new drugs and procedures with nephrotoxic potential are developed. Along with this, basic and clinical investigation into AKI prevention and treatment continues. Although only a single drug has been FDA approved for the treatment or prevention of AKI ("Osmitrol" or intravenous mannitol, approved on June 8, 1964), a number of novel targets and strategies are being investigated, with some promising signs.

In this textbook, we have invited leading clinicians, epidemiologists, basic scientists, and clinical trialists to provide an update on AKI. After reading their contributions, we hope you will share both their and our optimism and enthusiasm for a future in which AKI prevention and treatment will be yet another one of modern medicine's success stories.

Boston, MA, USA — Sushrut S. Waikar
Dublin, Ireland — Patrick T. Murray
Boston, MA, USA — Ajay K. Singh

Contents

Contributors

Alian A. Al-balas, MD Division of Nephrology, University of Alabama at Birmingham, Birmingham, AL, USA

Rashid Alobaidi, MD Division of Critical Care, Department of Pediatrics, Faculty of Medicine and Dentistry, University of Alberta, Edmonton, AB, Canada

Sean M. Bagshaw, MD, MSc Department of Critical Care Medicine, Faculty of Medicine and Dentistry, University of Alberta, Edmonton, AB, Canada

Justin M. Belcher, MD, PhD Section of Nephrology, Department of Internal Medicine, Yale University School of Medicine, New Haven, CT, USA

Frederic T. Billings IV, MD, MSc Department of Anesthesiology, Vanderbilt University, Nashville, TN, USA

Joseph V. Bonventre Renal Division and Engineering in Medicine Division, Department of Medicine, Brigham and Women's Hospital, Harvard Medical School, Boston, MA, USA

Division of Health Sciences and Technology, Harvard-Massachusetts Institute of Technology, Cambridge, MA, USA

Harvard Stem Cell Institute, Cambridge, MA, USA

Steven L. Chang Division of Urology, Department of Surgery, Brigham and Women's Hospital, Harvard Medical School, Boston, MA, USA

Paras Dedhia, MD Division of Nephrology, Department of Internal Medicine, Kidney CARE Program, University of Cincinnati, Cincinnati, OH, USA

Jeremy R. DeGrado, PharmD, BCPS Pharmacy Department, Brigham and Women's Hospital, Boston, MA, USA

Luca Di Lullo, MD, PhD Department of Nephrology and Dialysis, L. Parodi-Delfino Hospital, Colleferro, Italy

Zoltan H. Endre, BMedSci, MBBS, PhD, FRACP, FASN Department of Nephrology, Prince of Wales Hospital and Clinical School, University of New South Wales, Sydney, NSW, Australia

Jairam R. Eswara Division of Urology, Department of Surgery, Brigham and Women's Hospital, Harvard Medical School, Boston, MA, USA

David A. Ferenbach Department of Renal Medicine, Royal Infirmary of Edinburgh, Edinburgh, UK

MRC Centre of Inflammation Research, University of Edinburgh, Edinburgh, UK

Michael A. Ferguson, MD Division of Nephrology, Department of Medicine, Boston Children's Hospital, Harvard Medical School, Boston, MA, USA

Steven Gabardi, PharmD Department of Transplant Surgery, Brigham and Women's Hospital, Boston, MA, USA

Department of Pharmacy Services/Renal Division, Brigham and Women's Hospital, Boston, MA, USA

Harvard Medical School, Boston, MA, USA

James F. Gilmore, PharmD, BCPS Department of Pharmacy Services, Brigham and Women's Hospital, Boston, MA, USA

Glenda C. Gobe, BSc, MSc, PhD, GradDipEd School of Medicine, Centre for Kidney Disease Research, University of Queensland, Brisbane, QLD, Australia

Shruti Gupta, MD Division of Renal Medicine, Department of Medicine, Brigham and Women's Hospital, Boston, MA, USA

Benjamin Hohlfelder, PharmD Department of Pharmacy Services, Brigham and Women's Hospital, Boston, MA, USA

Elizabeth A. K. Hunt, MD Department of Pediatrics, Division of Pediatric Nephrology, University of Vermont Medical Center, Larner College of Medicine at UVM, Burlington, VT, USA

Vivekanand Jha, MD DM FAMS FRCP(London and Edin) George Institute for Global Health India, New Delhi, India

George Institute for Global Health, University of Oxford, UK

Jay L. Koyner, MD Section of Nephrology, Department of Medicine, University of Chicago, Chicago, IL, USA

Kelly V. Liang, MD Renal-Electrolyte Division, Department of Medicine, University of Pittsburgh School of Medicine, Pittsburgh, PA, USA

Randy L. Luciano, MD, PhD Section of Nephrology, Department of Internal Medicine, Yale University School of Medicine, New Haven, CT, USA

Colm C. Magee, MD, MPH, FRCPI Department of Nephrology, Beaumont Hospital, Dublin, Ireland

Alain Meyrier, MD, PhD Service de Néphrologie, Hôpital Georges Pompidou, Université Paris-Descartes Medical School, Paris, France

José A. Morfín, MD Division of Nephrology, Department of Internal Medicine, University of California Davis School of Medicine, Sacramento, CA, USA

Patrick T. Murray, MD, FASN, FRCPI, FJFICMI School of Medicine, University College Dublin, Dublin, Ireland

Patrick Niaudet, MD Department of Pediatric Nephrology, Hôpital Necker-Enfants Malades, Université Paris-Descartes, Paris, France

Sagar U. Nigwekar, MD, MMSc Department of Medicine/Nephrology, Massachusetts General Hospital, Boston, MA, USA

Jason B. O'Neal, MD Department of Anesthesiology, Vanderbilt University Medical Center, Nashville, TN, USA

Eoin D. O'Sullivan Department of Renal Medicine, Royal Infirmary of Edinburgh, Edinburgh, UK

MRC Centre of Inflammation Research, University of Edinburgh, Edinburgh, UK

Marlies Ostermann, PhD Department of Nephrology and Critical Care Medicine, King's College London, Guy's & St Thomas' Foundation Hospital, London, UK

Evan P. Owens, BS(Hons) Centre for Kidney Disease Research, The University of Queensland, Brisbane, QLD, Australia

Paul M. Palevsky, MD Renal Section, Medical Service, VA Pittsburgh Healthcare System, Pittsburgh, PA, USA

Renal-Electrolyte Division, Department of Medicine, University of Pittsburgh School of Medicine, Pittsburgh, PA, USA

Sreejith Parameswaran, MD, DM Department of Nephrology, Jawaharlal Institute of Postgraduate Medical Education and Research, Pondicherry, India

Chirag R. Parikh, MD, PhD Section of Nephrology, Department of Internal Medicine, Yale University School of Medicine, New Haven, CT, USA

Mark A. Perazella, MD, MS Section of Nephrology, Yale University School of Medicine, New Haven, CT, USA

Department of Medicine, Yale University, New Haven, CT, USA

Timothy J. Pianta, MBBS(Hons), FRACP, PhD Northern Clinical School, University of Melbourne, Epping, VIC, Australia

John R. Prowle, MA, MB, BChir, MSc, MD, FFICM Critical Care and Perioperative Medicine Research Group, William Harvey Research Institute, Barts and the London School of Medicine and Dentistry, Queen Mary University of London, London, UK

Valary T. Raup Division of Urology, Department of Surgery, Brigham and Women's Hospital, Harvard Medical School, Boston, MA, USA

Lynn Redahan, MB, BCh, BAO School of Medicine, University College Dublin, Dublin, Ireland

Claudio Ronco, MD, PhD International Renal Research Institute, S. Bortolo Hospital, Vicenza, Italy

Aparna Sharma, MD Section of Nephrology, Department of Medicine, University of Chicago, Chicago, IL, USA

Andrew D. Shaw, MB, FRCA, FCCM, FFICM, MMHC Department of Anesthesiology and Pain Medicine, University of Alberta, Edmonton, AB, Canada

Craig A. Stevens, PharmD Department of Pharmacy Services, Brigham and Women's Hospital, Boston, MA, USA

Charuhas V. Thakar, MD Division of Nephrology, Department of Internal Medicine, Kidney CARE Program, University of Cincinnati, Cincinnati, OH, USA

Ashita J. Tolwani, MD, MSc Division of Nephrology, University of Alabama at Birmingham, Birmingham, AL, USA

Sushrut S. Waikar, MD, MPH Division of Renal Medicine, Brigham and Women's Hospital, Harvard Medical School, Boston, MA, USA

Steven D. Weisbord, MD, MSc Renal-Electrolyte Division, Department of Medicine, VA Pittsburgh Healthcare System, University of Pittsburgh School of Medicine, Pittsburgh, PA, USA

Renal Section and Center for Health Equity Research and Promotion, VA Pittsburgh Healthcare System, Pittsburgh, PA, USA

Keith M. Wille, MD, MSPH Division of Pulmonary, Allergy, and Critical Care Medicine, University of Alabama at Birmingham, Birmingham, AL, USA

Part I

Epidemiology and Diagnosis

Epidemiology, Incidence, Risk Factors, and Outcomes of Acute Kidney Injury

1

Marlies Ostermann

1.1 Background

Acute kidney injury (AKI) is a syndrome which comprises many different types of renal disease. It is defined as an abrupt decline in kidney function. There are numerous different aetiologies, but the most common causes of AKI are sepsis, volume depletion, haemodynamic instability and nephrotoxic drugs. AKI is a frequent complication in hospitalised patients, especially in the intensive care unit (ICU). The exact incidence and prognosis depend on the specific patient population, the presence of comorbid factors and the overall severity of illness but also the criteria used to define AKI. There is increasing evidence that AKI is associated with serious short- and long-term medical problems, premature mortality and high healthcare costs.

The definition of AKI has evolved from the Risk, Injury, Failure, Loss, End-stage (RIFLE) criteria in 2004 to the AKI Network (AKIN) classification in 2007. In 2012, both were merged resulting in the Kidney Disease: Improving Global Outcomes (KDIGO) classification. Accordingly, AKI is diagnosed if serum creatinine increases by 0.3 mg/dL (26.5 μmol/L) or more in ≤48 h or rises to at least 1.5-fold from baseline within 7 days [1] (Table 1.1). AKI stages are defined by the maximum change of either serum creatinine or urine output. The importance of both criteria was confirmed in a study in >32,000 critically ill patients which showed that short- and long-term risk of death or renal replacement therapy (RRT) was greatest when patients met both criteria for AKI and when these abnormalities persisted for longer than 3 days [2].

Although serum creatinine is routinely used in clinical practice, it has important limitations which impact the diagnosis of AKI [3, 4] (Table 1.2). The serum creatinine concentration may take 24–36 h to rise after a definite renal insult [5]. Furthermore, creatinine generation depends on liver function and muscle bulk. Therefore, in patients with liver disease, muscle wasting and/or sepsis, a true fall in GFR may not be adequately reflected by the serum creatinine concentration. Serum creatinine can also change following exposure to certain drugs without a change in renal function. In addition, serum creatinine concentrations may be affected by the method used in the laboratory. Substances like bilirubin or drugs can interfere with certain analytical techniques, more commonly with Jaffe-based assays [4]. Finally, serum creatinine is measured as a concentration and therefore affected by variations in volume status. This means that the diagnosis of AKI may be delayed or missed in patients with rapid fluid accumulation.

M. Ostermann
Department of Nephrology and Critical Care Medicine, King's College London, Guy's & St Thomas' Foundation Hospital, London, UK
e-mail: Marlies.Ostermann@gstt.nhs.uk

S. S. Waikar et al. (eds.), *Core Concepts in Acute Kidney Injury*,
https://doi.org/10.1007/978-1-4939-8628-6_1

Table 1.1 KDIGO definition and classification of AKI (Diagnostic criteria for AKI and AKI staging system)

AKI is defined as any of the following:

- Increase in serum creatinine by ≥0.3 mg/dL (≥26.4 μmol/L) within 48 h
- Increase in serum creatinine to ≥1.5 times baseline, which is known or presumed to have occurred within the prior 7 days
- Urine volume < 0.5 mL/kg/h for 6 h

AKI stage	Serum creatinine criteria	Urine output criteria
AKI stage I	Increase of serum creatinine by ≥0.3 mg/dL (≥26.4 μmol/L) or Increase to 1.5—1.9 times from baseline	Urine output < 0.5 mL/kg/h for 6–12 h
AKI stage II	Increase of serum creatinine to 2.0—2.9 times from baseline	Urine output < 0.5 mL/kg/h for ≥12 h
AKI stage III	Increase of serum creatinine ≥3.0 times from baseline or Serum creatinine ≥4.0 mg/dL (≥354 μmol/L) or Treatment with RRT or In patients <18 years, decrease in estimated GFR to <35 mL/min per 1.73 m^2	Urine output < 0.3 mL/kg/h for ≥24 h or Anuria for ≥12 h

Abbreviations: *AKI* acute kidney injury, *GFR* glomerular filtration rate, *RRT* renal replacement therapy

Table 1.2 Potential pitfalls of AKI diagnosis based on creatinine and urine criteria

Clinical scenario	Consequence
Reduced production of creatinine (i.e. muscle wasting, liver disease, sepsis)	Delayed or missed diagnosis of AKI
Ingestion of substances which lead to increased generation of creatinine independent of renal function (i.e. creatine products, cooked meat)	Misdiagnosis of AKI
Administration of drugs which inhibit tubular secretion of creatinine (i.e. cimetidine, trimethoprim)	Misdiagnosis of AKI
Conditions associated with physiologically increased GFR (i.e. pregnancy)	Delayed diagnosis of AKI
Interference with laboratory technique of measuring creatinine (i.e. 5-fluorocytosine, cefoxitin, bilirubin)	Misdiagnosis/delayed diagnosis of AKI (depending on substance)
Rapid fluid accumulation	Delayed diagnosis of AKI (dilution of serum creatinine concentration)
Progressive CKD with gradual rise in serum creatinine	Misdiagnosis of AKI
Obesity	Overdiagnosis of AKI if actual weight is used when applying urine output criteria
Oliguria due to acute temporary release of ADH (i.e. post-operatively, nausea, pain)	Misdiagnosis of AKI

Abbreviations: *AKI* acute kidney injury, *ADH* antidiuretic hormone, *CKD* chronic kidney disease, *GFR* glomerular filtration rate

Another important limitation of all creatinine-based definitions of AKI is that they require a reference value to describe "baseline" renal function. Ideally, the reference value should reflect the patient's steady-state kidney function immediately before the episode of AKI. However, information on pre-hospital kidney function may not always be available. In this case, various methods are used to estimate renal function, including the application of in-patient results. Another approach is to assume that patients with missing results had normal baseline renal function. It is clear that these different methods can inflate as well as reduce the true incidence of AKI.

All current AKI classifications also include urine criteria. Urine output is an important clinical sign but, like creatinine, it is not renal specific. In fact, urine output may persist until renal function almost ceases. In contrast, oliguria may be an appropriate physiological response of functioning kidneys during periods of prolonged fasting, hypovolaemia, after surgery and following stress, pain or trauma. Finally, in obese patients, weight-based urine output criteria may be particularly misleading if urine output is calculated in mL/min/kg without adjusting for lean body weight.

These limitations of both serum creatinine and urine output need to be acknowledged when interpreting epidemiology data related to AKI.

1.2 Epidemiology

The reported incidence of AKI has increased in the last 20 years due to changes in population (ageing/comorbidities) and healthcare (increasing use of potentially nephrotoxic drugs, contrast media, high-risk interventions) but also increased awareness and recognition. In high-income countries, AKI affects between 7 and 22% of hospital in-patients. Older and critically ill patients are particularly at risk. A large, multinational meta-analysis of 154 studies published between 2004 and 2012 showed that the pooled incidence of AKI among hospitalised patients was 22% [6]. Patients with AKI had five times greater odds of death than those without AKI.

The International Society of Nephrology conducted a global snapshot study during a 10-week period in 2014 and collected the data of 4018 hospitalised patients with AKI from 8 geographical regions (North America, Latin America, Caribbean, Europe, Middle East, Asia, Oceania and Africa) [7]. The median age was 60 years with younger patients more commonly seen in lower-income countries. Chronic heart and liver diseases were more frequent in patients from high-income countries, whereas dehydration was the most common cause of AKI in lower-income countries. Twenty-two percent of all patients were treated with RRT. Mortality at 7 days was 12% in lower-income countries and 10% in high-income countries.

Acute kidney injury is particularly common during critical illness, affecting >50% of patients in the ICU of whom a quarter need RRT [8]. Hospital mortality appears to increase in a stepwise manner with increasing AKI severity.

Less is known about the true incidence of AKI in the community. The majority of data stems from hospital-only studies that identified patients who had an elevated serum creatinine at the time of hospital admission and were therefore assumed to have community-acquired AKI. For instance, an analysis of 15,976 patients admitted to hospital showed that 4.3% had AKI on admission to hospital compared to 2.1% of patients with hospital-acquired AKI [9]. Patients with AKI on admission were more likely to have AKI stage III but had a shorter length of stay in hospital than patients with hospital-acquired AKI. They also had better hospital survival (80.4% versus 57.2%, respectively) and survival 14 months later (55% versus 37%, respectively).

The incidence and outcome of patients with AKI in the community who are not admitted to hospital remain unclear. Studies are in progress to address this issue.

1.3 Risk Factors for the Development of AKI

In general, the risk for any disease represents the interaction between susceptibility (i.e. features intrinsic to the patient) and type and extent of exposure (i.e. causative factors) which may or may not be modifiable (Table 1.3). Typical exposures known to produce AKI in susceptible patients include sepsis; major surgery, in particular cardiovascular and emergency surgery; and nephrotoxic drugs. Typical risk factors which increase the susceptibility for AKI are age, pre-existing chronic kidney disease (CKD), left ventricular dysfunction, liver disease and proteinuria. A previous episode of AKI also increases the risk of a further event.

Table 1.3 Risk factors for AKI

Non-modifiable factors	Potentially modifiable factors
Older age	Use of nephrotoxic drugs
Female gender	Obesity
Genetics	Hyperuricaemia
CKD	Diabetes with proteinuria
Previous episode of AKI	Hypoalbuminaemia
Chronic heart disease	
Chronic liver disease	

Abbreviations: *AKI* acute kidney injury, *CKD* chronic kidney disease

The importance of proteinuria as a risk factor for AKI was highlighted in a prospective cohort of 11,200 participants in the Atherosclerosis Risk in Communities (ARIC) study [10]. Using a urine albumin-to-creatinine ratio <10 mg/g as a reference, the relative hazards of AKI after an average follow-up of 8 years, adjusted for age, gender, race, cardiovascular risk factors, and categories of estimated glomerular filtration rate (eGFR), were 1.9 [(95% confidence interval (CI) 1.4–2.6)], 2.2 (95% CI 1.6–3.0) and 4.8 (95% CI 3.2–7.2) for urine albumin-to-creatinine ratio groups of 11–29 mg/g, 30–299 mg/g and ≥300 mg/g, respectively.

Recent studies have identified several other nontraditional risk factors [11]:

(a) Hyperuricaemia: The risk of AKI from hyperuricaemia and intratubular uric acid crystallisation is well known in the context of tumour lysis syndrome. Hyperuricaemia has also been identified as a risk factor for AKI in patients undergoing cardiac surgery [12]. The potential underlying pathophysiological mechanisms appear to be related to renal vasoconstriction and increased oxidative stress.
(b) Hypoalbuminaemia: A meta-analysis of 11 observational studies including 2745 patients from various medical and surgical cohorts concluded that the adjusted odds ratio for AKI was 2.34 per 10 g/L decrement in serum albumin [13]. Subsequent studies showed similar results with no convincing evidence that albumin supplementation ameliorates the risk.
(c) Obesity: There is a consistent signal that the risk of AKI increases with rising body mass index (BMI) [14, 15]. The reported rates of AKI in patients undergoing bariatric surgery are between 6 and 8% which is significantly higher than following elective orthopaedic or general surgery. The exact reasons are not known, but obesity is often associated with traditional risk factors for AKI. In addition, drug dosing can be challenging in obese patients, and the risk of harm from nephrotoxic drugs is higher. However, it should also be acknowledged that reports showing links between obesity and AKI may be confounded by the fact that AKI is overdiagnosed if urine output is measured in mL/kg/h without adjusting for lean body weight (Table 1.2).
(d) Hydroxyethyl starch solutions: Starch solutions are effective volume expanders. Different preparations are available that vary with regard to mean molecular weight, molar substitution, concentration and substitution of hydroxyethyl for hydroxyl groups. There is clear evidence that they can deposit in the skin, liver, spleen and kidneys. Several randomised controlled trials and systematic reviews have concluded that their use is independently associated with an increased risk of AKI [16–20].
(e) Genetics: Evidence suggests that genetic factors play a very important role and influence patients' susceptibility to nephrotoxic exposures [21, 22].

Understanding an individual patient's susceptibility and risk profile is essential to prevent or ameliorate AKI through modification and avoidance of non-essential potentially nephrotoxic exposures.

1.4 CKD, CVD and ESRD as Possible Outcomes After an Episode of AKI

After an episode of AKI, there are four potential outcomes:

1. Full recovery of renal function to baseline:
2. Incomplete recovery of renal function resulting in de novo CKD
3. Exacerbation of pre-existing CKD and accelerated progression towards end-stage renal disease (ESRD)
4. Non-recovery of function leading directly to ESRD

It was previously assumed that patients who recovered kidney function after an episode of AKI had a favourable outcome. However, there is convincing evidence that this is not always the case. Complete recovery from severe AKI is far less common than previously assumed, and CKD

Table 1.4 Short- and long-term complications of AKI

Short-term complications	Long-term complications
Uraemia	Proteinuria
Fluid accumulation	CKD/ESRD
Dosing errors of renally excreted medications	Risk of cardiovascular morbidity
Non-recovery of renal function	Risk of strokes
Prolonged stay in hospital	Hypertension
Organ crosstalk (i.e. effects of AKI on distant organ systems)	Risk of fractures
Healthcare costs	Risk of infections/sepsis
	Recurrent AKI
	Premature mortality
	Healthcare costs
	Reduced quality of life

Abbreviations: *CKD* chronic kidney disease, *ESRD* end-stage renal disease

post AKI has now been recognised as a major public health problem [23–29] (Table 1.4).

AKI survivors represent a high-risk group facing significant chronic health problems, including CKD, cardiovascular and cerebrovascular events, infections and premature mortality (Table 1.5). Patients with diabetes, chronic vascular disease and pre-existing proteinuria and CKD are particularly vulnerable to the development of CKD after AKI. Other risk factors include older age and genetic predisposition.

AKI and CKD are clearly interlinked where CKD is a risk factor for AKI and AKI is associated with a long-term risk of CKD [30] (Fig. 1.1). A meta-analysis of 13 retrospective studies confirmed that patients with AKI had an almost 9 times higher risk of developing CKD, a 3 times greater risk of ESRD needing long-term dialysis and a 2 times higher risk of premature death compared to patients without AKI [26]. The risk of CKD and ESRD is particularly high in patients with more severe and more prolonged AKI. Follow-up data of the ATN study demonstrated that 24.6% of patients with AKI requiring RRT were still RRT dependent at 60 days [31]. Wald et al. compared 3769 adults with dialysis-dependent AKI to 13,598 matched controls who did not have acute dialysis [24]. After a median follow-up of 3 years, the incidence of

Table 1.5 Select studies demonstrating links between AKI and CKD

Study	Population	Effect of AKI on CKD
Ishani et al., 2009 [23]	233,803 hospitalised patients >67 years	Relative risk of ESRD 13.0
Wald et al., 2009 [24]	3769 patients with dialysis-dependent AKI versus 13,598 controls	Rate of ESRD In AKI patients: 2.63/100 person-years In controls: 0.9/100 person-years
Chawla et al., 2011 [25]	5351 patients with AKI	Development of CKD stage IV: 13.6%
Coca et al., 2012 [26]	>1,000,000 participants	Hazard ratio for new CKD 8.8 Hazard ratio for ESRD 3.1
Bucaloiu et al., 2012 [27]	1610 AKI patients without pre-existing CKD who recovered renal function within 90% of baseline eGFR compared to 3652 matched controls without AKI	Hazard ratio of de novo CKD during 3.3 year follow-up in AKI patients: 1.91
Heung et al., 2015 [28]	VA in-patients 17,049 patients with AKI 87,715 patients without AKI	Relative risk of new CKD III, IV or V AKI <3 days: 1.43 AKI 3–10 days: 2.0 AKI >10 days: 2.65

Abbreviations: *AKI* acute kidney injury, *CKD* chronic kidney disease, *ESRD* end-stage renal disease, *eGFR* estimated glomerular filtration rate

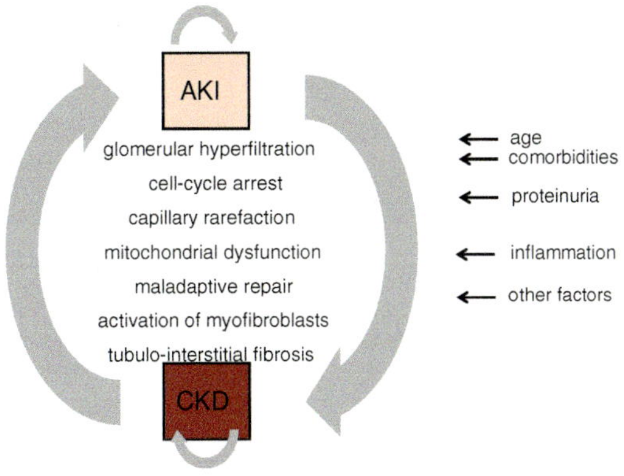

Fig. 1.1 Relationship between AKI and CKD. Abbreviations: *AKI* acute kidney injury, *CKD* chronic kidney disease

chronic dialysis in the AKI cohort was 2.63/100 person-years compared to 0.91/100 person-years among controls (adjusted HR, 3.23; 95% CI, 2.70–3.86).

Other long-term risks of AKI survivors are cardiovascular and cerebrovascular events, fractures, infections, gastrointestinal haemorrhage and premature mortality [32–36] (Fig. 1.2). Analysis of a large matched cohort study including 4869 patients of the Taiwan National Health Insurance Database who had recovered from dialysis-dependent AKI showed a significantly higher incidence of coronary events compared to matched controls without AKI (19.8 versus 10.3 per 1000 person-years, respectively), independent of the development of CKD [32]. In addition, survivors of AKI also had a higher incidence of strokes, bone fractures and de novo severe sepsis [33–35].

Quality of life (QoL) after AKI is another important outcome that has been investigated in several studies with mixed results. A systematic review including 18 studies concluded that health-related QoL of survivors of critical illness complicated by AKI was reduced when referenced to population norms but it was not significantly different from that of survivors without AKI [37]. Although physical limitations and disabilities were more commonly experienced by AKI patients, the impaired QoL was generally perceived as acceptable to patients.

Finally, the risk of premature death in patients who survived AKI is high, especially in those with more severe AKI. Follow-up analysis of the RENAL study, a multicentre RRT dosing study, showed that only one third of patients who had had acute RRT whilst in the ICU were alive 3.5 years later [38]. A prospective cohort evaluation of 2010 ICU patients in a tertiary care centre revealed that even survivors of AKI stage I had significantly lower 10-year survival rates than matched critically ill patients without AKI [39].

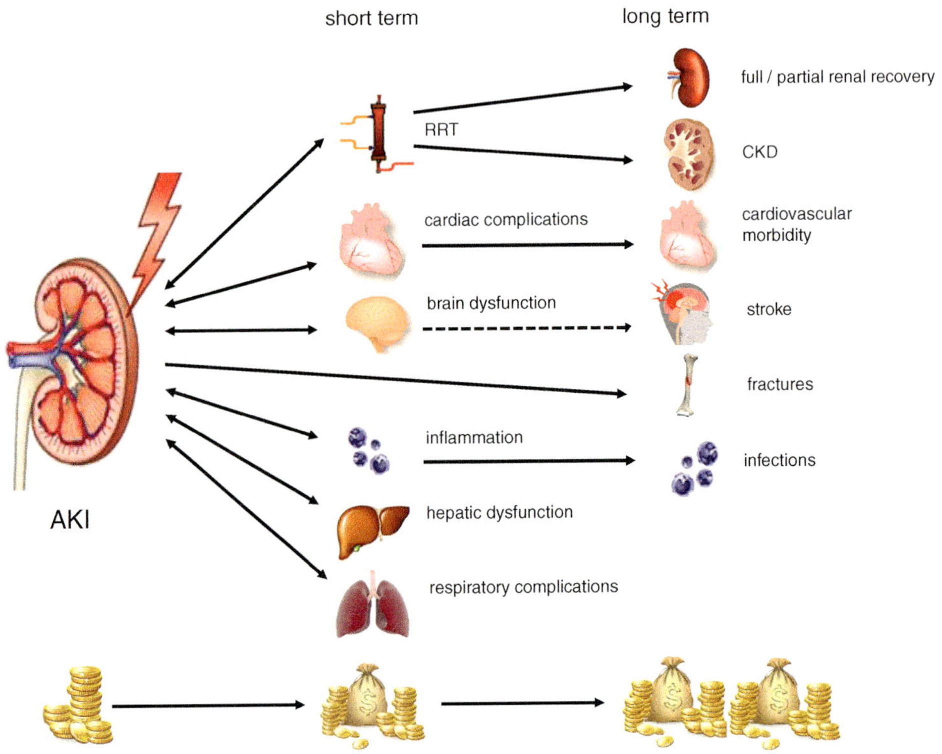

Fig. 1.2 Short- and long-term complications of acute kidney injury

1.5 Risk Factors for Poor Outcomes Following AKI

The reasons for the high risk of long-term complications and premature mortality after AKI are not fully understood but likely to be multifactorial, including pre-existing comorbidities and factors directly related to AKI per se [30]. In general, AKI occurs more frequently in an older population with a greater burden of recognised and unrecognised health problems in whom there may be a higher risk of adverse events anyway. In many patients, the factors that predisposed to AKI continue to exist after the episode of AKI has finished. For instance, Harel et al. followed survivors of dialysis-dependent AKI who had recovered renal function and showed that pre-existing CKD [hazard ratio (HR), 3.86; 95% CI, 2.99–4.98], hypertension (HR, 1.82; 95% CI, 1.28–2.58) and a higher Charlson comorbidity index score (HR, 1.10; 95% CI, 1.05–1.15/per unit) were significantly associated with risk of progression to ESRD [40].

The relationship between AKI and CKD also depends on the severity, duration, frequency and nature of AKI [41–43]. An analysis of 5351 patients with normal baseline renal function who had AKI whilst in hospital showed that severity of AKI was a strong predictor of CKD stage IV [42]. Advanced age, low serum albumin and the presence of diabetes were also predictive. Analysis of a Veterans' data set of over 3600 patients with diabetes revealed that in those with repeated episodes of AKI, each additional AKI event resulted in a doubling of the CKD risk [43].

The aetiology of AKI may also impact long-term renal sequelae. Patients with multifactorial AKI appear to have a higher risk of long-term CKD compared to those with single-cause AKI. However, more detailed work is necessary to investigate the link between specific aetiologies of AKI and risk of CKD.

1.6 Potential Pathogenetic Mechanisms for AKI: CKD Transition

In the aftermath of AKI, changes persist in the kidney, even if serum creatinine initially returns to baseline [44, 45]. Important processes involved in the pathophysiology and recovery from AKI play a role, including cell cycle arrest, maladaptive repair, recruitment of infiltrating inflammatory and stem cells, capillary rarefication, glomerular hyperfiltration and activation of myofibroblasts and fibrocytes [46] (Fig. 1.1).

1. *Endothelial injury and reduced capillary density*: Vascular density is reduced after an episode of AKI, resulting in activation of hypoxia-inducible pathways and promotion of pro-inflammatory and pro-fibrotic processes. In a vicious circle, capillary rarefaction, hypoxic signalling and tissue hypoxia may mutually reinforce each other leading to further damage and fibrosis.
2. *Glomerular hyperfiltration*: AKI can lead to a critical loss of nephron mass that exceeds the regenerative capability of the kidney to fully recovery. Hyperfiltration followed by hypertrophy of the residual glomeruli causes an increase in workload of tubular cells. This can lead to hypoxic signalling and stimulation of tubulo-interstitial fibrosis, the latter of which is a significant component in the development of CKD.
3. *Cell cycle arrest*: Mitotic arrest at the G2/M phase of the cell cycle in response to AKI is a natural, usually protective process. However, if prolonged, it can lead to maladaptive repair of damaged tubular cells and progressive fibrosis through the secretion of pro-fibrotic factors and the stimulation of myofibroblasts [44].
4. *Mitochondrial dysregulation*: In health, mitochondria constantly undergo regular fission and fusion. During cell injury, the dynamics are shifted to fission, a process that is associated with damage in the outer and inner membranes of the organelles and membrane leakage. A persistent disruption of mitochondrial homeostasis after AKI has been demonstrated which can lead to suboptimal cellular respiration, reduction in cellular adenosine triphosphate (ATP) levels and consequent tissue dysfunction, all contributing to the development of chronic cell damage.
5. *Maladaptive repair*: It has been shown that following an episode of AKI, dedifferentiated

tubular cells fail to redifferentiate during the repair phase and exhibit a persistent pro-fibrotic signal which leads to the activation of myofibroblasts [30, 42]. The range of change in response to tubular injury and the balance of full repair and maladaptive repair can comprise the entire spectrum of renal disease following AKI.

6. *Tubulo-interstitial inflammation/fibrosis*: Tubulo-interstitial fibrosis is a predominant feature of CKD following AKI. Tubular hypertrophy, reduced capillary density, recruitment of inflammatory cells and activation of fibroblasts play an important role in the pathogenesis [30]. Pro-fibrotic processes are initiated and maintained by ongoing production and secretion of a variety of peptides, including cytokines and growth factors. Although they are necessary for repair and tubule regeneration, these bioactive molecules have a stimulating effect on perivascular fibroblasts and the development of fibrosis.

A better understanding of the pathophysiological processes and key regulators is necessary to develop potential therapies and interventions.

Conclusions

Acute kidney injury is common and associated with serious short- and long-term complications and premature mortality. The underlying reasons are not fully understood, but pre-existing comorbidities and factors related to the pathophysiology of AKI per se play a role. More in-depth research is urgently required to identify the key factors and potential therapeutic interventions.

References

1. Kidney Disease: Improving Global Outcomes (KDIGO) Acute Kidney Injury Work Group. KDIGO clinical practice guideline for acute kidney injury. Kidney Int. 2012;2:1–138.
2. Kellum JA, Sileanu FE, Murugan R, Lucko N, Shaw AD, Clermont G. Classifying AKI by urine output versus serum creatinine level. J Am Soc Nephrol. 2015;26(9):2231–8.
3. Ostermann M. Diagnosis of acute kidney injury: Kidney Disease Improving Global Outcomes criteria and beyond. Curr Opin Crit Care. 2014;20(6):581–7.
4. Thomas M, Blaine C, Dawnay A, et al. The definition of acute kidney injury and its use in practice. Kidney Int. 2015;87(1):62–73.
5. Endre ZH, Pickering JW. New markers of acute kidney injury: giant leaps and baby steps. Clin Biochem Rev. 2011;32(2):121–4.
6. Susantitaphong P, Cruz DN, Cerda J, Abulfaraj M, Alqahtani F, Koulouridis I, et al. World incidence of AKI: a meta-analysis. Clin J Am Soc Nephrol. 2013;8(9):1482–93.
7. Mehta RL, Burdmann EA, Cerda J, et al. Recognition and management of acute kidney injury in the International Society of Nephrology 0by25 Global Snapshot: a multinational cross-sectional study. Lancet. 2016;387:2017–25.
8. Hoste E, Bagshaw SM, Bellomo R, et al. Epidemiology of acute kidney injury in critically ill patients: the multinational AKI-EPI study. Intensive Care Med. 2015;41(8):1411–23.
9. Wonnacott A, Meran S, Amphlett B, Talabani B, Phillips A. Epidemiology and outcomes in community-acquired versus hospital-acquired AKI. Clin J Am Soc Nephrol. 2014;9(6):1007–14.
10. Grams ME, Astor BC, Bash LD, Matsushita K, Wang Y, Coresh J. Albuminuria and estimated glomerular filtration rate independently associate with acute kidney injury. J Am Soc Nephrol. 2010;21(10):1757–64.
11. Varrier M, Ostermann M. Novel risk factors for acute kidney injury. Curr Opin Nephrol Hypertens. 2014;23:560–9.
12. Park SH, Shin WY, Lee EY, et al. The impact of hyperuricemia on in-hospital mortality and incidence of acute kidney injury in patients undergoing percutaneous coronary intervention. Circ J. 2011;75(3):692–7.
13. Wiedermann CJ, Wiedermann W, Joannidis M. Hypoalbuminemia and acute kidney injury: a meta-analysis of observational clinical studies. Intensive Care Med. 2010;36(10):1657–65.
14. Kumar AB, Bridget Zimmerman M, Suneja M. Obesity and post-cardiopulmonary bypass-associated acute kidney injury: a single-center retrospective analysis. J Cardiothorac Vasc Anesth. 2014;28(3):551–6.
15. Suneja M, Kumar AB. Obesity and perioperative acute kidney injury: a focused review. J Crit Care. 2014;29(4):694.e1–6.
16. Wiedermann CJ. Systematic review of randomized clinical trials on the use of hydroxyethyl starch for fluid management in sepsis. BMC Emerg Med. 2008;8:1.
17. Myburgh JA, Finfer S, Bellomo R, et al. Hydroxyethyl starch or saline for fluid resuscitation in intensive care. N Engl J Med. 2012;367(20):1901–11.
18. Perner A, Haase N, Guttormsen AB, et al. Hydroxyethyl starch 130/0.42 versus Ringer's acetate in severe sepsis. N Engl J Med. 2012;367(2):124–34.
19. Haase N, Perner A, Hennings LI, et al. Hydroxyethyl starch 130/0.38–0.45 versus crystalloid or albumin

in patients with sepsis: systematic review with meta-analysis and trial sequential analysis. BMJ. 2013;346:f839.
20. Zarychanski R, Abou-Setta AM, Turgeon AF, et al. Association of hydroxyethyl starch administration with mortality and acute kidney injury in critically ill patients requiring volume resuscitation: a systematic review and meta-analysis. JAMA. 2013;309(7):678–88.
21. Cardinal-Fernandez P, Ferruelo A, Martin-Pellicer A, et al. Genetic determinants of acute renal damage risk and prognosis: a systematic review. Med Intensiva. 2012;36(9):626–33.
22. Zhao B, Lu Q, Cheng Y, et al. A genome-wide association study to identify single-nucleotide polymorphisms for acute kidney injury. Am J Respir Crit Care Med. 2017;195(4):482–90.
23. Ishani A, Xue JL, Himmelfarb J, et al. Acute kidney injury increases risk of ESRD among elderly. J Am Soc Nephrol. 2009;20(1):223–8.
24. Wald R, Quinn RR, Luo J, et al. Chronic dialysis and death among survivors of acute kidney injury requiring dialysis. JAMA. 2009;302:1179–85.
25. Chawla LS, Amdur RL, Amodeo S, Kimmel PL, Palant CE. The severity of acute kidney injury predicts progression to chronic kidney disease. Kidney Int. 2011;79:1361–9.
26. Coca SG, Singanamala S, Parikh CR. Chronic kidney disease after acute kidney injury: a systematic review and meta-analysis. Kidney Int. 2012;81:442–8.
27. Bucaloiu ID, Kirchner HL, Norfolk ER, Hartle JE, Perkins RM. Increased risk of death and de novo chronic kidney disease following reversible acute kidney injury. Kidney Int. 2012;81:477–85.
28. Heung M, Steffick DE, Zivin K, et al. Acute kidney injury recovery pattern and subsequent risk of CKD: an analysis of Veterans Health Administration Data. Am J Kidney Dis. 2016;67(5):742–52.
29. Lewington AJ, Cerda J, Mehta RL. Raising awareness of acute kidney injury: a global perspective of a silent killer. Kidney Int. 2013;84(3):457–67.
30. Chawla LS, Eggers PW, Star RA, Kimmel PL. Acute kidney injury and chronic kidney disease as interconnected syndromes. N Engl J Med. 2014;371(1):58–66.
31. VA/NIH Acute Renal Failure Trial Network. Intensity of renal support in critically ill patients with acute kidney injury. N Engl J Med. 2008;359(1):7–20.
32. Wu VC, Wu CH, Huang TM, et al. Long-term risk of coronary events after AKI. J Am Soc Nephrol. 2014;25(3):595–605.
33. Wu VC, Wu PC, Wu CH, et al. The impact of acute kidney injury on the long-term risk of stroke. J Am Heart Assoc. 2014;3(4):e000933.
34. Wang WJ, Chao CT, Huang YC, et al. The impact of acute kidney injury with temporary dialysis on the risk of fracture. J Bone Miner Res. 2014;29(3):676–84.
35. Lai TS, Wang CY, Pan SC, et al. Risk of developing severe sepsis after acute kidney injury: a population-based cohort study. Crit Care. 2013;17(5):R231.
36. Wu PC, Wu CJ, Lin CJ, et al. Long-term risk of upper gastrointestinal hemorrhage after advanced AKI. Clin J Am Soc Nephrol. 2015;10(3):353–62.
37. Villeneuve PM, Clark EG, Sikora L, Sood MM, Bagshaw SM. Health-related quality-of-life among survivors of acute kidney injury in the intensive care unit: a systematic review. Intensive Care Med. 2016;42(2):137–46.
38. Gallagher M, Cass A, Bellomo R, et al. Long-term survival and dialysis dependency following acute kidney injury in intensive care: extended follow-up of a randomized controlled trial. PLoS Med. 2014;11(2):e1001601.
39. Linder A, Fjell C, Levin A, Walley KR, Russell JA, Boyd JH. Small acute increases in serum creatinine are associated with decreased long-term survival in the critically ill. Am J Respir Crit Care Med. 2014;189(9):1075–81.
40. Harel Z, Bell CM, Dixon SN, et al. Predictors of progression to chronic dialysis in survivors of severe acute kidney injury: a competing risk study. BMC Nephrol. 2014;15:114.
41. Ishani A, Nelson D, Clothier B, et al. The magnitude of acute serum creatinine increase after cardiac surgery and the risk of chronic kidney disease, progression of kidney disease and death. Arch Intern Med. 2011;171:226–33.
42. Chawla LS, Kimmel PL. Acute kidney injury and chronic kidney disease: an integrated clinical syndrome. Kidney Int. 2012;82:516–24.
43. Thakar CV, Christianson A, Himmelfarb J, Leonard AC. Acute kidney injury episodes and chronic kidney disease risk in diabetes mellitus. Clin J Am Soc Nephrol. 2011;6:2567–72.
44. Ferenbach DA, Bonventre JV. Acute kidney injury and chronic kidney disease: from the laboratory to the clinic. Nephrol Ther. 2016;12(12 Suppl):S41–8.
45. Ferenbach DA, Bonventre JV. Mechanisms of maladaptive repair after AKI leading to accelerated kidney ageing and CKD. Nat Rev Nephrol. 2015;11(5):264–76.
46. Varrier M, Forni LG, Ostermann M. Long-term sequelae from acute kidney injury: potential mechanisms for the observed poor renal outcomes. Crit Care. 2015;19(1):R102.

2 Definition and Classification of Acute Kidney Injury

Kelly V. Liang and Paul M. Palevsky

Acute kidney injury (AKI) is the sudden loss of kidney function, characterized by a rapid decline in the glomerular filtration rate (GFR), usually occurring over a period of hours to days. The loss of kidney function leads to the retention of metabolic waste products (e.g., urea and creatinine) and abnormalities of fluid, electrolyte, and acid-base homeostasis [1]. AKI is not a discrete disease; rather it is a heterogeneous syndrome associated with a broad constellation of pathophysiologic processes of variable severity and etiology. From a didactic standpoint, AKI is often subdivided into three broad pathophysiologic categories—prerenal AKI, intrinsic AKI, and post-renal AKI.

Prerenal AKI arises when hypoperfusion of the kidneys causes a reduction in glomerular filtration rate without causing overt parenchymal damage. Etiologies of prerenal AKI include both states of overt volume depletion and states of decreased effective arterial blood volume (EABV), as seen with heart failure, hepatic cirrhosis, and nephrotic syndrome. *Intrinsic AKI* encompasses multiple diseases involving the renal parenchyma including acute and rapidly progressive glomerulonephritis, acute interstitial nephritis, acute tubular injury, and acute vascular syndromes, such as seen with atheroembolic disease. The most common etiology of intrinsic AKI is acute tubular necrosis (ATN) resulting from ischemia-reperfusion injury, nephrotoxins, or sepsis. *Post-renal (obstructive) AKI* results from the acute obstruction of the urinary tract with either partial or complete obstruction to urinary flow. Although severe post-renal AKI requires obstruction of the bladder outlet or bilateral ureteral obstruction (or unilateral ureteral obstruction with an absent or nonfunctional contralateral kidney), lesser decrements in kidney function can be seen with unilateral ureteral obstruction, even in the presence of a normal contralateral kidney. Although this tripartite categorization conceptually is useful, considerable overlap may exist. For example, prerenal AKI may be associated with subclinical parenchymal injury, and prolonged prerenal or post-renal states may result in parenchymal damage.

The term AKI has now generally supplanted the older terminology of acute renal failure (ARF). This evolution in terminology reflects a recognition that the relationship between normal kidney function and overt organ failure is not

K. V. Liang
Renal-Electrolyte Division, Department of Medicine, University of Pittsburgh School of Medicine, Pittsburgh, PA, USA
e-mail: liangk@upmc.edu

P. M. Palevsky (✉)
Renal Section, Medical Service, VA Pittsburgh Healthcare System, Pittsburgh, PA, USA

Renal-Electrolyte Division, Department of Medicine, University of Pittsburgh School of Medicine, Pittsburgh, PA, USA
e-mail: palevsky@pitt.edu

S. S. Waikar et al. (eds.), *Core Concepts in Acute Kidney Injury*,
https://doi.org/10.1007/978-1-4939-8628-6_2

dichotomous but rather that small to modest acute decrements in kidney function are associated with adverse outcomes. Although the newer terminology emphasizes the graded aspect of acute kidney disease, this terminology is also imperfect. The term "injury" implies the presence of parenchymal organ damage, even though parenchymal injury is not characteristic of the acute decrement in kidney function associated with prerenal or post-renal AKI [2, 3]. Although the term AKI has sometimes been used interchangeably with ATN, these terms are not synonymous. While ATN is one of the most common forms of intrinsic AKI, particularly in critically ill patients, it represents only one of multiple etiologies of AKI. Furthermore, even in patients with a classic presentation of AKI in the setting of sepsis or ischemia-reperfusion injury, there may be a lack of concordance between the clinical syndrome of and the histopathologic findings described by the term ATN [4, 5].

2.1 Diagnosis and Staging of AKI

Prior to the last decade, there was no uniform operational definition of AKI. The AKI literature was characterized by a multitude of definitions, primarily based on a varying combination of absolute and relative changes in creatinine concentration in the blood. These definitions occasionally incorporated criteria based on urine output, with urine volumes of less than 400–500 mL/day defining oliguria and less than 100 mL/day classified as anuria [6]. The lack of consensus across these definitions limited understanding of the epidemiology of AKI and impeded comparisons across studies.

2.2 RIFLE Criteria

In 2002, the Acute Dialysis Quality Initiative (ADQI) group proposed the first of a series of three related consensus definitions of AKI. This definition, known by the acronym RIFLE (*Risk*, *Injury*, *Failure*, *Loss*, and *End-stage*), defined AKI utilizing three strata of criteria of increasing stringency based on relative change in creatinine concentration in the blood and duration of oliguria and two outcomes, based on duration of need for renal replacement therapy (Table 2.1). The first level (*Risk*) was defined as an increase in blood creatinine concentration to more than 1.5 times the baseline over no more than 7 days or the presence of oliguria, defined as a urine output of <0.5 mL/kg per hour, for more than 6 h. The second level (*Injury*) increased the stringency of the definition to an increase in creatinine concentration in the blood to more than two times the baseline or the presence of oliguria, again defined as a urine output of <0.5 mL/kg per hour, for more than 12 h. The third level (*Failure*) utilized even more stringent cutoffs, with the blood creatinine concentration needing to exceed more than three times the baseline value or, in patients with acute-on-chronic disease, increase by more than 0.5 mg/dL to a value of more than 4 mg/dL. The corresponding urine output criteria were oliguria, now defined as a urine output of <0.3 mL/kg per hour, for more than 24 h, and anuria for more than 12 h [7]. The concept underlying this three-tiered definition was that *Risk* would provide the most sensitive criteria and that each of the subsequent tiers would provide greater specificity at the expense of decreased sensitivity [8–10]. The final two tiers of the RIFLE criteria represented outcomes, with *Loss* defined as dialysis dependence for >4 weeks and *End-stage* as need for renal replacement therapy for more than 3 months.

In its original form, the *Risk*, *Injury*, and *Failure* categories also included criteria based on declines in eGFR of 25%, 50%, and 75%, respectively [9]. These eGFR criteria were subsequently dropped based on criticism that calculated eGFR should not be utilized as an index of kidney function in AKI since in the non-steady-state conditions that characterize AKI, creatinine levels in the blood do not correlate with glomerular filtration rate. Furthermore, even if the changes in blood creatinine concentration did correlate with calculated eGFR, the proposed decrements in eGFR did not correlate with the expected changes in eGFR associated with the 50%, 100%, and 200% increments in blood creatinine concentration (the corresponding decline in eGFR would be approximately 33%, 50%, and 67%, respectively, if blood creatinine was in steady state).

Table 2.1 RIFLE and AKIN and KDIGO criteria for diagnosis and staging of AKI

RIFLE class AKIN/KDIGO AKI stage	Blood creatinine criteria			Urine output criteria (common to all)
	RIFLE[a]	AKIN[b]	KDIGO	
RIFLE-Risk AKIN/KDIGO stage 1	Increase in creatinine to >1.5× baseline	Increase in creatinine to ≥0.3 mg/dL or Increase in creatinine to ≥150–200% of baseline	Increase in creatinine to ≥0.3 mg/dL within 48 h or increase in creatinine to ≥150–200% of baseline over <7 days	Urine output <0.5 mg/kg/h for >6 h
RIFLE-Injury AKIN/KDIGO stage 2	Increase in creatinine to >2× baseline	Increase in creatinine to >200–300% of baseline	Increase in creatinine to >200–300% of baseline	Urine output <0.5 mg/kg/h for >12 h
RIFLE-Failure AKIN/KDIGO stage 3	Increase in creatinine to >3× baseline or Increase in creatinine of ≥0.5 mg/dL to a value of ≥4 mg/dL	Increase in creatinine to >300% of baseline or Increase in creatinine to ≥4 mg/dL with an acute increase of ≥0.5 mg/dL or On RRT	Increase in creatinine to >300% of baseline or Increase in creatinine to ≥4 mg/dL with an acute increase of ≥0.3 mg/dL or Initiation of RRT or In patients <18 years, a decrease in eGFR to <35 mL/min per 1.73 m^2	Urine output <0.3 mg/kg/h for >24 h or Anuria for >12 h
RIFLE-Loss	Need for RRT for >4 weeks			
RIFLE-End-stage kidney disease	Need for RRT for >3 months			

Abbreviations: *AKI* acute kidney injury, *AKIN* Acute Kidney Injury Network, *KDIGO* Kidney Disease: Improving Global Outcomes, *RIFLE* Risk, Injury, Failure, Loss, End-stage disease, *RRT* renal replacement therapy, *eGFR* estimated glomerular filtration rate

[a]For RIFLE, the increase in blood creatinine concentration should be abrupt (within 7 days) and sustained (>24 h)

[b]For AKIN, AKI is defined as meeting the stage 1 criteria with the increase in blood creatinine concentration occurring in less than 48 h

2.3 Acute Kidney Injury Network (AKIN) Definition and Staging Criteria

The Acute Kidney Injury Network (AKIN) proposed modification to the RIFLE criteria. The most significant change proposed by AKIN was the addition of an absolute increase in blood creatinine concentration of ≥0.3 mg/dL to the >50% relative increase in blood creatinine concentration from the RIFLE-Risk criteria, specifying that these increases develop over no more than 48 h. This change was based on an epidemiologic study that demonstrated that an increase in blood creatinine concentration of 0.3–0.4 mg/dL was associated with an 80% increase in the odds of death during hospitalization [11]. In addition, AKIN introduced a more fundamental conceptual change. Unlike the original RIFLE concept of nested definitions of AKI characterized by increasing stringency, the AKIN criteria adopted a single definition, based on an increase in the creatinine concentration in blood of ≥0.3 mg/dL or ≥50% as compared to baseline developing over no more than 48 h or oliguria (0.5 mL/kg per hour) for more than 6 h. The *Injury* and *Failure* strata from the RIFLE criteria were transformed into subsequent "stages" of severity of AKI. In addition, initiation of renal replacement therapy was proposed as an additional criterion for stage 3 AKI. The AKIN criteria also eliminated the two outcome levels (*Loss* and *End-stage*) from the RIFLE criteria (Table 2.1).

2.4 Kidney Disease: Improving Global Outcomes (KDIGO) Classification

More recently, the Kidney Disease: Improving Global Outcomes (KDIGO) acute kidney injury workgroup proposed a revision to the AKIN definition and staging system as part of the KDIGO Clinical Practice Guidelines for Acute Kidney Injury. The KDIGO definition and staging system harmonizes several of the inconsistencies between the prior RIFLE and AKIN criteria. In the KDIGO definition, the urine output criteria, which were the same in RIFLE and AKIN, were retained without change. The increase in blood creatinine concentration of ≥0.3 mg/dL within 48 h that had been proposed by AKIN was retained, but the time frame for the ≥50% increase in blood creatinine concentration was extended to 7 days, as originally proposed in the RIFLE criteria. The concept of a single definition with three stages of severity was retained, with only minor modifications from the AKIN criteria (Table 2.1). One modification was that the minimum threshold change in blood creatinine concentration required to be classified as stage 3 based on a blood creatinine of >4 mg/dL was changed from ≥0.5 mg/dL to ≥0.3 mg/dL to be consistent with the underlying definition of AKI.

The KDIGO workgroup also recognized an important nosological conundrum created by the gap between the definition of AKI based on changes in blood creatinine concentration over less than 7 days duration and the definition of CKD based on the presence of kidney disease of more than 90-day duration. Patients with decrements in kidney function that were present for less than 90 days but that developed more gradually than required to meet the definition of AKI did not fall into either category. For this reason, the KDIGO workgroup introduced the term acute kidney diseases and disorders (AKD) defined as AKI or a GFR of <60 mL/min/1.73 m^2, a decline in eGFR of ≥35%, or an increase in the concentration of creatinine in the blood of ≥50% of less than 3-month duration.

2.5 AKI Definition and Staging in Pediatric Patients

The RIFLE criteria were modified for use in pediatric patients as the pRIFLE criteria [12]. The primary modifications to apply these criteria to children were the replacement of the blood creatinine concentration/eGFR criteria with declines in estimated creatinine clearance (eCrCl) calculated using the Schwartz formula, which better reflects the importance of weight-based calculations of renal function in children and alterations in the duration of oliguria to 8, 16, and 24 h, respectively (Table 2.2) [8, 12]. In addition, acute reduction in eCrCl to <35 mL/min/1.73 m^2 was added as a criterion for pRIFLE-Failure. In the KDIGO criteria, the only modification of the adult criteria for pediatric patients is the retention from the pRIFLE criteria of an acute reduction in eGFR (or eCrCl) to <35 mL/min/1.73 m^2 in patients <18 years in the criteria for stage 3 AKI.

2.6 Validation of AKI Definitions

Optimal validation of a definition of AKI would be based on an incontrovertible "gold standard" for the diagnosis. Unfortunately, such a standard

Table 2.2 Pediatric modified RIFLE (pRIFLE) criteria for diagnosis and classification of AKI in children

Class	eCCl	Urine output
Risk	eCCl decrease by >25%	Urine output <0.5 mL/kg/h for >8 h
Injury	eCCl decrease by >50%	Urine output <0.5 mL/kg/h for >16 h
Failure	eCCl decrease by >75% or eCCl <35 mL/min/1.73 m^2	Urine output <0.3 mL/kg/h for >24 h; or Anuria for >12 h
Loss	Persistent failure for >4 weeks	
End-stage kidney disease	Persistent failure for >3 months	

Abbreviations: *AKI* acute kidney injury, *eCrCl* estimated creatinine clearance using the Schwartz formula, *RIFLE* Risk, Injury, Failure, Loss, End-stage disease does not exist. The use of change in blood creatinine concentration as a marker for change in kidney function has substantial face validity. The reliability of the urine output criteria and the clinical evidence to support the specific thresholds selected were less robust. Cross validation of the different classification schemes has demonstrated expected differences in diagnosis and staging. For example, in an analysis of over 14,356 critically ill patients, 5093 (35%) were diagnosed with AKI using the RIFLE criteria as compared to 4093 (28%) using the AKIN definition and staging system [13]. Among the 9263 patients who were not diagnosed with AKI based on the RIFLE criteria, 504 (5%) were diagnosed as having AKI using the AKIN definition, while 1504 of the 10,263 patients (15%) who did not have AKI by the AKIN definition were classified as RIFLE-Risk (781 patients), RIFLE-Injury (452 patients), or RIFLE-Failure (271 patients).

The majority of studies assessing the validity of the AKI definitions have used mortality as their primary outcome. In the cross validation study cited above, increasing severity of AKI using either RIFLE or AKIN was associated with an increased risk of hospital mortality [13]. Similar findings have been observed across a wide range of clinical settings including sepsis, trauma, post-cardiac surgery, and hematopoietic cell transplant populations [2, 14–20]. Most recently, the Acute Kidney Injury-Epidemiologic Prospective Investigation (AKI-EPI) study prospectively evaluated the KDIGO definition and staging system among 1802 ICU patients in 97 intensive care units in 33 countries in North and South America, Europe, Africa, Asia, and Australia [21]. Increasing AKI severity was associated with progressively greater risk for in-hospital mortality when adjusted for other variables. The odds of death increased from 1.68 (95% CI 0.89–3.17; $p = 0.11$) with stage 1 AKI to 2.95 (95% CI 1.38–6.28; $p = 0.005$) with stage 2 AKI and 6.88 (95% CI 3.88–12.23; $p < 0.001$) with stage 3 AKI as compared to patients without AKI [21]. Patients developing AKI had worse kidney function at hospital discharge with an eGFR <60 mL/min/1.73 m^2 in 47.7% (95% CI 43.6–51.7) in those with AKI as compared to only 14.8% (95% CI 11.9–18.2) in those without AKI [21].

2.7 Limitations of the Current Definitions and Staging Criteria

The definitions of AKI are based on the long-standing clinical use of blood creatinine concentration as a marker of kidney function. Creatinine is an endogenous marker of glomerular filtration produced from muscle within an individual at a relatively constant rate and predominantly excreted in the urine primarily by filtration at the glomerulus. Thus, over relatively short periods of time, changes in the creatinine concentration in blood generally reflect reciprocal changes in glomerular filtration rate. Increases in blood creatinine concentration correspond to decrements in GFR, while decreases in creatinine concentration correspond to increases in GFR. There are, however, several important caveats to this relationship that need to be recognized. First, a small percentage of creatinine is excreted by tubular secretion with the percentage excreted by secretion increasing in patients with underlying kidney disease. Thus, medications such as trimethoprim and cimetidine that can interfere with creatinine secretion may raise blood creatinine levels in the absence of changes in kidney function. Second, several drugs, such as cefoxitin and flucytosine, and metabolic intermediates, such as acetoacetate, may interfere with colorimetric assays for creatinine, resulting in artifactual elevations. Third, serum creatinine concentrations may be affected by alterations in volume of distribution. Thus rapid fluid resuscitation may blunt the rise in creatinine levels in the blood despite marked impairment of kidney function. Fourth, creatinine production may be altered in acute illness. For example, studies have suggested that creatinine generation declines early in sepsis [22]. Thus, the use of definitions based on changes in blood creatinine concentration is subject to inherent limitations. Other markers, such as cystatin C, have been proposed as alternatives to creatinine in the assessment of kidney function [23–26], but are not widely used in clinical practice.

Separate from these more generic issues, several additional limitations regarding the consensus definitions have been raised. Since a definition that is based on change in a laboratory parameter requires a baseline value for comparison, one key issue in the use of these definitions is selection of the most appropriate baseline value for comparison. It has been suggested that in hospitalized patients, the ideal comparator should be a recent premorbid outpatient blood creatinine concentration; however, these values are often not available. In an analysis of alternative surrogate baseline creatinine measurements, Siew and colleagues found significant bidirectional misclassification associated with use of the first admission blood creatinine value, the lowest inpatient value, or back-calculation using an assumed eGFR of 75 mL/min/1.73 m^2 [27].

Using a threshold change in blood creatinine concentration of as little as 0.3 mg/dL is associated with several issues. Although small changes in blood creatinine concentration are associated with increased mortality risk and were the justification of the 0.3 mg/dL threshold, there remains uncertainty whether the mortality risk is mediated by these changes or whether small changes are merely a marker of diminished renal reserve and underlying vascular disease, either of which might be an independent mediator of mortality risk. Second, the significance of small changes in blood creatinine concentration varies based on the underlying level of kidney function. Thus, an increase in blood creatinine concentration from 0.7 to 1.0 mg/dL represents a much more significant change in kidney function than an increase from 3.2 to 3.5 mg/dL. While the first represents both a substantial absolute and relative decline in glomerular filtration, the latter may represent changes in glomerular filtration consistent within the range of normal biologic variability in patients with chronic kidney disease.

In addition, the use of small changes in serum creatinine to define AKI increases the likelihood of misclassification based on both inherent biological variability in blood creatinine concentration and errors in laboratory measurement. In a simulation analysis using known coefficients of laboratory and biological variability, use of a threshold of 0.3 mg/dL was associated with an 8% rate of incorrect diagnosis of AKI, with a markedly higher false-positive rate in individuals with a baseline blood creatinine concentration of ≥1.5 mg/dL (false-positive rate of AKI approximately 30%) as compared to individuals with a baseline blood creatinine concentration of <1.5 mg/dL (false-positive rate of AKI of approximately 2%) [28].

Another limitation that has been suggested is that the definitions were developed without regard to consideration of creatinine kinetics. In the setting of severe AKI, the initial rate of increase in the blood creatinine concentration is relatively independent of baseline kidney function although the time required to attain a fixed percent change in blood creatinine concentration is dependent on the baseline creatinine concentration [29]. Therefore, early in the course of AKI, absolute changes in blood creatinine concentration may be more readily detected than relative changes in concentration. Using a kinetic modeling approach, Waikar and colleagues simulated creatinine kinetics after AKI in the setting of normal baseline kidney function and stages 2, 3, and 4 CKD [29]. In their model, 24 h after a 90% reduction in GFR, the blood creatinine concentration increased 2.5-fold if baseline kidney function was normal but increased only by approximately 50% in an individual with a baseline eGFR of 15–30 mL/min/1.73 m^2. In contrast, the absolute increase in blood creatinine concentration was nearly identical (1.8–2.0 mg/dL) regardless of baseline kidney function. Qualitatively similar results were observed with a lesser acute reduction in kidney function [29]. Thus, based on creatinine kinetics, the use of graded absolute, rather than relative increases in blood creatinine concentration over 24 or 48 h, might provide a more robust diagnostic approach. In addition, these analyses suggest that a >0.3 mg/dL increase in creatinine concentration is an appropriate threshold for the diagnosis of AKI if the increase occurs over a 24-h interval but that the robustness of the definition is diminished if this increase occurs over 48 h.

Several limitations related to the urine output criteria also need to be noted. In settings outside of intensive care units, documentation of urine output is often unreliable. Furthermore, in retrospective epidemiologic studies, data on urine output is often missing, even in critically ill patients, limiting the diagnosis and staging of AKI entirely to changes in blood creatinine concentration. Several other limitations to use of urine output should be recognized. Urine output may be highly sensitive to volume resuscitation and diuretic administration. Oliguria may be the appropriate physiologic response to volume depletion, and the use of urine output as a marker of kidney dysfunction in an inadequately fluid resuscitated patient may be misleading [8]. Similarly, diuretic administration may decrease sensitivity of these criteria. The indexing of urine output to weight, while of critical importance in pediatric patients, decreases the reliability of these criteria in morbidly obese patients given the lack of a linear relationship between weight and urine volume in obesity. For example, in a patient who weighs 180 kg, a normal urine output of 1 L over 12 h would satisfy the criteria for stage 2 AKI. Further, it should be noted that only a small number of studies have correlated the urine output criteria for AKI with mortality and other adverse clinical outcomes and have found poor calibration between the urine output criteria and the blood creatinine criteria with regard to mortality risk [10].

Similar to the criteria for defining and staging chronic kidney disease (CKD), the definition and staging of AKI is independent of the underlying etiology of kidney dysfunction. Given the broad range of etiologies of AKI, with widely varying implications with regard to both management and prognosis, this is a significant limitation to these definition and staging criteria. The importance of identifying a specific etiology in the patient with AKI was explicitly recognized in the KDIGO Clinical Practice Guideline for AKI, which includes the guideline recommendation that "the cause of AKI should be determined whenever possible" immediately following the guideline statements encompassing the definition and staging of AKI.

Unlike the staging criteria for CKD, the staging of AKI is not clearly linked to the level of kidney function. Since blood levels of creatinine are not in steady state during AKI, there may be discordance between the time course of changes in creatinine concentration and underlying changes in kidney function. In a patient whose GFR acutely falls from near normal to <10 mL/min/1.73 m^2, blood creatinine concentration will progressively increase over several days. Applying the staging criteria prospectively will result in the appearance of worsening AKI. Given the lack of correlation between blood creatinine concentration and GFR, a patient may even progress with regard to AKI stage despite actual improvement in kidney function. This limitation is less significant when staging is applied retrospectively after resolution of the AKI episode. In addition, the staging does not take into consideration duration of AKI, which has been shown to be an independent predictor of mortality and other outcomes [30].

2.8 Use of AKI Definitions in Epidemiology and Clinical Research

The availability of a standardized AKI definition is invaluable to the conduct of epidemiologic studies. In the absence of a standardized definition, a wide array of criteria for the diagnosis of AKI were used, limiting the ability to compare the results of trials and trend rates of AKI over time. A standardized definition is also of potential benefit in identifying populations for inclusion in therapeutic trials of established AKI and as an endpoint in trials for the prevention of AKI. Unfortunately, there are limitations to the applicability of these definitions. As previously noted, data on urine output are often lacking in retrospective cohort studies, and prehospitalization creatinine measurements are often not available. However, despite these limitations, numerous epidemiologic studies utilizing these criteria have been undertaken across multiple patient populations. The availability of a standard definition may also improve administrative coding for AKI. Prior studies using administrative databases have underestimated the true period prevalence of AKI due to poor sensitivity of administrative coding for non-dialysis-requiring AKI [31].

2.9 Utility of AKI Definitions and Staging in Clinical Care

The utility and applicability of the AKI definitions and staging systems in clinical practice are less certain. The change in paradigm from acute renal failure to acute kidney injury has increased awareness of the importance of small changes in kidney function on patient outcomes, particularly in critically ill patients. What is less certain is the applicability of the definition and staging to clinical management. The KDIGO Clinical Practice Guidelines for AKI propose that patients with AKI be managed according to stage and cause as shown in Fig. 2.1 [3]. While this opinion-based recommendation is well intentioned, there are insufficient data to support this stage-based management approach. For example, the KDIGO guidelines suggest consideration of ICU admission and initiation of renal replacement therapy in patients with stage 2 AKI despite a paucity of evidence that applying such a strategy across all patients with AKI will improve outcomes. This recommendation could be considered to contradict the subsequent KDIGO recommendation regarding initiation of renal replacement therapy which recommends consideration of "...the broader clinical context, the presence of conditions that can be modified with RRT, and trends of laboratory tests—rather than single BUN and creatinine thresholds alone—when making the decision to start RRT" [3]. A stage-based management strategy may, however, assume greater clinical applicability if effective pharmacologic therapies for the treatment of AKI become available.

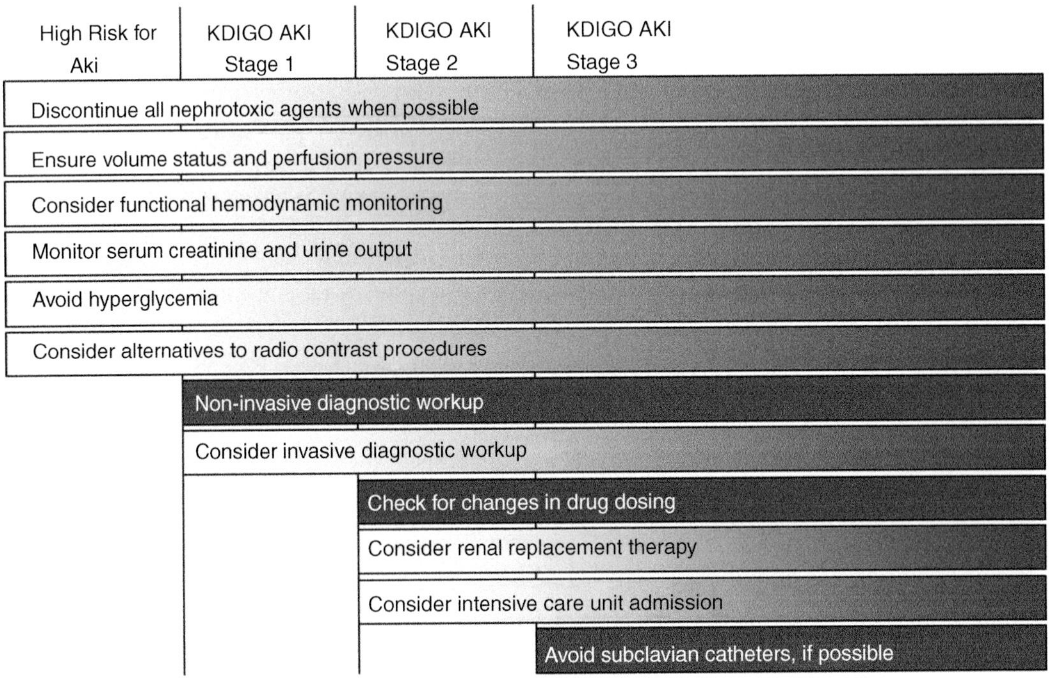

Fig. 2.1 Stage-based management of acute kidney injury (AKI) as proposed by the KDIGO Clinical Practice Guideline for Acute Kidney Injury. Shading of boxes indicates priority of action with solid shading indicating actions that are equally appropriate at all stages, while graded shading indicates increasing priority as severity of AKI increases. Adapted from KDIGO Clinical Practice Guideline for Acute Kidney Injury. *Kidney Int Suppl* 2012;2:1–138

References

1. Lameire N, Van Biesen W, Vanholder R. Acute renal failure. Lancet. 2005;365:417–30.
2. Mehta RL, Kellum JA, Shah SV, et al. Acute Kidney Injury Network (AKIN): report of an initiative to improve outcomes in acute kidney injury. Crit Care. 2007;11:R31.
3. Kidney Disease: Improving Global Outcomes (KDIGO) Acute Kidney Injury Work Group. KDIGO clinical practice guideline for acute kidney injury. Kidney Int Suppl. 2012;2:1–138.
4. Rosen S, Heyman SN. Difficulties in understanding human "acute tubular necrosis": limited data and flawed animal models. Kidney Int. 2001;60:1220–4.
5. Lameire N. The pathophysiology of acute renal failure. Crit Care Clin. 2005;21:197–210.
6. Klahr S, Miller SB. Acute oliguria. N Engl J Med. 1998;338:671–5.
7. Morgan DJ, Ho KM. A comparison of nonoliguric and oliguric severe acute kidney injury according to the risk injury failure loss end-stage (RIFLE) criteria. Nephron Clin Pract. 2010;115:c59–65.
8. Palevsky PM, Liu KD, Brophy PD, Chawla LS, Parikh CR, Thakar CV, Tolwani AJ, Waikar SS, Weisbord SD. KDOQI US commentary on the 2012 KDIGO clinical practice guideline for acute kidney injury. Am J Kidney Dis. 2013;61(5):649–72.
9. Bellomo R, Ronco C, Kellum JA, Mehta RL, Palevsky P, The ADQI Workgroup. Acute renal failure—definition, outcome measures, animal models, fluid therapy and information technology needs: the Second International Consensus Conference of the Acute Dialysis Quality Initiative (ADQI) Group. Crit Care. 2004;8:R204–12.
10. Ricci Z, Cruz D, Ronco C. The RIFLE criteria and mortality in acute kidney injury: a systematic review. Kidney Int. 2008;73(5):538–46.
11. Chertow GM, Burdick E, Honour M, Bonventre JV, Bates DW. Acute kidney injury, mortality, length of stay, and costs in hospitalized patients. J Am Soc Nephrol. 2005;16(11):3365–70.
12. Akcan-Arikan A, Zappitelli M, Loftis LL, Washburn KK, Jefferson LS, Goldstein SL. Modified RIFLE criteria in critically ill children with acute kidney injury. Kidney Int. 2007;71(10):1028–35.
13. Joannidis M, Metnitz B, Bauer P, Schusterschitz N, Moreno R, Druml W, Metnitz PG. Acute kidney injury in critically ill patients classified by AKIN versus RIFLE using the SAPS 3 database. Intensive Care Med. 2009;35(10):1692–702.
14. Lopes JA, Goncalves S, Jorge S, et al. Contemporary analysis of the influence of acute kidney injury after reduced intensity conditioning haematopoietic cell transplantation on long-term survival. Bone Marrow Transplant. 2008;42:619–26.
15. Bihorac A, Yavas S, Subbiah S, et al. Long-term risk of mortality and acute kidney injury during hospitalization after major surgery. Ann Surg. 2009;249:851–8.
16. Chen YC, Jenq CC, Tian YC, et al. Rifle classification for predicting in-hospital mortality in critically ill sepsis patients. Shock. 2009;31:139–45.
17. Perez Valdivieso JR, Bes-Rastrollo M, Monedero P, et al. Evaluation of the prognostic value of the risk, injury, failure, loss and end-stage renal failure (RIFLE) criteria for acute kidney injury. Nephrology (Carlton). 2008;13:361–6.
18. Bagshaw SM, George C, Gibney RT, et al. A multicenter evaluation of early acute kidney injury in critically ill trauma patients. Ren Fail. 2008;30:581–9.
19. Daher EF, Marques CN, Lima RS, et al. Acute kidney injury in an infectious disease intensive care unit—an assessment of prognostic factors. Swiss Med Wkly. 2008;138:128–33.
20. Cruz DN, Bolgan I, Perazella MA, et al. North East Italian Prospective Hospital Renal Outcome Survey on Acute Kidney Injury (NEiPHROS-AKI): targeting the problem with the RIFLE Criteria. Clin J Am Soc Nephrol. 2007;2:418–25.
21. Hoste EA, Bagshaw SM, Bellomo R, Cely CM, Colman R, Cruz DN, Edipidis K, Forni LG, Gomersall CD, Govil D, Honoré PM, Joannes-Boyau O, Joannidis M, Korhonen AM, Lavrentieva A, Mehta RL, Palevsky P, Roessler E, Ronco C, Uchino S, Vazquez JA, Vidal Andrade E, Webb S, Kellum JA. Epidemiology of acute kidney injury in critically ill patients: the multinational AKI-EPI study. Intensive Care Med. 2015;41(8):1411–23. Epub 2015 Jul 11.
22. Doi K, Yuen PS, Eisner C, Hu X, Leelahavanichkul A, Schnermann J, Star RA. Reduced production of creatinine limits its use as marker of kidney injury in sepsis. J Am Soc Nephrol. 2009;20(6):1217–21.
23. Herget-Rosenthal S, Marggraf G, Hüsing J, Göring F, Pietruck F, Janssen O, Philipp T, Kribben A. Early detection of acute renal failure by serum cystatin C. Kidney Int. 2004;66(3):1115–22.
24. Villa P, Jiménez M, Soriano MC, Manzanares J, Casasnovas P. Serum cystatin C concentration as a marker of acute renal dysfunction in critically ill patients. Crit Care. 2005;9(2):R139–43.
25. Wald R, Liangos O, Perianayagam MC, Kolyada A, Herget-Rosenthal S, Mazer CD, Jaber BL. Plasma cystatin C and acute kidney injury after cardiopulmonary bypass. Clin J Am Soc Nephrol. 2010;5(8):1373–9.
26. Ho J, Tangri N, Komenda P, Kaushal A, Sood M, Brar R, Gill K, Walker S, MacDonald K, Hiebert BM, Arora RC, Rigatto C. Urinary, plasma, and serum biomarkers' utility for predicting acute kidney injury associated with cardiac surgery in adults: a meta-analysis. Am J Kidney Dis. 2015;66(6):993–1005.
27. Siew ED, Matheny ME, Ikizler TA, Lewis JB, Miller RA, Waitman LR, Go AS, Parikh CR, Peterson JF. Commonly used surrogates for baseline renal function affect the classification and prognosis of acute kidney injury. Kidney Int. 2010;77(6):536–42.
28. Lin J, Fernandez H, Shashaty MG, Negoianu D, Testani JM, Berns JS, Parikh CR, Wilson FP. False-positive

rate of AKI using consensus creatinine-based criteria. Clin J Am Soc Nephrol. 2015;10(10):1723–31.
29. Waikar SS, Bonventre JV. Creatinine kinetics and the definition of acute kidney injury. J Am Soc Nephrol. 2009;20:672–9.
30. Coca SG, King JT Jr, Rosenthal RA, Perkal MF, Parikh CR. The duration of postoperative acute kidney injury is an additional parameter predicting long-term survival in diabetic veterans. Kidney Int. 2010;78(9):926–33.
31. Waikar SS, Wald R, Chertow GM, Curhan GC, Winkelmayer WC, Liangos O, Sosa MA, Jaber BL. Validity of international classification of diseases, ninth revision, clinical modification codes for acute renal failure. J Am Soc Nephrol. 2006;17(6):1688–94.

3 Diagnostic Approach: Differential Diagnosis, Physical Exam, Lab Tests, Imaging, and Novel Biomarkers

Aparna Sharma and Jay L. Koyner

Acute kidney injury (AKI) is a complex and common clinical syndrome that is classically defined as the abrupt loss of kidney function. The internationally accepted definitions and staging systems and epidemiology of AKI are discussed in Chap. 2 [1]. In this chapter we will discuss the differential diagnosis of AKI as well as the physical exam findings and laboratory tests that can be used when evaluating a patient with AKI. Finally, we will discuss the utility of the ever-expanding list of novel biomarkers that are associated with improvements in the diagnosis, risk stratification, and outcome prognostication of hospitalized patients with AKI [2].

3.1 Differential Diagnosis

Traditionally the differential diagnosis of AKI has been classified into prerenal, intrinsic renal/intrarenal, and post-renal causes [3] (Table 3.1). Classically this has allowed clinicians to think about the factors that affect renal function into those which occur before the kidney (prerenal), inside of the kidney, or after the kidney (post-renal—along the remainder of the genitourinary system). This anatomy-based classification system has been utilized for decades, and while more modern schemas have been suggested, the pre-, intra-, and post-renal remains a mainstay of clinical decision-making. Many clinicians believe that these distinctions are important as prerenal and post-renal causes of AKI may progress to becoming intrinsic/intrarenal AKI. Additionally, if diagnosed early, pre- and post-renal AKI may be readily reversible, with regard to changes in glomerular function/serum creatinine, and thus earlier diagnosis may not only mitigate the severity of the AKI but potentially the morbidity and mortality that are associated with it.

Prerenal causes of AKI result from impaired renal perfusion from either true intravascular volume depletion (e.g., GI losses, hemorrhage, or burns) or from decreases in the effective circulating volume (e.g., decompensated congestive heart failure with reduced ejection fraction or end-stage liver disease with cirrhosis). Additionally, several medications, which affect renal vascular autoregulation, have been associated with prerenal AKI. These include nonsteroidal anti-inflammatory drugs (NSAIDs) and calcineurin inhibitors (CNIs), angiotensin-converting enzyme inhibitors (ACE-I), and angiotensin II receptor blockers (ARBs), all of which modify renal vascular autoregulation. NSAIDs can cause afferent arteriole vasoconstriction, leading to fall in renal blood flow and thus a decline in glomerular filtration rate (GFR)/rise in creatinine. Similarly, CNIs including tacrolimus and cyclosporine have been

A. Sharma · J. L. Koyner (✉)
Section of Nephrology, Department of Medicine, University of Chicago, Chicago, IL, USA
e-mail: jkoyner@uchicago.edu

S. S. Waikar et al. (eds.), *Core Concepts in Acute Kidney Injury*,
https://doi.org/10.1007/978-1-4939-8628-6_3

Table 3.1 Classical differential diagnosis of AKI

AKI

Prerenal causes	Intrinsic renal causes	Post-renal causes
True volume depletion (diarrhea, vomiting, burns, hemorrhage, pancreatitis)	Processes involving renal microvasculature such as vasculitis, TTP, malignant hypertension, and renal atheroemboli	Bladder outlet obstruction including prostate disease in men and pelvic tumors
Renal artery stenosis	Processes affecting primarily glomeruli such as rapidly progressive glomerulonephritis	Ureteral: stones, stricture
Effective circulating volume depletion (decompensated heart failure, cardiac cirrhosis)	Processes affecting the tubulointerstitium such as acute tubular necrosis (ischemic or nephrotoxic), acute interstitial nephritis	Retroperitoneal fibrosis
Abdominal compartment syndrome		

The table displays the common causes of AKI along the prerenal, intrarenal, and post-renal classification. This traditional anatomic approach remains in clinical use despite disease processes crossing over in between categories. For example, persistently prolonged intravascular volume depletion in the setting of concomitant hypotension may lead to intrinsic tubular injury/tubular necrosis, or chronic urinary obstruction may eventually cause tubular loss and fibrosis leading to intrarenal manifestations

shown to cause renal arteriolar vasoconstriction leading to an increased association with AKI as measured by increases in serum creatinine. Additionally drugs which impact the renin-aldosterone system (e.g., ACE-I and ARBs) have been shown to alter renal hemodynamics and thus impact functional biomarkers of AKI (e.g., serum creatinine and cystatin C) but not biomarkers that report structural nephron injury/damage. Thus while ACE-I and ARBs lead to alterations of serum creatinine, the extent to which this is truly AKI remains under-investigated. This failing of currently available biomarker of AKI accounts for the growing push in nephrology to fundamentally change the manner in which we discuss the differential diagnosis of AKI (see new AKI paradigm below). The kidney has the capacity to autoregulate renal blood flow and GFR through changes in afferent and efferent arteriolar tone. However, prerenal conditions, if severe, can overwhelm these compensatory processes and lead to a dramatic fall in GFR. Furthermore in the setting of AKI, these autoregulatory mechanisms can be impaired leading to an exacerbation of initial injury following even mild decreases in blood pressure, eventually potentially converting to an intrarenal injury [4].

In the hospital setting, obstructive uropathy (post-renal) accounts for approximately 10% of cases of AKI [5]. Post-renal causes of AKI can result from obstruction anywhere along the urinary tract but is most commonly from bladder outlet obstruction as seen in prostatic hypertrophy in men [6]. It can also be seen in cases of pelvic masses and tumors compressing bilateral ureters [7]. Common obstructing tumors include those of the prostate, bladder, uterus, and cervix. A rare cause of obstructive uropathy is retroperitoneal fibrosis which may be idiopathic, but it can be associated with previous pelvic irradiation or malignancies such as lymphoma and a variety of solid tumors [8]. Importantly unilateral obstruction in those with two functioning kidneys is often not diagnosed through changes in GFR. Larger changes in GFR, in the setting of obstruction, often represent bilateral obstruction or the presence of a single functioning kidney (e.g., renal transplantation). Further information on post-renal AKI is presented in Chap. 16.

Intrarenal causes of AKI can be subdivided into processes affecting the glomeruli, intrarenal vasculature, or tubules/interstitium. The most common intrinsic cause of AKI is acute tubular necrosis (ATN), which accounts for roughly 75% of intrinsic AKI in hospitalized patients [5]. In one study done at 13 tertiary care hospitals in Spain, the incidence of ATN among all causes of AKI (including pre- and post-renal) was found to be 45% [9]. ATN is a clinical-pathologic syndrome of intrinsic acute renal injury that is secondary to ischemic (e.g., cardiac surgery or septic shock) or nephrotoxic insults. Common nephrotoxins include drugs such as aminoglycosides, cisplatin, tenofovir, or iodinated radiocontrast media as well as endogenous products such as the hemoglobin and myoglobin pigments that can damage nephrons in the setting of rhabdomyolysis leading to ATN. The histopathologic findings of ATN are frequently patchy. When present on a biopsy, ATN may subtly involve discrete cell injury in the proximal tubule, the collecting duct, and the medullary thick ascending limb without frank necrosis. Thus, the term ATN may often be a misnomer, and the term acute tubular injury may better reflect the physiopathologic dissociation often seen in this entity [10].

Other less common forms of intrinsic tubulointerstitial renal injury include acute urate nephropathy from tumor lysis syndrome, cast nephropathy in the setting of multiple myeloma, and acute phosphate nephropathy. Tumor lysis syndrome in oncology patients with a high tumor burden (e.g., leukemia or lymphoma) can lead to AKI from intratubular obstruction by urate crystals. Acute phosphate nephropathy can occur following the administration of a phosphate containing bowel preparation. Another more common intrinsic tubulointerstitial cause of AKI is acute interstitial nephritis (AIN). AIN is characterized by an inflammatory infiltration of the renal interstitium and is most commonly drug induced although it can be associated with autoimmune diseases and infectious processes. Common agents include antimicrobial agents (β-lactams, sulfonamides, quinolones, antiviral agents), antiulcer agents (proton-pump inhibitors, H2 antagonists), nonsteroidal anti-inflammatory drugs (NSAIDs), anticonvulsants, and allopurinol [11].

3.1.1 Rethinking the Differential Diagnosis of AKI

While the pre-, post-, and intrarenal paradigm of AKI has been a mainstay of clinical care, it remains an imperfect classification system with several subtypes of AKI crossing over anatomic categories. For example, persistently prolonged intravascular volume depletion (prerenal) in the setting of concomitant hypotension may lead to intrinsic tubular injury/ATN. Chronic urinary obstruction if left untreated may eventually cause tubular loss and fibrosis (intrarenal manifestations). These faults combined with the imperfections of serum creatinine and urine output as biomarkers of renal function and the emergence of newer kidney injury biomarkers have led to the development of a novel schema of AKI classification [12].

This revamped classification system has been proposed to classify patients based on the presence or absence of changes in functional (e.g., serum creatinine, serum cystatin C, urine output) and structural/injury biomarkers (e.g., neutrophil gelatinase-associated lipocalin (NGAL), interleukin 18 (IL-18) (Fig. 3.1), kidney injury molecule-1 (KIM-1)). Briefly, it is easy to understand that those without a change in functional or injury biomarkers do not have AKI, while those who have changes in both functional and injury biomarkers are akin to those with severe intrinsic AKI (e.g., ATN). Those with a change in functional biomarkers but no change in injury biomarkers can be potentially thought of as those with prerenal AKI, where there has been a drop in GFR in the absence of true tubular injury. Finally, those with changes in their injury biomarkers without a concomitant change in functional biomarkers may be viewed as having "subclinical AKI." This newer entity exists due to the inability of serum creatinine to adequately measure the underlying renal function in those with normal and near normal GFR. This concept of renal reserve [13] has led to several investigations which have demonstrated that in the absence of changes in urine output and serum creatinine,

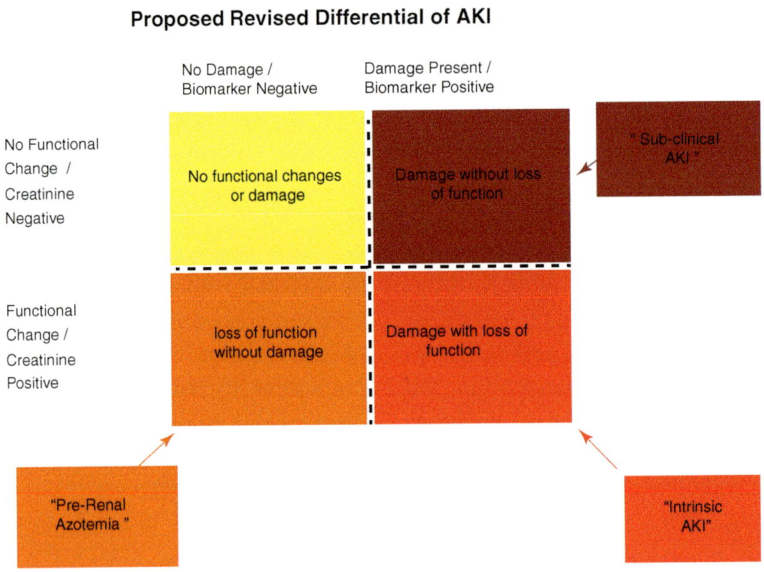

Fig. 3.1 Currently the definition of AKI is made exclusively through changes in urine output and/or serum creatinine, functional biomarkers of the kidney. The ADQI consensus meeting delineated a novel criteria for defining AKI in terms of changes in biomarkers of renal function (serum creatinine, urine output, serum cystatin) and biomarkers of kidney damage/injury (e.g., NGAL, TIMP-2*IGFBP7, IL-18). This paradigm allows for the combination of injury biomarkers with functional biomarkers and has proven useful in the discrimination of patients with AKI (Adapted from: Endre ZH, Kellum JA, Di Somma S, et al. Differential diagnosis of AKI in clinical practice by functional and damage biomarkers: workgroup statements from the tenth Acute Dialysis Quality Initiative Consensus Conference. *Contrib Nephrol.* 2013;182:30–44; used with permission)

those with increases in their injury biomarkers are at increased risk of needing renal replacement therapy (RRT) and death [14, 15]. The uses of these newer biomarkers and their clinical implications are discussed further in this chapter.

3.2 Physical Exam

The physical exam findings associated with AKI can involve almost every organ system. In the setting of AKI, the physical findings may be reflective of the AKI itself, i.e., a clinical manifestation of the decrease in GFR and associated retention of uremic toxins and/or total body fluid. However, the physical exam findings may also help the astute clinician identify the underlying etiology causing the AKI.

Hypotension may indicate a state of volume depletion and point toward a diagnosis of intravascular volume depletion/prerenal azotemia (change in biomarkers of glomerular function). However, if hypotension persists for long enough, it may progress to the point of ATN. Importantly, the absence of documented hypotension does not preclude AKI or more specifically ATN given the clinical entity of normotensive acute renal failure [16]. A lower mean arterial pressure (MAP) has been shown to increase the risk of developing severe/progressive AKI. In a multicenter prospective observational study of 423 Finnish subjects with sepsis, a MAP of less than 73 mmHg was associated with increased risk of progressive AKI (defined as a worsening of the Kidney Disease: Improving Global Outcomes (KDIGO) AKI criteria) [17]. Similarly, several other studies have demonstrated the importance of maintaining adequate renal perfusion pressures in the setting of AKI, with higher pressures being associated with decreased risk of adverse patient outcomes [18–22].

Overt neurologic signs and symptoms may occur in advanced kidney injury and may manifest as decreased mental acuity, asterixis, peripheral neuropathy, and seizures [23]. However, given the nonspecific nature of these signs, it is difficult to attribute a given neurologic sign to one specific source of AKI. The cardiovascular exam may reveal findings suggestive of fluid overload/congestive heart failure such as S3, pedal/sacral edema, and elevated JVD. A pericardial friction rub if present may be indicative of uremic pericarditis, which is traditionally an end-stage manifestation of severely decreased kidney function. The pulmonary exam may reveal coarse crackles that can suggest pulmonary edema due to volume overload but in rare instances may be associated with glomerular disease and result from pulmonary hemorrhage in the setting of an ANCA-associated vasculitis.

The dermatologic exam findings in AKI can be diverse and varied. They include livedo reticularis which may be suggestive of cholesterol emboli particularly in patients who have undergone recent endo-vascular procedures; however, livedo reticularis may also be seen in antiphospholipid antibody syndrome, cryoglobulinemia, and even calciphylaxis. Other dermatologic findings include palpable purpura which has been associated with leukocytoclastic vasculitis. Contrary to popular belief, AIN is infrequently associated with a rash; in a retrospective analysis of over 60 cases of biopsy-confirmed AIN, the incidence of rash at the time of presentation was found to be 21% [24]. Additionally, in this same case series, the incidence of AIN-associated uveitis (tubulointerstitial nephritis and uveitis syndrome (TINU)) was 7%.

The abdominal and genitourinary exams deserve close attention in the evaluation of a patient with AKI. A distended bladder may signify bladder outlet obstruction: a common cause of AKI particularly in elderly males with prostatic disease. The diagnosis of abdominal compartment syndrome (ACS) should be considered in any patient with a tense distended abdomen and concomitant oliguria. The clinical definition of ACS is intra-abdominal hypertension-induced new organ dysfunction without a strict intra-abdominal pressure threshold, since no intra-abdominal pressure can predictably diagnose ACS in all patients [25–27]. For clinical research purposes, ACS has been defined as a sustained intra-abdominal pressure greater than 20 mmHg, and this is different than intra-abdominal hypertension (IAH, defined as greater than 12 mmHg for research purposes). Both ACS and IAH have been associated with increased risk of AKI [28]. Finally, the presence of an abdominal bruit can indicate renal artery stenosis and can be indicative of AKI particularly in the setting of recent initiation of angiotensin-converting enzyme inhibitors or angiotensin receptor blocker use.

3.3 Lab Tests

3.3.1 Blood Tests

The laboratory evaluation of patients with AKI should be driven by their clinical presentation and their risk factors for kidney injury. Initial laboratory tests to be ordered include measurement of blood urea nitrogen (BUN) and serum creatinine, as well as other serum electrolytes, sodium, chloride, potassium, and bicarbonate (carbon dioxide) levels. These tests are important not only for the diagnosis but also for assessment of complications of AKI. In prerenal conditions resulting from enhanced salt and water avidity, the classic teaching is that there is a disproportionate increase in the ratio of BUN to creatinine (>20:1).The increase in BUN may stem from the presence of ADH that acts on distal tubules to increase urea transport from the luminal to the basolateral side. However, recent studies have demonstrated that the BUN to creatinine ratio is quite variable and higher ratios may not be indicative of prerenal etiologies [29]. In the setting of AKI, lab tests may show hyponatremia, due to decreased free water clearance in the setting of positive fluid balance. Hyponatremia is often found in the presence of AKI with several studies linking the two entities; in one prospective observational study of all patients admitted to an urban hospital with hyponatremia, AKI was evident in 32% of patients [30]. In a separate study of hyponatremia, AKI was present in 16% of the hospitalized cohort with AKI rates reaching over 20% in those older than 74 years [31]. Up to one third of the patients with severe AKI may develop dilution hyponatremia through decreased free water clearance, and this lab abnormality is associated with worse outcomes including an increased risk of death [32, 33].

Hyperkalemia is commonly seen and treated as a complication of AKI. In a multicenter observational study of 923 inpatients with hyperkalemia of >6.5 mEq/L, AKI was present in over 22% of those with normal baseline renal function and in over half (51.8%) of those with pre-existing chronic kidney disease [34]. In one study, hyperkalemia, although known to be a serious complication of AKI, had a smaller effect size/association with inpatient mortality than metabolic acidosis and cumulative fluid balance [35]. This result is likely due to the existence of standardized thresholds to define hyperkalemia and its risk as well as the rapid institution of several reliable therapeutic options for hyperkalemia (diuretics, RRT, and bicarbonate, among others). Such thresholds and treatment options are not as robust for volume overload or metabolic acidosis.

Metabolic acidosis is a common feature of both acute and chronic kidney injuries and results from the accumulation of anions such as urate, hippurate, phosphate, and other anions that are not routinely measured, such as sulfates. In a prospective randomized multicenter trial comparing high and low intensity of continuous RRT, severe acidosis, defined as a pH < 7.2, was present in 34.9% of subjects. Similarly in a post hoc analysis of the Finnish Acute Kidney Injury (FINNAKI) study, 52% of all subjects had a pH < 7.15 prior to the initiation of RRT, with acidosis being cited as the indication for RRT in 35.8% [36, 37]. Metabolic acidosis is thought to interfere with normal functioning of many processes in the body and contributes to adverse outcomes through the promotion of hemodynamic instability via decreased cardiac output and vasodilatation.

3.3.2 Urinary Test

Examination of urine sediment is a crucial component in formulating a differential diagnosis in the setting of AKI [38–40]. There is a growing body of evidence that suggests that urinalysis and the presence of renal tubular epithelial cells and cellular casts correlate with early diagnosis of AKI as well as AKI severity [38, 41–43]. Table 3.2 presents a summary of several of the recently published urinalysis score systems. A recent study demonstrated that a higher urine microscopy severity score, as measured by the increased presence of urinary granular and muddy brown casts, was associated with a greater than sevenfold increased risk of progressive AKI (i.e., a worsening of AKI clinical stage) [42]. However, despite the resurgence of interest in microscopic urinalysis, this clinical tool has not been well integrated into recent large-scale modern biomarker investigations [44–49]. Despite several published scoring systems, there have been no large-scale multicenter validation studies describing the performance of urine microscopy in the setting of hospital-based AKI [40–42].

In prerenal AKI, urine sediment exam may reveal hyaline casts (see Fig. 3.2a). Hyaline casts

Table 3.2 Summary of three previously published urinalysis severity scores: these scores have been shown to correlate well with severity of AKI and been specific for AKI

Study	Scoring system
Chawla et al. [41]	Grade 1: no casts or RTE Grade 2: at least 1 cast or RTE but <10% of LPF Grade 3: many casts or RTEs (between 10 and 90% of LPF) Grade 4: sheet of muddy brown casts and RTEs in >90% of LPF
Perazella et al. [42]	0 points: no casts or RTE seen 1 point each: 1–5 casts per LPF or 1–5 RTEs per HPF 2 points each: ≥6 casts per LPF or ≥6 RTEs per HPF
Bagshaw et al. [40]	0 points: no casts or RTE seen 1 point each: 1casts or 1 RTEs per HPF 2 points each: 2–4 casts or RTEs per HPF 3 points each: ≥ 5 casts or ≥ 5 RTEs per HPF

Several of these scores have been combined with biomarkers of tubular injury to improve prognostication of AKI and other adverse patient outcomes [40, 42, 43]
RTE renal tubule epithelial cells, *LPF* low-power field, *HPF* high-power field

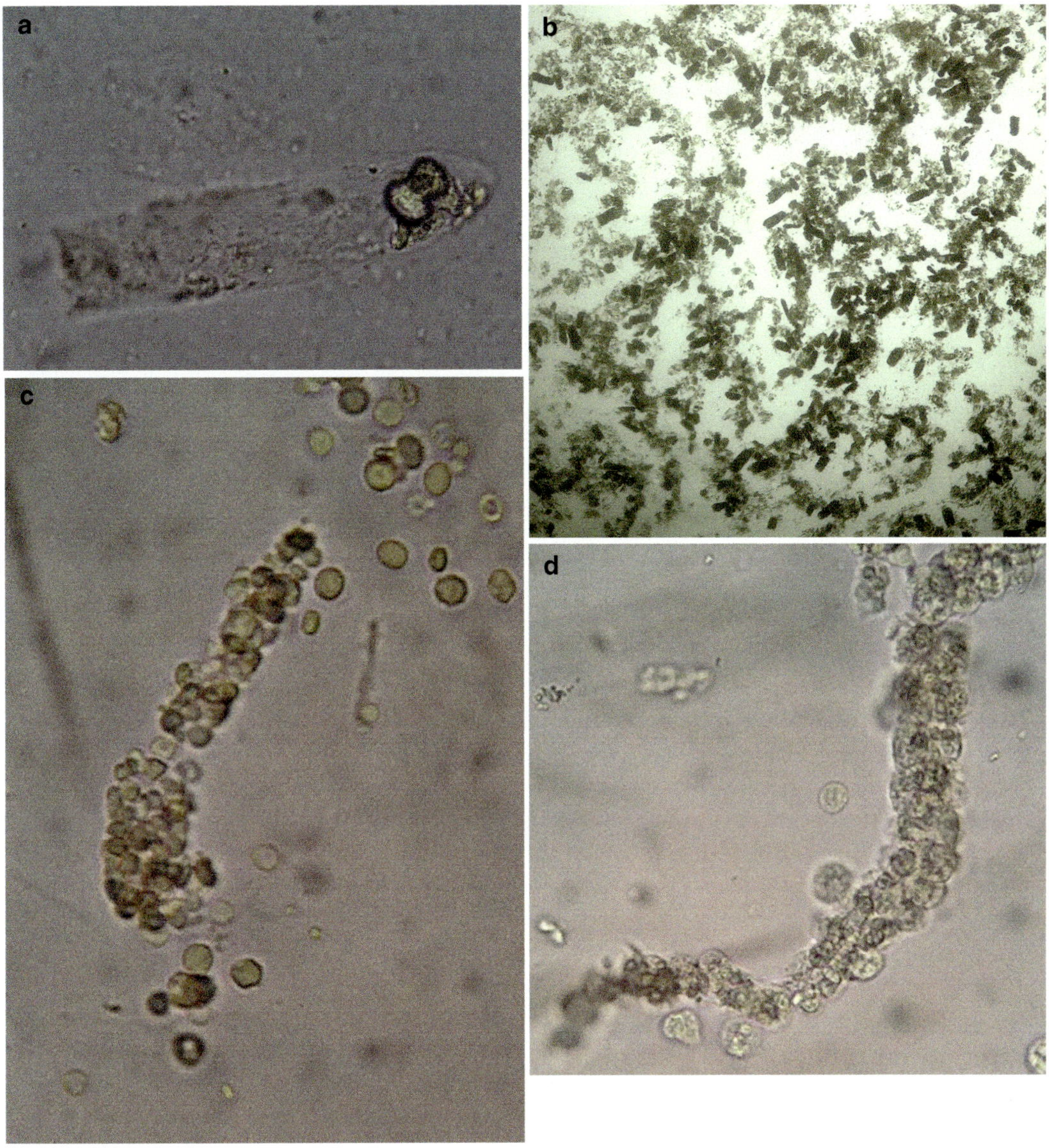

Fig. 3.2 (**a**) Hyaline cast at 400× power. These casts made of Tamm-Horsfall proteins are incredibly sticky and can collect elements in the tubule as seen by the calcium oxalate crystal attached to this hyaline cast. (**b**) Low-power field (40×) of ATN, with a large number of muddy brown casts. (**c**) RBC cast (400×)—where you can see the hyaline outline of the cast and the RBCs forming a multi-layer matrix on top of each other. (**d**) WBC cast (400×) in the setting of AIN. There are several nucleated white cells throughout the cast, and there are renal tubule epithelial cells in the background, which would be expected in the setting of AIN/active AKI. All photos are courtesy of Randy Luciano MD PhD, Yale University

are cylindrical molds of precipitated Tamm-Horsfall protein that are formed in the distal tubule. In ATN, muddy brown, coarse, granular casts are characteristically seen in addition to free renal tubular epithelial cells (Fig. 3.2b). Rapidly progressive glomerulonephritis (RPGN) is part of the differential diagnosis of AKI and is characterized by urine sediment containing RBC casts (Fig. 3.2c). These casts are composed of red cells in the matrix of Tamm-Horsfall protein. The presence of white blood cells (WBCs) in clumps and in casts, in the presence of bacteria, is suggestive of pyelonephritis, while the absence of bacteria suggests AIN (Fig. 3.2d). Importantly, while previously thought to be a useful tool, urine eosinophils are neither sensitive nor specific for AIN. In a recent retrospective study of renal biopsies with concomitant urine eosinophils ($n = 566$ biopsies, 91 of which had AIN), a cutoff of 1% provided a sensitivity of 30.8% and a specificity of 68.2% [50].

Urinary electrolyte indices such as the fractional excretions of sodium (FENa) and urea (FEUrea) have long been used by clinicians in order to differentiate etiologies of AKI. The FENa which measures the percentage of filtered sodium excreted by the kidney can be potentially helpful in differentiating decreased intravascular volume and renal perfusion (prerenal) from intrinsic tubular damage (e.g., ATN) [51]. Classically, a FENa below 1% suggests a prerenal etiology, where the kidney is acting appropriately to perceived paucity of renal perfusion by reabsorption of most of filtered sodium load [52, 53]. However, the clinical utility of FENa in critically ill patients with AKI has been challenged [54, 55]. A FENa below 1% can often be found in circumstances of established AKI (ATN) reflecting nonhomogeneous injury to the kidney parenchyma and preservation of tubular function in some regions. Additionally, the FENa may be below 1% in the setting of hepatorenal syndrome (see Chap. 7), radiocontrast administration (Chap. 6), urinary tract obstruction (Chap. 16), and sepsis (Chap. 10) [56–60]. Finally, several recent papers have explored the ability of the FENa to predict the future development of AKI (e.g., in the setting of cardiac surgery) or the presence of progressive AKI and determined that this biomarker is unable to predict any of these AKI outcomes in a significant fashion [61–63]. Similarly the FENa has not been shown to differentiate hepatorenal syndrome from ATN or prerenal AKI or predict AKI progression in those with cirrhosis and AKI [64, 65]. In the original paper by Schrier and colleagues, the FENa was evaluated in the absence of CKD (serum creatinine had to be less than 1.6 at baseline), those with oliguria (<500 ccs of urine per day), and in the absence of diuretics; however, in the decades since this original study, there have been broad acceptance and implementation of the FENa in a variety of AKI clinical setting despite a lack of wide-scale validation [52].

The FEUrea has been cited as a more precise method for discriminating early AKI in those receiving diuretics, which may impact the urinary sodium concentration rendering the FENa difficult to interpret. Importantly, should the urine sodium remain exceedingly low in the setting of active diuresis, this may point to the presence of intravascular volume depletion as the source of AKI. Regardless, a FEUrea of less than 35% has been thought to indicate prerenal AKI, whereas one above 35% is thought to be consistent with intrinsic AKI (ATN) [66]. However, FEUrea has been described in far fewer studies compared with FENa. In a study by Carvounis et al., a FEUrea less than 35% was evident in 90, 89, and 4% for prerenal, prerenal with diuretics, and ATN patients, respectively [67]. Additionally, as with the FENa, attempts to validate the FEUrea as a diagnostic/prognostic tool in the setting of early AKI have failed to demonstrate its clinical utility [61–63].

3.4 Imaging

A variety of imaging techniques have been used in the diagnosis and workup of patients with AKI. In this section we discuss the strengths and limitations of these modalities and then review newer methods for renal imaging.

Ultrasound is often the first-line imaging modality in the evaluation of AKI given its inexpensive nature, wide availability, and safety [68]. It is particularly helpful in diagnosing obstructive causes of AKI. In a study of 286 ultrasound exam reports for 63 consecutive patients who received 64 renal transplants, it was found that the sensitivity of detection of ureteral obstruction with ultrasound was 100% with a specificity of 91.9% [69]. In a large multicenter, pragmatic, comparative effectiveness trial, in 2759 patients with suspected nephrolithiasis, ultrasonography was associated with lower cumulative radiation exposure than initial computed tomography scan

(CT scan), without significant differences in high-risk diagnoses (such as obstructive AKI) with complications [70]. Importantly, the renal caliceal dilation that is a hallmark of ureteral obstruction is not specific to obstructive uropathy as it may be seen in pregnancy as well as diabetes insipidus [71, 72].

Ultrasound also provides information regarding kidney size, shape, anatomic location, and cortical echogenicity. Enlarged kidneys in the setting of AKI may suggest infiltrative diseases such as lymphoma or the presence of pre-existing diseases known to be associated with enlarged kidneys (e.g., HIV or diabetic nephropathy) but can also be seen in RPGN and AIN [73]. Doppler ultrasound can provide valuable information on renal blood flow. In one study of 41 individuals with kidney diseases, comparing Doppler US findings with biopsy results, kidneys with higher tubulointerstitial disease activity had higher resistive index compared to the kidneys with other forms of renal disease, including glomerular disease [74]. Importantly, ultrasound remains limited as a user-dependent tool, as images and their interpretation are only as good as those operating the modality.

Helical CT scan is another commonly used imaging modality for the diagnosis of obstructive AKI, especially in the setting of suspected nephrolithiasis. While CT scan is able to diagnose ureteral obstruction with accuracy on par with ultrasonography, it comes with the higher radiation exposure and is not able to be done at the bedside in unstable patients [70]. CT scans with iodinated contrast are to be avoided in the setting of AKI owing to the further risk of nephrotoxicity from the contrast.

Magnetic resonance imaging (MRI) without gadolinium is of limited utility in the workup of AKI. Imaging with gadolinium is limited in part by the concern of nephrogenic systemic fibrosis/nephrogenic fibrosing dermopathy (NSF/NFD). NSF has been associated with the gadolinium contrast agent particularly in pts with estimated glomerular filtration rates eGFR < 30 mL/min and as such is a concern for both those with AKI and those with end-stage renal disease (ESRD) [75]. However, newer non-gadolinium contrast agents have shown promise and safety in assessing renal blood flow [76]. This advance could improve care in the setting of ischemia-induced AKI while also improving patient safety in the setting of reduced kidney function in human studies.

Blood oxygen level-dependent magnetic resonance imaging (BOLD MRI) is a relatively new technique used to noninvasively measure intrarenal oxygenation and may have important implications in future research in the field of AKI [77]. BOLD MRI quantifies the differences in measurements of renal oxygenation based on changes in the magnetic properties of hemoglobin during its conversion from oxyhemoglobin to deoxyhemoglobin. The relationship between BOLD MRI signal intensity and renal oxygen tissue levels has been established by direct measurements of tissue partial pressure of oxygen (pO_2) utilizing oxygen-sensing microelectrodes and fiber-optic probes in experimental models of aortic occlusion. In swine and rat models of aortic occlusion/renal ischemia, medullary and cortical hypoxias were demonstrated during acute ischemia by BOLD MRI followed by an immediate return to baseline oxygenation after reperfusion [77–83]. In an observational study of BOLD MRI in renal transplant allografts performed by Han and colleagues, allografts with ATN had cortical and medullary hypoxia ($n = 7$) as compared with normal functioning allografts studied 10 days postoperatively [83]. However, based on this and other studies in the setting of contrast- and sepsis-associated AKI, the ideal cutoffs for the diagnosis of renal hypoxia and the associated AKI remain unclear [84]. The applicability of BOLD MRI in patients with AKI and more specifically critically ill patients however remains to be seen given that the modality is not point of care and the scans themselves take longer to perform than CT scans. However, in the future it may serve as a method to evaluate renal oxygenation and a trigger to initiate novel therapies aimed and reversing the effects of renal ischemia.

More recently, contrast-enhanced ultrasound (CEUS) has been investigated in animal and human models as a novel method to investigate renal microperfusion [85–88]. This technology utilizes the systemic infusion of gas-filled microbubbles to assess organ perfusion. Microbubbles have increased echogenicity compared to other tissues, and thus the presence of bubbles can readily identify areas of both ischemia and perfusion. Bonventre and colleagues demonstrated that this technique can be used to monitor changes in renal ischemia over time (24 h) and provide mapping of injured areas in a murine model of renal ischemia reperfusion [85]. CEUS has also been investigated in humans. Bellomo and colleagues performed scans in four patients with hepatorenal syndrome as a proof-of-concept report to estimate the effect of terlipressin on renal microcirculation [86]. This promising preliminary report, which detected increased perfusion in response to terlipressin, serves as a follow-up to their investigations of an ovine model [88]. This same group has reported a 36 scan investigation demonstrating that CEUS was feasible and well-tolerated and can detect decreased renal perfusion within the first 24 h following adult cardiac surgery [87]. We anticipate future investigations around the novel, noninvasive, and portal imaging modality and its ability to identify alterations in renal microcirculation.

While several other imagining modalities such as positron emission tomography (PET) and bioelectrical impedance analysis (BIA) have been explored in the setting of AKI, they remain beyond the scope of this chapter [89].

3.5 Novel Biomarkers

As discussed in Chap. 2, the internationally accepted KDIGO consensus definition of AKI relies on either serum creatinine, urine output, or both to define AKI. Thus the KDIGO criteria, like the consensus definitions before them, rely on long-standing imperfect markers of kidney function [90, 91]. Serum creatinine is not sensitive for the diagnosis of AKI, as there can be a large amount of tubular injury/nephron loss without a significant change in creatinine (e.g., living donor renal transplant and renal reserve). Additionally, creatinine is not 100% specific for renal tubular injury, as previously mentioned prerenal azotemia occurs when there is a change in creatinine in the absence of true tubular damage. Moreover, serum creatinine level can be affected by several clinical factors including muscle mass, age, race, and assay interference (caused by clinical factors such as hemolysis and lipemia as well as certain drugs) [92, 93]. Due to these shortcomings of serum creatinine as well as the ability to manipulate urine output through the use of diuretics, in 2005, the American Society of Nephrology Renal Research Report called for the standardization and discovery of new biomarkers of AKI as its highest research priority. Over the last decade, there has been a proliferation of studies focussing on the detection and validation of new biomarkers of AKI in a variety of different patient populations and clinical settings [2, 94–96].

An ideal AKI biomarker should fulfill several criteria including being highly sensitive and specific to renal injury and inexpensive to carry out and provide information regarding the underlying source of the AKI, AKI severity, and overall prognosis [97]. To date, there have been well over 30 candidate biomarkers for AKI identified and investigated with the characteristics and physiologic action of several of the most widely investigated biomarkers summarized in Table 3.3.

Biochemical biomarkers of AKI can be low molecular weight proteins that are present in the systemic circulation and undergo filtration, enzymes that are released by tubular cells into the urine after cell injury or inflammatory mediators released by renal cells or infiltrating inflammatory cells (markers of degree of damage and indicators of site of injury) [2, 94–96]. More recently functional biomarkers of AKI have been investigated but require large-scale validation [62, 89, 98]. Given that AKI is a heterogeneous complex clinical syndrome, investigations have attempted to focus on specific clinical scenarios (e.g., cardiac surgery/cardiopulmonary bypass, septic shock, end-stage liver disease). Each of these clinical settings has their own unique AKI fingerprint, and it is reasonable to expect that biomarkers that detect post-cardiopulmonary bypass AKI might be different from those for septic shock-associated AKI or AKI from hepatorenal syndrome.

Table 3.3 Characteristics and physiologic action for biomarkers of AKI

Category	Biomarker	Description	Physiologic action
GFR markers	Serum cystatin C	13 kDa protein produced at a constant rate with limited protein binding [94, 124]	Inhibitors of cysteine proteinases cathepsin H, B, and L and calpains [94, 124]. Freely filtered at the glomerulus reflecting underlying GFR, but levels are affected by corticosteroids, hyperthyroidism, hypertriglyceridemia, hyperbilirubinemia, and inflammation [125, 126]
Tubular injury markers	Urine cystatin C	13 kDa protein produced at a constant rate with limited protein binding [94, 124]	Freely filtered in glomerulus and degraded in proximal tubules, so in the absence of injury not present in urine [94]. Urinary level may increase with albuminuria through competitive inhibition of reabsorption [127]
	Interleukin-18 (IL-18)	IL-1 family cytokine precursor cleaved by caspase-1 to 17.2 kDa active form [128]	Induces IFN-ϒ and T-cell activation [128]. Urinary IL-18 found to be a marker of ATN in humans [129]
	Kidney injury molecule 1 (KIM-1)	40–70 kDa glycosylated transmembrane protein receptor expressed in proximal tubules, important in recognizing apoptotic cells [130, 131]	Upregulated after proximal tubule ischemic injury [130]. Expressed by immune cells to activate differentiation of T helper 1, 2, and 17 cells [132] FDA-approved for use in preclinical drug development
	Liver-type fatty acid-binding protein (L-FABP)	15 kDa protein expressed in proximal tubules [133]	Binds free fatty acids and transports them to mitochondria or peroxisomes. Found to be upregulated after ischemic injury [94, 134]. In mouse models found also a marker for COX-inhibitor and cisplatin-induced AKI [135, 136]
	Urinary NAG (*N*-acetyl-β-glucosaminidase)	~140 kDa proximal tubule enzyme, not renally filtered [94]	A sensitive urinary marker of loss of lysosomal integrity in proximal tubule and may reflect improvements in proximal tubular function. Inhibited by urea, industrial solvents, and heavy metals [94]. Not elevated with sepsis [137]
	Neutrophil gelatinase-associated lipocalin (NGAL)	25 kDa lipocalin protein covalently bound to gelatinase from neutrophils. May exist as monomer or dimer. Expressed in the lung, liver, and kidney [138]	Binds to free iron and assists in response to bacterial infection [139]. Upregulated in distal nephron in response to AKI but are also released from the liver and neutrophils in sepsis [140]. Assay differences due to different forms of NGAL [141]. Plasma levels may correlate with GFR/CKD
Cell cycle arrest	Tissue inhibitor metalloproteinase-2 and insulin-like growth factor-binding protein-7 (TIMP-2*IGFBP7)	TIMP-2 is part of the TIMP family of protease inhibitors expressed ubiquitously [142]. IGF-binding protein 7 is expressed in vascular endothelial cells and binds to insulin and insulin-like growth factor [143]	TIMP-2 inhibits matrix metalloproteinases, promoting fibrosis and blocking endothelial proliferation [144, 145]. IGFBP7 inhibits endothelial angiogenesis, among other functions [143, 146]. Both markers are linked to cell cycle arrest and are highly upregulated after kidney injury [44, 106]

Adapted and edited from: Chen LX, Koyner JL. Biomarkers in Acute Kidney Injury. *Critical care clinics*. 2015;31(4): 633–648; used with permission

Table 3.4 summarizes the findings of several large-scale multicenter studies that investigated the abilities of several biomarkers to detect clinical endpoints around AKI in a variety of clinical settings. Importantly, novel biomarkers have been investigated for more than just the ability to diagnose/detect AKI earlier than serum creatinine or urine output. Biomarkers have been

Table 3.4 Biomarker performance in detecting AKI from multicenter studies at a variety of clinical time points

	Perioperative AKI				Critically Ill			Emergency room		Liver disease with cirrhosis
	Pre-op AKI risk	Early post-op AKI	AKI progression	Long-term mortality	Early diagnosis of AKI	Type of AKI (transient vs. intrinsic)	Need for RRT	Early diagnosis of AKI	Type of AKI (transient vs. intrinsic)	AKI progression
Urine NGAL	N/A	+	–	+	+	+	+	+	+	+
Blood NGAL	–	+	+	?	–	?	–	?	?	N/A
Blood CysC	+	+	–	?	+	+	+	?	?	+
Urine CysC	N/A	–	–	–	+	+	+	+	+	
Urine IL-18	N/A	+	+	+	+	+	+	+	+	+
Urine KIM-1	N/A	+	–	+	+	–	–	+	+	+
Urine L-FABP	N/A	–	–	+	?	?	–	+	+	+
TIMP-2 IGFBP-7	N/A	+	+	?	+	?	+	?	?	N/A
Urine protein/ albumin	+	+	+	+	?	?	?	?	?	+

+ = data published displays the ability to detect this aspect of AKI
– = data published does not display the ability to detect this aspect of AKI
? = no large multicenter data published on this biomarker/aspect of AKI
N/A (not applicable) (a) Biomarkers of tubular injury have no role in preoperative risk screening
(b) Serum creatinine is intrinsic to the definitions of AKI being tested
Adapted and expanded from: Koyner JL, Parikh CR. Clinical Utility of Biomarkers of AKI in Cardiac Surgery and Critical Illness. *Clin J Am Soc Nephrol.* 2013;8(6):1034–1042; used with permission

shown to detect AKI severity, whether defined as the need for RRT or progressive AKI, help differentiate transient AKI from more intrinsic forms of kidney injury, and also predict short- and long-term mortality.

A seminal investigation by Mishra and colleagues demonstrated the role of plasma and urinary NGAL as a marker of kidney injury in 71 children undergoing cardiopulmonary bypass [99]. In this prospective observational single-center study, the 2-h post-bypass NGAL levels in urine and plasma predicted AKI (defined as a 50% increase from baseline), with an AUC of 0.998 for the urine NGAL and 0.91 for the plasma NGAL. This study, along with several other single-center investigations, served the basis for the formation and funding of the Translational Research Investigating Biomarker Endpoints for AKI (TRIBE-AKI). TRIBE-AKI performed a multicenter prospective observational study of over 1200 adults and over 300 children undergoing cardiac surgery and has measured several AKI biomarkers in the blood and urine. Several of their findings with regard to early AKI, progressive AKI, and long-term mortality are summarized in Table 3.4 [47–49, 100–102]. While other groups have investigated biomarkers in the setting of cardiac surgery, the TRIBE-AKI group remains the largest cohort to date. Ho and colleagues have recently published a meta-analysis of 28 published studies/cohorts around both urine and serum biomarkers of AKI concluding that several biomarkers, including NGAL, KIM-1, IL-18, NAG, and albuminuria, all possess modest discriminatory function when measured within 24 h of cardiac surgery [103]. This conclusion is based on their analyses of the myriad of aforementioned studies which demonstrate that these biomarkers provide a composite AUC of less than 0.75. As of the end of 2015, there is limited single-center data linking tissue inhibitor metalloproteinase-2 and insulin-like growth factor-binding protein-7 (TIMP-2*IGFBP7) with post-CV surgery AKI; we anticipate large-scale validation of this marker in this clinical setting in the near future [104–106].

While TIMP-2*IGFBP7 remains under-validated in the setting of cardiac surgery, these cell cycle arrest biomarkers have been investigated in the setting of mixed medical surgical ICU patients [44, 107–109]. In fact these markers have been cleared for marketing and clinical use by the US Food and Drug Administration for their ability to assist in the risk stratification of those at risk for the future development of severe (stage 2 or 3) AKI. Kashani and colleagues investigated these markers in a multicenter prospective observational study (derivation cohort (n = 622) and validation cohort (n = 744)) and demonstrated that they exhibited an AUC of 0.80 for the development of stage 2 AKI or higher within the next 12 h [44]. When measured alone, IGFBP7 and TIMP-2 exhibited an AUC of 0.76 and 0.79, respectively, with several other biomarkers (e.g., NGAL, KIM-1, IL-18) demonstrating a similarly modest ability to predict impending severe AKI. TIMP-2*IGFBP7 at the time of ICU arrival was also associated with 9-month long-term outcomes; in an adjusted analysis of 692 subjects, TIMP-2*IGFBP7 values demonstrated a stepwise increase in the long-term risk of death or dialysis in those with AKI [109].

Investigations around these most common biomarkers remain ongoing with studies looking to validate their use in other clinical settings as well as determine factors that impact their prognostic abilities. There remains uncertainty around the impact of baseline chronic kidney function and other clinical factors such as diabetes or sepsis on the individual biomarker performance [110–115]. Similarly it remains unclear if biomarkers measured at the time of AKI are associated with the long-term development of CKD, but this is also an area of current investigation [116].

Finally, investigators have begun to examine the utility of these new biomarkers of AKI in the context of the aforementioned revised differential diagnosis of AKI proposed by the Acute Dialysis Quality Initiative (Fig. 3.1). Several studies have demonstrated that elevation in damage biomarkers (e.g., KIM-1 or NGAL) in the absence of changes in functional markers (e.g., serum creatinine and urine output) (this correlates with the "subclinical AKI" group in Fig. 3.1) places patients at increased risk of adverse events such as the need for RRT or inpatient mortality [14,

15, 100]. Some of these same studies have demonstrated that the risk of "subclinical" AKI is similar to the risk for those who have increases in functional marker without the increase in damage markers (prerenal azotemia).

Haase and colleagues conducted a pooled, prospective study (n = 2322) that designated subjects as NGAL-positive or NGAL-negative and creatinine-positive or creatinine-negative. In this compilation of ten previously published biomarker cohorts, AKI (creatinine-positive) was defined by the RIFLE-Risk criteria (50% increase in serum creatinine). Subjects who were NGAL-negative-creatinine-positive had similar lengths of ICU and hospital stay compared to those who were NGAL-positive-creatinine-negative. Additionally, individuals who were NGAL-positive-creatinine-negative received RRT more than 16 times more often than those who were NGAL- and creatinine-negative [14]. NGAL-positive-creatinine-negative patients were also in the ICU and hospital longer and more likely to experience inpatient mortality compared to NGAL-negative creatinine-negative.

NGAL's clinical utility and this concept of "subclinical AKI" are further strengthened in a similar analysis by Nickolas et al. who investigated NGAL and KIM-1, among other biomarkers in an international, prospective, observational study of 1635 unselected emergency room patients. Using a cutoff of 104 ng/mL for urine NGAL and 1.4 mg/dL for serum creatinine, Nickolas demonstrated that 5.3% of those who had NGAL defined subclinical AKI (NGAL >104 ng/mL and a creatinine <1.4 mg/dL) received RRT or experienced inpatient mortality. This was not different from the 5.1% of those who were NGAL-negative-creatinine-positive who experienced the same composite endpoint but was significantly higher than those who had no elevation in either their serum creatinine or NGAL [15]. The authors demonstrated a similar trend for KIM-1 (cutoff 2.82 ng/mL) and creatinine with those patients with KIM-1 defined subclinical AKI (KIM-1 > 2.82 ng/mL, creatinine < 1.4 mg/dL) being at increased risk for the same composite endpoint. In this study, as in the Haase pooled analysis, those subjects who were biomarker-positive-creatinine-positive were at highest risk for all of the adverse patient outcomes, again demonstrating the strength of combining biomarkers with serum creatinine to improve AKI risk stratification [14, 15].

Finally, Basu and colleagues have investigated the utility of combining urine NGAL (cutoff of 200 ng/mg creatinine) and serum cystatin C (another functional marker, cutoff of 0.8 mg/L). In a cohort of 345 pediatric cardiac surgery subjects, they demonstrated that the composite of NGAL-positive/cystatin-positive outperformed the change in serum creatinine for both the development of severe AKI (defined as KDIGO stage 2 or higher) and persistent AKI (defined as lasting more than 48 h) [117]. Thus the combination of a glomerular function and tubular injury biomarker improved diagnostic precision over serum creatinine alone.

This idea of combining novel biomarkers with each other as well as with serum creatinine is attractive. Several studies have attempted to combine two or more biomarkers to improve their predictive capabilities for early and severe AKI [44, 49, 118–120]. While some studies have simply used the product of two biomarkers and then assessed the AUC, others have used techniques such as logistic regression to assess the AUC for two or more biomarkers. No consensus for the statistical methods for combining biomarkers exists, and this topic remains an area of continued investigation. More recent studies have acknowledged the premise that individual biomarkers will have their own specific kinetics and that combining biomarkers from different time points may improve their predictive capabilities [49]. As we learn more about the pathophysiologic and clinical factors that impact these new tests, our ability to combine them in a clinically meaningful manner will increase, and this in turn will lead to improved clinical care.

With data demonstrating a clear association between biomarker-positive-creatinine-negative patients and adverse outcomes, clinicians will increasingly face the challenge of caring for these patients. There is limited data on the how best to care for such patients; however, recent studies demonstrate a clear benefit of guideline-driven care in the setting of early AKI and biomarker-defined AKI [121–123]. Kolhe et al. investigated outcomes in a cohort of patients whose treating physicians received an interruptive electronic alert when those patients developed clinical AKI (AKIN and KDIGO definitions). This AKI alert was linked with a care bundle that followed simple guideline-based recommendations (assess history and examine patient, check a urinalysis, attempt to classify AKI, and treat the AKI) [122]. Completion of the AKI care bundle (which occurred in only 12.2%, $n = 306$) was associated with significantly improved patient outcomes including decreased progression to more severe AKI and lower inpatient mortality [122]. Similarly, Zarbock and colleagues conducted a single-center randomized controlled trial investigating the implementation of the KDIGO treatment guidelines in patients deemed to be high risk for AKI (as measured by a TIMP-2*IGFBP7 > 0.3) following adult cardiac surgery [123]. Biomarker-positive patients who were randomized to receive a KDIGO cardiac surgery care bundle (avoidance of nephrotoxins, discontinuation of renin-angiotensin agents for 48 h, volume management through a prespecified algorithm with a cardiac output monitoring catheter, avoidance of hyperglycemia, and strict monitoring of inputs and outputs) developed KDIGO AKI less frequently than those with elevated biomarkers receiving usual care (71.7% vs. 55.1%; $p = 0.004$). More specifically, those receiving the care bundle had fewer episodes of stage 2 and 3 AKI (29.7% vs. 44.9%) with an odds ratio (95%CI) of 0.52 (0.32–0.85) and $p = 0.009$ [123]. Thus while there are many exciting and novel therapeutics being investigated for the treatment (and prevention) of AKI, recent data demonstrate a clear benefit to simple guideline-driven interventions in the setting of early creatinine-based AKI as well as biomarker-defined AKI.

References

1. KDIGO. Kidney Disease: Improving Global Outcomes (KDIGO) Acute Kidney Injury Work Group. KDIGO clinical practice guideline for acute kidney injury. Kidney Int. 2012;2:1–138.
2. Koyner JL, Parikh CR. Clinical utility of biomarkers of AKI in cardiac surgery and critical illness. Clin J Am Soc Nephrol. 2013;8(6):1034–42.
3. Thadhani R, Pascual M, Bonventre JV. Acute renal failure. N Engl J Med. 1996;334(22):1448–60.
4. Kelleher SP, Robinette JB, Conger JD. Sympathetic nervous system in the loss of autoregulation in acute renal failure. Am J Physiol. 1984;246(4 Pt 2):F379–86.
5. Nolan CR, Anderson RJ. Hospital-acquired acute renal failure. J Am Soc Nephrol. 1998;9(4):710–8.
6. Sacks SH, Aparicio SA, Bevan A, Oliver DO, Will EJ, Davison AM. Late renal failure due to prostatic outflow obstruction: a preventable disease. BMJ. 1989;298(6667):156–9.
7. Humphreys BD, Soiffer RJ, Magee CC. Renal failure associated with cancer and its treatment: an update. J Am Soc Nephrol. 2005;16(1):151–61.
8. Thomas MH, Chisholm GD. Retroperitoneal fibrosis associated with malignant disease. Br J Cancer. 1973;28(5):453–8.
9. Liaño F, Pascual J. Epidemiology of acute renal failure: a prospective, multicenter, community-based study. Madrid Acute Renal Failure Study Group. Kidney Int. 1996;50(3):811–8.
10. Rosen S, Stillman IE. Acute tubular necrosis is a syndrome of physiologic and pathologic dissociation. J Am Soc Nephrol. 2008;19(5):871–5.
11. Perazella MA, Markowitz GS. Drug-induced acute interstitial nephritis. Nat Rev Nephrol. 2010;6(8):461–70.
12. Endre ZH, Kellum JA, Di Somma S, et al. Differential diagnosis of AKI in clinical practice by functional and damage biomarkers: workgroup statements from the tenth Acute Dialysis Quality Initiative Consensus Conference. Contrib Nephrol. 2013;182:30–44.
13. Bosch JP. Renal reserve: a functional view of glomerular filtration rate. Semin Nephrol. 1995;15(5):381–5.
14. Haase M, Devarajan P, Haase-Fielitz A, et al. The outcome of neutrophil gelatinase-associated lipocalin-positive subclinical acute kidney injury a multicenter pooled analysis of prospective studies. J Am Coll Cardiol. 2011;57(17):1752–61.
15. Nickolas TL, Schmidt-Ott KM, Canetta P, et al. Diagnostic and prognostic stratification in the emergency department using urinary biomarkers of nephron damage: a multicenter prospective cohort study. J Am Coll Cardiol. 2012;59(3):246–55.
16. Bellomo R, Kellum JA, Bagshaw SM. Normotensive ischemic acute renal failure. N Engl J Med. 2007;357(21):2205; author reply 2205–6.

17. Poukkanen M, Wilkman E, Vaara ST, et al. Hemodynamic variables and progression of acute kidney injury in critically ill patients with severe sepsis: data from the prospective observational FINNAKI study. Crit Care. 2013;17(6):R295.
18. Xue FS, Li RP, Wang SY. Association of intraoperative hypotension with postoperative acute kidney and myocardial injuries in noncardiac surgery patients. Anesthesiology. 2014;120(5):1278–80.
19. Walsh M, Devereaux PJ, Garg AX, et al. Relationship between intraoperative mean arterial pressure and clinical outcomes after noncardiac surgery: toward an empirical definition of hypotension. Anesthesiology. 2013;119(3):507–15.
20. Badin J, Boulain T, Ehrmann S, et al. Relation between mean arterial pressure and renal function in the early phase of shock: a prospective, explorative cohort study. Crit Care. 2011;15(3):R135.
21. Lehman LW, Saeed M, Moody G, Mark R. Hypotension as a risk factor for acute kidney injury in ICU patients. Comput Cardiol (2010). 2010;37:1095–8.
22. Raimundo M, Crichton S, Syed Y, et al. Low systemic oxygen delivery and BP and risk of progression of early AKI. Clin J Am Soc Nephrol. 2015;10(8):1340–9.
23. Meyer TW, Hostetter TH. Uremia. N Engl J Med. 2007;357(13):1316–25.
24. Clarkson MR, Giblin L, O'Connell FP, et al. Acute interstitial nephritis: clinical features and response to corticosteroid therapy. Nephrol Dial Transplant. 2004;19(11):2778–83.
25. Sugrue M. Abdominal compartment syndrome. Curr Opin Crit Care. 2005;11(4):333–8.
26. Bailey J, Shapiro MJ. Abdominal compartment syndrome. Crit Care. 2000;4(1):23–9.
27. Malbrain ML, Deeren D, De Potter TJ. Intra-abdominal hypertension in the critically ill: it is time to pay attention. Curr Opin Crit Care. 2005;11(2):156–71.
28. Kirkpatrick AW, Roberts DJ, De Waele J, et al. Intra-abdominal hypertension and the abdominal compartment syndrome: updated consensus definitions and clinical practice guidelines from the World Society of the Abdominal Compartment Syndrome. Intensive Care Med. 2013;39(7):1190–206.
29. Uchino S, Bellomo R, Goldsmith D. The meaning of the blood urea nitrogen/creatinine ratio in acute kidney injury. Clin Kidney J. 2012;5(2):187–91.
30. Adams D, de Jonge R, van der Cammen T, Zietse R, Hoorn EJ. Acute kidney injury in patients presenting with hyponatremia. J Nephrol. 2011;24(6):749–55.
31. Turgutalp K, Ozhan O, Gok Oguz E, et al. Clinical features, outcome and cost of hyponatremia-associated admission and hospitalization in elderly and very elderly patients: a single-center experience in Turkey. Int Urol Nephrol. 2013;45(1):265–73.
32. Uchino S, Bellomo R, Ronco C. Intermittent versus continuous renal replacement therapy in the ICU: impact on electrolyte and acid-base balance. Intensive Care Med. 2001;27(6):1037–43.
33. Funk GC, Lindner G, Druml W, et al. Incidence and prognosis of dysnatremias present on ICU admission. Intensive Care Med. 2010;36(2):304–11.
34. An JN, Lee JP, Jeon HJ, et al. Severe hyperkalemia requiring hospitalization: predictors of mortality. Crit Care. 2012;16(6):R225.
35. Libório AB, Leite TT, Neves FM, Teles F, Bezerra CT. AKI complications in critically ill patients: association with mortality rates and RRT. Clin J Am Soc Nephrol. 2015;10(1):21–8.
36. Vaara ST, Reinikainen M, Wald R, Bagshaw SM, Pettila V. Timing of RRT based on the presence of conventional indications. Clin J Am Soc Nephrol. 2014;9(9):1577–85.
37. Bellomo R, Cass A, Cole L, et al. Intensity of continuous renal-replacement therapy in critically ill patients. N Engl J Med. 2009;361(17):1627–38.
38. Perazella MA, Coca SG, Kanbay M, Brewster UC, Parikh CR. Diagnostic value of urine microscopy for differential diagnosis of acute kidney injury in hospitalized patients. Clin J Am Soc Nephrol. 2008;3(6):1615–9.
39. Perazella MA. The urine sediment as a biomarker of kidney disease. Am J Kidney Dis. 2015;66(5):748–55.
40. Bagshaw SM, Haase M, Haase-Fielitz A, Bennett M, Devarajan P, Bellomo R. A prospective evaluation of urine microscopy in septic and non-septic acute kidney injury. Nephrol Dial Transplant. 2012;27(2):582–8.
41. Chawla LS, Dommu A, Berger A, Shih S, Patel SS. Urinary sediment cast scoring index for acute kidney injury: a pilot study. Nephron Clin Pract. 2008;110(3):c145–50.
42. Perazella MA, Coca SG, Hall IE, Iyanam U, Koraishy M, Parikh CR. Urine microscopy is associated with severity and worsening of acute kidney injury in hospitalized patients. Clin J Am Soc Nephrol. 2010;5(3):402–8.
43. Schinstock CA, Semret MH, Wagner SJ, et al. Urinalysis is more specific and urinary neutrophil gelatinase-associated lipocalin is more sensitive for early detection of acute kidney injury. Nephrol Dial Transplant. 2013;28(5):1175–85.
44. Kashani K, Al-Khafaji A, Ardiles T, et al. Discovery and validation of cell cycle arrest biomarkers in human acute kidney injury. Crit Care. 2013;17(1):R25.
45. Endre ZH, Walker RJ, Pickering JW, et al. Early intervention with erythropoietin does not affect the outcome of acute kidney injury (the EARLYARF trial). Kidney Int. 2010;77(11):1020–30.
46. Ralib A, Pickering JW, Shaw GM, et al. Test characteristics of urinary biomarkers depend on quantitation method in acute kidney injury. J Am Soc Nephrol. 2012;23(2):322–33.
47. Parikh CR, Coca SG, Thiessen-Philbrook H, et al. Postoperative biomarkers predict acute kidney injury and poor outcomes after adult cardiac surgery. J Am Soc Nephrol. 2011;22(9):1748–57.

48. Parikh CR, Devarajan P, Zappitelli M, et al. Postoperative biomarkers predict acute kidney injury and poor outcomes after pediatric cardiac surgery. J Am Soc Nephrol. 2011;22(9):1737–47.
49. Parikh CR, Thiessen-Philbrook H, Garg AX, et al. Performance of kidney injury molecule-1 and liver fatty acid-binding protein and combined biomarkers of AKI after cardiac surgery. Clin J Am Soc Nephrol. 2013;8(7):1079–88.
50. Muriithi AK, Nasr SH, Leung N. Utility of urine eosinophils in the diagnosis of acute interstitial nephritis. Clin J Am Soc Nephrol. 2013;8(11):1857–62.
51. Espinel CH, Gregory AW. Differential diagnosis of acute renal failure. Clin Nephrol. 1980;13(2):73–7.
52. Miller TR, Anderson RJ, Linas SL, et al. Urinary diagnostic indices in acute renal failure: a prospective study. Ann Intern Med. 1978;89(1):47–50.
53. Espinel CH. The FENa test. Use in the differential diagnosis of acute renal failure. JAMA. 1976;236(6):579–81.
54. Bagshaw SM, Langenberg C, Bellomo R. Urinary biochemistry and microscopy in septic acute renal failure: a systematic review. Am J Kidney Dis. 2006;48(5):695–705.
55. Pru C, Kjellstrand CM. The FENa test is of no prognostic value in acute renal failure. Nephron. 1984;36(1):20–3.
56. Jones LW, Weil MH. Water, creatinine and sodium excretion following circulatory shock with renal failure. Am J Med. 1971;51(3):314–8.
57. Vaz AJ. Low fractional excretion of urine sodium in acute renal failure due to sepsis. Arch Intern Med. 1983;143(4):738–9.
58. Langenberg C, Wan L, Bagshaw SM, Egi M, May CN, Bellomo R. Urinary biochemistry in experimental septic acute renal failure. Nephrol Dial Transplant. 2006;21(12):3389–97.
59. Fang LS, Sirota RA, Ebert TH, Lichtenstein NS. Low fractional excretion of sodium with contrast media-induced acute renal failure. Arch Intern Med. 1980;140(4):531–3.
60. Van Biesen W, Yegenaga I, Vanholder R, et al. Relationship between fluid status and its management on acute renal failure (ARF) in intensive care unit (ICU) patients with sepsis: a prospective analysis. J Nephrol. 2005;18(1):54–60.
61. Koyner JL, Bennett MR, Worcester EM, et al. Urinary cystatin C as an early biomarker of acute kidney injury following adult cardiothoracic surgery. Kidney Int. 2008;23:23.
62. Koyner JL, Davison DL, Brasha-Mitchell E, et al. Furosemide stress test and biomarkers for the prediction of AKI severity. J Am Soc Nephrol. 2015;26(8):2023–31.
63. Koyner JL, Vaidya VS, Bennett MR, et al. Urinary biomarkers in the clinical prognosis and early detection of acute kidney injury. Clin J Am Soc Nephrol. 2010;5(12):2154–65.
64. Belcher JM, Sanyal AJ, Peixoto AJ, et al. Kidney biomarkers and differential diagnosis of patients with cirrhosis and acute kidney injury. Hepatology (Baltimore, Md). 2014;60(2):622–32.
65. Belcher JM, Garcia-Tsao G, Sanyal AJ, et al. Urinary biomarkers and progression of AKI in patients with cirrhosis. Clin J Am Soc Nephrol. 2014;9(11):1857–67.
66. Kaplan AA, Kohn OF. Fractional excretion of urea as a guide to renal dysfunction. Am J Nephrol. 1992;12(1–2):49–54.
67. Carvounis CP, Nisar S, Guro-Razuman S. Significance of the fractional excretion of urea in the differential diagnosis of acute renal failure. Kidney Int. 2002;62(6):2223–9.
68. Kalantarinia K. Novel imaging techniques in acute kidney injury. Curr Drug Targets. 2009;10(12):1184–9.
69. Gottlieb RH, Voci SL, Cholewinski SP, et al. Sonography: a useful tool to detect the mechanical causes of renal transplant dysfunction. J Clin Ultrasound. 1999;27(6):325–33.
70. Smith-Bindman R, Aubin C, Bailitz J, et al. Ultrasonography versus computed tomography for suspected nephrolithiasis. N Engl J Med. 2014;371(12):1100–10.
71. Anderson IH, Jones GR, Standen JR. Ultrasonographic assessment of hydronephrosis of pregnancy. J Can Assoc Radiol. 1983;34(1):29–31.
72. Stevens S, Brown BD, McGahan JP. Nephrogenic diabetes insipidus: a cause of severe nonobstructive urinary tract dilatation. J Ultrasound Med. 1995;14(7):543–5.
73. Pozzi Mucelli R, Bertolotto M, Quaia E. Imaging techniques in acute renal failure. Contrib Nephrol. 2001;132:76–91.
74. Platt JF, Ellis JH, Rubin JM, DiPietro MA, Sedman AB. Intrarenal arterial Doppler sonography in patients with nonobstructive renal disease: correlation of resistive index with biopsy findings. AJR Am J Roentgenol. 1990;154(6):1223–7.
75. Abu-Alfa AK. Nephrogenic systemic fibrosis and gadolinium-based contrast agents. Adv Chronic Kidney Dis. 2011;18(3):188–98.
76. Choyke PL, Kobayashi H. Functional magnetic resonance imaging of the kidney using macromolecular contrast agents. Abdom Imaging. 2006;31(2):224–31.
77. Juillard L, Lerman LO, Kruger DG, et al. Blood oxygen level-dependent measurement of acute intrarenal ischemia. Kidney Int. 2004;65(3):944–50.
78. Pedersen M, Dissing TH, Mørkenborg J, et al. Validation of quantitative BOLD MRI measurements in kidney: application to unilateral ureteral obstruction. Kidney Int. 2005;67(6):2305–12.
79. Zhang JL, Morrell G, Rusinek H, et al. Measurement of renal tissue oxygenation with blood oxygen level-dependent MRI and oxygen transit modeling. Am J Physiol Renal Physiol. 2014;306(6):F579–87.
80. Li LP, Ji L, Santos E, Dunkle E, Pierchala L, Prasad P. Effect of nitric oxide synthase inhibition on intrarenal oxygenation as evaluated by blood oxygen-

ation level-dependent magnetic resonance imaging. Invest Radiol. 2009;44(2):67–73.
81. Arakelyan K, Cantow K, Hentschel J, et al. Early effects of an x-ray contrast medium on renal T(2) */T(2) MRI as compared to short-term hyperoxia, hypoxia and aortic occlusion in rats. Acta Physiol (Oxf). 2013;208(2):202–13.
82. Alford SK, Sadowski EA, Unal O, et al. Detection of acute renal ischemia in swine using blood oxygen level-dependent magnetic resonance imaging. J Magn Reson Imaging. 2005;22(3):347–53.
83. Han F, Xiao W, Xu Y, et al. The significance of BOLD MRI in differentiation between renal transplant rejection and acute tubular necrosis. Nephrol Dial Transplant. 2008;23(8):2666–72.
84. Zhou HY, Chen TW, Zhang XM. Functional magnetic resonance imaging in acute kidney injury: present status. Biomed Res Int. 2016;2016:2027370.
85. Fischer K, Meral FC, Zhang Y, et al. High-resolution renal perfusion mapping using contrast-enhanced ultrasonography in ischemia-reperfusion injury monitors changes in renal microperfusion. Kidney Int. 2016;89(6):1388–98.
86. Schneider AG, Schelleman A, Goodwin MD, Bailey M, Eastwood GM, Bellomo R. Contrast-enhanced ultrasound evaluation of the renal microcirculation response to terlipressin in hepato-renal syndrome: a preliminary report. Ren Fail. 2015;37(1):175–9.
87. Schneider AG, Goodwin MD, Schelleman A, Bailey M, Johnson L, Bellomo R. Contrast-enhanced ultrasound to evaluate changes in renal cortical perfusion around cardiac surgery: a pilot study. Crit Care. 2013;17(4):R138.
88. Schneider AG, Calzavacca P, Schelleman A, et al. Contrast-enhanced ultrasound evaluation of renal microcirculation in sheep. Intensive Care Med Exp. 2014;2(1):33.
89. Okusa MD, Jaber BL, Doran P, et al. Physiological biomarkers of acute kidney injury: a conceptual approach to improving outcomes. Contrib Nephrol. 2013;182:65–81.
90. Bellomo R, Ronco C, Kellum JA, Mehta RL, Palevsky P. Acute renal failure—definition, outcome measures, animal models, fluid therapy and information technology needs: the Second International Consensus Conference of the Acute Dialysis Quality Initiative (ADQI) Group. Crit Care. 2004;8(4):R204–12.
91. Mehta RL, Kellum JA, Shah SV, et al. Acute Kidney Injury Network: report of an initiative to improve outcomes in acute kidney injury. Crit Care. 2007;11(2):R31.
92. Baum N, Dichoso CC, Carlton CE. Blood urea nitrogen and serum creatinine. Physiology and interpretations. Urology. 1975;5(5):583–8.
93. Ducharme MP, Smythe M, Strohs G. Drug-induced alterations in serum creatinine concentrations. Ann Pharmacother. 1993;27(5):622–33.
94. Charlton JR, Portilla D, Okusa MD. A basic science view of acute kidney injury biomarkers. Nephrol Dial Transplant. 2014;29(7):1301–11.
95. Chen LX, Koyner JL. Biomarkers in acute kidney injury. Crit Care Clin. 2015;31(4):633–48.
96. Vanmassenhove J, Vanholder R, Nagler E, Van Biesen W. Urinary and serum biomarkers for the diagnosis of acute kidney injury: an in-depth review of the literature. Nephrol Dial Transplant. 2013;28(2):254–73.
97. Ostermann M, Philips BJ, Forni LG. Clinical review: biomarkers of acute kidney injury: where are we now? Crit Care. 2012;16(5):233.
98. Chawla LS, Davison DL, Brasha-Mitchell E, et al. Development and standardization of a furosemide stress test to predict the severity of acute kidney injury. Crit Care. 2013;17(5):R207.
99. Mishra J, Dent C, Tarabishi R, et al. Neutrophil gelatinase-associated lipocalin (NGAL) as a biomarker for acute renal injury after cardiac surgery. Lancet. 2005;365(9466):1231–8.
100. Coca SG, Garg AX, Thiessen-Philbrook H, et al. Urinary biomarkers of AKI and mortality 3 years after cardiac surgery. J Am Soc Nephrol. 2014;25(5):1063–71.
101. Koyner JL, Garg AX, Coca SG, et al. Biomarkers predict progression of acute kidney injury after cardiac surgery. J Am Soc Nephrol. 2012;23(5):905–14.
102. Zappitelli M, Coca SG, Garg AX, et al. The association of albumin/creatinine ratio with postoperative AKI in children undergoing cardiac surgery. Clin J Am Soc Nephrol. 2012;7(11):1761–9.
103. Ho J, Tangri N, Komenda P, et al. Urinary, plasma, and serum biomarkers' utility for predicting acute kidney injury associated with cardiac surgery in adults: a meta-analysis. Am J Kidney Dis. 2015;66(6):993–1005.
104. Pilarczyk K, Edayadiyil-Dudasova M, Wendt D, et al. Urinary [TIMP-2]*[IGFBP7] for early prediction of acute kidney injury after coronary artery bypass surgery. Ann Intensive Care. 2015;5(1):50.
105. Meersch M, Schmidt C, Van Aken H, et al. Validation of cell-cycle arrest biomarkers for acute kidney injury after pediatric cardiac surgery. PLoS One. 2014;9(10):e110865.
106. Meersch M, Schmidt C, Van Aken H, et al. Urinary TIMP-2 and IGFBP7 as early biomarkers of acute kidney injury and renal recovery following cardiac surgery. PLoS One. 2014;9(3):e93460.
107. Bihorac A, Chawla LS, Shaw AD, et al. Validation of cell-cycle arrest biomarkers for acute kidney injury using clinical adjudication. Am J Respir Crit Care Med. 2014;189(8):932–9.
108. Hoste EA, McCullough PA, Kashani K, et al. Derivation and validation of cutoffs for clinical use of cell cycle arrest biomarkers. Nephrol Dial Transplant. 2014;29(11):2054–61.
109. Koyner JL, Shaw AD, Chawla LS, et al. Tissue inhibitor metalloproteinase-2 (TIMP-2) IGF-binding protein-7 (IGFBP7) levels are associated with adverse long-term outcomes in patients with AKI. J Am Soc Nephrol. 2015;26(7):1747–54.

110. Endre ZH, Pickering JW, Walker RJ, et al. Improved performance of urinary biomarkers of acute kidney injury in the critically ill by stratification for injury duration and baseline renal function. Kidney Int. 2011;79(10):1119–30.
111. Koyner JL, Coca SG, Thiessen-Philbrook H, et al. Urine biomarkers and perioperative acute kidney injury: the impact of preoperative estimated GFR. Am J Kidney Dis. 2015;66(6):1006–14.
112. Chou KM, Lee CC, Chen CH, Sun CY. Clinical value of NGAL, L-FABP and albuminuria in predicting GFR decline in type 2 diabetes mellitus patients. PLoS One. 2013;8(1):e54863.
113. Conway BR, Manoharan D, Manoharan D, et al. Measuring urinary tubular biomarkers in type 2 diabetes does not add prognostic value beyond established risk factors. Kidney Int. 2012;82(7):812–8.
114. Bagshaw SM, Langenberg C, Haase M, Wan L, May CN, Bellomo R. Urinary biomarkers in septic acute kidney injury. Intensive Care Med. 2007;9:9.
115. Parikh CR, Abraham E, Ancukiewicz M, Edelstein CL. Urine IL-18 is an early diagnostic marker for acute kidney injury and predicts mortality in the intensive care unit. J Am Soc Nephrol. 2005;16(10):3046–52.
116. Go AS, Parikh CR, Ikizler TA, et al. The assessment, serial evaluation, and subsequent sequelae of acute kidney injury (ASSESS-AKI) study: design and methods. BMC Nephrol. 2010;11:22.
117. Basu RK, Wong HR, Krawczeski CD, et al. Combining functional and tubular damage biomarkers improves diagnostic precision for acute kidney injury after cardiac surgery. J Am Coll Cardiol. 2014;64(25):2753–62.
118. Krawczeski CD, Goldstein SL, Woo JG, et al. Temporal relationship and predictive value of urinary acute kidney injury biomarkers after pediatric cardiopulmonary bypass. J Am Coll Cardiol. 2011;58(22):2301–9.
119. Katagiri D, Doi K, Honda K, et al. Combination of two urinary biomarkers predicts acute kidney injury after adult cardiac surgery. Ann Thorac Surg. 2012;93(2):577–83.
120. Katagiri D, Doi K, Matsubara T, et al. New biomarker panel of plasma neutrophil gelatinase-associated lipocalin and endotoxin activity assay for detecting sepsis in acute kidney injury. J Crit Care. 2013;28(5):564–70.
121. Kolhe NV, Reilly T, Leung J, et al. A simple care bundle for use in acute kidney injury: a propensity score matched cohort study. Nephrol Dial Transplant. 2016;31(11):1846–54.
122. Kolhe NV, Staples D, Reilly T, et al. Impact of compliance with a care bundle on acute kidney injury outcomes: a prospective observational study. PLoS One. 2015;10(7):e0132279.
123. Meersch M, Schmidt C, Hoffmeier A, et al. Prevention of cardiac surgery-associated AKI by implementing the KDIGO guidelines in high risk patients identified by biomarkers: the PrevAKI randomized controlled trial. Intensive Care Med. 2017;43(11):1551–61.
124. Zhang Z, Lu B, Sheng X, Jin N. Cystatin C in prediction of acute kidney injury: a systemic review and meta-analysis. Am J Kidney Dis. 2011;58(3):356–65.
125. Herget-Rosenthal S, Bökenkamp A, Hofmann W. How to estimate GFR-serum creatinine, serum cystatin C or equations? Clin Biochem. 2007;40(3–4):153–61.
126. Séronie-Vivien S, Delanaye P, Piéroni L, Mariat C, Froissart M, Cristol J-P. Cystatin C: current position and future prospects. Clin Chem Lab Med. 2008;46:1664.
127. Nejat M, Hill JV, Pickering JW, Edelstein CL, Devarajan P, Endre ZH. Albuminuria increases cystatin C excretion: implications for urinary biomarkers. Nephrol Dial Transplant. 2012;27(Suppl 3):iii96–iii103.
128. Dinarello CA, Novick D, Kim S, Kaplanski G. Interleukin-18 and IL-18 binding protein. Front Immunol. 2013;4:289.
129. Parikh CR, Jani A, Melnikov VY, Faubel S, Edelstein CL. Urinary interleukin-18 is a marker of human acute tubular necrosis1. Am J Kidney Dis. 2004;43(3):405–14.
130. Ichimura T, Bonventre JV, Bailly V, et al. Kidney injury molecule-1 (KIM-1), a putative epithelial cell adhesion molecule containing a novel immunoglobulin domain, is up-regulated in renal cells after injury. J Biol Chem. 1998;273(7):4135–42.
131. Bonventre JV. Kidney injury molecule-1: a translational journey. Trans Am Clin Climatol Assoc. 2014;125:293–9.
132. Ichimura T, Brooks CR, Bonventre JV. Kim-1/Tim-1 and immune cells: shifting Sands. Kidney Int. 2012;81(9):809–11.
133. Maatman RG, van de Westerlo EM, van Kuppevelt TH, Veerkamp JH. Molecular identification of the liver- and the heart-type fatty acid-binding proteins in human and rat kidney. Use of the reverse transcriptase polymerase chain reaction. Biochem J. 1992;288(Pt 1):285–90.
134. Yamamoto T, Noiri E, Ono Y, et al. Renal L-type fatty acid–binding protein in acute ischemic injury. J Am Soc Nephrol. 2007;18(11):2894–902.
135. Tanaka T, Noiri E, Yamamoto T, et al. Urinary human L-FABP is a potential biomarker to predict COX-inhibitor-induced renal injury. Nephron Exp Nephrol. 2008;108(1):e19–26.
136. Negishi K, Noiri E, Sugaya T, et al. A role of liver fatty acid-binding protein in cisplatin-induced acute renal failure. Kidney Int. 2007;72(3):348–58.
137. Yamashita T, Doi K, Hamasaki Y, Matsubara T, et al. Evaluation of urinary tissue inhibitor of metalloproteinase-2 in acute kidney injury: a prospective observational study. Crit Care. 2014;18(6):716. https://www.ncbi.nlm.nih.gov/pubmed/25524453
138. Kjeldsen L, Johnsen A, Sengelov H, Borregaard N. Isolation and primary structure of NGAL, a novel protein associated with human neutrophil

gelatinase. J Biol Chem. 1993;268(0021–9258 (Print)):10425–32.
139. Haase-Fielitz A, Haase M, Devarajan P. Neutrophil gelatinase-associated lipocalin as a biomarker of acute kidney injury: a critical evaluation of current status. Ann Clin Biochem. 2014;51(Pt 3):335–51.
140. Singer E, Markó L, Paragas N, et al. Neutrophil gelatinase-associated lipocalin: pathophysiology and clinical applications. Acta Physiol (Oxf). 2013;207(4):663–72.
141. Martensson J, Bellomo R. The rise and fall of NGAL in acute kidney injury. Blood Purif. 2014;37:304–10.
142. Chang C, Werb Z. The many faces of metalloproteases: cell growth, invasion, angiogenesis and metastasis. Trends Cell Biol. 2001;11(11):S37–43.
143. Tamura K, Hashimoto K, Suzuki K, Yoshie M, Kutsukake M, Sakurai T. Insulin-like growth factor binding protein-7 (IGFBP7) blocks vascular endothelial cell growth factor (VEGF)-induced angiogenesis in human vascular endothelial cells. Eur J Pharmacol. 2009;610(1–3):61–7.
144. Mazanowska O, Żabińska M, Kościelska-Kasprzak K, et al. Increased plasma matrix metalloproteinase-2 (MMP-2), tissue inhibitor of proteinase-1 (TIMP-1), TIMP-2, and urine MMP-2 concentrations correlate with proteinuria in renal transplant recipients. Transplant Proc. 2014;46(8):2636–9.
145. Seo D-W, Li H, Qu C-K, et al. Shp-1 mediates the antiproliferative activity of tissue inhibitor of metalloproteinase-2 in human microvascular endothelial cells. J Biol Chem. 2006;281(6):3711–21.
146. Hwa V, Oh Y, Rosenfeld RG. The insulin-like growth factor-binding protein (IGFBP) superfamily. Endocr Rev. 1999;20(6):761–87.

Part II

Pathophysiology

Overview of Pathophysiology of Acute Kidney Injury: Human Evidence, Mechanisms, Pathological Correlations and Biomarkers and Animal Models

4

Timothy J. Pianta, Glenda C. Gobe, Evan P. Owens, and Zoltan H. Endre

Abbreviations

AKI	Acute kidney injury
ATI	Acute tubular injury
ATN	Acute tubular necrosis
Bax	B-cell lymphoma 2/Bcl-2-associated X protein
CKD	Chronic kidney disease
CXCl16	Chemokine ligand 16
EDHF	Endothelium-derived hyperpolarising factor
ER	Endoplasmic reticulum
ESKD	End-stage kidney disease
FENa	Fractional excretion of sodium
GFR	Glomerular filtration rate
GST	Glutathione *S*-transferase
HR	Hazard ratio
ICAM-1	Intercellular adhesion molecule-1
ICU	Intensive care unit
IGFBP7	Insulin-like growth factor-binding protein 7
IL	Interleukin
im	Intramuscular
ip	Intraperitoneal
iv	Intravenous
KIM-1	Kidney injury molecule-1
L-FABP	Liver-associated fatty acid-binding protein
LPS	Lipopolysaccharide
MCP-1	Monocyte chemotactic protein-1
MIF	Migration inhibitory factor
MPT	Mitochondria permeability transition
NGAL	Neutrophil gelatinase-associated lipocalin
NO	Nitric oxide
NOS	Nitric oxide synthase

T. J. Pianta
Northern Clinical School, University of Melbourne, Epping, VIC, Australia
e-mail: timothy.pianta@nh.org.au

G. C. Gobe
School of Medicine, Centre for Kidney Disease Research, University of Queensland, Brisbane, QLD, Australia
e-mail: g.gobe@uq.edu.au

E. P. Owens
Centre for Kidney Disease Research, The University of Queensland, Brisbane, QLD, Australia
e-mail: evan.owens@uq.edu.au

Z. H. Endre (✉)
Department of Nephrology, Prince of Wales Hospital and Clinical School, University of New South Wales, Sydney, NSW, Australia
e-mail: zoltan.endre@unsw.edu.au; z.endre@unsw.edu.au

S. S. Waikar et al. (eds.), *Core Concepts in Acute Kidney Injury*,
https://doi.org/10.1007/978-1-4939-8628-6_4

PIDD	p53-induced protein with death domain
PUMA-α[alpha]	p53 upregulated modulator of apoptosis-α[alpha]
ROS	Reactive oxygen species
SCr	Serum creatinine
TBARS	Thiobarbituric acid-reacting substances
TGF	Transforming growth factor
TIMP-2	Tissue inhibitor of metalloproteinases-2
TNF-α[alpha]	Tumour necrosis factor-α[alpha]
VEGF	Vascular endothelial growth factor

4.1 Introduction: Evidence of the Human Significance of Acute Kidney Injury

Acute kidney injury (AKI) is the consensus term for acute kidney failure, previously termed acute renal failure, and is an important global clinical problem with adverse effects on patient prognosis and healthcare costs [1, 2]. AKI is a syndrome of multifactorial origin characterised by rapid loss of kidney function and oliguria. Depending on the definition used, AKI has been estimated to occur in 3–30% of hospitalised patients [1, 3, 4] and up to 60% of critically ill patients [5–8] with severe AKI that requires dialysis complicating the care of more than 5% of patients who require intensive care [8]. The scale of the problem is enormous. Recent large-scale meta-analyses, utilising the consensus Kidney Disease: Improving Global Outcomes (KDIGO) definition and incorporating data from over 49 million subjects, confirm that 1 in 5 adults and 1 in 3 children worldwide experience AKI during a hospital episode of care [9], with 2% of hospital admissions and 11% of all AKI requiring dialysis [10].

Mortality and morbidity associated with AKI are high. Using the Acute Kidney Injury Network (AKIN) staging of AKI (Table 4.1), the pooled AKI-associated all-cause mortality rate was 23.0% (95% CI, 21.3–24.8) and increased with higher stages of severity amongst 110 studies that used the KDIGO-equivalent AKI definition [9]. For AKI stages 1–3, the odds ratios (OR) for mortality versus no-AKI were, respectively, 3.37 (95% CI, 2.43–4.68), 7.52 (95% CI, 5.03–11.27) and 13.19 (95% CI, 8.39–20.76). For patients who required dialysis, the OR for mortality was 24.08 (95% CI, 12.62–45.95) [9]. Thus mortality

Table 4.1 Classification and staging of acute kidney injury

	Serum creatinine	Urine output
RIFLE classification		
Risk	Serum creatinine increase to >1.5-fold	<0.5 mL/kg/h for 6 h
Injury	Serum creatinine increase to >2.0-fold	<0.5 mL/kg/h for 12 h
Failure	Serum creatinine increase to >3.0-fold OR serum creatinine ≥354 μ[mu]mol/L (≥4 mg/dL) with an acute increase of at least 44 μ[mu]mol/L (0.5 mg/dL)	Anuria for 12 h
AKIN staging		
1	Serum creatinine increase ≥26.5 μ[mu]mol/L (0.3 mg/dL) OR increase to 1.5–2.0-fold from baseline	<0.5 mL/kg/h for 6 h
2	Serum creatinine increase 2.0–3.0-fold from baseline	<0.5 mL/kg/h for 12 h
3	Serum creatinine increase to 3.0-fold OR GFR decrease >75% from baseline OR serum creatinine ≥354 μ[mu]mol/L (≥4 mg/dL) with an acute increase of at least 44 μ[mu]mol/L (0.5 mg/dL) OR need for renal replacement therapy	<0.3 mL/kg/h for 24 h OR anuria for 12 h OR need for renal replacement therapy

RIFLE risk, injury, failure, loss, end-stage kidney disease, *AKIN* acute kidney injury network, *GFR* glomerular filtration rate
Adapted from KDIGO. KDIGO Clinical Practice Guideline for Acute Kidney Injury. Kidney International Supplements. 2012;2:1–143; used with permission

rates of 45–55% were observed in recent large intensive care unit (ICU)-based trials [11, 12].

Although it was originally assumed that most survivors of an episode of AKI recover, it is now clear that adults who experience AKI have a ninefold increased risk of developing chronic kidney disease (CKD), a threefold increased risk of developing end-stage kidney disease (ESKD) and a twofold increased long-term mortality risk compared with those without AKI [13]. Children are also at risk of CKD after an episode of AKI although the risk is lower [1, 14]. For example, Pannu and colleagues [15] evaluated renal recovery after AKI between 2002 and 2007 in a large population-based cohort study in Canada (n = 190,714). They utilised a definition of AKI equivalent to stage 2, that is, a twofold increase between prehospital and peak in-hospital serum creatinine (SCr), and assessed recovery using the value of SCr closest to 90 days after AKI. They evaluated all-cause mortality and the combined renal outcome of sustained doubling of SCr or progression to ESKD. Of the 3.7% of the participants (n = 7014) who developed AKI, 62.7% (n = 4400) survived 90 days. Recovery could be assessed in 3231 patients with a median follow-up of 34 months; of these AKI survivors, 30.8% (n = 1268) died, and 2.1% (n = 85) progressed to kidney failure. When AKI participants who recovered to within 25% of baseline SCr were used as the reference group (adjusted mortality hazard ratio/HR, 1.26; 95% CI, 1.10–1.43), participants who did not recover kidney function had a fourfold higher risk for mortality and adverse renal outcomes (adjusted renal outcomes HR, 4.13; 95% CI, 3.38–5.04). The mortality HR increased sharply when participants failed to recover to within 55% of baseline.

AKI is associated with septic shock, major surgery, cardiogenic shock, hypovolaemia, nephrotoxic drugs, liver disease (hepato-renal syndrome), obstruction and other multiple factors [8]. This review will examine the pathophysiology of AKI, including the human evidence, mechanisms, pathological correlations and animal models. Mechanisms that might contribute to failure to recover kidney function are highlighted, along with clinico-pathological correlations that allow development or use of novel biomarkers that diagnose AKI early, or herald non-recovery. Most examples cited are from human studies.

4.2 Defining Acute Kidney Injury

4.2.1 Traditional Acute Kidney Injury Descriptors

The traditional "anatomical flow" model divides AKI aetiology into prerenal, renal (intrinsic) and postrenal causes. While useful, this construct has been challenged [16, 17]. Historically, prerenal AKI (or "prerenal azotemia") was regarded as distinct from "intrinsic" AKI which included acute tubular necrosis (ATN, otherwise known as acute tubular injury, ATI, discussed below). Prerenal AKI is commonly attributed to a transient decrease in the effective perfusion of the kidney from volume depletion or relative hypotension [18] and defined by prompt improvement after fluid resuscitation ("volume responsiveness" or "reversibility"), along with preservation of renal tubular function, as typified by sodium reabsorption, typically a fractional excretion of sodium (FENa) of <1% [16]. However, recent studies show that patients with prerenal AKI (defined using KDIGO criteria plus a duration less than 48 h and preservation of tubular function, FENa <1.0%) had increased urinary concentrations of protein biomarkers that indicate cellular damage [16, 17]. These studies suggest that prerenal AKI is not a reversible loss of function without cellular damage but simply the mild end of a continuum of renal injury. Furthermore, other prerenal conditions, including cardiorenal syndromes, present with similar laboratory findings, yet management requires fluid restriction. Consequently, the "prerenal" nomenclature cannot be used to suggest clinical management. We have previously suggested that it is preferable to describe AKI according to specific aetiology and duration (transient or persistent) [19].

Similarly, postrenal AKI (alternatively "acute obstructive AKI", or "postrenal azotemia") was recognised as a transient decrease in kidney function from acute obstruction to urinary outflow and characterised by prompt improvement following alleviation of mechanical obstruction [20]. Recent consensus statements suggest that functional impairment follows intrinsic kidney damage [19, 21] and preclinical studies usually confirm this. For example, in acute ureteric obstruction, structural injury detected by increases in the damage biomarker, kidney injury molecule-1 (KIM-1), occurred before detectable functional change [22]. The precise sequence of functional impairment and kidney damage with urinary outflow obstruction remains to be delineated [21]. The third historical anatomical construct is "intrinsic" AKI, whereby acute damage within the kidneys causes rapid loss of function. This is further divided into conditions primarily affecting glomerulus, tubules and interstitium (sometimes considered together as the "tubulointerstitium") and non-glomerular vessels (sometimes further divided into microvasculature and larger vessels such as arterioles).

While accumulated evidence suggests these distinctions are arbitrary, they are sometimes helpful in delineating the cause of AKI. For example, "glomerular" causes (e.g. acute glomerulonephritis) are recognised by the presence of proteinuria and/or haematuria [23]. Acute (tubulo)interstitial nephritis is typically oligosymptomatic but may be suggested by constitutional symptoms such as fever, rash, joint pain and peripheral eosinophilia [24]. Thrombotic microangiopathies, recognised histologically by endothelial abnormalities, thrombosis of the glomerular capillaries and arterioles and sometimes myocyte proliferation and onion skinlike thickening of small arteries, are suspected through an association with systemic features such as microangiopathic haemolytic anaemia or thrombocytopaenia [25]. Even amongst well-recognised syndromes, there is considerable overlap. Histological features of tubulointerstitial injury frequently accompany glomerulonephritis and are the most important histological determinant of long-term outcome [8, 26, 27]. Thrombotic microangiopathies are typically complicated by pathological changes to glomeruli and tubules in addition to peritubular capillaries and arterioles [28]. Acute interstitial nephritis can be accompanied by glomerulopathy [29].

4.2.2 Functional Descriptors: Serum Creatinine, SCr, and Oliguria

As surrogates of glomerular filtration rate (GFR), SCr and oliguria are intuitive markers of global kidney function, notionally representing failed clearance of nitrogenous waste and insufficient urine output to facilitate obligate solute excretion. Although the relationship between impaired GFR and urine output is complex, oliguria is easily detected in catheterised patients. SCr estimation is standardised [30] and familiar to all physicians, and there is a "dose-response" relationship change between perturbations in SCr and the risk of adverse outcomes, including death [31]. Consequently, consensus diagnostic criteria recognise that AKI following even a small, absolute (0.3 mg/dL or 26.5 μmol/L) increase in SCr reflects the risk of a more severe functional disturbance [32, 33].

However, the increased recognition of the importance of AKI has not yet translated into improved outcomes for affected patients [21]. Amongst the reasons are the limitations of both increased creatinine and oliguria as biomarkers of AKI. Multiple factors are responsible for the delay between renal insult and the recognition of reduced GFR, which adversely affects the prompt recognition and timely management of AKI [34].

First, if AKI can be attributed to a single insult, there is a delay before a decrease in GFR which has been termed the "injury evolution time" [34]. Second, even an abrupt fall in GFR will produce a gradual, exponential increase in SCr with an inevitable lag before SCr reaches a threshold for detection and longer before the extent of reduced GFR can be accurately calculated (three to five times the new half-life). As GFR falls, the half-life of SCr, which is approximately 4 h when GFR is normal, increases by the reciprocal of the decline in GFR. In response to an abrupt alteration in GFR, SCr will increase slowly, often taking up to 72 h to reach steady state, at which time it is again a surrogate for GFR. Staggered or continuing renal injury extends the time to reach the new steady state. Third, although small increases of SCr are associated with increased cohort mortality [32], this is of less significance if baseline

SCr is increased. Small increases are also difficult to recognise due to intra-person variability from biological and analytical factors and inter-patient variability. In healthy individuals, the intra-person variability in SCr averages 8% [35]. Variability is increased by factors such as intravenous fluid replacement [36], altered creatinine generation and release, drugs affecting tubular creatinine secretion [37] and chronic conditions, including diabetes and cardiovascular disease [38]. Analytical variability is increased by use of the Jaffe reaction compared to enzymatic assay [39], use of multiple laboratories [40] and time [40]. Furthermore, baseline SCr is frequently unavailable and difficult to estimate. Baseline SCr is affected by GFR, age, sex, race and body mass. The back-calculation of baseline creatinine using such formula as the Modification of Diet in Renal Disease and an assumed estimated GFR (eGFR) of 75 or 100 mL/min/1.73m^2 has become widespread for post hoc analysis in research. This results in misclassification of AKI in research [41] and has similar limitations in clinical management.

The use of oliguria to diagnose AKI also remains open to further refinement. While typically defined by urine output <0.5 mL/kg/h over a minimum of 6 h [32], others suggest this definition is too liberal. Ralib, Pickering and colleagues [36] observed that a 6-h urine output of<0.3 mL/kg/h was better associated with dialysis requirements, in-hospital and 1-year mortality. In individuals, clinical adjudication needs to include the effects of drugs (e.g., diuretics), fluid balance and obesity. In early goal-directed therapy for shock, protocols have typically randomised patients to haemodynamic targets or central venous oxygen saturation versus standard care [11, 42] rather than urine output targets, and a similar hemodynamic intervention in high-risk subjects after cardiac surgery reduced the frequency of AKI [43]. Several interventions, which have targeted oliguria, such as low-dose dopamine, did not reduce renal dysfunction or death [44]. A recent meta-analysis [45] evaluating perioperative fluid management strategies targeting oliguria was limited by a non-standard definition of AKI. Guidelines [32] only recommend that oliguria "serve as the starting point for further evaluation [of] patients recognized to be at increased risk" of AKI.

4.3 Aetiology of Acute Kidney Injury

Uchino et al [8] reported that, in 1726 ICU patients, AKI was associated with septic shock in 48%, major surgery in 34%, cardiogenic shock in 27%, hypovolaemia in 26%, potentially nephrotoxic drugs in 20%, liver disease (hepato-renal syndrome) in 6%, obstruction in 2% and other factors in 12%. Several studies report sepsis and cardiac surgery as prominent risk factors for AKI in hospitalised patients [8, 26] (Table 4.2). The majority of cases of AKI are attributed to ATI, also known as ATN. Authors have increasingly rejected "ATN"

Table 4.2 Aetiology of acute kidney injury categorised by setting

Contributing factor			Setting	
		Community	Hospital	ICU
Sepsis or septic shock		~12	24–73	48
Major surgery		N/A	25	34
Hypoperfusion				
	Reduced circulating blood volume	53–60	26–36	26
	Cardiogenic shock	Unclear	Unclear	27
	Chronic liver disease	Unclear	Unclear	6
Nephrotoxicant drugs		6–19	17–27	20
Kidney obstruction		~11	<5%	2
Other		Unclear	Unclear	12

Data derived from [8, 50–52]
ICU: intensive care unit

as a misnomer [46]. ATI reflects that, even in the absence of overt cell death, tubular injury may still occur, recognisable by histological features such as loss of epithelial brush border, or cytoplasmic vacuolisation [46, 47], or induction of injury mechanisms or cellular dysfunction. Molecular studies have established that cell death in AKI is due to both unprogrammed and accidental cell death (necrosis) and that there are distinct mechanisms of programmed cell death including apoptosis, necroptosis and mitochondrial permeability transition—summarised by Linkermann and Green and others [48, 49]. Even the term "ATI" may be misleading, with increasing awareness of the roles of endothelial injury, altered renal microvasculature and local and systemic inflammatory responses in AKI development.

The three most common causes of AKI are ischaemia-reperfusion injury, systemic or localised inflammation such as in sepsis and after surgery and nephrotoxic injury (Table 4.2). Sepsis, surgery and (some) nephrotoxicant drugs are more prominent in hospital-acquired AKI than community-acquired AKI [8, 26]. Obstruction and hypovolaemia are more prominent in community-acquired AKI [8, 48, 50–53]. Some causes of AKI are more prevalent in specific geographical settings. For example, herbicide and pesticide self-poisoning [54] and snakebite [55] are frequent causes of AKI in Sri-Lanka but infrequent in more developed countries.

In contrast to general belief, renal ischaemia may not be central to the pathogenesis of sepsis-induced AKI [47]. For example, in a sheep model, sepsis caused an increase of renal blood flow and SCr, and, although nonselective nitric oxide synthase (NOS) inhibition normalised blood flow, it did not correct SCr [56]. Alternative mechanisms of injury in sepsis include heterogeneity in renal blood flow (with some capillaries underperfused, while others have apparently normal blood flow [57]), direct injury including bacterial toxins and cytokines and hypoxia in the absence of overt hypoperfusion [58].

The incidence of AKI is much greater following cardiac than after noncardiac surgery. Following noncardiac surgery, AKI incidence is approximately 1% [59] and approximately 9% in those patients requiring ICU support [60]. The incidence of AKI in cardiac surgery is between 10 and 40% [61–65]. The pathophysiology of AKI after major surgery, particularly cardiac surgery, is conceived as multifactorial via a combination of hemodynamic instability and impaired cardiac output leading to ischaemia-reperfusion injury with a systemic inflammatory response associated with surgery and particularly cardiopulmonary bypass [66]. Perioperative sepsis and nephrotoxic drug exposures may contribute.

4.4 Pathophysiology of Acute Kidney Injury

Although most AKI is probably due to ATI, biopsy series typically report higher proportions of acute glomerulonephritis, interstitial nephritis and thrombotic microangiopathy than epidemiological series [50], which probably reflects sampling bias. Firstly, because there is no specific therapeutic intervention available, clinicians rarely confirm the diagnosis of ATI by biopsy. Whereas, since specific therapies exist for acute glomerulonephritis [23], interstitial nephritis [67] and thrombotic microangiopathy [28, 68], therapy is often guided by biopsy. Secondly, biopsies allow only limited sampling of tissue and typically focus on the cortex and glomeruli. This leads to underappreciation of ATI since the histological changes of acute tubular injury may be greater in the outer medulla than in cortex and may be focal due to regional variations in blood flow [69]. Thirdly, in contrast to standardised histopathological diagnoses such as renal allograft rejection [70], widely adopted consensus criteria for the histological diagnosis of ATI are lacking. This leads to high interobserver variability in diagnosis. Fourthly, there is a poor correlation between changes in GFR and histological injury in AKI. Differences in the timing, severity or even presence of classic histological injury and functional change are repeatedly demonstrated in animal studies. For example, in toxicant-induced AKI, histological injury typically precedes substantial functional change, particularly where injury is mild [71, 72]. While challenged by recent research [16, 17, 73], it remains possible that severe reductions in GFR could occur with minimal observable renal histological abnormalities, particularly where autoregulation is modified or glomerular capillary pressure is reduced without change in renal blood flow, such as that occurs during renin-angiotensin blockade. However, it is doubtful if such physiological modifications are identical to those characterising typical volume depletion.

4.4.1 Tubular Injury and Linked Biomarkers

In most models of ischaemia-reperfusion and hypoxic injury and many cytotoxic models, tubular epithelial cell damage is most prominent in the S3 segment of the proximal tubule [74]. Cellular damage is marked by a loss of cytostructural integrity and cell polarity with mislocation of proteins, such as Na^+/K^+ATP-ase, adhesion proteins and β[beta]1-integrin on the cell membrane [75]. Shedding of the brush border is accompanied by release of a number of preformed proteins in the tubular cell membrane such as alkaline phosphatase, γ[gamma]-glutamyl transpeptidase and α[alpha]-glutathione *S*-transferase [76].

Even sublethal cellular injury can result in loss of critical kidney function. Proximal tubular dysfunction can be recognised by glucosuria and enhanced excretion of amino acids suggesting impaired sodium-dependent glucose and amino acid transport. When accompanied by proximal renal tubular acidosis, hyperphosphaturia, hypouricaemia and aminoaciduria, this generalised proximal dysfunction is designated the Fanconi syndrome [77]. Recent studies have identified distinct nonesterified fatty acids and triglycerides in serum, urine and kidney tissue following tubular injury [78].

Many low molecular weight proteins are recycled from the glomerular filtrate in the proximal tubule for recirculation or tubular lysosomal digestion [79]. Some of these urinary proteins have gained prominence as biomarkers of kidney damage, including neutrophil gelatinase-associated lipocalin (NGAL), cystatin C and liver-associated fatty acid-binding protein (L-FABP). Disruption to the glomerular filtration barrier will increase the protein load presented to the proximal tubule. While proteinuria and albuminuria are considered hallmarks of glomerular injury, proximal tubular injury can impair protein endocytosis through the megalin-cubilin system [80]. Both glomerular and tubular injury can therefore result in increased concentrations of large proteins such as albumin, β[beta]2-microglobulin or total protein and low molecular weight proteins such as cystatin C, NGAL and others. Through competition for megalin-cubilin transport, albuminuria itself increases the urinary concentration of other low molecular weight proteins such as NGAL and cystatin C [17]. It is therefore interesting that urinary albumin has received regulatory qualification as a marker of proximal tubular injury in animal toxicity studies [72] while urinary β[beta]2-macroglobulin, total protein and cystatin C were qualified as markers of glomerular injury [81, 82]. Not surprisingly, aspects of this pathophysiology remain under intense debate [80, 83–86].

Cellular injury activates a large number of genes and proteins including those involved in the cell cycle. Insulin-like growth factor-binding protein 7 (IGFBP7) and tissue inhibitor of metalloproteinases-2 (TIMP-2) are proteins that mediate G_1 cell cycle arrest. IGFBP7 triggers increased expression of p53 and p21 and TIMP-2 increases p27. These have been mainly investigated as inhibitors of tumour growth but are associated with AKI in numerous clinical settings, and measurement in urine is now FDA-approved as biomarkers of AKI risk (stage ≥ 2) [87–89].These proteins block cyclin-dependent protein kinase complexes required for progression through the G1/S checkpoint. This may be reno-protective in AKI by preventing replication of damaged cells [88], although direct evidence is lacking. G1 cell cycle arrest can also be triggered by DNA damage and transforming growth factor (TGF)-β[beta] release by other pathways [90].

Cell death in AKI may follow unprogrammed or accidental cell death (necrosis) and several distinct pathways of programmed cell death including apoptosis, necroptosis and mitochondrial permeability transition pore discharge—see Linkermann and Green [48, 49]. Autophagic cell death and mitotic catastrophe also participate. The risk of cell death increases with increasing severity or duration of injury. While good evidence of these different modes of cellular death is available in renal cellular models, only low-level evidence is available from in vivo studies and human tissue [49].

4.4.2 Apoptosis and Mitochondrial Associations

Activation of several mitochondrial mechanisms results in apoptosis. Direct cytotoxic DNA damage triggers phosphorylation of p53, which in turn triggers pro-apoptotic gene pathways such as the PIDD (p53-induced protein with death domain) and Bcl-2/Bax (B-cell lymphoma 2/Bcl-2-associated X protein) families. For instance, induction of PUMA-α[alpha] (p53 upregulated modulator of apoptosis-α[alpha]) is pro-apoptotic, since PUMA-α[alpha] neutralises the anti-apoptotic protein Bcl-XL, freeing Bax to translocate across the mitochondrial membrane and release apoptotic factors, such as cytochrome C [91, 92]. p53 and the Bcl-2 pathway are implicated ischaemia-reperfusion-induced AKI [93–95]. Mitochondrial function is essential for formation of endogenous antioxidants including α[alpha]-lipoic acid [96] and ubiquinone [97]. Depletion of ATP, such as that occurs in ischaemic AKI [98, 99], or direct toxic mitochondrial injury [82] can impact the mitochondrial respiratory chain. As well, nephrotoxic agents such as cisplatin can directly react with glutathione or related antioxidants, and the consequent depletion or inactivation of antioxidants may shift the cellular redox status, leading to the intracellular accumulation of endogenous reactive oxygen species (ROS) [87]. Renal toxicants also directly induce ROS formation in microsomes via the cytochrome p450 system [100].

Because of their highly reactive nature, ROS target and modify many molecules in cells including lipids, proteins and DNA, resulting in cellular stress. This can induce apoptosis via p53-dependent mechanisms. Accumulation of unfolded or misfolded proteins at the endoplasmic reticulum (ER) leads to ER stress, which also induces apoptosis—via caspase-12 activation [101]. The detection of molecules modified by ROS may be useful biomarkers of oxidative stress in AKI. Tissue concentrations of thiobarbituric acid-reacting substances (TBARS), including malondialdehyde, have been reported as a marker of kidney lipid peroxidation [102, 103], and plasma TBARS have been reported as a biomarker of delayed graft function [104].

4.4.3 Necrosis and Necroptosis

Necrosis is cell death caused by catastrophic loss of cellular energy [105]. The cells usually die as a contiguous mass, they lyse, and an inflammatory reaction is usually initiated. Some of the necrotic debris that is released into the tubular lumen includes preformed brush border enzymes, including alkaline phosphatase and γ[gamma]-GT, and cytoplasmic enzymes including α[alpha]-glutathione *S*-transferase (GST) and π[pi]-GST isomers in the proximal and distal tubular epithelial cells, respectively. These form part of a panel of biomarker assays to indicate necrosis has occurred in AKI [76]. Regulated (programmed) necrosis, or necroptosis, has also been proposed as a distinct form of necrosis [48, 49]. Initially it was described as being initiated by tumour necrosis factor receptor-1 ligation and inhibited by the receptor-interacting protein-targeting chemical necrostatin-1. Other necroptosis triggers known to initiate apoptosis have been described: FAS/CD95, TNF-related apoptosis-inducing ligand receptor, toll-like receptor 3/4, etoposide and ischaemia-reperfusion injury. Necroptotic pathways may involve the mitochondria permeability transition (MPT) pore. Upon opening of the MPT, proteins are released that may induce apoptosis, but if apoptosis is inhibited, a necroptotic cell death mode may be initiated. Mitotic catastrophe may also occur. This is a mechanism of cell death initiated by perturbations of the mitotic apparatus during the M phase of the cell cycle and paralleled by some degree of mitotic arrest, ultimately leading to cell death or senescence.

4.4.4 Autophagic Cell Death

Autophagy, or "self-eating", is a mechanism of cell survival whereby stressed cells reduce their size and recycle cell molecules from effete cell parts via lysosomal digestion. Autophagic cell death is a feature of progression of autophagy whereby enough essential cell organelles are removed via phagocytosis that the cell cannot survive. Its role in AKI has recently been described [106]. This mode of cell death is characterised by massive cytoplasmic vacuolisation and initiation of some specific death pathways, such as autophagy (atg) genes and beclin-1. Whether autophagic cell death constitutes a distinct cell death programme or merely a survival mechanism against stress remains under debate, and the use of this term should be limited to instances where the mode of cell death has been proven.

4.4.5 Relationship Between Tubular Damage and Reduced GFR

Even in AKI models where histological injury to glomeruli is minimal, such as collapse of the glomerular tuft, a substantial reduction in GFR may occur. The pathological events linking tubular injury and loss of function remain uncertain, despite the fundamental nature of this relationship to clinical practice. In AKI, reduced GFR is at least partly mediated by a reduced transcapillary hydraulic pressure gradient and intratubular obstruction. Tubular backleak may also be important [47, 107]. A reduced transcapillary hydraulic pressure gradient is mediated by increased angiotensin II production leading to vasoconstriction of afferent and efferent glomerular arterioles, tubuloglomerular feedback, dysregulated autoregulation and microcirculatory obstruction and dysfunction. In AKI inadequate sodium reabsorption in the injured proximal tubule increases solute delivery to the distal nephron and swelling of the salt-sensing macula densa which generates tubuloglomerular feedback via adenosine-mediated afferent arteriolar vasoconstriction and thereby decreases single nephron GFR. Although tubuloglomerular feedback appears preserved in AKI, excess nitric oxide and probably endothelium-derived hyperpolarising factor produce endothelial dysfunction and antagonise autoregulation [108]. The relative extent to which dysfunction of glomerular and peritubular microcirculatory networks and obstruction by resident and migratory leucocytes contribute to the loss of GFR is unclear [109].

Tubular backleak and obstruction occur with severe injury. Injured tubular cells are desquamated, leaving the basement membrane as the only barrier between glomerular filtrate and the peritubular interstitium. The increase in permeability results in leakage of filtrate into the interstitium. Detached cells and debris combine with proteins present in the tubular lumen such as uromodulin to form casts that can obstruct the tubule and increase intratubular pressure worsening backleak. Despite these observations, at least one study of transplanted kidneys suggested that vascular factors rather than tubular obstruction is the major cause of reduced GFR after kidney ischaemia [107].

4.4.6 Endothelial and Vascular Injury

Under normal conditions, endothelial cells maintain a vasodilator, antithrombotic and anti-inflammatory state [110]. They are major determinants of vascular tone and leukocyte adhesion in AKI. Cell adhesion molecules, such as intercellular adhesion molecule-1 (ICAM-1), are constitutively expressed in the vasa recta of normal animals. In AKI, expression of as ICAM-1 is increased in injured vascular endothelial cells, as are counter-receptors on leucocytes resulting in leucocyte activation and transmigration [111]. Amongst the many effects of leucocytes is obstruction of the renal microvasculature and postcapillary venules. Apart from their rheological properties, leucocytes reduce renal blood flow by releasing vasoactive cytokines including tumour necrosis factor-α[alpha] (TNF-α[alpha]) [112], numerous interleukins [110] and endothelin [113]. These chemicals can augment vasoconstriction caused by an imbalance between vasoconstrictors and vasodilators. Reduced release of nitric oxide (NO) and other vasodilatory substances, and increased expression of endothelin by the damaged endothelial cell, is seen in ischaemic and toxic models of AKI [114, 115] and is related to reduced expression of such molecules as endothelial NOS [114]. Reduced responsiveness to vasodilators such as NO, acetylcholine and bradykinin has been demonstrated [115–118]. These circulatory changes trigger activation of the sympathetic system, which induces increased renin-angiotensin-aldosterone activity [119], and further escalate renal vasoconstriction. The effect of vasoconstriction is further exacerbated by vascular compression due to interstitial oedema [120].

Although total renal blood flow is frequently reduced in AKI, regional changes in blood flow appear more important in a variety of AKI models including both classic ischaemic and toxic models [121] and may also be important in sepsis-induced AKI. Outer medullary blood flow is reduced disproportionately to the reduction in total flow in animal models of ischaemic AKI [69], and relative hypoperfusion may also play a role in the greater susceptibility of the S3 segment to toxicant-induced AKI, such as seen following cisplatin exposure [121].

4.4.7 Inflammation and the Immune Response

The complex innate and adaptive immune responses that contribute to AKI have been extensively reviewed and will only be briefly summarised here. Components of the innate immune systems include neutrophils, monocytes-macrophages, immature dendritic cells, natural killer cells and natural killer T cells and are responsible for response to injury in a nonantigen-specific fashion. The adaptive component, activated by specific antigens, is initiated within hours and lasts more than several days after injury. These mechanisms include maturation of dendritic cells as antigen-presenting cells [122], T lymphocyte proliferation and activation [123] and T-cell-B-cell interactions. Complement activation is an important player, bridging the innate and adaptive immune response systems. In AKI it is predominantly activated via the alternative pathway and results in significant deposition of the complement activation product C3d along tubular basement membranes [124].

Participant cells in the inflammatory response are derived from extrinsic and intrinsic sources. Importantly, renal parenchyma including tubular epithelium is an active participant in the inflammatory response, with upregulation of several pro-inflammatory molecules including NGAL [116–118], KIM-1 [125, 126], interleukin (IL)-18 [127] and, as discussed above, TNF-α[alpha] [92]. Experimental evidence also implicates renal epithelium as an important but not exclusive source of such cytokines as monocyte chemotactic protein-1 (MCP-1) [128], macrophage migration inhibitory factor (MIF) [118, 129] and chemokine ligand 16 (CXCL16) [130]. Nuclear factor-κB is a key regulator of the expression of such genes although it frequently functions in concert with other transcription factors, including activator protein-1 and the nuclear factor of IL-6 [131]. These biomarkers will receive further attention later in the review.

Numerous anti-inflammatory pathways are stimulated in AKI and provide a brake to the many pro-inflammatory positive feedback loops initiated with AKI. These include induction of heme oxygenase 1 and IL-10 [132, 133]. Heme oxygenase 1 limits free heme accumulation and iron-induced injury, ROS generation and oxidative stress and therefore inhibits autophagy and apoptosis [132]. IL-10 inhibits the synthesis of several cytokines, including interferon-γ[gamma], IL-2 and TNF-α[alpha] produced by activated macrophages and by helper T cells [133].

Interorgan "crosstalk"—the interaction between remote organs and kidneys—may help explain the development of some AKI and partially explains the association of sepsis and major surgery with AKI [134, 135]. Similarly, AKI appears to mediate distant organ dysfunction and possibly explains the association between AKI and mortality. AKI is associated with increased circulating concentrations of numerous cytokines including pro-inflammatory IL-6, IL-8, as well as anti-inflammatory molecules such as IL-10 [135]. The effect of AKI on distant organs is beyond the scope of this review, but these effects appear to be mediated by many of the pathways listed above including oxidative stress and pro-apoptotic pathways, by changes in levels of soluble factors such as cytokines and chemokines and by leukocyte activation and trafficking [134].

4.5 Biomarkers

Fundamentally, it has been recognised that even if reduced GFR could be detected instantly, clinically significant kidney damage may occur without loss of GFR [21]. Firstly, the temporal role of injury evolution time has been discussed above. Secondly, due to the segmental nature of AKI within kidneys, even if functional impairment does occur in some nephrons, compensatory hyperfiltration in remaining functional nephron units may mean that total GFR is unchanged [136]. The role of renal reserve in AKI remains ill-defined. Thirdly, even in the absence of an overt systemic illness, AKI is marked by local and systemic inflammation, immune dysregulation and changes to systemic vascular tone as discussed. Selective failure of other kidney functions may be disproportional to the loss of GFR. Complications of AKI may include hyperkalaemia, acidosis and volume overload. Other complications include anaemia, platelet dysfunction and pathological bleeding, dysregulation of phosphate and calcium balance, hypomagnesaemia or hyperglycaemia and dysregulation of insulin metabolism. These events rather than impaired GFR appear to produce adverse pathophysiological consequences, probably including yet unrecognised problems associated with an increased risk of morbidity or mortality.

The weaknesses of current renal functional markers in diagnosis of AKI are widely recognised [32, 137] and have led to an explosion of preclinical and clinical research involving novel AKI biomarkers. Numerous strategies, including metabolomics, genomics and proteomics have been employed to discover candidate biomarkers, while numerous other known "traditional" biomarkers including proteins, nucleic acids and clinical parameters have been revisited. Of these, several protein biomarkers in blood and urine appear to be best placed to improve the diagnosis and management of AKI.

In this light, the 10th Acute Dialysis Quality Initiative (ADQI) workgroup in 2013 proposed a new diagnostic paradigm which permits the diagnosis of AKI based on recognition of loss of function, kidney damage or both [21]. According to this paradigm, available biomarkers can be classified as representing changes in renal function ("functional biomarkers") and those reflecting kidney damage ("damage biomarkers"). The functional biomarkers are surrogates of GFR and include traditional markers such as SCr, and urine output, and more novel markers such as serum cystatin C. Better-known examples of damage biomarkers include KIM-1, NGAL and IL-18 and have been studied in serum and urine.

Several authors [21, 76, 138] have discussed the potential role of novel AKI biomarkers. These include complementing or replacing SCr in the early diagnosis of AKI [21, 138], in prognosis [21, 138, 139] or as endpoints of clinical trials [140]. Analogous to the use of SCr and proteinuria to identify patients with CKD and thus an increased risk of AKI, novel biomarkers might also help in risk stratification [138] and clinical trial enrichment [141]. Damage biomarkers may also have a unique role in evaluating patients already diagnosed with AKI, specifically in evaluating the differential diagnosis of AKI [19], in determining the time course or "phase" of injury [21, 137] and in the "biomonitoring" of therapeutic interventions [142].

4.5.1 Damage Biomarkers for Early Diagnosis of AKI

NGAL, a member of the lipocalin superfamily, is induced in the distal tubule in response to a variety of kidney injuries [116, 117]. It modifies iron traffic in kidney injury by forming complexes with iron-binding siderophores. Endocytic delivery of a lipocalin-siderophore-iron complex resulted in amelioration of injury in an ischaemic AKI model [116]. Since the endocytic receptor megalin is responsible for binding and endocytosis of NGAL, increased urinary NGAL may also signal proximal tubular dysfunction [143]. The role of NGAL in crosstalk between distal and adjacent proximal tubules remains to be elucidated [117]. Since its recognition as one of the most highly upregulated genes following AKI [118], urinary and serum concentrations of NGAL have been the most extensively evaluated novel AKI biomarker.

KIM-1 is an epithelial cell receptor that enables proximal tubule cells to recognise and phagocytose necrotic debris such as apoptotic cells, necrotic cells and oxidised lipoproteins, potentially limiting the inflammatory response. KIM-1 has been presented as the most highly upregulated protein in the proximal tubule of the kidney after acute or chronic insults [144]. KIM-1 (also known as T-cell immunoglobulin domain and mucin domain protein 1 and hepatitis A virus cellular receptor 1) is a type 1 membrane glycoprotein which contains an extracellular immunoglobulin- and mucin-like domain, with *N*- and *O*-glycosylation sites. It has a transmembrane domain and short intracellular domain with intracellular tyrosine phosphorylation sites. KIM-1 has several effects on lymphocytes including T-cell activation [123] and influences the commitment of alloactivated T cells to regulatory and effector phenotypes [145]. The shed ectodomain of KIM-1 can be detected in urine following AKI [125].

IL-18 is a cytokine product of caspase-1 produced by bone marrow-derived, resident leukocytes and renal parenchyma including tubular epithelial cells, podocytes and mesangial cells in response to AKI. Although inhibition of IL-18 has resulted in amelioration of ischaemic AKI [127], it activates both inflammation-suppressing and pro-injury pathways in experimental toxic AKI [146].

Various other apparently pro-inflammatory genes and proteins can be detected in multiple experimental models of AKI. These include MCP-1 [147], MIF [148, 149] and CXCL16 [130] and numerous other cytokines [47]. Inhibition studies demonstrate that many of these numerous mechanisms are overlapping and redundant [150].

Incorporating damage biomarkers into AKI diagnosis can potentially overcome the major weaknesses of SCr and oliguria for early diagnosis of AKI. First, a damage biomarker that rapidly signals the onset kidney injury could overcome the delay in AKI diagnosis due to the combination of "injury evolution time" and the slow elevation of SCr after kidney failure. Several kidney damage biomarkers including KIM-1, NGAL, L-FABP and IL-18 may be elevated before an increase in SCr [138]. Second, damage biomarkers can diagnose clinically significant AKI in the absence of functional change. Damage biomarkers have been used to identify patients with increased risk of adverse outcomes, in the absence of diagnostic increases in SCr and in the absence of azotemia or oliguria [36, 151, 152]. Haase, Devarajan [151] reported a multicentre pooled analysis including 2322 critically ill patients from 10 separate studies. Approximately one fifth of patients had a significant elevation in either urinary or serum NGAL but did not have elevation in SCr sufficient to meet RIFLE criteria for AKI [153]. This subgroup of NGAL-positive-creatinine-negative subjects encountered a substantial increase in hospital stay, dialysis requirement, ICU stay and mortality. Similarly, in a multicentre prospective cohort study of 1635 emergency department patients, patients with increased urinary NGAL or KIM-1 but low SCr at hospital admission were at increased risk of dialysis or death [152]. Md Ralib, Pickering [36] reported that fluid resuscitation following cardiac arrest can mask elevations in SCr and thus AKI. Patients with increased urinary cystatin C, plasma NGAL or urinary NGAL but unchanged SCr (biomarker-positive, creatinine-negative) had increased risk of mortality. This preliminary evidence suggests that combining functional and damage biomarkers allows for a graded assessment of prognosis. Following a potential kidney insult, patients with no evidence of a significant reduction in GFR or of significant kidney damage appear at lowest risk of morbidity and mortality. Patients with either reduced function or kidney damage but not both appear at intermediate risk.

Patients with both damaged and reduced function are at greatest risk. In Fig. 4.1, the combination of kidney functional and damage biomarkers may simultaneously provide a simple method to stratify patients with AKI in terms of both prognosis (e.g. at presentation represented by colour) [36, 151, 152] and injury progression and resolution over time (represented by arrows) [21]. This approach might also permit using the time sequence of changes in functional or damage markers to determine the duration and progress of AKI. For example, some causes of AKI (e.g. renal obstruction) are thought to be purely functional at first but are characterised by a combination of damage and dysfunction if not promptly and effectively reversed. Conversely, in other causes of AKI (e.g. toxin-induced AKI), damage is expected to precede a change in function. Such cases of AKI are expected to proceed from no functional changes or damage (damage biomarker +/functional biomarker −), to damage without loss of function (damage biomarker +/functional biomarker −), through to damage with loss of function (damage biomarker +/functional biomarker +). According to this paradigm, recovery might involve normalisation of damage biomarkers prior to functional biomarkers, or vice versa (Fig. 4.1).

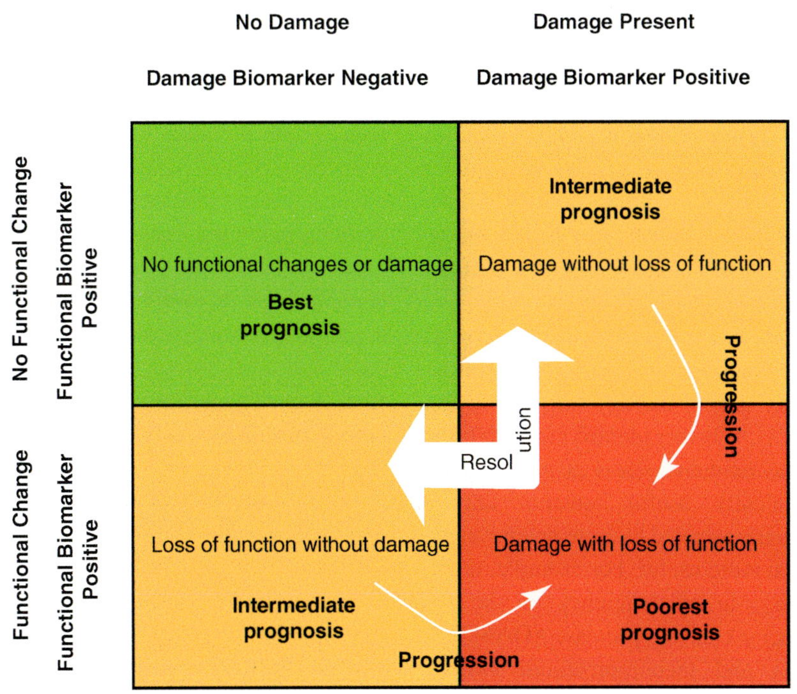

Fig. 4.1 A proposed framework for evaluating acute kidney injury (AKI) based on functional and damage biomarkers. The combination of kidney functional and damage biomarkers may simultaneously provide a simple method to stratify patients with AKI in terms of prognosis and injury progression and resolution over time (represented by arrows). This approach might also permit using the time sequence of changes in functional or damage markers to determine the duration and progress of AKI. *Adapted from* Murray P, Mehta R, Shaw A, Ronco C, Endre Z, Kellum J, et al. Potential use of biomarkers in acute kidney injury: report and summary of recommendations from the 10th Acute Dialysis Quality Initiative consensus conference. Kidney International. 2014;85:513–21 and McCullough P, Bouchard J, Waikar S, Siew E, Endre Z, Goldstein S, et al. Implementation of novel biomarkers in the diagnosis, prognosis, and management of acute kidney injury: executive summary from the tenth consensus conference of the Acute Dialysis Quality Initiative (ADQI). Contributions to Nephrology. 2013;182:5–12

4.6 Novel Roles for Damage Biomarkers in Acute Kidney Injury

4.6.1 Differential Diagnosis

The differential association of different damage biomarkers to aetiology or pathophysiological mechanisms underlying AKI may permit their use in differential diagnosis of AKI (see [19]. Although this application remains experimental for the syndrome currently known as acute tubular injury, as discussed above, this is already well established in clinical practice for some causes of AKI. For example, AKI due to glomerular disease such as glomerulonephritis is suggested by the presence of proteinuria or haematuria or both. Preclinical studies have implied site specificity for several kidney damage biomarkers. For instance, renal papillary antigen-1 demonstrated high specificity for collecting duct injury and is approved as a marker of distal tubule injury in rodent kidney toxicity studies [154], while urinary cystatin C and β[beta]2-microglobulin have been approved as markers of glomerular injury [81].

Identifying a predominant pathophysiological mechanism in cases of AKI is even more attractive, as it may permit therapy targeted to that mechanism [21]. Whether identifying such broad mechanisms as oxidative stress or inflammation will be clinically useful remains unclear. Biomarkers better targeted to more precise mechanisms may be more useful. For example, recognition of the role of deficiency of the von Willebrand factor-cleaving protease ADAMTS13 (a disintegrin and metalloproteinase with a thrombospondin type 1 motif, member 13) has transformed the diagnosis and management of thrombotic microangiopathy [25].

4.6.2 Biomonitoring Treatment Success or Failure

Using biomarkers as physiological goals to which therapy can be targeted has been called "delineation of the functional space" [21]. Analogous to the current use of arterial blood pressure monitoring or pulse oximetry, novel biomarkers could provide a feedback loop linking alterations in renal homeostasis, biomarker expression and therapeutic intervention. For example, this has been illustrated for experimental nephrotoxic AKI induced by cisplatin [155]. While real-time GFR will provide timely functional assessment, the absence of baseline information will still re. Further research is required to determine which strategies are best suited for evaluation in specific circumstances and disease states [21].

4.7 Recovery and Renal Reserve

The repair process after kidney injury involves a regeneration phase in which injured or dead cells are replaced by cells of the same lineage. If regeneration of the tubular epithelium is incomplete, a fibrotic phase may be initiated in which connective tissues replace normal kidney parenchymal tissue [156]. AKI can result in incomplete repair and persistent tubulointerstitial inflammation, with proliferation of fibroblasts and excessive deposition of extracellular matrix, a common feature of many kinds of kidney diseases and a primary determinant of progression to ESKD. The efficiency of tubular epithelial cells to proliferate and regenerate lost cells is crucial for repair and enables recovery from AKI. This is often determined by expression of cell cycle regulatory proteins p53, p21 and p16. These proteins have been implicated in repair in ischaemic and cisplatin-induced toxic AKI animal models, deteriorating renal transplants and chronic-diseased native kidneys in humans [156]. Modulating these cell cycle regulatory proteins may impact on severity of AKI from multiple causes. Cell cycle arrest or dysregulation may also be linked with progression to fibrosis and CKD. The release of TIMP-2 and IGFBP7 is understood to mark cell cycle arrest in AKI, and the measurement of the product of urinary TIMP-2 and urinary IGFBP7 concentrations was the first urinary biomarker granted regulatory approval to aid risk assessment for AKI in intensive care units [87].

The kidneys can maintain function by compensatory hyperfiltration and hypertrophy even while there is significant injury. This is one of the reasons people with early CKD are not detected. Renal reserve explains maintenance of GFR in the presence of renal injury or nephron loss. Recovery is facilitated by migration of viable epithelial cells, which help to cover denuded areas of the basement membrane. Histologically, regeneration is marked by basophilia and increased mitosis with increased expression of cell proliferation biomarkers such as Ki-67. Several molecules including clusterin appear to facilitate renal recovery and protect from fibrosis [157, 158]. Clusterin is a secreted heterodimer glycoprotein found in numerous physiological fluids, and its expression is upregulated in response to AKI in a variety of models [81, 158–160]. Clusterin appears to be involved in regulating tubular epithelial cell migration. In normal physiology, clusterin appears to maintain intercellular and cell-matrix interactions [115, 161]. In a clusterin knockout model, clusterin expression was associated with upregulation of a variety of genes required to protect cell cycle progression and renal recovery in ischaemia-reperfusion injury [158]. However, in vitro, clusterin suppressed tubular epithelial cell migration in the same study. Taken together these data suggest that successful cell migration is a complex function that requires active regulation.

4.7.1 Maladaptive Healing and Chronic Kidney Disease

AKI and CKD are interconnected syndromes (reviewed by [90, 162]). The presence of CKD is a major risk factor for AKI, and the progression to CKD is common after AKI. Pathologically, maladaptive or incomplete repair after AKI can result in the histological hallmarks of CKD including tubular atrophy, interstitial fibrosis and loss of capillary density. Perpetuation of defects in tubular proliferation contributes to tubular apoptosis and "dropout" [162]. DNA damage is a trigger for failed progression through the G_2/M phase of the cell cycle. Unlike G1/S arrest, which appears to protect kidneys, G_2/M phase arrest appears maladaptive [90]. During sustained cell cycle arrest, tubular epithelium develops a secretory phenotype and, in concert with macrophages, releases increased profibrotic growth factors such as IL-13, arginase and TGF-β[beta]1. This results in increased myofibroblast deposition and proliferation and deposition of extracellular matrix [90]. Persistently high expression of NGAL and KIM-1 4 weeks after experimental AKI suggests a possible role for these genes in the transition from AKI to CKD [113]. The role of epithelial to mesenchymal (phenotypical) transformation in this process remains under debate [163]. Capillary rarefaction is associated with impaired GFR both directly [164] and indirectly via hypertension [165] which is a feature of, and risk factor for, CKD.

Vascular endothelial growth factor (VEGF), and in particular VEGF-A, is an important molecule in the regulation of angiogenesis following AKI and has mitogenic and anti-apoptotic properties [166]. However contradictory evidence clouds the precise role of VEGF in the pathogenesis AKI. For instance, while VEGF expression was decreased in numerous models of AKI [112, 166], [167] increased urinary VEGF was reported in patients with AKI [168].

4.8 Animal Models

As mentioned previously, the cause of AKI is typically multifactorial. Table 4.3 lists preclinical animal models of AKI that are in common use. The three most prominent models involve ischaemia-reperfusion injury, systemic or localised inflammation such as that occurs in sepsis and after surgery and toxicity due to exogenous factors such as nephrotoxic drugs. The best-studied animal models of AKI seek to mimic these three causes of AKI [169]. The most commonly used is ischaemia-reperfusion induced by acute occlusion of the renal artery plus reperfusion. Much of the understanding of AKI mechanisms is inferred from such models. However, many authors have lamented the simplicity of these models and their inadequacy for modelling more complex clinical conditions including cardiogenic shock or sepsis [58]. The seemingly "uncomplicated" models of ischaemia-reperfusion

Table 4.3 List of preclinical animal models for AKI

Model	Method
Ischaemia-reperfusion	Clamping of both renal arteries in rats for 45–60 min followed by varying times of reperfusion. Unilateral renal artery clamping may also be used, with or without contralateral nephrectomy
Sepsis	Ligation of caecum and punctured three times
Sepsis	Administration of LPS 2.5–15 mg/kg single dose *ip*
Drug toxicity	Gentamicin dose of 100 mg/kg, *ip* for 5 days
Drug toxicity	Cisplatin dose range 5–60 mg/kg, *ip* single dose (up to 100 mg/kg)
Radiocontrast media	Diatrizoate single dose range 2–10 mL/kg, *iv*
	Ioxaglate dose 1 mL/min, intra-aortic injection for 3 min
	Iohexol dose range 1.5–3 g of iodine/kg, *ip* injection
	Sodium iothalamate dose 6 mL/kg intra-aortic administration for 2–3 min
NSAIDs	Acetaminophen dose range 375–3000 mg/kg, *ip* single dose
	Diclofenac sodium dose 15 mg/kg, *ip* injection for 3 days
Glycerol	Single dose 8 mg/kg, *im*
Osmotic nephrosis	Sucrose, single dose 4–27% w/v *ip*
Ifosfamide	Dose range 50–1100 mg/kg, *ip* 1–5 days
Uranium	Uranyl nitrate dose range 0.5–25 mg/kg
	Uranyl acetate single dose 5 mg/kg, *sc*
Mercuric chloride	Dose range 1–10 mg/kg *ip* and 10 mg/kg *sc*
Folic acid	Single dose 250 mg/kg, *iv*
Ferric nitrilo-triacetate	Dose range 1–15 mg of iron/kg, *ip*

LPS lipopolysaccharide, *ip* intraperitoneal, *iv* intravenous, *im* intramuscular

injury have been able to define many mechanisms and molecular pathways involved in AKI. They have demonstrated that AKI is mediated by a complex series of events which overlap in space and time with similarly complex repair mechanisms [47]. Nevertheless, renal oxygenation is critically impaired in AKI beyond the initiation of injury [170]. The major events in ischaemia-reperfusion-induced AKI include endothelial injury and vasoconstriction; inflammation including activation of the complement cascade, induction of an inflammatory phenotype in tubular cells and activation of proliferation of numerous resident and migratory leucocyte subtypes; tubular epithelial injury, including loss of cellular polarity, cellular adhesion and the cellular brush border and apoptosis and necrosis; and also simultaneous upregulation of endogenous inhibitors of inflammation including epithelial cell heme oxygenase-1 [47]. Furthermore, crosstalk in which extrarenal injury can trigger organ injury and vice versa [134] may account for some of the association between AKI and increased mortality.

Despite differences, animal models have been able to demonstrate that AKI from ischaemia-reperfusion injury, and toxicant-induced AKI, share many common injury mechanisms, although the sequence and, possibly, the relative importance of each mechanism may vary. For example, in ischaemia-reperfusion injury, endothelial injury, with accompanying vasoconstriction and adhesion of leucocytes to vascular endothelium and migration to the interstitium, appears to precede tubular injury, apoptosis and necrosis [47]. The injured tubular epithelium releases pro-inflammatory cytokines and chemokines, which help to amplify endothelial injury, leucocyte adhesion or migration and tubular injury. By contrast, in toxicant-induced AKI, tubular dysfunction, apoptosis and necrosis are considered primary events with the consequent local pro-inflammatory signals leading to endothelial injury and systemic inflammation, thereby amplifying tubular injury. However, it is apparent that even these distinctions, particularly between inflammation and cellular injury, are arbitrary. For example, TNF-α[alpha] which is produced by injured tubular epithelial cells can act simultaneously: intracellularly via the death receptor pathway to induce apoptosis in the cell of origin;

in a paracrine fashion, to induce death of neighbouring tubular cells in a process called fratricide [171]; to injure vascular endothelium including glomerular endothelium [112]; and to amplify local and systemic inflammation.

Conclusion

AKI is important. It affects approximately one fifth of all hospitalised adults and one third of hospitalised children and is associated with excess mortality. AKI is also associated with maladaptive healing and the development of CKD, which in turn is a risk factor for further AKI. Important causes of AKI include sepsis, hypovolaemia and hypotension, nephrotoxic drugs and surgery. However multiple causes are frequently present in the same patient, and acute tubular injury is probably underrepresented in biopsy series. The syndrome is currently defined clinically by the recognition of impaired function, namely, by elevated SCr or oliguria, but this is a flawed paradigm. Traditional constructs including prerenal AKI have been challenged by evidence demonstrating that cellular injury may occur without functional impairment and vice versa.

Animal models have helped elucidate many of the cellular events of AKI but potentially lack sufficient accuracy or complexity to translate to human AKI. Important events include tubular epithelial injury, including loss of cellular polarity, cellular adhesion and the cellular brush border and apoptosis and necrosis; endothelial injury and vasoconstriction; inflammation including complement activation, induction of an inflammatory phenotype in tubular cells and activation of proliferation of numerous resident and migratory leucocyte subtypes; but also simultaneous upregulation of endogenous inhibitors of inflammation.

Proteins or other molecules that appear in greater or lesser concentrations in plasma or urine after the initiation of kidney injury represent distinct physiological or pathological processes in the pathway of acute kidney injury. Collectively, these molecules represent potential kidney damage biomarkers. Recent consensus criteria propose the definition of AKI by either impaired function, or the detection of kidney damage biomarkers. Potential kidney damage biomarkers include urinary or plasma KIM-1, NGAL and IL-18, although to date only the product of urinary TIMP-2 and urinary IGFBP7 concentrations has obtained regulatory approval in the USA for clinical use. Expanding the use of novel biomarkers will hopefully lead to better recognition and in turn management of this deadly condition.

References

1. Lameire N, Bagga A, Cruz D, De Maeseneer J, Endre Z, Kellum J, et al. Acute kidney injury: an increasing global concern. Lancet. 2013;382:170–9.
2. Palevsky P. Renal support in acute kidney injury—how much is enough? N Engl J Med. 2009;361:1699–701.
3. Uchino S, Bellomo R, Goldsmith D, Bates S, Ronco C. An assessment of the RIFLE criteria for acute renal failure in hospitalized patients. Crit Care Med. 2006;34(7):1913.
4. Wonnacott A, Meran S, Amphlett B, Talabani B, Phillips A. Epidemiology and outcomes in community-acquired versus hospital-acquired AKI. Clin J Am Soc Nephrol. 2014;9:1007–14.
5. Bagshaw S, Laupland K, Doig C, Mortis G, Fick G, Mucenski M, et al. Prognosis for long-term survival and renal recovery in critically ill patients with severe acute renal failure: a population based study. Crit Care. 2005;9:R700–R9.
6. Hoste E, Schurgers M. Epidemiology of acute kidney injury: how big is the problem? Crit Care Med. 2008;36:S146–S51.
7. Lo L, Go A, Chertow G, McCulloch C, Fan D, Ordoñez J, et al. Dialysis-requiring acute renal failure increases the risk of progressive chronic kidney disease. Kidney Int. 2009;76:893–9.
8. Uchino S, Kellum J, Bellomo R, Doig G, Morimatsu H, Morgera S, et al. Acute renal failure in critically ill patients. J Am Med Assoc. 2005;294:813–8.
9. Susantitaphong P, Cruz D, Cerda J, Abulfaraj M, Alqahtani F, Koulouridis I, et al. World incidence of AKI: a meta-analysis. Clin J Am Soc Nephrol. 2013;8:1482–93.
10. Mehta R, Cerdá J, Burdmann E, Tonelli M, García-García G, Jha V, et al. International Society of Nephrology's 0by25 initiative for acute kidney injury (zero preventable deaths by 2025): a human rights case for nephrology. Lancet. 2015;385:2616–43.
11. Investigators TP. A randomized trial of protocol-based care for early septic shock. N Engl J Med. 2014;370:1683–93.

12. VA/NIH Acute Renal Failure Trial Network, Palevsky P, Zhang J, O'Connor T, Chertow G, Crowley S, et al. Intensity of renal support in critically ill patients with acute kidney injury. N Engl J Med. 2008;359:7–20.
13. Coca S, Yusuf B, Shlipak M, Garg A, Parikh C. Long-term risk of mortality and other adverse outcomes after acute kidney injury: a systematic review and meta-analysis. Am J Kidney Dis. 2009;53:961–73.
14. Mammen C, Al Abbas A, Skippen P, Nadel H, Levine D, Collet J-P, et al. Long-term risk of CKD in children surviving episodes of acute kidney injury in the intensive care unit: a prospective cohort study. Am J Kidney Dis. 2012;59:523–30.
15. Pannu N, James M, Hemmelgarn B, Klarenbach S, Network AKD. Association between AKI, recovery of renal function, and long-term outcomes after hospital discharge. Clin J Am Soc Nephrol. 2013;8(2):194–202. https://doi.org/10.2215/CJN.06480612.
16. Doi K, Katagiri D, Negishi K, Hasegawa S, Hamasaki Y, Fujita T, et al. Mild elevation of urinary biomarkers in prerenal acute kidney injury. Kidney Int. 2012;82:1114–20.
17. Nejat M, Pickering J, Devarajan P, Bonventre J, Edelstein C, Walker R, et al. Some biomarkers of acute kidney injury are increased in pre-renal acute injury. Kidney Int. 2012;81:1254–62.
18. Koyner J, Garg A, Thiessen-Philbrook H, Coca S, Cantley L, Peixoto A, et al. Adjudication of etiology of acute kidney injury: experience from the TRIBE-AKI multi-center study. BMC Nephrol. 2014;15:1–9.
19. Endre Z, Kellum J, Di Somma S, Doi K, Goldstein S, Koyner J, et al. Differential diagnosis of AKI in clinical practice by functional and damage biomarkers: workgroup statements from the tenth Acute Dialysis Quality Initiative Consensus Conference. Contrib Nephrol. 2013;182:30–44.
20. Hamdi A, Hajage D, Van Glabeke E, Belenfant X, Vincent F, Gonzalez F, et al. Severe post-renal acute kidney injury, post-obstructive diuresis and renal recovery. BJU Int. 2012;110:E1027–E34.
21. Murray P, Mehta R, Shaw A, Ronco C, Endre Z, Kellum J, et al. Potential use of bioma5rkers in acute kidney injury: report and summary of recommendations from the 10th Acute Dialysis Quality Initiative consensus conference. Kidney Int. 2014;85:513–21.
22. Sabbisetti V, Waikarm S, Antoine D, Smiles A, Wang C, Ravisankar A, et al. Blood kidney injury molecule-1 is a biomarker of acute and chronic kidney injury and predicts progression to ESRD in type I diabetes. J Am Soc Nephrol. 2014;25:2177–86.
23. KDIGO, Kidney Disease Improving Global Outcomes Acute Kidney Injury Work Group. KDIGO clinical practice guideline for acute kidney injury. Kidney Int Suppl. 2012;2:1–143.
24. Praga M, González E. Acute interstitial nephritis. Kidney Int. 2010;77:956–61.
25. George J, Nester C. Syndromes of thrombotic microangiopathy. N Engl J Med. 2014;371:654–66.
26. Liangos O, Wald R, O'Bell J, Price L, Pereira B, Jaber B. Epidemiology and outcomes of acute renal failure in hospitalized patients: a national survey. Clin J Am Soc Nephrol. 2006;1:43–51.
27. Quintana L, Peréz N, De Sousa E, Rodas L, Griffiths M, Solé M, et al. ANCA serotype and histopathological classification for the prediction of renal outcome in ANCA-associated glomerulonephritis. Nephrol Dial Transplant. 2014;29:1764–9.
28. Ruggenenti P, Noris M, Remuzzi G. Thrombotic microangiopathy, hemolytic uremic syndrome, and thrombotic thrombocytopenic purpura. Kidney Int. 2001;60:831–46.
29. Porile J, Bakris G, Garella S. Acute interstitial nephritis with glomerulopathy due to nonsteroidal anti-inflammatory agents: a review of its clinical spectrum and effects of steroid therapy. J Clin Pharmacol. 1990;30:468–75.
30. Levey A, Stevens L, Schmid C, Zhang Y, Castro A, Feldman H, et al. A new equation to estimate glomerular filtration rate. Ann Intern Med. 2009;150:604–12.
31. Chertow G, Burdick E, Honour M, Bonventre J, Bates D. Acute kidney injury, mortality, length of stay, and costs in hospitalized patients. J Am Soc Nephrol. 2005;16:3365–70.
32. KDIGO. KDIGO clinical practice guideline for acute kidney injury. Kidney Int Suppl. 2012;2:1–141.
33. Mehta R, Kellum J, Shah S, Molitoris B, Ronco C, Warnock D, et al. Acute Kidney Injury Network: report of an initiative to improve outcomes in acute kidney injury. Crit Care. 2007;11:1–8.
34. Pickering J, Endre Z. GFR shot by RIFLE: errors in staging acute kidney injury. Lancet. 2009;373:1318–9.
35. Selvin E, Juraschek S, Eckfeldt J, Levey A, Inker L, Coresh J. Within-person variability in kidney measures. Am J Kidney Dis. 2013;61:716–22.
36. Md Ralib A, Pickering J, Shaw G, Endre Z. The urine output definition of acute kidney injury is too liberal. Crit Care. 2013;17:1–11.
37. Pianta T, Buckley N, Peake P, Endre Z. Clinical use of biomarkers for toxicant-induced acute kidney injury. Biomark Med. 2013;7:441–56.
38. Perkins R, Kirchner H, Hartle J, Bucaloiu I. Estimated glomerular filtration rate variability and risk of end-stage renal disease among patients with Stage 3 chronic kidney disease. Clin Nephrol. 2013;80:256–62.
39. Drion I, Cobbaert C, Groenier K, Weykamp C, Bilo H, Wetzels J, et al. Clinical evaluation of analytical variations in serum creatinine measurements: why laboratories should abandon Jaffe techniques. BMC Nephrol. 2012;13:1–8.
40. Joffe M, Hsu C, Feldman H, Weir M, Landis J, Hamm L, et al. Variability of creatinine measurements in clinical laboratories: results from the CRIC study. Am J Nephrol. 2010;31:426–35.

41. Pickering J, Endre Z. Back-calculating baseline creatinine with MDRD misclassifies acute kidney injury in the intensive care unit. Clin J Am Soc Nephrol. 2010;5:1165–73.
42. Rivers E, Nguyen B, Havstad S, Ressler J, Muzzin A, Knoblich B, et al. Early goal-directed therapy in the treatment of severe sepsis and septic shock. N Engl J Med. 2001;345:1368–77.
43. Meersch M, Schmidt C, Hoffmeier A, Van Aken H, Wempe C, Gerss J, Zarbock A. Prevention of cardiac surgery-associated AKI by implementing the KDIGO guidelines in high risk patients identified by biomarkers: the PrevAKI randomized controlled trial. Intensive Care Med. 2017;43(11):1551–61. https://doi.org/10.1007/s00134-016-4670-3.
44. Friedrich J, Adhikari N, Herridge M, Beyene J. Meta-analysis: low-dose dopamine increases urine output but does not prevent renal dysfunction or death. Ann Intern Med. 2005;142:510–24.
45. Egal M, Erler N, de Geus H, van Bommel J, Groeneveld J. Targeting oliguria reversal in goal-directed hemodynamic management does not reduce renal dysfunction in perioperative and critically ill patients: a systematic review and meta-analysis. Anesth Analg. 2016;122:173–85.
46. Famulski K, de Freitas D, Kreepala C, Chang J, Sellares J, Sis B, et al. Molecular phenotypes of acute kidney injury in kidney transplants. J Am Soc Nephrol. 2012;23:948–58.
47. Bonventre J, Yang L. Cellular pathophysiology of ischemic acute kidney injury. J Clin Invest. 2011;121:4210–21.
48. Linkermann A, Green D. Necroptosis. N Engl J Med. 2014;370:455–65.
49. Sancho-Martínez S, López-Novoa J, López-Hernández F. Pathophysiological role of different tubular epithelial cell death modes in acute kidney injury. Clin Kidney J. 2015;8:548–59.
50. Chu R, Li C, Wang S, Zou W, Liu G, Yang L. Assessment of KDIGO definitions in patients with histopathologic evidence of acute renal disease. Clin J Am Soc Nephrol. 2014;9:1175–82.
51. Obialo C, Okonofua E, Tayade A, Riley L. Epidemiology of de novo acute renal failure in hospitalized African Americans: comparing community-acquired vs hospital-acquired disease. Arch Intern Med. 2000;160:1309–13.
52. Schissler M, Zaidi S, Kumar H, Deo D, Brier M, McLeish K. Characteristics and outcomes in community-acquired versus hospital-acquired acute kidney injury. Nephrology (Carlton). 2013;18:183–7.
53. Wang Y, Cui Z, Fan M. Hospital-acquired and community-acquired acute renal failure in hospitalized Chinese: a ten-year review. Ren Fail. 2007;29:163–8.
54. Roberts D, Wilks M, Roberts M, Swaminathan R, Mohamed F, Dawson A, et al. Changes in the concentrations of creatinine, cystatin C and NGAL in patients with acute paraquat self-poisoning. Toxicol Lett. 2011;202:69–74.
55. Maduwage K, Isbister G, Silva A, Bowatta S, Mendis S, Gawarammana I. Epidemiology and clinical effects of hump-nosed pit viper (Genus: Hypnale) envenoming in Sri Lanka. Toxicon. 2013;61:11–5.
56. Ishikawa K, Bellomo R, May C. The impact of intrarenal nitric oxide synthase inhibition on renal blood flow and function in mild and severe hyperdynamic sepsis. Crit Care Med. 2011;39:770–6.
57. Spronk P, Ince C, Gardien M, Mathura K, Oudemans-van Straaten H, Zandstra D. Nitroglycerin in septic shock after intravascular volume resuscitation. Lancet. 2002;360:1395–6.
58. Bellomo R, Kellum J, Ronco C. Acute kidney injury. Lancet. 2012;380:756–66.
59. Kheterpal S, Tremper K, Englesbe M, O'Reilly M, Shanks A, Fetterman D, et al. Predictors of postoperative acute renal failure after noncardiac surgery in patients with previously normal renal function. Anesthesiology. 2007;107:892–902.
60. Kheterpal S, Tremper K, Heung M, Rosenberg A, Englesbe M, Shanks A, et al. Development and validation of an acute kidney injury risk index for patients undergoing general surgery: results from a national data set. Anesthesiology. 2009;110:505–15.
61. Bastin A, Ostermann M, Slack A, Diller G, Finney S, Evans T. Acute kidney injury after cardiac surgery according to risk/injury/failure/loss/end-stage, acute kidney injury network, and kidney disease: improving global outcomes classifications. J Crit Care. 2013;28:389–96.
62. Brown J, Kramer R, Coca S, Parikh C. Duration of acute kidney injury impacts long-term survival following cardiac surgery. Ann Thorac Surg. 2012;90:1–14.
63. Ginès P, Schrier R. Renal failure in cirrhosis. N Engl J Med. 2009;361:1279–90.
64. Ho J, Reslerova M, Gali B, Nickerson P, Rush D, Sood M, et al. Serum creatinine measurement immediately after cardiac surgery and prediction of acute kidney injury. Am J Kidney Dis. 2012;59:196–201.
65. Swaminathan M, Hudson C, Phillips-Bute B, Patel U, Mathew J, Newman M, et al. Impact of early renal recovery on survival after cardiac surgery-associated acute kidney injury. Ann Thorac Surg. 2010;89:1098–104.
66. Gallagher S, Jones D, Kapur A, Wragg A, Harwood S, Mathur R, et al. Remote ischemic preconditioning has a neutral effect on the incidence of kidney injury after coronary artery bypass graft surgery. Kidney Int. 2015;87:473–81.
67. Gonzálezm E, Gutiérrez E, Galeano C, Chevia C, de Sequera P, Bernis C, et al. Early steroid treatment improves the recovery of renal function in patients with drug-induced acute interstitial nephritis. Kidney Int. 2008;73:940–6.
68. Legendre C, Licht C, Muus P, Greenbaum L, Babu S, Bedrosian C, et al. Terminal complement inhibitor eculizumab in atypical hemolytic-uremic syndrome. N Engl J Med. 2013;368:2169–81.

69. Karlberg L, Norlén B, Ojteg G, Wolgast M. Impaired medullary circulation in postischemic acute renal failure. Acta Physiol Scand. 1983;118:11–7.
70. Mengel M, Sis B, Haas M, Colvin R, Halloran P, Racusen L, et al. Banff 2011 Meeting report: new concepts in antibody-mediated rejection. Am J Transplant. 2012;12:563–70.
71. Vaidya V, Ozer J, Dieterle F, Collings F, Ramirez V, Troth S, et al. Kidney injury molecule-1 outperforms traditional biomarkers of kidney injury in preclinical biomarker qualification studies. Nat Biotechnol. 2010;28:478–85.
72. Yu Y, Jin H, Holder D, Ozer J, Villarreal S, Shughrue P, et al. Urinary biomarkers trefoil factor 3 and albumin enable early detection of kidney tubular injury. Nat Biotechnol. 2010;28:470–7.
73. Bellomo R, Bagshaw S, Langenberg C, Ronco C. Pre-renal azotemia: a flawed paradigm in critically ill septic patients? Contrib Nephrol. 2007;156:1–9.
74. Endre Z, Ratcliffe P, Tange J, Ferguson D, Radda G, John L. Erythrocytes alters the pattern of renal hypoxic injury: predominance of proximal tubular injury with moderate hypoxia. Clin Sci. 1989;76:19–29.
75. Zuk A, Bonventre J, Brown D, Matlin K. Polarity, integrin, and extracellular matrix dynamics in the postischemic rat kidney. Am J Physiol. 1998;275:C711–C31.
76. Westhuyzen J, Endre Z, Reece G, Reith D, Saltissi D, Morgan T. Measurement of tubular enzymuria facilitates early detection of acute renal impairment in the intensive care unit. Nephrol Dial Transplant. 2003;118:543–51.
77. Choudhury D, Ahmed Z. Drug-associated renal dysfunction and injury. Nat Clin Pract Nephrol. 2006;2:80–91.
78. Portilla D, Li S, Nagothu K, Megyesi J, Kaissling B, Schnackenberg L, et al. Metabolomic study of cisplatin-induced nephrotoxicity. Kidney Int. 2006;69:2194–204.
79. Christensen E, Verroust P, Nielsen R. Receptor-mediated endocytosis in renal proximal tubule. Pflugers Arch. 2009;458:1039–48.
80. Christensen E, Birn H, Rippe B, Maunsbach A. Controversies in nephrology: renal albumin handling, facts, and artifacts! Kidney Int. 2007;72:1192–4.
81. Dieterle F, Perentes E, Cordier A, Roth D, Verdes P, Grenet O, et al. Urinary clusterin, cystatin C, β2-microglobulin and total protein as markers to detect drug-induced kidney injury. Nat Biotechnol. 2010;28:463–9.
82. Ma S, Nishikawa M, Hyoudou K, Takahashi R, Ikemura M, Kobayashi Y, et al. Combining cisplatin with cationized catalase decreases nephrotoxicity while improving antitumor activity. Kidney Int. 2007;72:1474–82.
83. Kaseda R, Iino N, Hosojima M, Takeda T, Hosaka K, Kobayashi A, et al. Megalin-mediated endocytosis of cystatin C in proximal tubule cells. Biochem Biophys Res Commun. 2007;357:1130–4.
84. Russo L, Sandoval R, Campos S, Molitoris B, Comper W, Brown D. Impaired tubular uptake explains albuminuria in early diabetic nephropathy. J Am Soc Nephrol. 2009;20:489–94.
85. Russo L, Sandoval R, McKee M, Osicka T, Collins A, Brown D, et al. The normal kidney filters nephrotic levels of albumin retrieved by proximal tubule cells: retrieval is disrupted in nephrotic states. Kidney Int. 2007;71:504–13.
86. Siddik Z. Cisplatin: mode of cytotoxic action and molecular basis of resistance. Oncogene. 2003;22:7265–79.
87. Endre Z, Pickering J. Acute kidney injury: cell cycle arrest biomarkers win race for AKI diagnosis. Nat Rev Nephrol. 2014;10(12):683–5.
88. Kashani K, Al-Khafaji A, Ardiles T, Artigas A, Bagshaw S, Bell M, et al. Discovery and validation of cell cycle arrest biomarkers in human acute kidney injury. Crit Care. 2013;1:1–12.
89. Meersch M, Schmidt C, Van Aken H, Martens S, Rossaint J, Singbartl K, et al. Urinary TIMP-2 and IGFBP7 as early biomarkers of acute kidney injury and renal recovery following cardiac surgery. PLoS One. 2014;9:1–9.
90. Canaud G, Bonventre J. Cell cycle arrest and the evolution of chronic kidney disease from acute kidney injury. Nephrol Dial Transplant. 2015;30:575–83.
91. Lee Y, Bae S, Won N, Pyo H, Kwon Y. Alpha-lipoic acid attenuates cisplatin-induced tubulointerstitial injuries through inhibition of mitochondrial bax translocation in rats. Nephron Exp Nephrol. 2009;113:e104–e12.
92. Pabla N, Dong Z. Cisplatin nephrotoxicity: mechanisms and renoprotective strategies. Kidney Int. 2008;73:994–1007.
93. Gobé G, Zhang X, Willgoss D, Schoch E, Hogg N, Endre Z. Relationship between expression of Bcl-2 genes and growth factors in ischemic acute renal failure in the rat. J Am Soc Nephrol. 2000;11:454–67.
94. Johnson D, Pat B, Vesey D, Guan Z, Endre Z, Gobe G. Delayed administration of darbepoetin or erythropoietin protects against ischemic acute renal injury and failure. Kidney Int. 2006;69:1806–13.
95. Molitoris B, Sandoval R, Campos S, Ashush H, Fridman E, Brafman A, et al. siRNA targeted to p53 attenuates ischemic and cisplatin-induced acute kidney injury. J Am Soc Nephrol. 2009;20:1754–64.
96. Jordan S, Cronan J. A new metabolic link: the acyl carrier protein of lipid synthesis donates lipoic acid to the pyruvate dehydrogenase complex in *Escherichia coli* and mitochondria. J Biol Chem. 1997;272:17903–6.
97. Kozlov A, Gille L, Staniek K, Nohl H. Dihydrolipoic acid maintains ubiquinone in the antioxidant active form by two-electron reduction of ubiquinone and one-electron reduction of ubisemiquinone. Arch Biochem Biophys. 1999;363:148–54.

98. Wang Z, Gall J, Bonegio R, Havasi A, Hunt C, Sherman M, et al. Induction of heat shock protein 70 inhibits ischemic renal injury. Kidney Int. 2011;79:861–70.
99. Ratcliffe P, Moonen C, Endre Z, Blackledge M, Ledingham J, Radda G. 31P nuclear magnetic resonance in the investigation of renal ischemia during hypotension. Contrib Nephrol. 1987;56:152–8.
100. Liu H, Baliga R. Cytochrome P450 2E1 null mice provide novel protection against cisplatin-induced nephrotoxicity and apoptosis. Kidney Int. 2003;63:1687–96.
101. Liu H, Baliga R. Endoplasmic reticulum stress-associated caspase 12 mediates cisplatin-induced LLC-PK1 cell apoptosis. J Am Soc Nephrol. 2005;16:1985–92.
102. Abdel-latif R, Morsy M, El-Moselhy M, Khalifa M. Sildenafil protects against nitric oxide deficiency-related nephrotoxicity in cyclosporine A treated rats. Eur J Pharmacol. 2013;705:126–34.
103. Yu M, Xue J, Li Y, Zhang W, Ma D, Liu L, et al. Resveratrol protects against arsenic trioxide-induced nephrotoxicity by facilitating arsenic metabolism and decreasing oxidative stress. Arch Toxicol. 2013;87:1025–35.
104. Fonseca I, Reguengo H, Almeida M, Dias L, Martins L, Pedroso S, et al. Oxidative stress in kidney transplantation: malondialdehyde is an early predictive marker of graft dysfunction. Transplantation. 2014;97:1058–65.
105. Gobe G, Harmon B. Apoptosis: morphological criteria and other assays. Encyclopedia of life science. Chichester: Wiley; 2008.
106. Kaushal G, Shah S. Autophagy in acute kidney injury. Kidney Int. 2016;89:779–91.
107. Alejandro V, Scandling JJ, Sibley R, Dafoe D, Alfrey E, Deen W, et al. Mechanisms of filtration failure during postischemic injury of the human kidney. A study of the reperfused renal allograft. J Clin Invest. 1995;95:820–31.
108. Guan Z, Gobé G, Willgoss D, Endre Z. Renal endothelial dysfunction and impaired autoregulation after ischemia-reperfusion injury result from excess nitric oxide. Am J Physiol Renal Physiol. 2006;291:F619–F28.
109. Ergin B, Kapucu A, Demirci-Tansel C, Ince C. The renal microcirculation in sepsis. Nephrol Dial Transplant. 2015;30:169–77.
110. Sprague A, Khalil R. Inflammatory cytokines in vascular dysfunction and vascular disease. Biochem Pharmacol. 2009;78:539–52.
111. Kelly K, Williams WJ, Colvin R, Meehan S, Springer T, Gutierrez-Ramos J, et al. Intercellular adhesion molecule-1-deficient mice are protected against ischemic renal injury. J Clin Invest. 1996;97:1056–63.
112. Xu C, Chang A, Hack B, Eadon M, Alper S, Cunningham P. TNF-mediated damage to glomerular endothelium is an important determinant of acute kidney injury in sepsis. Kidney Int. 2014;85:72–81.
113. Ko G, Grigoryev D, Linfert D, Jang H, Watkins T, Cheadle C, et al. Transcriptional analysis of kidneys during repair from AKI reveals possible roles for NGAL and KIM-1 as biomarkers of AKI-to-CKD transition. Am J Physiol Renal Physiol. 2010;289:F1472–F83.
114. Bae E, Lee J, Ma S, Kim I, Frøkiaer J, Nielsen S, et al. Alpha-Lipoic acid prevents cisplatin-induced acute kidney injury in rats. Nephrol Dial Transplant. 2009;24:2692–700.
115. Kwon O, Hong S, Ramesh G. Diminished NO generation by injured endothelium and loss of macula densa nNOS may contribute to sustained acute kidney injury after ischemia-reperfusion. Am J Physiol Renal Physiol. 2009;296:F25–33.
116. Mori K, Lee H, Rapoport D, Drexler I, Foster K, Yang J, et al. Endocytic delivery of lipocalin-siderophore-iron complex rescues the kidney from ischemia-reperfusion injury. J Clin Invest. 2005;115:610–21.
117. Paragas N, Qiu A, Zhang Q, Samstein B, Deng S, Schmidt-Ott K, et al. The Ngal reporter mouse detects the response of the kidney to injury in real time. Nat Med. 2011;17:216–22.
118. Supavekin S, Zhang W, Kucherlapati R, Kaskel F, Moore L, Devarajan P. Differential gene expression following early renal ischemia/reperfusion. Kidney Int. 2003;63:1714–24.
119. Efrati S, Berman S, Hamad R, Siman-Tov Y, Ilgiyaev E, Maslyakov I, et al. Effect of captopril treatment on recuperation from ischemia/reperfusion-induced acute renal injury. Nephrol Dial Transplant. 2012;27:136–45.
120. Molitoris B, Sutton T. Endothelial injury and dysfunction: role in the extension phase of acute renal failure. Kidney Int. 2004;66:496–9.
121. Salman I, Ameer O, Sattar M, Abdullah N, Yam M, Najim H, et al. Characterization of renal hemodynamic and structural alterations in rat models of renal impairment: role of renal sympathoexcitation. J Nephrol. 2011;24:68–77.
122. John R, Nelson P. Dendritic cells in the kidney. J Am Soc Nephrol. 2007;18:2628–35.
123. Umetsu S, Lee W, McIntire J, Downey L, Sanjanwala B, Akbari O, et al. TIM-1 induces T cell activation and inhibits the development of peripheral tolerance. Nat Immunol. 2005;6:447–54.
124. Thurman J, Lucia M, Ljubanovic D, Holers V. Acute tubular necrosis is characterized by activation of the alternative pathway of complement. Kidney Int. 2005;67:524–30.
125. Han W, Bailly V, Abichandani R, Thadhani R, Bonventre J. Kidney Injury Molecule-1 (KIM-1): a novel biomarker for human renal proximal tubule injury. Kidney Int. 2002;62:237–44.
126. Ichimura T, Asseldonk E, Humphreys B, Gunaratnam L, Duffield J, Bonventre J. Kidney injury molecule-1 is a phosphatidylserine receptor that confers a phagocytic phenotype on epithelial cells. J Clin Invest. 2008;118:1657–68.

127. Wu H, Craft M, Wang P, Wyburn K, Chen G, Ma J, et al. IL-18 contributes to renal damage after ischemia-reperfusion. J Am Soc Nephrol. 2008;19:2331–41.
128. Chen H, Lai P, Lan Y, Cheng C, Zhong W, Lin Y, et al. Exosomal ATF3 RNA attenuates pro-inflammatory gene MCP-1 transcription in renal ischemia-reperfusion. J Cell Physiol. 2014;229:1202–11.
129. Imamura K, Nishihira J, Suzuki M, Yasuda K, Sasaki S, Kusunoki Y, et al. Identification and immunohistochemical localization of macrophage migration inhibitory factor in human kidney. Biochem Mol Biol Int. 1996;40:1233–42.
130. Izquierdo M, Sanz A, Mezzano S, Blanco J, Carrasco S, Sanchez-Niño M, et al. TWEAK (tumor necrosis factor-like weak inducer of apoptosis) activates CXCL16 expression during renal tubulointerstitial inflammation. Kidney Int. 2012;81:1098–107.
131. Barnes P, Karin M. Nuclear factor-kappaB: a pivotal transcription factor in chronic inflammatory diseases. N Engl J Med. 1997;336:1066–71.
132. Bolisetty S, Traylor A, Kim J, Joseph R, Ricart K, Landar A, et al. Heme oxygenase-1 inhibits renal tubular macroautophagy in acute kidney injury. J Am Soc Nephrol. 2010;21:1702–12.
133. Grigoryev D, Liu M, Hassoun H, Cheadle C, Barnes K. H R. The local and systemic inflammatory transcriptome after acute kidney injury. J Am Soc Nephrol. 2008;19:547–58.
134. Li X, Hassoun H, Santora R, Rabb H. Organ cross-talk: the role of the kidney. Curr Opin Crit Care. 2009;15:481–7.
135. Simmons E, Himmelfarb J, Sezer M, Chertow G, Mehta R, Paganini E, et al. Plasma cytokine levels predict mortality in patients with acute renal failure. Kidney Int. 2004;65:1357–65.
136. Pickering J, Endre Z. New metric for assessing diagnostic potential of candidate biomarkers. Clin J Am Soc Nephrol. 2012;7:1355–64.
137. Endre Z, Pickering J, Walker R. Clearance and beyond: the complementary roles of GFR measurement and injury biomarkers in acute kidney injury (AKI). Am J Physiol Renal Physiol. 2011;301:F697–707.
138. Coca S, Yalavarthy R, Concato J, Parikh C. Biomarkers for the diagnosis and risk stratification of acute kidney injury: a systematic review. Kidney Int. 2008;73:1008–16.
139. Cruz DD, Bagshaw S, Maisel A, Lewington A, Thadhani R, Chakravarthi R, et al. Use of biomarkers to assess prognosis and guide management of patients with acute kidney injury. Contrib Nephrol. 2013;182:45–64.
140. Murray P. Acute kidney injury biomarkers and endpoints for clinical trials. Contrib Nephrol. 2011;171:208–12.
141. Food and Drug Administration/Centre for Drug Evaluation and Research. Enrichment strategies. Small Business Chronicles. 2013;10:1–2.
142. Okusa M, Jaber BL, Doran P, Duranteau J, Yang L, Murray P, Mehta R, et al. Physiological biomarkers of acute kidney injury: a conceptual approach to improving outcomes. Contrib Nephrol. 2013;182:65–81.
143. Hvidberg V, Jacobsen C, Strong R, Cowland J, Moestrup S, Borregaard N. The endocytic receptor megalin binds the iron transporting neutrophil-gelatinase-associated lipocalin with high affinity and mediates its cellular uptake. FEBS Lett. 2005;579(3):773–7.
144. Bonventre J. Kidney Injury Molecule-1: a translational journey. Trans Am Clin Climatol Assoc. 2014;125:293–9.
145. Degauque N, Mariat C, Kenny J, Zhang D, Gao W, Vu M, et al. Immunostimulatory Tim-1-specific antibody deprograms Tregs and prevents transplant tolerance in mice. J Clin Invest. 2008;118:735–41.
146. Nozaki Y, Kinoshita K, Yano T, Asato K, Shiga T, Hino S, et al. Signaling through the interleukin-18 receptor α[alpha] attenuates inflammation in cisplatin-induced acute kidney injury. Kidney Int. 2012;82:892–902.
147. Zager R, Johnson A, Lund S. Uremia impacts renal inflammatory cytokine gene expression in the setting of experimental acute kidney injury. Am J Renal Physiol. 2009;297:F961–F70.
148. Hong M-Y, Tseng C-C, Chuang C-C, Chen C-L, Lin S-H, Lin C-F. Urinary macrophage migration inhibitory factor serves as a potential biomarker for acute kidney injury in patients with acute pyelonephritis. Mediat Inflamm. 2012;2012:1–9.
149. Rice E, Tesch G, Cao Z, Cooper M, Metz C, Bucala R, et al. Induction of MIF synthesis and secretion by tubular epithelial cells: a novel action of angiotensin II. Kidney Int. 2003;63:1265–75.
150. Mount P, Gleich K, Tam S, Fraser S, Choy S-W, Dwyer K, et al. The outcome of renal ischemia-reperfusion injury is unchanged in AMPK-β1 deficient mice. PLoS One. 2012;7(1):e29887.
151. Haase M, Devarajan P, Haase-Fielitz A, Bellomo R, Cruz D, Wagener G, et al. The outcome of neutrophil gelatinase-associated lipocalin-positive subclinical acute kidney injury: a multicenter pooled analysis of prospective studies. J Am Coll Cardiol. 2011;57:1752–61.
152. Nickolas T, Schmidt-Ott K, Canetta P, Forster C, Singer E, Sise M, et al. Diagnostic and prognostic stratification in the emergency department using urinary biomarkers of nephron damage: a multicenter prospective cohort study. J Am Coll Cardiol. 2012;59:246–55.
153. Bellomo R, Ronco C, Kellum J, Mehta R, Palevsky P, Acute Dialysis Quality Initiative Workgroup. Acute renal failure—definition, outcome measures, animal models, fluid therapy and information technology needs: the Second International Consensus Conference of the Acute Dialysis Quality Initiative (ADQI) Group. Crit Care. 2004;8:R204–R12.

154. Harpur E, Ennulat D, Hoffman D, Betton G, Gautier J, Riefke B, et al. Biological qualification of biomarkers of chemical-induced renal toxicity in two strains of male rat. Toxicol Sci. 2011;122:235–52.
155. Pianta TJ, Succar L, Davidson T, Buckley NA, Endre ZH. Monitoring treatment of acute kidney injury with damage biomarkers. Toxicol Lett. 2017;268:63–70. https://doi.org/10.1016/j.toxlet.2017.01.001.
156. Yang L, Besschetnova T, Brooks C, Shah J, Bonventre J. Epithelial cell cycle arrest in G2/M mediates kidney fibrosis after injury. Nat Med. 2010;16:535–43.
157. Jung G, Kim M, Jung Y, Kim H, Park I, Min B, et al. Clusterin attenuates the development of renal fibrosis. J Am Soc Nephrol. 2012;23:73–85.
158. Nguanm C, Guan Q, Gleave M, Du C. Promotion of cell proliferation by clusterin in the renal tissue repair phase after ischemia-reperfusion injury. Am J Physiol Renal Physiol. 2014;306:F724–F33.
159. Hidaka S, Kränzlin B, Gretz N, Witzgall R. Urinary clusterin levels in the rat correlate with the severity of tubular damage and may help to differentiate between glomerular and tubular injuries. Cell Tissue Res. 2002;310:289–96.
160. Yoshida T, Kurella M, Beato F, Min H, Ingelfinger J, Stears R, et al. Monitoring changes in gene expression in renal ischemia-reperfusion in the rat. Kidney Int. 2002;61:1646–54.
161. Correa-Rotter R, Hostetter T, Nath K, Manivel J, Rosenberg M. Interaction of complement and clusterin in renal injury. J Am Soc Nephrol. 1992;3:1172–9.
162. Chawla L, Eggers P, Star R, Kimmel P. Acute kidney injury and chronic kidney disease as interconnected syndromes. N Engl J Med. 2014;371:58–66.
163. Kriz W, Kaissling B, Hir ML. Epithelial-mesenchymal transition (EMT) in kidney fibrosis: fact or fantasy? J Clin Invest. 2011;121:468–74.
164. Hohenstein B, Renk S, Lang K, Daniel C, Freund M, Léon C, et al. P2Y1 gene deficiency protects from renal disease progression and capillary rarefaction during passive crescentic glomerulonephritis. J Am Soc Nephrol. 2007;18:494–505.
165. Johnson R, Gordon K, Suga S, Duijvestijn A, Griffin K, Bidani A. Renal injury and salt-sensitive hypertension after exposure to catecholamines. Hypertension. 1999;34:151–9.
166. Kanellis J, Paizis K, Cox A, Stacker S, Gilbert R, Cooper M, et al. Renal ischemia-reperfusion increases endothelial VEGFR-2 without increasing VEGF or VEGFR-1 expression. Kidney Int. 2002;61:1696–706.
167. Basile D, Fredrich K, Chelladurai B, Leonard E, Parrish A. Renal ischemia reperfusion inhibits VEGF expression and induces ADAMTS-1, a novel VEGF inhibitor. Am J Physiol Renal Physiol. 2008;294:F928–F36.
168. Vaidya V, Waikar S, Ferguson M, Collings F, Sunderland K, Gioules C, et al. Urinary biomarkers for sensitive and specific detection of acute kidney injury in humans. Clin Transl Sci. 2008;1:200–8.
169. de Caestecker M, Humphreys B, Liu K, Fissell W, Cerda J, Nolin T, et al. Bridging translation by improving preclinical study design in AKI. J Am Soc Nephrol. 2015;26:2905–16.
170. Ricksten S-E, Bragadottir G, Redfors B. Renal oxygenation in clinical acute kidney injury. Crit Care. 2013;17:1–10.
171. Linkermann A, Himmerkus N, Rölver L, Keyser K, Steen P, Bräsen J, et al. Renal tubular Fas ligand mediates fratricide in cisplatin-induced acute kidney failure. Kidney Int. 2011;79:169–78.

Tubular Physiology in Acute Kidney Injury: Cell Signalling, Injury and Inflammation

5

David A. Ferenbach, Eoin D. O'Sullivan, and Joseph V. Bonventre

5.1 Introduction

Acute kidney injury (AKI) is a highly prevalent and devastating clinical problem, one for which new treatments and prophylactic therapies are urgently required. In order to understand and devise novel interventions, a complete understanding of the changes seen in renal physiology in response to acute insults is required. This chapter will discuss the alterations seen in cell polarity, the cell–cell signalling in the tubular compartment and the function of the enzyme heme oxygenase-1 (HO-1) in experimental AKI. Furthermore, the role of acute inflammation in AKI will be considered, including the roles played by cytokine release, inflammatory leukocytes, toll-like receptors (TLRs) and complement activation on disease initiation and progression (Fig. 5.1). Much of our understanding of this area is based on experimental models of acute kidney injury in rodents such as cisplatin nephrotoxicity and renal ischaemia/reperfusion injury. While these models provide valuable information of putative pathophysiological changes within the injured kidney, it must be borne in mind that in the clinical setting, patients with AKI are usually advanced in age, with multiple comorbidities and renal insults, and where human data exists, this will also be discussed.

5.2 Cell Polarity in AKI

Tubular cell polarity is of fundamental importance to normal renal function. The maintenance of luminal and basolateral membrane specificity is central to providing vectorial and selective molecule transport. During tubulogenesis, epithelia coordinate the polarity of individual cells in relation to their neighbouring cells and matrix to create spatially and functionally distinct membranes. This coordination occurs largely through orientating signals from cell–cell and cell–matrix interactions.

The essential structures in determining cell polarity include specific surface membrane

D. A. Ferenbach · E. D. O'Sullivan
MRC Centre of Inflammation Research, University of Edinburgh, Edinburgh, UK

Department of Renal Medicine, Royal Infirmary of Edinburgh, Edinburgh, UK
e-mail: david.ferenbach@ed.ac.uk

J. V. Bonventre (✉)
Renal Division and Engineering in Medicine Division, Department of Medicine, Brigham and Women's Hospital, Harvard Medical School, Boston, MA, USA

Division of Health Sciences and Technology, Harvard-Massachusetts Institute of Technology, Cambridge, MA, USA

Harvard Stem Cell Institute, Cambridge, MA, USA
e-mail: joseph_bonventre@hms.harvard.edu; rgerstein@bwh.harvard.edu

S. S. Waikar et al. (eds.), *Core Concepts in Acute Kidney Injury*,
https://doi.org/10.1007/978-1-4939-8628-6_5

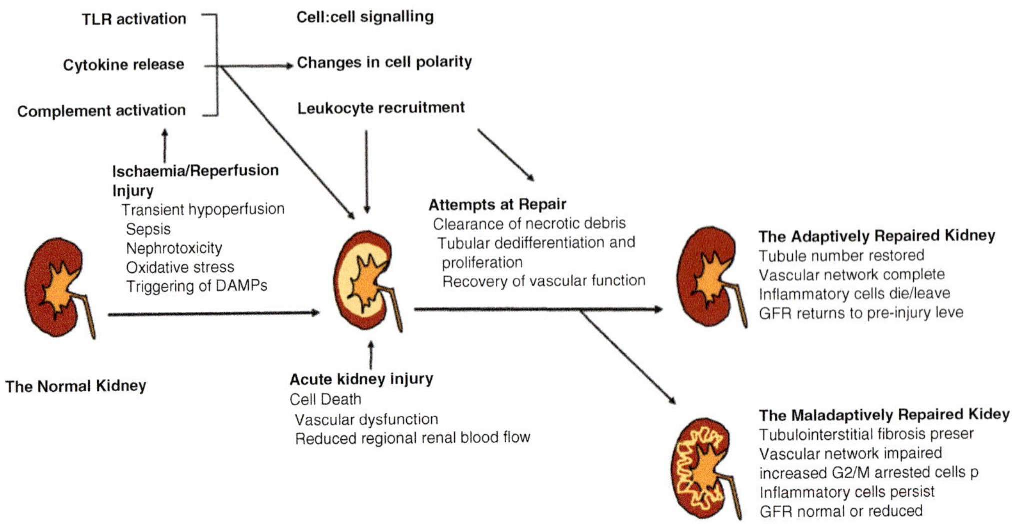

Fig. 5.1 Acute kidney injury. This diagram illustrates the various topics covered in this chapter and their approximate timings and roles in the initiation, propagation and subsequent repair of the injured kidney

domains, a number of junctional complexes (tight junctions, gap junctions, adherens junctions and desmosomes) and the actin cytoskeleton [1].

5.2.1 Acute Injury

There is a loss of cell polarity in acute renal injury [2–6]. Much of our current understanding stems from in vivo ischaemia/reperfusion injury (IRI) models and in vitro models of cultured tubular cells, which allow variable degrees of injury and ATP depletion [7, 8]. An important response to tubular injury is the redistribution of key structural proteins between the apical surface and basolateral membrane. Both actin and the actin-binding protein, villin, have been shown to migrate from the apical to the basolateral plasma membrane within 1 h of reperfusion following ischaemic injury [9]. The tubular apical cytoskeleton is exquisitely sensitive to hypoxia, and assembly of actin and intracellular microfilaments diminishes rapidly as ATP levels are reduced [9–12]. Furthermore, in IRI models, fragmentation of the microtubule network itself has been described [13]. Human studies are consistent with the observations in rodents. In human transplant allograft studies, redistributed cytoskeletal proteins are seen in injured kidneys [14].

Ischaemic injury and ATP depletion in vitro and in vivo also disrupt the epithelial tight junctions [15, 16]. Depleting ATP causes tight junctions to aggregate intracellularly and to form insoluble particulate complexes [17, 18]. β[beta]$_1$-integrins, which mediate epithelial matrix and cell–cell adhesion, migrate to the apical surface during ischaemic injury [19]. The now apically expressed β[beta]$_1$-integrins remain functional and may contribute to abnormal epithelial cell adhesion within the tubule following desquamation [20]. These free tubular cells may adhere to each other and to exocytosed cytoplasmic contents and result in tubular blockage, raising intratubular pressure and resulting in increased "backleak" (see below) of glomerular filtrate from tubular lumen into peritubular capillaries [21]. Loss of these junctional proteins and resultant cytoskeletal change disrupts the molecular anchors, leading to exfoliation of tubular cells into the lumen [22–25].

In humans, posttransplant allograft biopsies of injured kidneys demonstrate redistribution of the Na+/K+-ATPase from the basolateral membrane to both the apical membrane and cytoplasm [3, 26–28]. The Na+/K+-ATPase is thought to be crucial in tight junction formation in addition to its functions in sodium reabsorption [29]. The loss of epithelial cells and Na+/K+-ATPase reduces overall tubular reabsorptive capacity. When the increased sodium load is sensed at the macula densa, this triggers tubuloglomerular feedback, reducing blood flow to the glomerulus and further decreasing effective GFR. The loss of epithelial continuity leads to tubular filtrate translocating paracellularly into the renal interstitium and renal venous system. This phenomenon results in reduced effective glomerular filtration and is known as "backleak" [14, 22, 30, 31].

Recovery of polarity following ischaemic injury requires reassembly of the tight junction catenin components. While milder injury may allow reuse of preformed catenins, more severe ischaemia may require synthesis of new proteins in the endoplasmic reticulum [15]. In some models of injury, reorganisation of the tubular microstructure can be observed as early as 24-h post-reperfusion [13].

5.3 Cell Signalling in AKI

5.3.1 Arachidonic Acid Metabolites

While three pathways of arachidonic acid metabolism exist, cyclooxygenase (COX)-generated compounds are believed to be the most important for renal tubule–tubule signalling [32]. It is worth noting that other arachidonic acid metabolites (e.g. epoxyeicosatrienoic acids or 20-hydroxyeicosatetraenoic acid derived from the P450 system) can alter epithelial sodium transport, glomerular haemodynamics and vascular reactivity and have anti-inflammatory effects [33, 34]. Both COX1 and COX2 enzymes produce PG compounds in the normal and diseased kidney, with ischaemia and vasoconstriction both reported to produce acute increases in levels of vasodilatory PGE_2 and PGI_2 [35]. Levels of COX2 increase in response to renal insults, ageing, diabetes [36], heart failure [37] and lithium treatment [38], with COX2 inhibition reported to be protective [39]. The metabolites of COX1 and COX2 have important roles within the kidney, regulating blood flow, affecting the release of renin and mediating NaCl excretion [40]. Supporting this, agonists of the PGE_2 receptor have lessened renal injury after experimental mercuric chloride-induced AKI [41], while a clinical trial of the PGI_2 analog Iloprost lessened contrast-induced AKI in patients [42]. While these functions fulfil important physiologic roles, increased levels of COX metabolites are seen in disease states and likely contribute to inflammatory injury. COX2-derived prostanoids are renal vasodilators [43], and the inhibition of this effect by non-steroidal anti-inflammatory drugs likely contributes to their nephrotoxicity [44].

Three studies of 20-HETE antagonism or supplementation have been published with conflicting results [45–47], with the most recent papers agreeing that inhibition of 20-HETE improves vascular tone and renal function after murine experimental IRI [45, 46]. Resolvins, protectins and maresins produced via the degradation of omega-3 fatty acids and docosahexaenoic acid have all been reported to promote the resolution of the inflammation following the acute phase of renal injury [48], with their administration to mice mitigating the adverse effects of experimental IRI [49].

5.3.2 Adenosine Triphosphate (ATP)

While ATP is generated within mitochondria and is predominantly intracellular, it is recognised also to be a paracrine signal that acts among renal tubules [50, 51]. At one-thousandth of the intracellular concentration, extracellular ATP (eATP) mediates autocrine and paracrine signalling between renal tubular cells. ATP ligates two families of purinergic receptors—ionotropic (P2X) and metabotropic (P2Y) [52]. When released by dying renal cells in AKI, ATP functions as a danger-associated molecular pattern (DAMP) and elicits immunostimulatory responses in leukocytes [53].

In the mouse, P2X7 receptor inhibition protects against IRI, with protection also seen in the unilateral ureteric obstruction (UUO) model of renal injury and fibrosis in rats [54, 55].

5.3.3 Nitric Oxide

Nitric oxide (NO) is generated in tissues by nitric oxide synthase (NOS) with all three NOS enzymes present within the tubular cells of the kidney [56]. NOS3 is expressed in cells of the proximal convoluted tubule (PCT), thick ascending limb (TAL) and collecting duct (CD) and NOS2 within PCT, TAL, distal convoluted tubule (DCT) and CD cells, while NOS1 is found at low levels in the TAL and CD. Tubular epithelial NO exerts autocrine and paracrine effects promoting natriuresis and diuresis and conveys signals to the adjacent vasculature [57]. Physiologic renal NO release has beneficial effects on renal haemodynamics and function. Renal NO levels decline with advancing stages of CKD [58].

Studies of experimental IRI demonstrate that pre-induction of NO ameliorates disease severity, while co-treatment with NO inhibitors abolishes protection [59]. Potentiating tubular NO production merits investigation as a translational protective therapy for acute and chronic renal injury [60].

5.3.4 Dopamine

Renal dopamine is generated within the cells of the PCT and secreted through the apical and basolateral membranes exhibiting local paracrine effects and hormonal actions via the blood stream on distal nephron segments [61]. Dopamine signals via five known receptors, broadly grouped into D_1-like (D_1 and D_5 receptors) and D_2-like (D_2, D_3 and D_4) groups. In the kidney, the D_1 receptor family is expressed throughout the nephron, juxtaglomerular apparatus and vasculature [62].

In experimental IRI in animals, dopamine has been associated with improved urine output and renal function. However, attempts to translate this into clinical practice have been unsuccessful, with no beneficial effect on rates of death/AKI or dialysis after cardiac surgery seen after dopamine infusion in multiple small studies (reviewed in [63]).

5.3.5 Angiotensin II

Angiotensin II (ATII) is synthesised and released from the proximal tubule and impacts renal water and electrolyte uptake in addition to other sides of production and effects on the vasculature. ATII stimulates sodium uptake by the cells of the PCT, TAL and the CD [64]. In health, ATII augments salt and water uptake via the tubular AT_1 receptor with the renal AT_1R, a driver of systemic hypertension [65]. Via hormonal or paracrine signalling, ATII also induces proliferation, hypertrophy, inflammation and matrix production by tubular cells [66]—all features common to progressive renal disease. Additionally, ATII mediates tubule–tubule crosstalk indirectly via interstitial pericytes and fibrocytes [67]. Recent work has shown that in murine experimental IRI, ATII levels increase in the aftermath of injury, although its vasoconstrictive actions appear to be antagonised by the presence of reactive oxygen species [68].

5.3.6 Bradykinin

The nine-amino acid peptide bradykinin has effects on the heart, kidney and systemic blood vessels [69]. Bradykinin is synthesised in the kidney by the TAL and CD with secretion occurring across apical and basolateral membranes [70]. Bradykinin's effects occur predominantly at a local tissue level, influencing blood pressure via release of NO and prostaglandins [69]. Through interaction with bradykinin B_1 and B_2 receptors, bradykinin promotes diuresis and natriuresis.

Bradykinin B_1 receptors are expressed by differentiating renal tubules [71] and mediate potentially pro-inflammatory effects, with B_1 receptor KO mice normotensive and protected from inflammation and AKI [72]. Both kinin receptor inhibition and kinin B_1 and B_2 receptor knockout mice are protected against cisplatin-induced AKI [73, 74], with B_1 receptor antagonists also reducing fibrosis after experimental UUO presumably due to inhibition of bradykinin's pro-inflammatory actions, including promotion of migration of immune cells to injured tissue [75].

5.4 Heme Oxygenase-1

Although the constitutively expressed enzymes heme oxygenase-2 and oxygenase-3 provide some basal metabolic activity, the predominant route of mammalian heme metabolism is via the inducible enzyme heme oxygenase-1 (HO-1). While removing a source of oxidative stress and generating free iron, the other products of heme metabolism, biliverdin and carbon monoxide (CO), are all recognised to possess immunomodulatory, antiapoptotic and in the case of CO vasoactive properties [76–79]. HO-1 induction is also coupled to increased availability of ferritin, leading to prompt conjugation and removal of free iron—removing another source of potential oxidative stress.

5.4.1 Heme Oxygenase and the Kidney

Our current knowledge of the role of HO-1 in renal disease is largely based on experience of animal models of kidney disease, with additional insights from limited studies performed in human renal biopsy material. Such human data would support HO-1 as being a component of the response of the tubulo-interstitial compartment to injury, with tubular induction of HO-1 in response to injury correlating with reduced markers of oxidative stress [80]. These findings are consistent with the first reported case of human HO-1 deficiency, which was characterised by systemic inflammation, haemolysis and nephropathy with progressive tubulo-interstitial inflammation [81]. Consistent with this, the HO-1 −/− mouse demonstrates exaggerated iron accumulation in the kidney under physiologic conditions with heightened susceptibility to AKI following models of IRI, rhabdomyolysis and cisplatin-induced AKI [82–84].

As the principal route of free heme conjugation in the event of tissue injury, HO-1 is induced in a range of organs in response to IRI. Such upregulation has been demonstrated in the rodent kidney in response to experimental IRI [85], human renal allografts (maximal in organs subject to delayed graft function) [86] and cardiac surgery (maximal in patients with AKI) [87]. Renal HO-1 can be induced by diverse noxious stimuli including hypoxia, LPS administration and bile duct ligation, all of which result in protection against a subsequent, more severe experimental IRI insult—implicating HO-1 induction as a potential mediator of the phenomenon of ischaemic preconditioning [88].

In general, chemical upregulation of HO-1 prior to the induction or renal injury results in functional and structural protection against IRI, while inhibition of HO-1 activity results in an abolition of protected phenotype and often an augmented pattern of injury. Such approaches are not without caveats, as the widely used HO-1 inducer, hemin, is itself a pro-oxidant and the HO-1 inhibiting protoporphyrin compounds almost ubiquitously impact the activity of inducible nitric oxide synthase [89].

The mechanisms underlying the protected phenotypes reproducibly seen by HO-1 induction are likely multifactorial (Fig. 5.2). Three broad areas have been identified as downstream targets of HO-1: the maintenance of renal blood flow, the promotion of cell survival and the modulation of immune phenotype in response to renal injury.

5.4.2 Renal Blood Flow and the Microcirculation

Chemical inhibition of HO activity results in reduced medullary blood flow, supporting a role for HO-1 in the maintenance of medullary perfusion [90]. HO-1 induction in renal transplantation in rats increased capillary flow and diameter of intrarenal vessels when assessed by intravital microscopy [91]. Carbon monoxide has important effects on the circulation—via its potent vasodilatory effects and the inhibition of platelet aggregation [92]. Micropuncture studies have demonstrated that HO-1 induction via stannous mesoporphyrin resulted in the abolition of tubuloglomerular feedback-induced afferent arteriolar vasoconstriction, with the effect reproducible by the administration of either a CORM or exogenous biliverdin—implicating both heme metab-

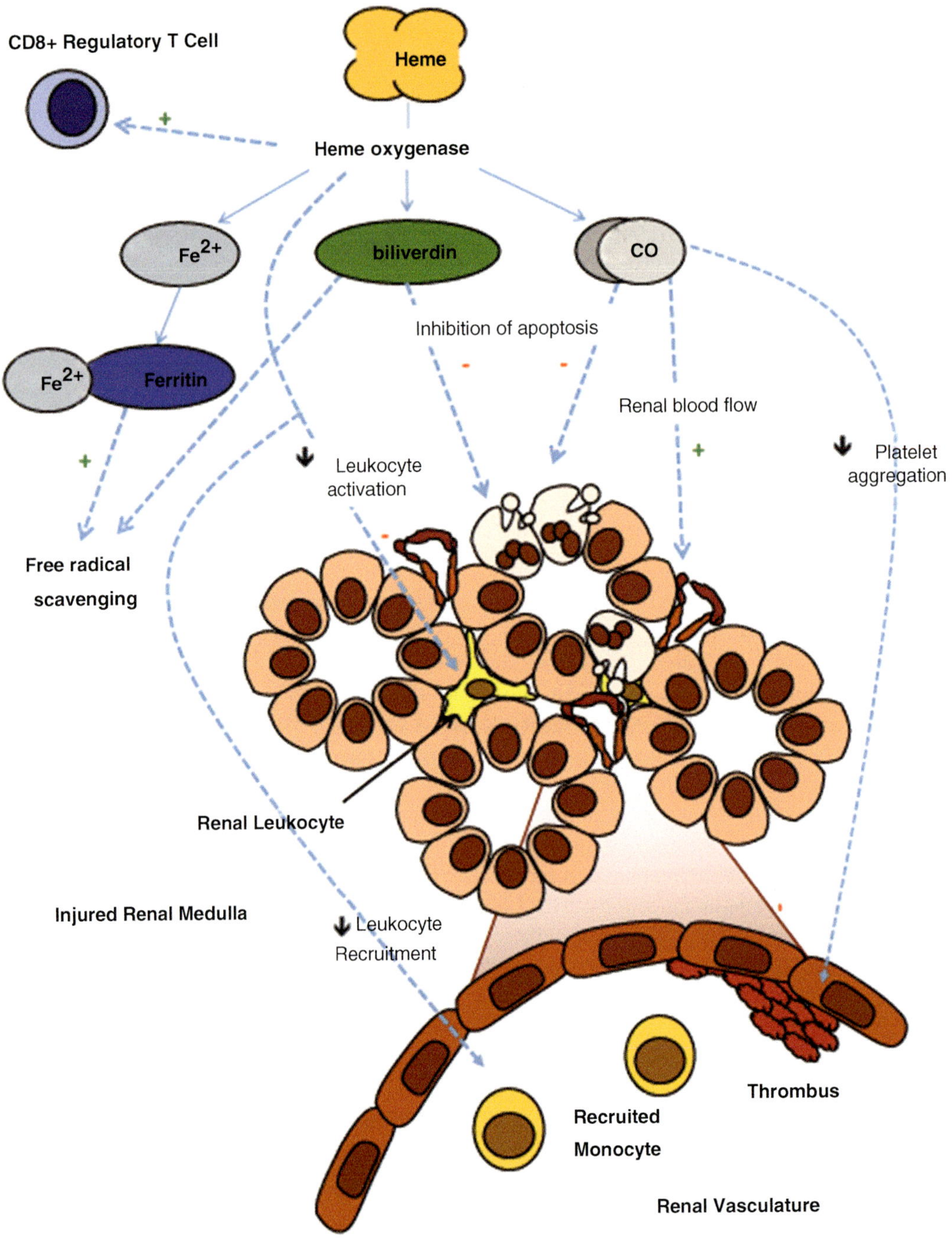

Fig. 5.2 Current working hypothesis of putative actions of HO-1 in acute kidney injury. HO-1 and the downstream metabolites of heme exhibit pleiotropic effects on the inflammatory response, the cell survival and the microcirculation, all of which are of potential importance in mediating its potential protective effects after IRI (dashed arrows)

olites in the mediation of this effect [93]. Studies combining inhaled CO with infused bilirubin in rat renal transplantation demonstrated synergistic effects on both graft survival and on GFR and blood flow rates [94].

5.4.3 Cell Apoptosis and Survival

A consistent pattern of reduced cell death is present throughout the studies of HO-1 upregulation, while HO-1 inhibition/genetic depletion results in increased levels of apoptosis/necrosis and impaired autophagy, jeopardising cell survival after AKI [95]. The pleiotropic effects of HO-1 make the dissection of the exact mechanism of this survival benefit problematic. It remains possible that protection is related to a secondary phenomenon due to improved perfusion and reduced immune activation. Mitochondrial dysfunction is a feature of IRI, and mice with transgenic overexpression of HO-1 within these organelles are protected from experimental IRI [96]. In vitro evidence from studies of tubular epithelial cell culture has implicated HO-1 as promoting cell survival by induction of the cyclin-dependent kinase inhibitor p21 [97].

5.4.4 Effects of HO-1 on Immune Phenotype

It is now widely accepted that HO-1 may act as a 'molecular brake' on the activation, recruitment and amplification of immune responses (reviewed in [76]). Overexpression of HO-1 results in reduced expression of leukocyte adhesion molecules and reduced activity of the NF-κ[kappa]B pathway. Constitutively HO-1-deficient animals exhibit increased levels of monocyte chemoattractant protein (MCP-1) [82]. HO-1 has been shown to be a target antigen for CD8+ regulatory T cells, resulting in modulation of cellular immune responses [98]. Given the recognised role of lymphocyte populations in determining susceptibility to IRI, this adds an additional 'extra-enzymatic' arm to the immunomodulatory properties of HO-1.

Studies in aged mice demonstrated reduced levels of renal HO-1 after IRI, with dosing of the HO-1 inducer heme arginate protective. Of note, this effect was lost when HO-1-expressing macrophages were pharmacologically depleted—implicating the myeloid cell as an important target of HO-1's effects [99]. Further studies have borne out the importance of myeloid cell HO-1 expression, with animals where HO-1 deficiency is restricted to myeloid cells, exhibiting delayed recovery and increased fibrosis after IRI [100]. Studies in HO-1 −/− mice injected with a bacterial artificial chromosome containing functional human HO-1 demonstrate protection from subsequent IRI, again validating the potential role of this protein in human AKI [101].

5.4.5 Candidate Pharmacological Inducers of HO-1

Given the accumulating experimental evidence for the beneficial effects of HO-1 in renal injury, induction of HO-1 in the clinical setting is under active investigation. While statins have been shown to induce HO-1 in vitro [102], data in recent large prospective clinical trials have not shown alterations in rates of acute kidney injury [103]. The lipid-lowering agent probucol has HO-1-inducing activity in animal models [104]; however its clinical utility has been limited by its undesired effect of lowering HDL levels. The compound heme arginate (HA) has HO-1-inducing properties [105], is stable at injectable pH [106] and is licenced and available for the treatment of acute porphyria [107]. As such, HA represents a promising translational agent for HO-1 induction in man, with clinical studies currently ongoing [108].

5.5 Cytokine Release in AKI

The release of cytokines by injured/necrotic renal cells or resident leukocytes is a well-recognised component of early AKI. Subsequent signals produced by recruited leukocytes contribute to further inflammation and tissue damage [109]. A wide range of cytokines and chemokines has been detected in experimental animal models of AKI, with chemokine release occurring in both intrinsic renal cells and recruited leukocytes in response to reactive oxygen species, cytokine release, nuclear factor κ[kappa]B (NF-κ[kappa]B) activation and ligation of TLRs (summarised in Table 5.1) [110].

The exact roles for each cytokine have been harder to define. An example of this is the case of IL-18 where studies in septic AKI and cisplatin-induced AKI show different outcomes to those seen with IRI [111–113] when the effects of IL-18 blockade have been investigated. These differences may reflect the different pathways of importance in the various experimental models of kidney injury or indeed the relative efficacy and off-target effects of blocking sera vs. genetic ablation in the models used. It is also worth noting that despite various successful interventions

Table 5.1 Cytokine/chemokine release and receptor expression in experimental AKI

Cytokine/receptor	Role in AKI	Therapeutic studies
IL-1 α[alpha], IL-1β[beta], IL-1R	Upregulated in response to experimental AKI. IL-1β[beta] is cleaved by caspase-1 to active form	Caspase-1-deficient mice are protected from cisplatin-induced AKI [221], but IL-1β[beta] inhibition had no effect on cisplatin injury [112]. Blockade/deficiency of IL-1R protects against cisplatin but not IRI [222]
IL-2	Upregulated in response to experimental AKI	
IL-6/IL-6R	Both cytokine and soluble receptors are increased in experimental AKI	Inhibition of IL-6 had no effect on pathogenesis of cisplatin-induced injury [112]. IL-6-deficient mice are protected from $MgCl_2$-induced renal injury [223]
IL-10	Produced by M2 macrophages and stimulate epithelial cell proliferation	IL-10 is acutely reduced in patients following D+HUS [196]
IL-18	Upregulated in response to experimental AKI. Cleaved by caspase-1 to active form	Caspase-1-deficient mice are protected from IRI [224]. IL-18 blockade protects against IRI [224] but not against cisplatin-induced injury [112]
IL-22	Secreted by macrophages in response to TLR4 ligation in recovery phase of injury [200]	
TNF-α[alpha]	Secreted by resident dendritic cells after IRI [134]. Capable of inducing necroptosis	TNF-α is increased in patients at d1 following D+HUS [196]. Blockade of TNF-α[alpha] or its signalling protects in multiple animal models of AKI [225–227]
Interferon-γ[gamma]	Upregulated in response to experimental AKI. Capable of inducing necroptosis	
Transforming growth factor-β[beta]	Upregulated in response to experimental AKI. Expressed by senescent tubular cells [120]	Production by tubular cells in the aftermath of renal injury is implicated in the progression of post-AKI fibrosis [124, 125]
CCL2	Increased in IRI	Induction after IRI is suppressed by methylprednisolone therapy [228]
CCR1	Facilitates leukocyte infiltration in experimental AKI [131]	Pharmacological antagonism reduced myeloid infiltration after IRI [131]
CX_3CL1	Increased in response to IRI and cisplatin nephropathy [229]	
CX_3CR1	Expressed by resident renal phagocytes	CX3CR1 blockade using antibodies reduced macrophage infiltration and IRI injury [229], but inhibition or deficiency had no effect on cisplatin injury [230]
CXCL1	Neutrophil chemoattractant. Levels increased in rodent AKI [203]	Use of a CXCL1 blocking antibody reduced neutrophil ingress and injury levels in murine IRI [138]
CXCR1/2	Receptors for CXCL1	CXCR2 inhibitor treatment reduced IRI-related renal dysfunction in rats [231]

targeting cytokine signalling in rodent models of AKI, no therapies have yet proved successful in clinical trials, reinforcing the limitations of current in vivo experimentation in modelling the multifaceted aetiologies of AKI in man.

5.5.1 Factors Released by Injured/Necrotic Cells in Early AKI

Hypoxia and reoxygenation in the kidney can induce apoptosis or regulated necrosis ('necroptosis') via diverse mechanisms including consequent to mitochondrial injury [114]. While apoptosis is considered a non-inflammatory mode of cell death, necrotic death results in the release of damage-associated molecular patterns (DAMPs), including alarmins and cytokines in the early aftermath of acute renal injury, all of which are capable of inducing further regulated cell death in the parenchymal cell pool [115, 116]. As indicated previously, release of free heme moieties in the context of cell stress acts as an additional source of oxidative damage to neighbouring cells, with the potential for further propagation of cellular injury and death if it is not metabolised via the induction of protective HO-1 [117].

Both the tumour necrosis factor (TNF-α[alpha]) and interferon-γ[gamma] have recently been shown to be capable of inducing necroptosis [118], while TNF-α[alpha] and interleukin-18 can induce neutrophil cell death via neutrophil extracellular traps (NETosis) [119]. The release of extracellular histones (a DAMP) has also been shown in experimental murine systems to be capable of inducing necrotic cell death within the kidney [119].

5.5.2 Cytokine Production in Senescent or G2/M-Arrested Tubular Cells

Paracrine signalling is a recognised feature of senescent tubular cells expressing p16INK4a [120]. These cells accumulate with ageing and renal injury. They produce TGF-β[beta],HGF, IGF-1 and VEGF and promote fibrogenesis and further senescence and are associated with impaired tubular proliferation. Studies in both progeroid and wild-type aged mice demonstrate that depletion of p16INK4a+ve senescent cells delays ageing and increases healthy lifespan [121, 122].

Transgenic mice expressing the simian diphtheria toxin receptor allow the study of the effects of selective, repeated tubular injury on the kidney signalling, function and scarring. Repeated tubular injury results in tubular, vascular and glomerular loss with increased fibrosis [123]. The response of tubular cells to acute injury, including expression of TGF-β[beta] acting in a paracrine and autocrine way, has been implicated as important in determining fibrotic outcomes and eventual glomerulosclerosis [124, 125].

Our group has demonstrated that models of severe and progressive renal injury (including severe IRI) show accumulation of tubular cells in the G2/M phase of the cell cycle [126]. These cells adopt a pro-fibrotic profile in vivo and in vitro, secreting growth factors including connective tissue growth factor (CTGF) and TGF-β[beta]1 in addition to increased collagen 4 α[alpha] 1 and 1 α[alpha] 1 mRNA [126] (Fig. 5.3). Thus, cell cycle arrest can induce paracrine signalling from tubular cells themselves, which can be a key component of the fibrotic response to renal injury, a hypothesis supported by recent reports from other laboratories [127–129]. Pharmacological inhibition of G2/M-arrested cells reduced fibrosis, whereas increases in the G2/M-arrested proportion of cells in the cell cycle exacerbated fibrosis [127–129].

5.6 Inflammation in AKI

There is a growing body of evidence suggesting that the disruption of renal architecture and function seen in acute tubular necrosis may have a more prominent inflammatory aetiology than initially believed [130]. Renal IRI is associated with the production of numerous proinflammatory cytokines and chemokines from the kidney, which are chemotactic for leukocytes, including macro-

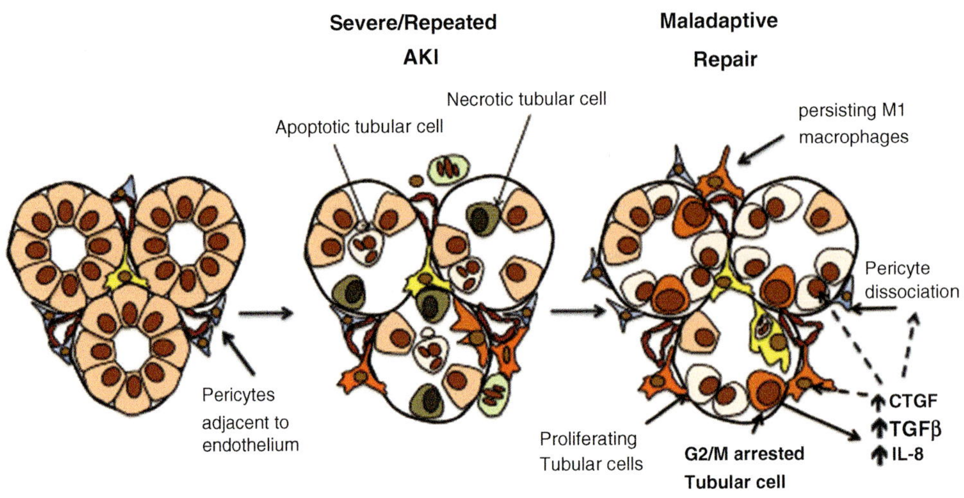

Fig. 5.3 Paracrine effects of the secretory phenotype seen in G2/M-arrested tubular epithelial cells. The proportion of tubular cells in the G2/M phase of the cell cycle increases in response to severe or sustained renal injuries. These cells produce factors, including CTGF and TGF-β[beta]1. These exert paracrine effects on both neighbouring tubular cells as well as on the phenotypes and numbers of interstitial cells, endothelial cells and macrophages. There is deposition of collagen and other matrix material within the kidney

phage inflammatory protein 1 α[alpha] (MIP-1α[alpha]), monocyte chemotactic protein-1 (MCP-1), regulated upon activation normal T-cell expressed and secreted (RANTES), interleukins 1 and 6, the CXC cytokine KC and tumour necrosis factor-α[alpha] (TNF-α[alpha]) [131–136]. Several types of leukocytes have been implicated as potentially pathogenic and are discussed below.

5.6.1 Neutrophils

The neutrophil has been identified as infiltrating early into the post-ischaemic kidney [137] and is often measured as a surrogate of tissue injury severity [110]. However studies employing anti-neutrophil strategies have not shown consistent protection. Part of the explanation for differences may relate to the species studied (e.g. rat vs. mouse) and incomplete neutrophil depletion strategies. It is possible that the volume of neutrophil recruitment is a marker of injury severity rather than the driver of the process. While blocking cytokines or integrins to reduce neutrophil ingress have demonstrated functional protection in animal models [138, 139], two different depleting antibody approaches failed to protect the post-ischaemic kidney from injury despite alterations in neutrophil number [140, 141]. Additional recent work studying experimental cisplatin nephropathy showed no change in renal injury levels despite 90% neutrophil depletion [142]. Transplanted kidneys from aged animals demonstrate higher levels of tubular injury, despite neutrophil influx equivalent to younger kidneys [143], and a multicentre human renal transplant trial showed no benefit from neutrophil inhibition via ICAM-1 blockade [144]. As such any role for the neutrophil as the major effector of renal IRI remains unproven and controversial [145].

5.6.2 Lymphocytes

A number of studies have presented results demonstrating the involvement of the lymphocytes, components of the adaptive immune system, in the initiation of IRI. Several studies have demonstrated profound functional protection from IRI in rodent models with either genetic or pharmacologic depletion of T lymphocytes, [146–150], with a similar magnitude of protection seen in μ[mu]MT mice lacking B lymphocytes [151].

The actual effector mechanisms underlying the pathogenic role of lymphocytes in IRI remains unclear, although IFN γ[gamma] production by

CD4+ cells has been implicated [146]. Wild-type serum, but not cell transfer into μ[mu]MT animals, restores the injury phenotype, suggesting a soluble factor originating in B lymphocytes [151]. The complexity of the system is emphasised by the conflicting data relating to the RAG-1 knockout (KO) mouse. Although the mouse is deficient in both T and B lymphocytes, there is no resultant protection from IRI [152]. Interestingly, injury is ameliorated by adoptive transfer of wild-type lymphocytes [147].

Studies have reported the key role played by T regulatory lymphocytes (Tregs) in determining the recovery from ischaemic renal injury [153]. Tregs are present in augmented numbers within the post-ischaemic kidney at both 3 and 10 days post-injury. Furthermore, when anti-CD25 antibodies were employed to deplete Tregs in vivo in the recovery phase of IRI, there were a persistence of structural injury and a reduction of tubular proliferation in both cortical and medullary compartments.

5.6.3 Macrophages

The macrophage (MΦ[phi]) is well characterised as a key effector cell in several models of renal inflammation [154–156]. Furthermore, in a model of lymphocyte-mediated injury such as renal transplantation, it has been demonstrated that targeting MΦ[phi] for depletion enhances allograft survival [155]. It is known that MΦ[phi] enters the kidney in the aftermath of IRI [137], and recent studies have demonstrated that ablation of renal MΦ[phi] can improve outcome in models of renal IRI [157, 158], glomerulonephritis [159] and fibrosis [160].

The role of the MΦ[phi] in renal IRI remains incompletely understood. One report of their depletion in rats showed improved long-term recovery after IRI [161]. This stands in contrast to evidence from other renal models in mice showing that depletion of MΦ[phi] prevented repair in mice after IRI [162]. Thus MΦ[phi] represents key contributors to the successful resolution of renal inflammation but if persisting can contribute to renal fibrosis (reviewed in [163, 164]).

Macrophages have conventionally been described as either classically ('M1') or alternatively ('M2') activated in response to stimuli. Classically activated MΦ[phi] was thought to arise in response to interferon-gamma and LPS stimulation, produce NO and had been demonstrated to be pathogenic to renal cells both in vitro and in vivo [165–168]. Alternatively activated macrophages were thought to be induced by IL-4, IL-10 and IL-13 and stimulate cellular proliferation and collagen deposition [169, 170]. However, more complete characterisation of the various functional states of tissue MΦ[phi] has confounded attempts to subdivide these cells into two discrete-activated subgroups. A recently proposed revision to this classification scheme again suggests a more fluid 'spectrum' of activation states based on cytokine profile [171] (summarised in Fig. 5.4). Briefly, this variability allows for macrophages to respond to various environmental and cytokine cues to adopt features of 'classical activation', 'regulatory' and 'wound healing'

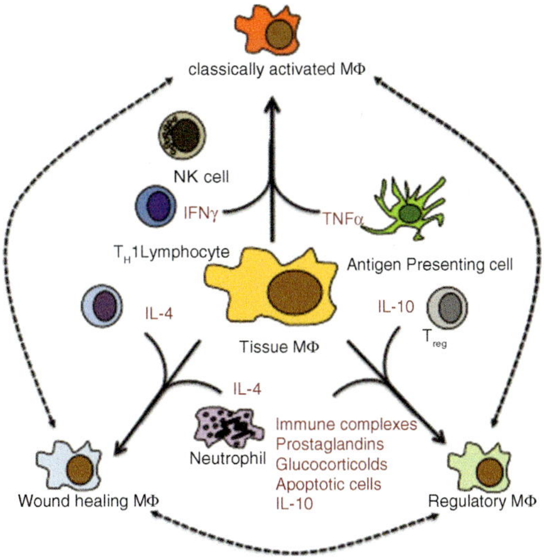

Fig. 5.4 This diagram summarises the proposed classification of macrophage phenotype proposed by Mosser and Edwards. Solid black arrows indicate cellular/cytokine stimuli for each polarisation, and dotted lines indicate the plasticity which exists between all activation states. Adapted from Mosser DM, Edwards JP. Exploring the full spectrum of macrophage activation. Nat Rev Immunol. 2008 Dec;8(12):958–69. PubMed PMID: 19029990. Pubmed Central PMCID: 2724991. Epub 2008/11/26. eng.; used with permission

MΦ[phi] subsets, with provision for further alteration in the expressed characteristics on the basis of subsequent interactions.

There is circumstantial evidence supporting a role for classically activated MΦ[phi] in the evolution of renal IRI. T-cell-derived IFN-γ[gamma] is of documented importance in IRI pathogenesis [146]—a cytokine associated with classical activation of MΦ[phi]. Classically activated MΦ[phi] has been shown to be pathogenic to renal cells both in vitro and in vivo [165–168]. It is recognised that MΦ[phi] phenotype is modified within a hypoxic microenvironment, such as a tumour [172] or an ischaemic organ [173].

Previous work has demonstrated the pathogenic significance of MΦ[phi]-derived nitric oxide (NO) production as a death signal for resident renal cells both in vitro and in vivo [166, 167]. NO is implicated in the evolution of renal injury [174], and it is interesting that inhibition of NO generation has also been shown to be protective in models of IRI [175–177]. The leukocyte Fc receptor is recognised as an important mechanism for MΦ[phi] interaction with deposited immunoglobulins, an important step in the initiation and progression of renal inflammation [178, 179]. Activating FcR knockout mice exhibit reduced infarct size in models of cerebral ischaemia [180].

Until recently, a widely accepted view of the resident mononuclear phagocyte system held MΦ[phi] and dendritic cells (DC) as clearly distinct in terms of cellular function while occupying overlapping anatomical sites in peripheral tissues and the reticuloendothelial system. In practice, distinguishing between macrophages and dendritic cells has relied on the use of cell surface markers thought to be specific to either cell. The progressive refinement and increasing number of available markers have served to complicate rather than simplify our understanding of the renal mononuclear phagocyte system.

Increasing the characterisation of both the surface markers expressed by MΦ[phi] and DC, and further characterisation of the functional capabilities and phenotypic plasticity of both cells, has led to an ongoing blurring of the previously accepted 'unique' characteristics of each lineage [181]. It is now recognised that activated macrophages can demonstrate antigen presentation and co-stimulatory capacity [182], while DCs are capable of NO production and cytotoxicity [183, 184]. This has led to the emergence of an alternative conceptual view where a common myeloid progenitor gives rise to a spectrum of mature cells within tissues adapted to diverse roles with overlapping functions, rather than two functionally distinct lineages [185, 186].

5.7 Toll-Like Receptors in the Kidney and AKI

5.7.1 Toll-Like Receptors in the Kidney

The toll gene was first described in *Drosophila melanogaster* in 1985 [187]. Toll-like receptors (TLRs) have been identified in humans and multiple vertebrate and invertebrate species in subsequent years [188, 189]. In humans and experimental mice, TLRs are expressed by cells of the innate immune system, including macrophages, dendritic cells and natural killer cells, along with some epithelial, endothelial and mesenchymal cell populations. TLRs comprise a range of receptors to various pathogen-associated molecular patterns, which when triggered activate the innate immune response. In the kidney, epithelial and mesenchymal cells express TLRs 1 to 4 and 6, with similar expression patterns seen in both mice and humans [190].

5.7.2 TLR Activation in Response to Acute Kidney Injury

It has been demonstrated at both a transcriptional and protein level that TLR2 and TLR4 are upregulated in the rodent kidney in the aftermath of experimental IRI [191] and can be found at markedly increased levels at 5-day post-injury [192]. In the context of the acutely injured kidney, damage-associated molecular patterns (DAMPs) and alarmins released from necrotic renal cells are capable of ligating TLRs, activating MyD88-dependent and MyD88-independent signalling leading to NF-κ[kappa]B expression and a rapid activation and recruitment of innate immune cells [53].

Supporting the importance of TLR2 signalling in the evolution of IRI, studies using various approaches to block TLR2 signalling in one or more of the kidney and leukocyte populations demonstrated that renal TLR2 deficiency was sufficient to protect the kidney from both inflammation and injury [193]. Similarly, TLR −/− mice demonstrated reduced numbers of renal neutrophils and chemokines in the aftermath of injury and a reduced degree of renal injury and dysfunction after IRI [194], with chimeric mice suggesting an equal contribution from renal and leukocyte-derived TLR4 activation. TLRs are also triggered by both DAMPs and PAMPs in sepsis-induced AKI, with LPS triggering inflammatory activation via TLR4, a situation where TLR4−/− mice exhibit marked protection [189]. Haemolytic uraemic syndrome with associated diarrhoea (D + HUS) is a significant cause of AKI, particularly in the paediatric population. There is experimental evidence that the recognised nephrotoxicity of Shiga toxin in this disease is augmented by the presence of bacterial LPS [195] with studies in man demonstrating much higher TLR4 positivity in neutrophils in acute D + HUS patients [196].

5.7.3 Ligands Responsible for TLR Activation in the Kidney

The endogenous ligands activating inflammatory signalling via TLR ligation remain incompletely understood. Potential TLR4 ligands biglycan, HMGB1 and hyaluronan are all increased in the aftermath of experimental IRI [197]. Studies using chimeric animals with TLR4 deficiencies in either kidneys or leukocytes suggest that HMGB1 is released from injured intrinsic renal cells and activates leukocytes via TLR4 ligation [198]. Supporting this, blockade of HMGB1 via antibody administration protects against experimental IRI [199].

TLR signalling via DAMPs such as HMGB1 results in inflammatory macrophage activation and immune-mediated tissue damage in the early ‘amplification’ phase of kidney injury [53]. Subsequent macrophage phenotypic switching from pro-inflammatory M1 to a pro-repair M2 polarisation state has been shown to be a vital part of successful renal repair after experimental injury [162]. These pro-repair macrophages secrete IL-22 via a mechanism requiring TLR4 ligation [200]—suggesting that these pathways could have dual roles of importance in both injury and repair phases.

5.8 Complement Activation in the Kidney in AKI

5.8.1 The Complement System in Health and Disease

The complement pathway is an ancient, highly conserved component of innate immunity [201]. It is a complex system, which can be activated via three cascades, namely, the classical, alternate and lectin pathways. Complement activity is regulated by over 40 genes, but despite this complexity, each pathway ultimately converges on C3 and C5 cleaving them to form soluble C3a, C3b, C5a and C5b.

A key downstream effect of C3a and C5a is the generation of a pro-inflammatory and chemotactic environment. C3a and C5a bind to G protein-coupled anaphylatoxin receptors C3aR and C5aR1 which increase production of co-stimulatory molecules and interleukin 6 [202]. C3b or C4b may opsonise cell surfaces for macrophages and lead to the production of macrophage inflammatory protein-2 and keratinocyte-derived chemokine [203].

The second major effect of C5 cleavage is the ability of C5b to catalyse the formation of the C5b-9 membrane attack complex. The membrane attack complex can insert itself into cell membranes leading to cell lysis and contributing to an inflammatory milieu by activating intracellular pathways and synthesis of pro-inflammatory eicosanoids [204].

5.8.2 Activation of Complement in Acute Kidney Injury

The complement system is a dynamic equilibrium where there is a balance between continuous complement activation and regulation. Within the human kidney, there is continuous C3 activation, as demonstrated by C3d staining along the basement membranes of Bowman's capsule and renal tubules in normal kidneys [205]. This activation is regulated by a variety of proteins including factor H, decay-accelerating factor, membrane cofactor protein, C4-binding protein and complement receptor 1-related gene/protein y [206].

Complement plays an important role in various disease processes, which affect the kidney and lead to acute injury. Complement activity is central in atypical haemolytic uraemic syndrome, ANCA-associated vasculitis and anti-glomerular basement membrane disease [207]. It is unclear whether the role of complement in these specific processes is novel or reflects the broader role of complement in AKI. Thus IRI is used experimentally as a generic injury model from which to draw broader conclusions.

In AKI, the renal microenvironment shifts the balance towards complement activation. Following ischaemia reperfusion, there is upregulation of tubular cell production of C3, which activates local complement [208–210]. Compounding this increased activation, ischaemic tubules lose their regulatory surface molecules [211, 212]. Other factors contributing to complement activation may include an acidic environment, circulating pathogens, vascular congestion, exposed intracellular antigens and microparticles [207, 213–216].

During AKI, complement activation occurs primarily through the alternative pathway [152, 217, 218]. Kidneys from patients with acute tubular necrosis had increased C3d deposition along a greater number of tubules than normal, but C4d was absent supporting the central role of alternative pathway activation [205]. In murine experimental IRI, in contrast to the heart, intestine and lung, tubular epithelial cells were the main structures damaged by complement-mediated attack, and the renal vasculature was spared [219]. The formation of the membrane attack complex may also contribute to the damaging effect of complement on the kidney [219].

Inhibiting complement remains an attractive avenue of potential intervention with inhibition reducing IRI-induced renal damage in murine models [205, 212, 220]. Difficulties in translating complement inhibition to human studies include the challenges of tissue penetration to the level of the tubule, the uncertainties surrounding timing and intensity of complement inhibition and the potential for serious adverse effects, most crucially infection [207].

Acknowledgements DAF is funded by Intermediate Clinical Fellowship 100171MA from the Wellcome Trust. JVB is funded by grants DK039773 and DK072381 from the NIH.

References

1. Epstein FH, Fish EM, Molitoris BA. Alterations in epithelial polarity and the pathogenesis of disease states. N Engl J Med. 1994;330:1580–8.
2. Thadhani R, Pascual M, Bonventre JV. Acute renal failure. N Engl J Med. 1996;334:1448–60.
3. Alejandro VSJ, Nelson WJ, Huie P, Sibley RK, Dafoe D, Kuo P, et al. Postischemic injury, delayed function and Na+/K+-ATPase distribution in the transplanted kidney. Kidney Int. 1995;48:1308–15.
4. Bonventre JV. Mechanisms of ischemic acute renal failure. Kidney Int. 1993;43:1160–78.
5. Lieberthal W. Biology of acute renal failure: therapeutic implications. Kidney Int. 1997;52:1102–15.
6. Sheridan AM, Bonventre JV. Cell biology and molecular mechanisms of injury in ischemic acute renal failure. Curr Opin Nephrol Hypertens. 2000;9:427–34.
7. Bush KT, Keller SH, Nigam SK. Genesis and reversal of the ischemic phenotype in epithelial cells. J Clin Invest. 2000;106:621–6. PubMed PMID: 10974012.
8. Lieberthal W, Nigam SK, Huie P, Sibley RK, Dafoe D, Kuo P, et al. Acute renal failure. II. Experimental models of acute renal failure: imperfect but indispensable. Am J Physiol Renal Physiol. 2000;278:F1–F12. PubMed PMID: 10644651.
9. Brown D, Lee R, Bonventre JV. Redistribution of villin to proximal tubule basolateral membranes after ischemia and reperfusion. Am J Physiol. 1997;273:F1003–12. PubMed PMID: 9435690.
10. Kellerman PS, Bogusky RT. Microfilament disruption occurs very early in ischemic proximal tubule cell injury. Kidney Int. 1992;42:896–902.

11. Molitoris BA, Falk SA, Dahl RH. Ischemia-induced loss of epithelial polarity. Role of the tight junction. J Clin Invest. 1989;84:1334–9.
12. Shelden EA, Weinberg JM, Sorenson DR, Edwards CA, Pollock FM. Site-specific alteration of actin assembly visualized in living renal epithelial cells during ATP depletion. J Am Soc Nephrol. 2002;13:2667–80.
13. Abbate M, Bonventre JV, Brown D. The microtubule network of renal epithelial cells is disrupted by ischemia and reperfusion. Am J Physiol. 1994;267:F971–8. PubMed PMID: 7810705.
14. Kwon O, Nelson WJ, Sibley R, Huie P, Scandling JD, Dafoe D, et al. Backleak, tight junctions, and cell- cell adhesion in postischemic injury to the renal allograft. J Clin Invest. 1998;101:2054–64.
15. Bush KT, Tsukamoto T, Nigam SK. Selective degradation of E-cadherin and dissolution of E-cadherin-catenin complexes in epithelial ischemia. Am J Physiol Renal Physiol. 2000;278:F847–52. PubMed PMID: 10807598.
16. Fish EM, Molitoris BA. Alterations in epithelial polarity and the pathogenesis of disease states. N Engl J Med. 1994;330:1580–8. PubMed PMID: 8177249.
17. Duan Y, Gotoh N, Yan Q, Du Z, Weinstein AM, Wang T, et al. Shear-induced reorganization of renal proximal tubule cell actin cytoskeleton and apical junctional complexes. Proc Natl Acad Sci U S A. 2008;105:11418–23. PubMed PMID: 18685100.
18. Tsukamoto T, Nigam SK. Tight junction proteins form large complexes and associate with the cytoskeleton in an ATP depletion model for reversible junction assembly. J Biol Chem. 1997;272:16133–9. PubMed PMID: 9195909.
19. Zuk A, Bonventre JV, Brown D, Matlin KS. Polarity, integrin, and extracellular matrix dynamics in the postischemic rat kidney. Am J Physiol. 1998;275:C711–31. PubMed PMID: 9730955.
20. Lieberthal W, McKenney JB, Kiefer CR, Snyder LM, Kroshian VM, Sjaastad MD. Beta1 integrin-mediated adhesion between renal tubular cells after anoxic injury. J Am Soc Nephrol. 1997;8(2):175–83. PubMed PMID: 9048335.
21. Molitoris BA. Actin cytoskeleton in ischemic acute renal failure. Kidney Int. 2004;66(2):871–83. PubMed PMID: 15253754.
22. Donohoe JF, Venkatachalam MA, Bernard DB, Levinsky NG. Tubular leakage and obstruction after renal ischemia: structural-functional correlations. Kidney Int. 1978;13:208–22.
23. Bonventre JV, Colvin RB. Adhesion molecules in renal disease. Curr Opin Nephrol Hypertens. 1996;5(3):254–61. PubMed PMID: 8737861. Epub 1996/05/01. eng.
24. Noiri E, Romanov V, Forest T, Gailit J, DiBona GF, Miller F, et al. Pathophysiology of renal tubular obstruction: therapeutic role of synthetic RGD peptides in acute renal failure. Kidney Int. 1995;48:1375–85.
25. Tanner GA, Sophasan S. Kidney pressures after temporary renal artery occlusion in the rat. Am J Physiol. 1976;230(4):1173–81. PubMed PMID: 1267015.
26. Kwon O, Corrigan G, Myers BD, Sibley R, Scandling JD, Dafoe D, et al. Sodium reabsorption and distribution of Na+/K+-ATPase during postischemic injury to the renal allograft. Kidney Int. 1999;55:963–75.
27. Molitoris BA, Dahl R, Geerdes A. Cytoskeleton disruption and apical redistribution of proximal tubule Na(+)-K(+)-ATPase during ischemia. Am J Physiol. 1992;263:F488–95. PubMed PMID: 1329535.
28. Wald FA, Figueroa Y, Oriolo AS, Salas PJI. Membrane repolarization is delayed in proximal tubules after ischemia-reperfusion: possible role of microtubule-organizing centers. Am J Physiol Renal Physiol. 2003;285:F230–40. PubMed PMID: 12709392.
29. Rajasekaran AK, Rajasekaran SA. Role of Na-K-ATPase in the assembly of tight junctions. Am J Physiol Renal Physiol. 2003;285:F388–96. PubMed PMID: 12890662.
30. Moran SM, Myers BD. Pathophysiology of protracted acute renal failure in man. J Clin Invest. 1985;76:1440–8.
31. Myers BD, Chui F, Hilberman M, Michaels AS. Transtubular leakage of glomerular filtrate in human acute renal failure. Am J Physiol. 1979;237:F319–25. PubMed PMID: 495725.
32. Arendshorst WJ, Bello-Reuss E. The kidney. In: Bradshaw RA, Dennis EA, editors. Handbook of cell signaling. Oxford: Elsevier; 2010. p. 2707–31.
33. Imig JD. Epoxyeicosatrienoic acids, hypertension, and kidney injury. Hypertension. 2015;65(3):476–82. PubMed PMID: 25583156. Pubmed Central PMCID: 4326585.
34. Schnermann J. Concurrent activation of multiple vasoactive signaling pathways in vasoconstriction caused by tubuloglomerular feedback: a quantitative assessment. Annu Rev Physiol. 2015;77:301–22. PubMed PMID: 25668021.
35. McCullough PA, Tumlin JA. Prostaglandin-based renal protection against contrast-induced acute kidney injury. Circulation. 2009;120(18):1749–51. PubMed PMID: 19841295.
36. Jia Z, Sun Y, Liu S, Liu Y, Yang T. COX-2 but not mPGES-1 contributes to renal PGE2 induction and diabetic proteinuria in mice with type-1 diabetes. PLoS One. 2014;9(7):e93182. PubMed PMID: 24984018. Pubmed Central PMCID: 4077725.
37. Rubattu S, Mennuni S, Testa M, Mennuni M, Pierelli G, Pagliaro B, et al. Pathogenesis of chronic cardiorenal syndrome: is there a role for oxidative stress? Int J Mol Sci. 2013;14(11):23011–32. PubMed PMID: 24264044. Pubmed Central PMCID: 3856103.
38. Rao R, Zhang MZ, Zhao M, Cai H, Harris RC, Breyer MD, et al. Lithium treatment inhibits renal GSK-3 activity and promotes cyclooxygenase 2-dependent polyuria. Am J Physiol Renal Physiol. 2005;288(4):F642–9. PubMed PMID: 15585669.

39. Jia Z, Zhang Y, Ding G, Heiney KM, Huang S, Zhang A. Role of COX-2/mPGES-1/prostaglandin E2 cascade in kidney injury. Mediat Inflamm. 2015;2015:147894. PubMed PMID: 25729216. Pubmed Central PMCID: 4333324.
40. Harris RC, Zhang MZ. Cyclooxygenase metabolites in the kidney. Compr Physiol. 2011;1(4):1729–58. PubMed PMID: 23733687.
41. Vukicevic S, Simic P, Borovecki F, Grgurevic L, Rogic D, Orlic I, et al. Role of EP2 and EP4 receptor-selective agonists of prostaglandin E(2) in acute and chronic kidney failure. Kidney Int. 2006;70(6):1099–106. PubMed PMID: 16871242.
42. Spargias K, Adreanides E, Demerouti E, Gkouziouta A, Manginas A, Pavlides G, et al. Iloprost prevents contrast-induced nephropathy in patients with renal dysfunction undergoing coronary angiography or intervention. Circulation. 2009;120(18):1793–9. PubMed PMID: 19841299.
43. Eskildsen MP, Hansen PB, Stubbe J, Toft A, Walter S, Marcussen N, et al. Prostaglandin I2 and prostaglandin E2 modulate human intrarenal artery contractility through prostaglandin E2-EP4, prostacyclin-IP, and thromboxane A2-TP receptors. Hypertension. 2014;64(3):551–6. PubMed PMID: 24914192.
44. Curiel RV, Katz JD. Mitigating the cardiovascular and renal effects of NSAIDs. Pain Med. 2013;14(Suppl 1):S23–8. PubMed PMID: 24255997.
45. Roman RJ, Akbulut T, Park F, Regner KR. 20-HETE in acute kidney injury. Kidney Int. 2011;79(1):10–3. PubMed PMID: 21157458. Pubmed Central PMCID: PMC3146060.
46. Hoff U, Lukitsch I, Chaykovska L, Ladwig M, Arnold C, Manthati VL, et al. Inhibition of 20-HETE synthesis and action protects the kidney from ischemia/reperfusion injury. Kidney Int. 2011;79(1):57–65. PubMed PMID: 20962739. Pubmed Central PMCID: PMC3813968.
47. Park F, Sweeney WE Jr, Jia G, Akbulut T, Mueller B, Falck JR, et al. Chronic blockade of 20-HETE synthesis reduces polycystic kidney disease in an orthologous rat model of ARPKD. Am J Physiol Renal Physiol. 2009;296(3):F575–82. PubMed PMID: 19129252. Pubmed Central PMCID: PMC2660198.
48. Hong S, Lu Y. Omega-3 fatty acid-derived resolvins and protectins in inflammation resolution and leukocyte functions: targeting novel lipid mediator pathways in mitigation of acute kidney injury. Front Immunol. 2013;4:13. PubMed PMID: 23386851. Pubmed Central PMCID: 3558681.
49. Duffield JS, Hong S, Vaidya VS, Lu Y, Fredman G, Serhan CN, et al. Resolvin D series and protectin D1 mitigate acute kidney injury. J Immunol. 2006;177(9):5902–11. PubMed PMID: 17056514.
50. Schwiebert EM, Zsembery A. Extracellular ATP as a signaling molecule for epithelial cells. Biochim Biophys Acta. 2003;1615(1–2):7–32. PubMed PMID: 12948585.
51. Solini A, Usuelli V, Fiorina P. The dark side of extracellular ATP in kidney diseases. J Am Soc Nephrol. 2015;26(5):1007–16. PubMed PMID: 25452669. Pubmed Central PMCID: 4413770.
52. Howarth AR, Conway BR, Bailey MA. Vascular and inflammatory actions of P2X receptors in renal injury. Auton Neurosci. 2015;191:135–40. PubMed PMID: 25998687.
53. Rosin DL, Okusa MD. Dangers within: DAMP responses to damage and cell death in kidney disease. J Am Soc Nephrol. 2011;22(3):416–25. PubMed PMID: 21335516. Pubmed Central PMCID: PMC4493973.
54. Menzies RI, Howarth AR, Unwin RJ, Tam FW, Mullins JJ, Bailey MA. Inhibition of the purinergic P2X7 receptor improves renal perfusion in angiotensin-II-infused rats. Kidney Int. 2015;88(5):1079–87. PubMed PMID: 26108066.
55. Yan Y, Bai J, Zhou X, Tang J, Jiang C, Tolbert E, et al. P2X7 receptor inhibition protects against ischemic acute kidney injury in mice. Am J Physiol Cell Physiol. 2015;308(6):C463–72. PubMed PMID: 25588875. Pubmed Central PMCID: 4360025.
56. Baylis C. Nitric oxide synthase derangements and hypertension in kidney disease. Curr Opin Nephrol Hypertens. 2012;21(1):1–6. PubMed PMID: 22048724. Pubmed Central PMCID: 3277934.
57. Horita S, Nakamura M, Shirai A, Yamazaki O, Satoh N, Suzuki M, et al. Regulatory roles of nitric oxide and angiotensin II on renal tubular transport. World J Nephrol. 2014;3(4):295–301. PubMed PMID: 25374825. Pubmed Central PMCID: 4220364.
58. Baylis C. Nitric oxide deficiency in chronic kidney disease. Am J Physiol Renal Physiol. 2008;294(1):F1–9. PubMed PMID: 17928410.
59. Koul V, Kaur A, Singh AP. Investigation of the role of nitric oxide/soluble guanylyl cyclase pathway in ascorbic acid-mediated protection against acute kidney injury in rats. Mol Cell Biochem. 2015;406(1–2):1–7. PubMed PMID: 26142728.
60. Amaral JH, Ferreira GC, Pinheiro LC, Montenegro MF, Tanus-Santos JE. Consistent antioxidant and antihypertensive effects of oral sodium nitrite in DOCA-salt hypertension. Redox Biol. 2015;5:340–6. PubMed PMID: 26119848. Pubmed Central PMCID: 4491646.
61. Choi MR, Kouyoumdzian NM, Rukavina Mikusic NL, Kravetz MC, Roson MI, Rodriguez Fermepin M, et al. Renal dopaminergic system: pathophysiological implications and clinical perspectives. World J Nephrol. 2015;4(2):196–212. PubMed PMID: 25949933. Pubmed Central PMCID: 4419129.
62. Carey RM. The intrarenal renin-angiotensin and dopaminergic systems: control of renal sodium excretion and blood pressure. Hypertension. 2013;61(3):673–80. PubMed PMID: 23407646. Pubmed Central PMCID: 3577093.
63. Patel NN, Rogers CA, Angelini GD, Murphy GJ. Pharmacological therapies for the prevention of acute kidney injury following cardiac surgery: a systematic review. Heart Fail Rev. 2011;16(6):553–67. PubMed PMID: 21400231.

64. Carey RM. The intrarenal renin-angiotensin system in hypertension. Adv Chronic Kidney Dis. 2015;22(3):204–10. PubMed PMID: 25908469.
65. Crowley SD, Gurley SB, Herrera MJ, Ruiz P, Griffiths R, Kumar AP, et al. Angiotensin II causes hypertension and cardiac hypertrophy through its receptors in the kidney. Proc Natl Acad Sci U S A. 2006;103(47):17985–90. PubMed PMID: 17090678. Pubmed Central PMCID: 1693859.
66. Macconi D, Remuzzi G, Benigni A. Key fibrogenic mediators: old players. Renin-angiotensin system. Kidney Int Suppl. 2014;4(1):58–64. PubMed PMID: 26312151. Pubmed Central PMCID: 4536968.
67. Schrimpf C, Teebken OE, Wilhelmi M, Duffield JS. The role of pericyte detachment in vascular rarefaction. J Vasc Res. 2014;51(4):247–58. PubMed PMID: 25195856. Pubmed Central PMCID: 4476411.
68. Huang Q, Wang Q, Zhang S, Jiang S, Zhao L, Yu L, et al. Increased hydrogen peroxide impairs angiotensin II contractions of afferent arterioles in mice after renal ischemia-reperfusion injury. Acta Physiol. 2016;218(2):136–45. PubMed PMID: 27362287.
69. Campbell DJ, Kladis A, Duncan AM. Bradykinin peptides in kidney, blood, and other tissues of the rat. Hypertension. 1993;21(2):155–65. PubMed PMID: 8428778.
70. Mamenko M, Zaika O, Pochynyuk O. Direct regulation of ENaC by bradykinin in the distal nephron. Implications for renal sodium handling. Curr Opin Nephrol Hypertens. 2014;23(2):122–9. PubMed PMID: 24378775. Pubmed Central PMCID: 4114036.
71. Bulut OP, Dipp S, El-Dahr S. Ontogeny of bradykinin B1 receptors in the mouse kidney. Pediatr Res. 2009;66(5):519–23. PubMed PMID: 19581823. Pubmed Central PMCID: 2783398.
72. Kayashima Y, Smithies O, Kakoki M. The kallikrein-kinin system and oxidative stress. Curr Opin Nephrol Hypertens. 2012;21(1):92–6. PubMed PMID: 22048723. Pubmed Central PMCID: 3657726.
73. Estrela GR, Wasinski F, Almeida DC, Amano MT, Castoldi A, Dias CC, et al. Kinin B1 receptor deficiency attenuates cisplatin-induced acute kidney injury by modulating immune cell migration. J Mol Med. 2014;92(4):399–409. PubMed PMID: 24357263.
74. Estrela GR, Wasinski F, Bacurau RF, Malheiros DM, Camara NO, Araujo RC. Kinin B2 receptor deletion and blockage ameliorates cisplatin-induced acute renal injury. Int Immunopharmacol. 2014;22(1):115–9. PubMed PMID: 24975837.
75. Huart A, Klein J, Gonzalez J, Buffin-Meyer B, Neau E, Delage C, et al. Kinin B1 receptor antagonism is equally efficient as angiotensin receptor 1 antagonism in reducing renal fibrosis in experimental obstructive nephropathy, but is not additive. Front Pharmacol. 2015;6:8. PubMed PMID: 25698969. Pubmed Central PMCID: 4313587.
76. Wagener FA, Volk HD, Willis D, Abraham NG, Soares MP, Adema GJ, et al. Different faces of the heme-heme oxygenase system in inflammation. Pharmacol Rev. 2003;55(3):551–71. PubMed PMID: 12869663.
77. Akagi R, Takahashi T, Sassa S. Cytoprotective effects of heme oxygenase in acute renal failure. Contrib Nephrol. 2005;148:70–85. PubMed PMID: 15912028.
78. Lai IR, Ma MC, Chen CF, Chang KJ. The protective role of heme oxygenase-1 on the liver after hypoxic preconditioning in rats. Transplantation. 2004;77(7):1004–8. PubMed PMID: 15087761.
79. Vera T, Henegar JR, Drummond HA, Rimoldi JM, Stec DE. Protective effect of carbon monoxide-releasing compounds in ischemia-induced acute renal failure. J Am Soc Nephrol. 2005;16(4):950–8. PubMed PMID: 15728782.
80. Morimoto K, Ohta K, Yachie A, Yang Y, Shimizu M, Goto C, et al. Cytoprotective role of heme oxygenase (HO)-1 in human kidney with various renal diseases. Kidney Int. 2001;60(5):1858–66. PubMed PMID: 11703604.
81. Koizumi S. Human heme oxygenase-1 deficiency: a lesson on serendipity in the discovery of the novel disease. Pediatr Int. 2007;49(2):125–32. PubMed PMID: 17445026.
82. Pittock ST, Norby SM, Grande JP, Croatt AJ, Bren GD, Badley AD, et al. MCP-1 is up-regulated in unstressed and stressed HO-1 knockout mice: pathophysiologic correlates. Kidney Int. 2005;68(2):611–22. PubMed PMID: 16014038.
83. Shiraishi F, Curtis LM, Truong L, Poss K, Visner GA, Madsen K, et al. Heme oxygenase-1 gene ablation or expression modulates cisplatin-induced renal tubular apoptosis. Am J Physiol Renal Physiol. 2000;278(5):F726–36. PubMed PMID: 10807584. Epub 2000/05/12. eng.
84. Nath KA, Haggard JJ, Croatt AJ, Grande JP, Poss KD, Alam J. The indispensability of heme oxygenase-1 in protecting against acute heme protein-induced toxicity in vivo. Am J Pathol. 2000;156(5):1527–35. PubMed PMID: 10793064.
85. Maines MD, Mayer RD, Ewing JF, McCoubrey WK Jr. Induction of kidney heme oxygenase-1 (HSP32) mRNA and protein by ischemia/reperfusion: possible role of heme as both promotor of tissue damage and regulator of HSP32. J Pharmacol Exp Ther. 1993;264(1):457–62. PubMed PMID: 8423544.
86. Ollinger R, Kogler P, Biebl M, Sieb M, Sucher R, Bosmuller C, et al. Protein levels of heme oxygenase-1 during reperfusion in human kidney transplants with delayed graft function. Clin Transpl. 2008;22(4):418–23. PubMed PMID: 18261117.
87. Billings FT 4th, Yu C, Byrne JG, Petracek MR, Pretorius M. Heme oxygenase-1 and acute kidney injury following cardiac surgery. Cardiorenal Med. 2014;4(1):12–21. PubMed PMID: 24847330. Pubmed Central PMCID: PMC4024967.

88. Nath KA. Heme oxygenase-1: a provenance for cytoprotective pathways in the kidney and other tissues. Kidney Int. 2006;70(3):432–43. PubMed PMID: 16775600.
89. Appleton SD, Chretien ML, McLaughlin BE, Vreman HJ, Stevenson DK, Brien JF, et al. Selective inhibition of heme oxygenase, without inhibition of nitric oxide synthase or soluble guanylyl cyclase, by metalloporphyrins at low concentrations. Drug Metab Dispos. 1999;27(10):1214–9. PubMed PMID: 10497150.
90. Zou AP, Billington H, Su N, Cowley AW Jr. Expression and actions of heme oxygenase in the renal medulla of rats. Hypertension. 2000;35(1 Pt 2):342–7. PubMed PMID: 10642322.
91. Holzen JP, August C, Bahde R, Minin E, Lang D, Heidenreich S, et al. Influence of heme oxygenase-1 on microcirculation after kidney transplantation. J Surg Res. 2008;148(2):126–35. PubMed PMID: 18456280.
92. Chlopicki S, Olszanecki R, Marcinkiewicz E, Lomnicka M, Motterlini R. Carbon monoxide released by CORM-3 inhibits human platelets by a mechanism independent of soluble guanylate cyclase. Cardiovasc Res. 2006;71(2):393–401. PubMed PMID: 16713591.
93. Ren Y, D'Ambrosio MA, Wang H, Liu R, Garvin JL, Carretero OA. Heme oxygenase metabolites inhibit tubuloglomerular feedback (TGF). Am J Physiol Renal Physiol. 2008;295(4):F1207–12. PubMed PMID: 18715939. Pubmed Central PMCID: 2576153. Epub 2008/08/22. eng.
94. Nakao A, Neto JS, Kanno S, Stolz DB, Kimizuka K, Liu F, et al. Protection against ischemia/reperfusion injury in cardiac and renal transplantation with carbon monoxide, biliverdin and both. Am J Transplant. 2005;5(2):282–91. PubMed PMID: 15643987.
95. Bolisetty S, Traylor AM, Kim J, Joseph R, Ricart K, Landar A, et al. Heme oxygenase-1 inhibits renal tubular macroautophagy in acute kidney injury. J Am Soc Nephrol. 2010;21(10):1702–12. PubMed PMID: 20705711. Pubmed Central PMCID: PMC3013546.
96. Bolisetty S, Traylor A, Zarjou A, Johnson MS, Benavides GA, Ricart K, et al. Mitochondria-targeted heme oxygenase-1 decreases oxidative stress in renal epithelial cells. Am J Physiol Renal Physiol. 2013;305(3):F255–64. PubMed PMID: 23720344. Pubmed Central PMCID: PMC3742869.
97. Inguaggiato P, Gonzalez-Michaca L, Croatt AJ, Haggard JJ, Alam J, Nath KA. Cellular overexpression of heme oxygenase-1 up-regulates p21 and confers resistance to apoptosis. Kidney Int. 2001;60(6):2181–91. PubMed PMID: 11737592. Epub 2001/12/12. eng.
98. Andersen MH. Identification of heme oxygenase-1-specific regulatory CD8+ T cells in cancer patients. J Clin Invest. 2009;119(8):2245–56.
99. Ferenbach DA, Nkejabega NC, McKay J, Choudhary AK, Vernon MA, Beesley MF, et al. The induction of macrophage hemeoxygenase-1 is protective during acute kidney injury in aging mice. Kidney Int. 2011;79(9):966–76. PubMed PMID: 21248714. Epub 2011/01/21. Eng.
100. Hull TD, Kamal AI, Boddu R, Bolisetty S, Guo L, Tisher CC, et al. Heme oxygenase-1 regulates myeloid cell trafficking in AKI. J Am Soc Nephrol. 2015;26(9):2139–51. PubMed PMID: 25677389. Pubmed Central PMCID: PMC4552119.
101. Kim J, Zarjou A, Traylor AM, Bolisetty S, Jaimes EA, Hull TD, et al. In vivo regulation of the heme oxygenase-1 gene in humanized transgenic mice. Kidney Int. 2012;82(3):278–91. PubMed PMID: 22495295. Pubmed Central PMCID: PMC3396739.
102. Ali F, Zakkar M, Karu K, Lidington EA, Hamdulay SS, Boyle JJ, et al. Induction of the cytoprotective enzyme heme oxygenase-1 by statins is enhanced in vascular endothelium exposed to laminar shear stress and impaired by disturbed flow. J Biol Chem. 2009;284(28):18882–92. PubMed PMID: 19457866. Pubmed Central PMCID: PMC2707208.
103. Billings FT 4th, Hendricks PA, Schildcrout JS, Shi Y, Petracek MR, Byrne JG, et al. High-dose perioperative atorvastatin and acute kidney injury following cardiac surgery: a randomized clinical trial. JAMA. 2016;315(9):877–88. PubMed PMID: 26906014. Pubmed Central PMCID: PMC4843765.
104. Wu BJ, Kathir K, Witting PK, Beck K, Choy K, Li C, et al. Antioxidants protect from atherosclerosis by a heme oxygenase-1 pathway that is independent of free radical scavenging. J Exp Med. 2006;203(4):1117–27. PubMed PMID: 16606673.
105. Kubulus D, Rensing H, Paxian M, Thierbach JT, Meisel T, Redl H, et al. Influence of heme-based solutions on stress protein expression and organ failure after hemorrhagic shock. Crit Care Med. 2005;33(3):629–37. PubMed PMID: 15753757.
106. Tenhunen R, Tokola O, Linden IB. Haem arginate: a new stable haem compound. J Pharm Pharmacol. 1987;39(10):780–6. PubMed PMID: 2891815.
107. Ventura P, Cappellini MD, Rocchi E. The acute porphyrias: a diagnostic and therapeutic challenge in internal and emergency medicine. Intern Emerg Med. 2009;4(4):297–308. PubMed PMID: 19479318.
108. Thomas RA, Czopek A, Bellamy CO, McNally SJ, Kluth DC, Marson LP. Hemin preconditioning upregulates heme oxygenase-1 in deceased donor renal transplant recipients: a randomized, controlled, phase IIB trial. Transplantation. 2016;100(1):176–83. PubMed PMID: 26680374.
109. Bonventre JV, Yang L. Cellular pathophysiology of ischemic acute kidney injury. J Clin Invest. 2011;121(11):4210–21. PubMed PMID: 22045571. Pubmed Central PMCID: 3204829.
110. Mulay SR, Holderied A, Kumar SV, Anders HJ. Targeting inflammation in so-called acute kidney injury. Semin Nephrol. 2016;36(1):17–30. PubMed PMID: 27085732.
111. He Z, Lu L, Altmann C, Hoke TS, Ljubanovic D, Jani A, et al. Interleukin-18 binding pro-

tein transgenic mice are protected against ischemic acute kidney injury. Am J Physiol Renal Physiol. 2008;295(5):F1414–21. PubMed PMID: 18753296. Pubmed Central PMCID: 2584896. Epub 2008/08/30. eng.
112. Faubel S, Lewis EC, Reznikov L, Ljubanovic D, Hoke TS, Somerset H, et al. Cisplatin-induced acute renal failure is associated with an increase in the cytokines interleukin (IL)-1beta, IL-18, IL-6, and neutrophil infiltration in the kidney. J Pharmacol Exp Ther. 2007;322(1):8–15. PubMed PMID: 17400889.
113. Wang W, Faubel S, Ljubanovic D, Mitra A, Falk SA, Kim J, et al. Endotoxemic acute renal failure is attenuated in caspase-1-deficient mice. Am J Physiol Renal Physiol. 2005;288(5):F997–1004. PubMed PMID: 15644489.
114. Linkermann A, Brasen JH, Darding M, Jin MK, Sanz AB, Heller JO, et al. Two independent pathways of regulated necrosis mediate ischemia-reperfusion injury. Proc Natl Acad Sci U S A. 2013;110(29):12024–9. PubMed PMID: 23818611. Pubmed Central PMCID: PMC3718149.
115. Linkermann A, Green DR. Necroptosis. N Engl J Med. 2014;370(5):455–65. PubMed PMID: 24476434. Pubmed Central PMCID: PMC4035222.
116. Linkermann A, Hackl MJ, Kunzendorf U, Walczak H, Krautwald S, Jevnikar AM. Necroptosis in immunity and ischemia-reperfusion injury. Am J Transplant. 2013;13(11):2797–804. PubMed PMID: 24103029.
117. Ferenbach DA, Kluth DC, Hughes J. Hemeoxygenase-1 and renal ischaemia-reperfusion injury. Nephron Exp Nephrol. 2010;115(3):e33–7. PubMed PMID: 20424481. Epub 2010/04/29. eng.
118. Friedmann Angeli JP, Schneider M, Proneth B, Tyurina YY, Tyurin VA, Hammond VJ, et al. Inactivation of the ferroptosis regulator Gpx4 triggers acute renal failure in mice. Nat Cell Biol. 2014;16(12):1180–91. PubMed PMID: 25402683. Pubmed Central PMCID: PMC4894846.
119. Kumar SV, Kulkarni OP, Mulay SR, Darisipudi MN, Romoli S, Thomasova D, et al. Neutrophil extracellular trap-related extracellular histones cause vascular necrosis in severe GN. J Am Soc Nephrol. 2015;26(10):2399–413. PubMed PMID: 25644111. Pubmed Central PMCID: PMC4587690.
120. Yang H, Fogo AB. Cell senescence in the aging kidney. J Am Soc Nephrol. 2010;21(9):1436–9. PubMed PMID: 20705707. Epub 2010/08/14. eng.
121. Baker DJ, Wijshake T, Tchkonia T, Lebrasseur NK, Childs BG, van de Sluis B, et al. Clearance of p16(Ink4a)-positive senescent cells delays ageing-associated disorders. Nature. 2011;479(7372):232–6. PubMed PMID: 22048312. Epub 2011/11/04. Eng.
122. Baker DJ, Childs BG, Durik M, Wijers ME, Sieben CJ, Zhong J, et al. Naturally occurring p16(Ink4a)-positive cells shorten healthy lifespan. Nature. 2016;530(7589):184–9. PubMed PMID: 26840489. Pubmed Central PMCID: 4845101.
123. Grgic I, Campanholle G, Bijol V, Wang C, Sabbisetti VS, Ichimura T, et al. Targeted proximal tubule injury triggers interstitial fibrosis and glomerulosclerosis. Kidney Int. 2012;82(2):172–83. PubMed PMID: 22437410. Epub 2012/03/23. eng.
124. Venkatachalam MA, Weinberg JM, Kriz W, Bidani AK. Failed tubule recovery, AKI-CKD transition, and kidney disease progression. J Am Soc Nephrol. 2015;26(8):1765–76. PubMed PMID: 25810494. Pubmed Central PMCID: 4520181.
125. Lan R, Geng H, Polichnowski AJ, Singha PK, Saikumar P, McEwen DG, et al. PTEN loss defines a TGF-beta-induced tubule phenotype of failed differentiation and JNK signaling during renal fibrosis. Am J Physiol Renal Physiol. 2012;302(9):F1210–23. PubMed PMID: 22301622. Pubmed Central PMCID: 3362177. Epub 2012/02/04. eng.
126. Yang L, Besschetnova TY, Brooks CR, Shah JV, Bonventre JV. Epithelial cell cycle arrest in G2/M mediates kidney fibrosis after injury. Nat Med. 2010;16(5):535–43, 1p following 143. PubMed PMID: 20436483. Epub 2010/05/04. eng.
127. Tang J, Liu N, Tolbert E, Ponnusamy M, Ma L, Gong R, et al. Sustained activation of EGFR triggers renal fibrogenesis after acute kidney injury. Am J Pathol. 2013;183(1):160–72. PubMed PMID: 23684791. Pubmed Central PMCID: 3702747.
128. Cianciolo Cosentino C, Skrypnyk NI, Brilli LL, Chiba T, Novitskaya T, Woods C, et al. Histone deacetylase inhibitor enhances recovery after AKI. J Am Soc Nephrol. 2013;24(6):943–53. PubMed PMID: 23620402. Pubmed Central PMCID: 3665399. Epub 2013/04/27. eng.
129. Wu CF, Chiang WC, Lai CF, Chang FC, Chen YT, Chou YH, et al. Transforming growth factor beta-1 stimulates profibrotic epithelial signaling to activate pericyte-myofibroblast transition in obstructive kidney fibrosis. Am J Pathol. 2013;182(1):118–31. PubMed PMID: 23142380. Pubmed Central PMCID: 3538028.
130. Bonventre JV, Zuk A. Ischemic acute renal failure: an inflammatory disease? Kidney Int. 2004;66(2):480–5. PubMed PMID: 15253693.
131. Furuichi K, Gao JL, Horuk R, Wada T, Kaneko S, Murphy PM. Chemokine receptor CCR1 regulates inflammatory cell infiltration after renal ischemia-reperfusion injury. J Immunol. 2008;181(12):8670–6. PubMed PMID: 19050287. Pubmed Central PMCID: PMC2633769.
132. Furuichi K, Gao JL, Murphy PM. Chemokine receptor CX3CR1 regulates renal interstitial fibrosis after ischemia-reperfusion injury. Am J Pathol. 2006;169(2):372–87. PubMed PMID: 16877340.
133. Furuichi K, Wada T, Iwata Y, Kitagawa K, Kobayashi K, Hashimoto H, et al. CCR2 signaling contributes to ischemia-reperfusion injury in kidney. J Am Soc Nephrol. 2003;14(10):2503–15. PubMed PMID: 14514728.
134. Dong X, Swaminathan S, Bachman LA, Croatt AJ, Nath KA, Griffin MD. Resident dendritic cells

are the predominant TNF-secreting cell in early renal ischemia-reperfusion injury. Kidney Int. 2007;71(7):619–28. PubMed PMID: 17311071. Epub 2007/02/22. eng.
135. Jang HR, Ko GJ, Wasowska BA, Rabb H. The interaction between ischemia-reperfusion and immune responses in the kidney. J Mol Med. 2009;87(9):859–64. PubMed PMID: 19562316.
136. Daemen MA, de Vries B, van't Veer C, Wolfs TG, Buurman WA. Apoptosis and chemokine induction after renal ischemia-reperfusion. Transplantation. 2001;71(7):1007–11. PubMed PMID: 11349710.
137. Ysebaert DK, De Greef KE, Vercauteren SR, Ghielli M, Verpooten GA, Eyskens EJ, et al. Identification and kinetics of leukocytes after severe ischaemia/reperfusion renal injury. Nephrol Dial Transplant. 2000;15(10):1562–74. PubMed PMID: 11007823.
138. Miura M, Fu X, Zhang QW, Remick DG, Fairchild RL. Neutralization of Gro alpha and macrophage inflammatory protein-2 attenuates renal ischemia/reperfusion injury. Am J Pathol. 2001;159(6):2137–45. PubMed PMID: 11733364. Pubmed Central PMCID: PMC1850606.
139. Kelly KJ, Williams WW Jr, Colvin RB, Bonventre JV. Antibody to intercellular adhesion molecule 1 protects the kidney against ischemic injury. Proc Natl Acad Sci U S A. 1994;91(2):812–6. PubMed PMID: 7904759.
140. Paller MS. Effect of neutrophil depletion on ischemic renal injury in the rat. J Lab Clin Med. 1989;113(3):379–86. PubMed PMID: 2926243.
141. Thornton MA, Winn R, Alpers CE, Zager RA. An evaluation of the neutrophil as a mediator of in vivo renal ischemic-reperfusion injury. Am J Pathol. 1989;135(3):509–15. PubMed PMID: 2782382. Pubmed Central PMCID: 1879883.
142. Tadagavadi RK, Gao G, Wang WW, Gonzalez MR, Reeves WB. Dendritic cell protection from cisplatin nephrotoxicity is independent of neutrophils. Toxins. 2015;7(8):3245–56. PubMed PMID: 26295408. Pubmed Central PMCID: PMC4549748.
143. Jang HR, Park JH, Kwon GY, Park JB, Lee JE, Kim DJ, et al. Aging has small effects on initial ischemic acute kidney injury development despite changing intrarenal immunologic micromilieu in mice. Am J Physiol Renal Physiol. 2016;310(4):F272–83. PubMed PMID: 26661651.
144. Salmela K, Wramner L, Ekberg H, Hauser I, Bentdal O, Lins LE, et al. A randomized multicenter trial of the anti-ICAM-1 monoclonal antibody (enlimomab) for the prevention of acute rejection and delayed onset of graft function in cadaveric renal transplantation: a report of the European Anti-ICAM-1 Renal Transplant Study Group. Transplantation. 1999;67(5):729–36. PubMed PMID: 10096530.
145. Friedewald JJ, Rabb H. Inflammatory cells in ischemic acute renal failure. Kidney Int. 2004;66(2):486–91. PubMed PMID: 15253694.
146. Burne MJ, Daniels F, El Ghandour A, Mauiyyedi S, Colvin RB, O'Donnell MP, et al. Identification of the CD4(+) T cell as a major pathogenic factor in ischemic acute renal failure. J Clin Invest. 2001;108(9):1283–90. PubMed PMID: 11696572.
147. Burne-Taney MJ, Yokota-Ikeda N, Rabb H. Effects of combined T- and B-cell deficiency on murine ischemia reperfusion injury. Am J Transplant. 2005;5(6):1186–93. PubMed PMID: 15888022.
148. Yokota N, Daniels F, Crosson J, Rabb H. Protective effect of T cell depletion in murine renal ischemia-reperfusion injury. Transplantation. 2002;74(6):759–63. PubMed PMID: 12364852.
149. Rabb H, Daniels F, O'Donnell M, Haq M, Saba SR, Keane W, et al. Pathophysiological role of T lymphocytes in renal ischemia-reperfusion injury in mice. Am J Physiol Renal Physiol. 2000;279(3):F525–31. PubMed PMID: 10966932.
150. Rabb H. The T cell as a bridge between innate and adaptive immune systems: implications for the kidney. Kidney Int. 2002;61(6):1935–46. PubMed PMID: 12028434.
151. Burne-Taney MJ, Ascon DB, Daniels F, Racusen L, Baldwin W, Rabb H. B cell deficiency confers protection from renal ischemia reperfusion injury. J Immunol. 2003;171(6):3210–5. PubMed PMID: 12960350.
152. Park P, Haas M, Cunningham PN, Bao L, Alexander JJ, Quigg RJ. Injury in renal ischemia-reperfusion is independent from immunoglobulins and T lymphocytes. Am J Physiol Renal Physiol. 2002;282(2):F352–7. PubMed PMID: 11788450.
153. Gandolfo MT, Jang HR, Bagnasco SM, Ko GJ, Agreda P, Satpute SR, et al. Foxp3+ regulatory T cells participate in repair of ischemic acute kidney injury. Kidney Int. 2009;76(7):717–29. PubMed PMID: 19625990.
154. Erwig LP, Kluth DC, Rees AJ. Macrophages in renal inflammation. Curr Opin Nephrol Hypertens. 2001;10(3):341–7. PubMed PMID: 11342795.
155. Jose MD, Ikezumi Y, van Rooijen N, Atkins RC, Chadban SJ. Macrophages act as effectors of tissue damage in acute renal allograft rejection. Transplantation. 2003;76(7):1015–22. PubMed PMID: 14557746.
156. Kluth DC, Erwig LP, Rees AJ. Multiple facets of macrophages in renal injury. Kidney Int. 2004;66(2):542–57. PubMed PMID: 15253705.
157. Day YJ, Huang L, Ye H, Linden J, Okusa MD. Renal ischemia-reperfusion injury and adenosine 2A receptor-mediated tissue protection: role of macrophages. Am J Physiol Renal Physiol. 2005;288(4):F722–31. PubMed PMID: 15561971.
158. Jo SK, Sung SA, Cho WY, Go KJ, Kim HK. Macrophages contribute to the initiation of ischaemic acute renal failure in rats. Nephrol Dial Transplant. 2006;21(5):1231–9. PubMed PMID: 16410269. Epub 2006/01/18. eng.
159. Duffield JS, Tipping PG, Kipari T, Cailhier JF, Clay S, Lang R, et al. Conditional ablation of macrophages halts progression of crescentic glomerulonephritis. Am J Pathol. 2005;167(5):1207–19. PubMed PMID: 16251406.

160. Henderson NC, Mackinnon AC, Farnworth SL, Kipari T, Haslett C, Iredale JP, et al. Galectin-3 expression and secretion links macrophages to the promotion of renal fibrosis. Am J Pathol. 2008;172(2):288–98. PubMed PMID: 18202187.
161. Ko GJ, Boo CS, Jo SK, Cho WY, Kim HK. Macrophages contribute to the development of renal fibrosis following ischaemia/reperfusion-induced acute kidney injury. Nephrol Dial Transplant. 2008;23(3):842–52. PubMed PMID: 17984109. Epub 2007/11/07. eng.
162. Lee S, Huen S, Nishio H, Nishio S, Lee HK, Choi BS, et al. Distinct macrophage phenotypes contribute to kidney injury and repair. J Am Soc Nephrol. 2011;22(2):317–26. PubMed PMID: 21289217. Epub 2011/02/04. eng.
163. Ricardo SD, van Goor H, Eddy AA. Macrophage diversity in renal injury and repair. J Clin Invest. 2008;118(11):3522–30. PubMed PMID: 18982158.
164. Rogers NM, Ferenbach DA, Isenberg JS, Thomson AW, Hughes J. Dendritic cells and macrophages in the kidney: a spectrum of good and evil. Nat Rev Nephrol. 2014;10(11):625–43. PubMed PMID: 25266210.
165. Duffield JS, Erwig LP, Wei X, Liew FY, Rees AJ, Savill JS. Activated macrophages direct apoptosis and suppress mitosis of mesangial cells. J Immunol. 2000;164(4):2110–9. PubMed PMID: 10657665.
166. Ikezumi Y, Atkins RC, Nikolic-Paterson DJ. Interferon-gamma augments acute macrophage-mediated renal injury via a glucocorticoid-sensitive mechanism. J Am Soc Nephrol. 2003;14(4):888–98. PubMed PMID: 12660323.
167. Kipari T, Cailhier JF, Ferenbach D, Watson S, Houlberg K, Walbaum D, et al. Nitric oxide is an important mediator of renal tubular epithelial cell death in vitro and in murine experimental hydronephrosis. Am J Pathol. 2006;169(2):388–99. PubMed PMID: 16877341.
168. Qi F, Adair A, Ferenbach D, Vass DG, Mylonas KJ, Kipari T, et al. Depletion of cells of monocyte lineage prevents loss of renal microvasculature in murine kidney transplantation. Transplantation. 2008;86(9):1267–74. PubMed PMID: 19005409. Epub 2008/11/14. eng.
169. Binger KJ, Gebhardt M, Heinig M, Rintisch C, Schroeder A, Neuhofer W, et al. High salt reduces the activation of IL-4- and IL-13-stimulated macrophages. J Clin Invest. 2015;125(11):4223–38. PubMed PMID: 26485286. Pubmed Central PMCID: 4639967.
170. Kim MG, Kim SC, Ko YS, Lee HY, Jo SK, Cho W. The role of M2 macrophages in the progression of chronic kidney disease following acute kidney injury. PLoS One. 2015;10(12):e0143961. PubMed PMID: 26630505. Pubmed Central PMCID: 4667939.
171. Mosser DM, Edwards JP. Exploring the full spectrum of macrophage activation. Nat Rev Immunol. 2008;8(12):958–69. PubMed PMID: 19029990. Pubmed Central PMCID: 2724991. Epub 2008/11/26. eng.
172. Lewis C, Murdoch C. Macrophage responses to hypoxia: implications for tumor progression and anti-cancer therapies. Am J Pathol. 2005;167(3):627–35. PubMed PMID: 16127144.
173. Murdoch C, Muthana M, Lewis CE. Hypoxia regulates macrophage functions in inflammation. J Immunol. 2005;175(10):6257–63. PubMed PMID: 16272275.
174. Anders HJ, Frink M, Linde Y, Banas B, Wornle M, Cohen CD, et al. CC chemokine ligand 5/RANTES chemokine antagonists aggravate glomerulonephritis despite reduction of glomerular leukocyte infiltration. J Immunol. 2003;170(11):5658–66. PubMed PMID: 12759447.
175. Ling H, Edelstein C, Gengaro P, Meng X, Lucia S, Knotek M, et al. Attenuation of renal ischemia-reperfusion injury in inducible nitric oxide synthase knockout mice. Am J Physiol. 1999;277(3 Pt 2):F383–90. PubMed PMID: 10484522.
176. Noiri E, Peresleni T, Miller F, Goligorsky MS. In vivo targeting of inducible NO synthase with oligodeoxynucleotides protects rat kidney against ischemia. J Clin Invest. 1996;97(10):2377–83. PubMed PMID: 8636419.
177. Walker LM, Walker PD, Imam SZ, Ali SF, Mayeux PR. Evidence for peroxynitrite formation in renal ischemia-reperfusion injury: studies with the inducible nitric oxide synthase inhibitor L-N(6)-(1-Iminoethyl)lysine. J Pharmacol Exp Ther. 2000;295(1):417–22. PubMed PMID: 10992009.
178. Tarzi RM, Davies KA, Claassens JW, Verbeek JS, Walport MJ, Cook HT. Both Fcgamma receptor I and Fcgamma receptor III mediate disease in accelerated nephrotoxic nephritis. Am J Pathol. 2003;162(5):1677–83. PubMed PMID: 12707052.
179. Tarzi RM, Davies KA, Robson MG, Fossati-Jimack L, Saito T, Walport MJ, et al. Nephrotoxic nephritis is mediated by Fcgamma receptors on circulating leukocytes and not intrinsic renal cells. Kidney Int. 2002;62(6):2087–96. PubMed PMID: 12427132.
180. Komine-Kobayashi M, Chou N, Mochizuki H, Nakao A, Mizuno Y, Urabe T. Dual role of Fcgamma receptor in transient focal cerebral ischemia in mice. Stroke. 2004;35(4):958–63. PubMed PMID: 14988576.
181. Ferenbach D, Hughes J. Macrophages and dendritic cells: what is the difference? Kidney Int. 2008;74(1):5–7. PubMed PMID: 18560360.
182. Martinez-Pomares L, Gordon S. Antigen presentation the macrophage way. Cell. 2007;131(4):641–3. PubMed PMID: 18022354.
183. Serbina NV, Salazar-Mather TP, Biron CA, Kuziel WA, Pamer EG. TNF/iNOS-producing dendritic cells mediate innate immune defense against bacterial infection. Immunity. 2003;19(1):59–70. PubMed PMID: 12871639.
184. Stary G, Bangert C, Tauber M, Strohal R, Kopp T, Stingl G. Tumoricidal activity of TLR7/8-

activated inflammatory dendritic cells. J Exp Med. 2007;204(6):1441–51. PubMed PMID: 17535975.
185. Auffray C, Fogg DK, Narni-Mancinelli E, Senechal B, Trouillet C, Saederup N, et al. CX3CR1+ CD115+ CD135+ common macrophage/DC precursors and the role of CX3CR1 in their response to inflammation. J Exp Med. 2009;206(3):595–606. PubMed PMID: 19273628. Pubmed Central PMCID: 2699130. Epub 2009/03/11. eng.
186. Hume DA. Macrophages as APC and the dendritic cell myth. J Immunol. 2008;181(9):5829–35. PubMed PMID: 18941170. Epub 2008/10/23. eng.
187. Anderson KV, Jurgens G, Nusslein-Volhard C. Establishment of dorsal-ventral polarity in the Drosophila embryo: genetic studies on the role of the Toll gene product. Cell. 1985;42(3):779–89. PubMed PMID: 3931918.
188. Medzhitov R, Preston-Hurlburt P, Janeway CA Jr. A human homologue of the Drosophila Toll protein signals activation of adaptive immunity. Nature. 1997;388(6640):394–7. PubMed PMID: 9237759.
189. Poltorak A, He X, Smirnova I, Liu MY, Van Huffel C, Du X, et al. Defective LPS signaling in C3H/HeJ and C57BL/10ScCr mice: mutations in Tlr4 gene. Science. 1998;282(5396):2085–8. PubMed PMID: 9851930.
190. Tsuboi N, Yoshikai Y, Matsuo S, Kikuchi T, Iwami K, Nagai Y, et al. Roles of toll-like receptors in C-C chemokine production by renal tubular epithelial cells. J Immunol. 2002;169(4):2026–33. PubMed PMID: 12165529.
191. Kim BS, Lim SW, Li C, Kim JS, Sun BK, Ahn KO, et al. Ischemia-reperfusion injury activates innate immunity in rat kidneys. Transplantation. 2005;79(10):1370–7. PubMed PMID: 15912106.
192. Wolfs TG, Buurman WA, van Schadewijk A, de Vries B, Daemen MA, Hiemstra PS, et al. In vivo expression of Toll-like receptor 2 and 4 by renal epithelial cells: IFN-gamma and TNF-alpha mediated up-regulation during inflammation. J Immunol. 2002;168(3):1286–93. PubMed PMID: 11801667.
193. Leemans JC, Stokman G, Claessen N, Rouschop KM, Teske GJ, Kirschning CJ, et al. Renal-associated TLR2 mediates ischemia/reperfusion injury in the kidney. J Clin Invest. 2005;115(10):2894–903. PubMed PMID: 16167081. Pubmed Central PMCID: PMC1201659.
194. Pulskens WP, Teske GJ, Butter LM, Roelofs JJ, van der Poll T, Florquin S, et al. Toll-like receptor-4 coordinates the innate immune response of the kidney to renal ischemia/reperfusion injury. PLoS One. 2008;3(10):e3596. PubMed PMID: 18974879. Pubmed Central PMCID: PMC2570789.
195. Palermo M, Alves-Rosa F, Rubel C, Fernandez GC, Fernandez-Alonso G, Alberto F, et al. Pretreatment of mice with lipopolysaccharide (LPS) or IL-1beta exerts dose-dependent opposite effects on Shiga toxin-2 lethality. Clin Exp Immunol. 2000;119(1):77–83. PubMed PMID: 10606967. Pubmed Central PMCID: PMC1905548.
196. Valles PG, Melechuck S, Gonzalez A, Manucha W, Bocanegra V, Valles R. Toll-like receptor 4 expression on circulating leucocytes in hemolytic uremic syndrome. Pediatr Nephrol. 2012;27(3):407–15. PubMed PMID: 21969092.
197. Goligorsky MS. TLR4 and HMGB1: partners in crime? Kidney Int. 2011;80(5):450–2. PubMed PMID: 21841835.
198. Chen J, Hartono JR, John R, Bennett M, Zhou XJ, Wang Y, et al. Early interleukin 6 production by leukocytes during ischemic acute kidney injury is regulated by TLR4. Kidney Int. 2011;80(5):504–15. PubMed PMID: 21633411. Pubmed Central PMCID: PMC3394593.
199. Li J, Gong Q, Zhong S, Wang L, Guo H, Xiang Y, et al. Neutralization of the extracellular HMGB1 released by ischaemic damaged renal cells protects against renal ischaemia-reperfusion injury. Nephrol Dial Transplant. 2011;26(2):469–78. PubMed PMID: 20679140.
200. Kulkarni OP, Hartter I, Mulay SR, Hagemann J, Darisipudi MN, Kumar Vr S, et al. Toll-like receptor 4-induced IL-22 accelerates kidney regeneration. J Am Soc Nephrol. 2014;25(5):978–89. PubMed PMID: 24459235. Pubmed Central PMCID: PMC4005301.
201. Anders HJ. Four danger response programs determine glomerular and tubulointerstitial kidney pathology: clotting, inflammation, epithelial and mesenchymal healing. Organogenesis. 2012;8(2):29–40. PubMed PMID: 22692229. Pubmed Central PMCID: PMC3429510.
202. Strainic MG, Shevach EM, An F, Lin F, Medof ME. Absence of signaling into CD4+ cells via C3aR and C5aR enables autoinductive TGF-β[beta]1 signaling and induction of Foxp3+ regulatory T cells. Nat Immunol. 2012;14:162–71.
203. Thurman JM, Lenderink AM, Royer PA, Coleman KE, Zhou J, Lambris JD, et al. C3a is required for the production of CXC chemokines by tubular epithelial cells after renal ishemia/reperfusion. J Immunol. 2007;178:1819–28. PubMed PMID: 17237432.
204. Morgan BP. Regulation of the complement membrane attack pathway. Crit Rev Immunol. 1999;19:173–98. PubMed PMID: 10422598.
205. Thurman JM, Scott Lucia M, Ljubanovic D, Michael Holers V. Acute tubular necrosis is characterized by activation of the alternative pathway of complement. Kidney Int. 2005;67:524–30.
206. Brar JE, et al. Complement activation in the tubulointerstitium: Aki, ckd, and in between. Kidney International. 2014;86:663–6.
207. McCullough JW, Renner B, Thurman JM. The role of the complement system in acute kidney injury. Semin Nephrol. 2013;33:543–56. PubMed PMID: 24161039.
208. Pratt JR, Basheer SA, Sacks SH. Local synthesis of complement component C3 regulates acute renal transplant rejection. Nat Med. 2002;8:582–7. PubMed PMID: 12042808.
209. Takada M, Nadeau KC, Shaw GD, Marquette KA, Tilney NL. The cytokine-adhesion molecule cascade

in ischemia/reperfusion injury of the rat kidney. Inhibition by a soluble P-selectin ligand. J Clin Invest. 1997;99:2682–90. PubMed PMID: 9169498.
210. Farrar CA, Zhou W, Lin T, Sacks SH. Local extravascular pool of C3 is a determinant of postischemic acute renal failure. FASEB J. 2006;20(2):217–26. PubMed PMID: 16449793.
211. Renner B, Coleman K, Goldberg R, Amura C, Holland-Neidermyer A, Pierce K, et al. The complement inhibitors Crry and factor H are critical for preventing autologous complement activation on renal tubular epithelial cells. J Immunol (Baltimore, Md: 1950). 2010;185:3086–94. PubMed PMID: 20675597.
212. Thurman JM, Ljubanović D, Royer PA, Kraus DM, Molina H, Barry NP, et al. Altered renal tubular expression of the complement inhibitor Crry permits complement activation after ischemia/reperfusion. J Clin Invest. 2006;116:357–68. PubMed PMID: 16444293.
213. Bonventre JV. Complement and renal ischemia-reperfusion injury. Am J Kidney Dis. 2001;38:430–3.
214. Elward K, Griffiths M, Mizuno M, Harris CL, Neal JW, Morgan BP, et al. CD46 plays a key role in tailoring innate immune recognition of apoptotic and necrotic cells. J Biol Chem. 2005;280:36342–54. PubMed PMID: 16087667.
215. Isenman DE, Kells DI, Cooper NR, Müller-Eberhard HJ, Pangburn MK. Nucleophilic modification of human complement protein C3: correlation of conformational changes with acquisition of C3b-like functional properties. Biochemistry. 1981;20:4458–67. PubMed PMID: 7284336.
216. Mason J, Torhorst J, Welsch J. Role of the medullary perfusion defect in the pathogenesis of ischemic renal failure. Kidney Int. 1984;26:283–93.
217. Thurman JM, Ljubanovic D, Edelstein CL, Gilkeson GS, Holers VM. Lack of a functional alternative complement pathway ameliorates ischemic acute renal failure in mice. J Immunol. 2003;170(3):1517–23. PubMed PMID: 12538716.
218. Thurman JM, Holers VM. The central role of the alternative complement pathway in human disease. J Immunol. 2006;176(3):1305–10. ubMed PMID: 16424154.
219. Zhou W, Farrar CA, Abe K, Pratt JR, Marsh JE, Wang Y, et al. Predominant role for C5b-9 in renal ischemia/reperfusion injury. J Clin Invest. 2000;105:1363–71. PubMed PMID: 10811844.
220. De Vries B, Matthijsen RA, Wolfs TGAM, Van Bijnen AAJHM, Heeringa P, Buurman WA. Inhibition of complement factor C5 protects against renal ischemia-reperfusion injury: inhibition of late apoptosis and inflammation. Transplantation. 2003;75:375–82. PubMed PMID: 12589162.
221. Faubel S, Ljubanovic D, Reznikov L, Somerset H, Dinarello CA, Edelstein CL. Caspase-1-deficient mice are protected against cisplatin-induced apoptosis and acute tubular necrosis. Kidney Int. 2004;66(6):2202–13. PubMed PMID: 15569309.
222. Akcay A, Nguyen Q, Edelstein CL. Mediators of inflammation in acute kidney injury. Mediat Inflamm. 2009;2009:137072. PubMed PMID: 20182538. Pubmed Central PMCID: PMC2825552.
223. Nechemia-Arbely Y, Barkan D, Pizov G, Shriki A, Rose-John S, Galun E, et al. IL-6/IL-6R axis plays a critical role in acute kidney injury. J Am Soc Nephrol. 2008;19(6):1106–15. PubMed PMID: 18337485. Pubmed Central PMCID: PMC2396933.
224. Melnikov VY, Ecder T, Fantuzzi G, Siegmund B, Lucia MS, Dinarello CA, et al. Impaired IL-18 processing protects caspase-1-deficient mice from ischemic acute renal failure. J Clin Invest. 2001;107(9):1145–52. PubMed PMID: 11342578. Pubmed Central PMCID: PMC209282.
225. Ramesh G, Reeves WB. TNF-alpha mediates chemokine and cytokine expression and renal injury in cisplatin nephrotoxicity. J Clin Invest. 2002;110(6):835–42. PubMed PMID: 12235115. Pubmed Central PMCID: PMC151130.
226. Knotek M, Rogachev B, Wang W, Ecder T, Melnikov V, Gengaro PE, et al. Endotoxemic renal failure in mice: role of tumor necrosis factor independent of inducible nitric oxide synthase. Kidney Int. 2001;59(6):2243–9. PubMed PMID: 11380827.
227. Adachi T, Sugiyama N, Yagita H, Yokoyama T. Renal atrophy after ischemia-reperfusion injury depends on massive tubular apoptosis induced by TNFalpha in the later phase. Med Mol Morphol. 2014;47(4):213–23. PubMed PMID: 24407718.
228. Poon M, Megyesi J, Green RS, Zhang H, Rollins BJ, Safirstein R, et al. In vivo and in vitro inhibition of JE gene expression by glucocorticoids. J Biol Chem. 1991;266(33):22375–9. PubMed PMID: 1939262.
229. Oh DJ, Dursun B, He Z, Lu L, Hoke TS, Ljubanovic D, et al. Fractalkine receptor (CX3CR1) inhibition is protective against ischemic acute renal failure in mice. Am J Physiol Renal Physiol. 2008;294(1):F264–71. PubMed PMID: 18003857.
230. Lu LH, Oh DJ, Dursun B, He Z, Hoke TS, Faubel S, et al. Increased macrophage infiltration and fractalkine expression in cisplatin-induced acute renal failure in mice. J Pharmacol Exp Ther. 2008;324(1):111–7. PubMed PMID: 17932247.
231. Cugini D, Azzollini N, Gagliardini E, Cassis P, Bertini R, Colotta F, et al. Inhibition of the chemokine receptor CXCR2 prevents kidney graft function deterioration due to ischemia/reperfusion. Kidney Int. 2005;67(5):1753–61. PubMed PMID: 15840022.

Part III

Clinical Syndromes

6 Contrast-Associated Acute Kidney Injury

Steven D. Weisbord

6.1 Pathophysiology of CA-AKI

Several pathophysiological processes triggered by intravascular contrast administration result in renal tubular epithelial cell damage and acute kidney injury. These include vasoconstriction that results in mismatch of oxygen supply and demand in the renal medulla, direct toxicity to tubular epithelial cells, and generation of oxygen-free radicals that augment renal injury (Fig. 6.1).

6.1.1 Vasoconstriction and Medullary Hypoxia

Following the intravascular administration of iodinated contrast, blood flow to the renal medulla decreases, resulting in diminished oxygenation in a region of the kidney parenchyma with marginal oxygen reserve under normal circumstances [1, 2]. Concurrently, iodinated contrast increases oxygen requirements by leading to active transport in the distal nephron. Thus, concominant reductions in oxygen delivery and increases in oxygen demand in the outer renal medulla lead to tissue hypoxia and tubular epithelial cell injury.

6.1.2 Direct Tubular Toxicity and Generation of Reactive Oxygen Species

Tubular epithelial cell injury also results from the direct cytotoxicity of iodinated contrast and indirectly through the effects of reactive oxygen species (ROS) [3–8]. Intravascular iodinated contrast is filtered at the glomerulus and enters the tubular lumen where it has directly toxic effects that lead to necrosis of tubular epithelial cells [5–7, 9]. The generation of oxygen-free radicals in the kidney following contrast administration is also associated with renal injury [10–14]. Endothelial damage related to oxygen-free radicals and reparative effects can further aggravate tissue hypoxia and epithelial cell damage [11, 15–17]. Thus, direct and indirect toxic effects of iodinated contrast collectively contribute to epithelial cell injury, tubular necrosis, and AKI.

S. D. Weisbord
Renal Section and Center for Health Equity Research and Promotion, VA Pittsburgh Healthcare System, Pittsburgh, PA, USA

Renal-Electrolyte Division, Department of Medicine, University of Pittsburgh School of Medicine, Pittsburgh, PA, USA
e-mail: weisbordsd@upmc.edu

S. S. Waikar et al. (eds.), *Core Concepts in Acute Kidney Injury*,
https://doi.org/10.1007/978-1-4939-8628-6_6

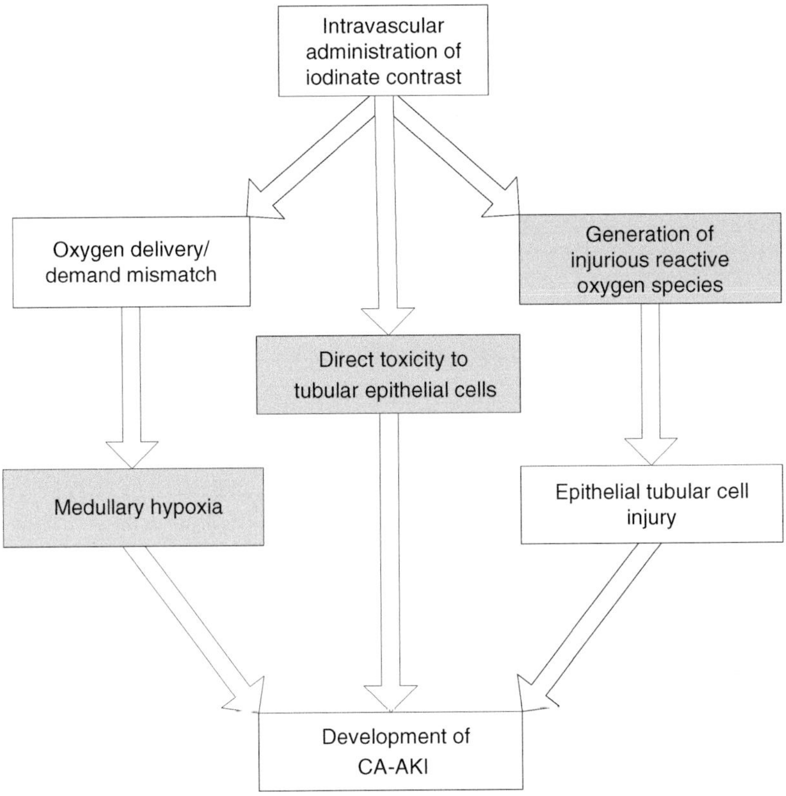

Fig. 6.1 Pathophysiology of contrast-associated acute kidney injury. Pathophysiology of contrast-induced acute kidney injury involves medully hypoxia, direct toxicity to tubular epithelial cells, and effects of injurious reactive oxygen species

6.2 Incidence of CA-AKI

The incidence of CA-AKI varies based on patient and procedural characteristics and criteria used to define the development of renal injury. Among patients with a baseline estimated glomerular filtration rate (eGFR) less than 60 ml/min/1.73 m^2, Weisbord and colleagues reported incident rates of CA-AKI, defined by an increase in serum creatinine (SCr) of ≥25%, of 13.2%, 8.5%, and 6.5% following non-emergent non-coronary angiography, coronary angiography, and contrast-enhanced computed tomography, respectively [18]. In a study of 1111 hospitalized patients who underwent contrast-enhanced procedures, the incidence of CA-AKI, defined as an increase in SCr of ≥0.5 mg/dL within 1–5 days, was as high as 44% among diabetic patients with underlying kidney disease [19]. D'Elia et al. defined CA-AKI using a larger increment in SCr of at least 1.0 mg/dL and found that 33% of patients with kidney disease developed this condition following angiography [20]. However, the aforementioned study by Weisbord et al. documented a considerably lower rate of CA-AKI (0.3–3.8%), defined by an increase in SCr of at least 1.0 mg/dL [18].

Identifying precise incidence estimates of CA-AKI is confounded by changes in SCr that occur independently of iodinated contrast administration. This was demonstrated in a study by Bruce et al. that compared the incidence of AKI, defined by an increase in SCr ≥0.5 mg/dL or decrease in eGFR ≥25%, among 11,588 patients who underwent computed tomography scans either with (N = 5790) or without (N = 7484) iodinated contrast [21]. Among subjects with CKD, the incidence of AKI following computed tomography without contrast (8.8%) was comparable to that following contrast-enhanced computed tomography (9.7% with iso-osmolal iodixanol and 9.9% with low-osmolal iohexol). A series of more recent observational studies have questioned the nephrotoxicity of iodinated contrast by demonstrating comparable rates of AKI among patients who underwent procedures with and without intravascular iodinated contrast [22–26]. A meta-analysis by McDonald and colleagues that included 13 studies with a total of 25,950 patients demonstrated that the risk of AKI following procedures with intravascular contrast administration was similar to the risk following procedures that did not utilize contrast (relative risk = 0.79, 95% CI: 0.62–1.02) [27]. Similarly, Wilhelm-Leen and colleagues compared the incidence of AKI in a very large population of hospitalized patients who did and did not undergo contrast-enhanced procedures [26]. In adjusted analyses, the incidence of AKI was lower (5.1%) among patients who received intravascular contrast compared with those who did not (5.6%; adjusted odds ratio 0.93; 95% CI: 0.88–0.97). However, careful examination of these studies demonstrates methodological limitations related to study design and unmeasured confounding that call into question the conclusion that contrast may not be nephrotoxic. What is clear is that baseline fluctuation in SCr and causal factors unrelated to iodinated contrast should be considered when estimating the incidence of AKI following contrast-enhanced procedures, particularly when defined by small increments in SCr.

6.3 Risk Factors for CA-AKI

6.3.1 Patient-Related Risk Factors

There are well-recognized patient-related and procedure-related risk factors for CA-AKI. (Table 6.1) Patient-associated risk factors include conditions and clinical states that reduce the capacity of the kidneys to effectively counteract the hemodynamic and microcirculatory effects of iodinated contrast administration. Underlying impairment in kidney function is the most important patient-related risk factor for CA-AKI, with an inverse relationship between the level of kidney function and degree of risk [28]. D'Elia et al. demonstrated a markedly higher incidence of CA-AKI among azotemic patients compared to non-azotemic patients (33% vs. 2%) and found that baseline kidney disease was the only clinical risk factor for CA-AKI among hospitalized patients undergoing angiography [20]. In a large cohort of patients who underwent angiography, McCullough et al. demonstrated a strong association of baseline renal insufficiency with risk of CA-AKI [29]. Contrary to popular belief, the presence of diabetes in patients with intact kidney function does not appear to confer an increased risk for CA-AKI [20, 29–32]. However, diabetes substantially amplifies risk in patients with underlying kidney disease as demonstrated by Rudnick et al. in the Iohexol Cooperative Study. This trial of 1196 patients found that post-angiography increments in SCr of ≥1.0 mg/dL developed in none of the 359 patients without diabetes or underlying CKD, in less than 1% of patients with diabetes and intact kidney function, in 6% of non-diabetics with impaired renal function, yet in 20% of diabetics with renal impairment [30]. These findings indicate that diabetes significantly amplifies the risk of CA-AKI in the setting of underlying kidney disease, but does not increase the risk in patients with intact kidney function. Of note, elevated serum glucose concentration at the time of contrast administration was shown in one study to be associated with an increased risk of CA-AKI among non-diabetic patients, but not in diabetics [33]. The clinical significance of this observation warrants determination in future studies.

Table 6.1 Risk factors for CA-AKI

Patient associated	Procedure associated
Renal impairment	High-osmolal contrast media
Diabetes mellitus[a]	Large contrast volume
Reduced absolute intravascular volume	Multiple sequential procedures
Reduced effective intravascular volume	Intra-arterial contrast administration
Concomitant nephrotoxic agents	

[a]Amplifies risk in patients with kidney disease

Patients with absolute (e.g., GI losses) or effective (e.g., heart failure) intravascular volume depletion are at increased risk for CA-AKI as the associated reduction in renal blood flow can magnify the effect of contrast-induced renal vasoconstriction [34, 35]. Similarly, the risk for CA-AKI is increased in patients consuming selective and non-selective non-steroidal anti-inflammatory medications, which inhibit vasodilatory prostaglandins in the kidney [36]. There are a series of other patient-related factors, including older age, hypertension, anemia, and proteinuria that have been associated with increased risk for CA-AKI in some studies, yet each is closely correlated with kidney disease, confounding confirmation of their independent association with CA-AKI [37–40].

6.3.2 Procedure-Related Risk Factors

Factors related to the performance of contrast-enhanced procedures are also associated with risk for CA-AKI. The administration of large volumes of contrast is associated with increased risk although the threshold volume beyond which at-risk patients are likely to experience renal injury has not been definitively determined [29, 41]. Similarly, higher doses of iodine are associated with increased risk for CA-AKI although the importance of iodine dose relative to contrast volume remains unclear [42, 43]. The performance of multiple consecutive contrast-enhanced procedures over a short period of time also appears to confer risk for CA-AKI. Finally, the use of high-osmolal contrast media is linked with an increased risk for CA-AKI [30, 44].

The risk for CA-AKI appears to be higher following intra-arterial contrast administration than intravenous (IV) administration. Although no large clinical trials have directly compared risk for CA-AKI based on procedure type and route of contrast administration, an observational analysis by Weisbord et al. demonstrated lower rates of CA-AKI following computed tomography (6.5%) than coronary (8.5%) and non-coronary angiography (13.2%) in patients with CKD [18]. However, this study did not adjust for differences in clinical risk factors such as diabetes mellitus, heart failure, or severity of CKD; or in differential application of preventive interventions such as IV fluids. Dissimilarity in underlying comorbidity and utilization of preventive care may explain the findings of this study.

6.4 Outcomes Associated with CA-AKI

6.4.1 Adverse Short-Term Outcomes Associated with CA-AKI

Multiple studies have reported that CA-AKI is associated with increased risk for short-term mortality (Table 6.2) [29, 45–49]. McCullough et al. found a significantly higher rate of in-hospital mortality among patients who developed CA-AKI following percutaneous coronary intervention compared to patients who did not develop CA-AKI (7.1% vs. 1.1%, $p < 0.0001$) [29]. Other large observational studies and several clinical trials also demonstrated higher short-term mortality rates among patients who developed CA-AKI [45–49]. As part of a clinical trial investigating N-acetylcysteine, Marenzi and colleagues reported that subjects with CA-AKI experienced a higher incidence of in-hospital death compared with patients without CA-AKI

Table 6.2 Association of CA-AKI with short-term mortality

Study authors	(*N*)	CA-AKI definition	Adjusted Odds Ratio	95% Confidence Interval
Levy et al.	357	↑ SCr ≥25% to ≥2.0 mg/dL	5.5	2.9–13.2
Gruberg et al.	439	↑ SCr >25%	3.9	2.0–7.6
Shema et al.	1111	↑ SCr ≥50% or ↓ eGFR ≥25%	3.9	1.2–12.0
McCullough et al.	1826	↑ SCr >25%	6.6	3.3–12.9
From et al.	3236	↑ SCr ≥25% or ≥ 0.5 mg/dL	3.4	2.6–4.4
Rihal et al.	7586	↑ SCr >0.5 mg/dL	10.8	6.9–17.0
Bartholomew et al.	20,479	↑ SCr ≥1.0 mg/dL	22	16–31
Weisbord et al.	27,608	↑ SCr 0.25–0.5 mg/dL	1.8	1.4–2.5

(26% vs. 1.4%, $p < 0.001$) [50]. Similarly, a clinical trial by Maioli et al. that compared IV sodium bicarbonate with IV sodium chloride documented a significantly higher in-hospital mortality rate among patients with CA-AKI compared with patients without CA-AKI (11.1% vs. 0.2%, $p = 0.001$) [51]. CA-AKI is also associated with increased length of hospital stay as demonstrated in a study by Adolph et al. that found that patients who developed this complication had an average prolongation in hospitalization of 2 days [52]. Extended hospital length of stay translates into higher healthcare costs as shown in a decision analysis by Subramanian et al. that estimated an increase in hospital-related costs of more than $10,000 with the development of CA-AKI [53].

6.4.2 Long-Term Outcomes Associated with CA-AKI

CA-AKI is also associated with increased long-term mortality (Table 6.3) [49, 54–58]. A study by Solomon and colleagues demonstrated a higher than threefold increased risk of death, stroke, myocardial infarction, and/or end-stage renal disease at 1-year among patients who developed post-angiography CA-AKI [57]. Harjai et al. documented an independent association of post-angiography CA-AKI with increased risk of death at 24 months (HR = 2.6; 95% CI: 1.5–4.4) [55]. Brown et al. examined outcomes in 7856 patients and found that either transient or persistent post-angiography decrements in kidney function were associated with a two- to threefold increase in long-term mortality [58]. In a smaller study of 78 patients, Goldenberg et al. documented that post-angiography CA-AKI that recovered to baseline was associated with a greater than twofold increase in mortality after 5 years of follow-up (HR = 2.66, 95% CI 1.72–4.46) [54].

CA-AKI also associates with an acceleration in the rate of progression of underlying CKD [51, 54, 59, 60]. Goldenberg et al. demonstrated that patients who manifested transient CA-AKI experienced a larger loss of kidney function 2 years following angiography than patients without CA-AKI (Δ eGFR -20 ± 11 ml/min/1.73 m^2 vs. -6 ± 16 ml/min/1.73 m^2, $p = 0.02$) [54]. James et al. found that patients who developed CA-AKI following coronary angiography lost kidney function over 3 months more rapidly than patients who did not develop CA-AKI (loss of eGFR 0.8 ml/min/1.73 m^2/year vs. 0.2 ml/min/1.73 m^2/year) [59]. In this study, CA-AKI was also associated with an increased risk of mortality and end-stage renal disease over 3 years of follow-up [60].

6.4.3 Potential Clinical Implications of Data Associating CA-AKI with Adverse Outcomes

While the aforementioned studies demonstrated associations of CA-AKI with serious, adverse short- and long-term outcomes, the causal nature of these associations remains unproven. It is plausible that CA-AKI represents a marker of patients with more hemodynamic instability and less renal reserve that places them at increased risk for adverse short- and long-term events, rather than a mediator of such outcomes. This possibility is particularly relevant in light of the

Table 6.3 Association of CA-AKI with long-term mortality

Study authors	(*N*)	CA-AKI definition	Follow-up (months)	Adjusted Hazard Ratio	95% Confidence Interval
Goldenberg et al.	78	↑SCr ≥0.5 mg/dL or ≥25%	60	2.7	1.7–4.5
Solomon et al.	294	↑SCr ≥0.3 mg/dL	12	3.2[a]	1.1–8.7
Harjai et al.	985	↑SCr ≥0.5 mg/dL	24	2.6	1.5–4.4
Roghi et al.	2860	↑SCr ≥0.5 mg/dL	24	1.8	1.0–3.4
Rihal et al.	7075	↑ SCr >0.5 mg/dL	6	b	b
Brown et al.	7856	↑SCr ≥0.5 mg/dL	90	3.1	2.4–4.0

[a]Denotes incident rate ratio of death, cerebrovascular accident, MI, ESRD
[b]6-month mortality 9.8% v. 2.3% ($p < 0.0001$)

growing evidence documenting the practice of "renalism," which denotes the under-performance of indicated diagnostic and/or therapeutic contrast-enhanced procedures in patients with kidney disease out of concern, in the case of angiography, for adverse renal outcomes. Chertow et al. initially described "renalism" in an observational study of over 57,000 patients with acute myocardial infarction, demonstrating that the presence of CKD was associated with an approximately 50% decrease in the performance of coronary angiography after adjustment for the appropriateness of this procedure [61]. Percutaneous revascularization was also less commonly utilized in those with CKD (54.7% vs. 62.0%, $p < 0.0001$), while mortality at 1 year was nearly twice as common among patients with CKD who did not undergo coronary angiography compared with patients with CKD who did undergo angiography. Concern for the risk of CA-AKI was a hypothesized explanation for the under-utilization of angiography and revascularization in subjects with CKD.

There have since been several other studies documenting renalism related to the performance of coronary angiography in patients with CKD and acute coronary syndrome (ACS) (Table 6.4) [62–65]. A study by Han et al. of approximately 45,000 patients found that subjects with CKD were nearly 50% less likely to undergo coronary angiography than those without CKD [62]. In a study by Nauta et al. that included patients with even more emergent presentations characterized by ST elevation myocardial infarction, rates of percutaneous revascularization were lower in subjects with stage 4 CKD compared to those without CKD, while thrombolysis was used more commonly in this patient group. These findings are of particular importance in light of data documenting a survival advantage with the performance of coronary angiography and revascularization in those with CKD. In the initial study of renalism by Chertow et al., patients with CKD deemed appropriate for angiography experienced a nearly 50% decrease in 1-year mortality (adjust OR = 0.58; 95% CI: 0.50–0.67) with the performance of this procedure. More recently, James et al. compared short- and long-term outcomes among patients presenting with non-ST elevation ACS who received either conservative or early invasive management. Among patients with stage 3 CKD, early invasive management consisting of coronary angiography was associated with a slightly higher rate of in-hospital AKI (risk ratio 1.42; 95% CI 1.18–1.71), a comparable rate of end-stage renal disease (risk ratio 1.53; 95% CI 0.62–3.75), yet considerably lower long-term mortality (risk ratio 0.61; 95% CI 0.46–0.79) compared with conservative management [66].

Collectively, these data suggest that indicated coronary procedures are under-utilized in patients with CKD, likely related to provider concern for the development of CA-AKI; however, the performance of indicated angiographic procedures

Table 6.4 Studies reporting under-utilization of coronary angiography in patients with CKD

Authors	Presenting condition	Patients (*N*)	Patients with CKD (%)	Angiography/revascularization CKD v. no CKD (%)
Chertow et al.	MI	57,284	26.3	25.2 v. 46.8
Han et al.	NSTE ACS	45,343	14.5	47.6 v. 73.8
Goldenberg et al.	NSTE ACS	13,141	31.8	49.9 v. 67.7
Szummer et al.	MI	57,477	33.3	33.2 v. 58.4[a]
Nauta et al.	MI	12,087	25[b]	NR[c]

[a]Denotes % patients with non-ST elevation MI who underwent revascularization by CKD status, defined as eGFR <60 ml/min/1.73 m^2

[b]CKD defined based on eGFR <60 ml/min/1.73 m^2

[c]Procedure rates not reported

in patients with CKD and ACS is associated with lower mortality. The clinical relevance of these observations is brought into focus by the lack of sound data confirming a causal link between the development of CA-AKI and adverse short- and long-term outcomes. These findings underscore the need to definitively determine the causal effects of CA-AKI on patient-centered outcomes and the importance of establishing and implementing effective interventions for the prevention of this iatrogenic condition.

6.5 Prevention of CA-AKI

6.5.1 Overview

CA-AKI is one of the few preventable forms of AKI as its risk factors are well characterized, the timing of renal insult is known in advance, and most contrast-enhanced procedures are performed on a non-emergent basis allowing sufficient time to implement preventive care. Identifying high-risk patients based on underlying risk factors informs the appropriate use of alternative imaging procedures that do not involve the administration of iodinated contrast, but that provide comparable diagnostic yield. Once a determination is made that intravascular iodinated contrast is required, evidence-based preventive care to mitigate risk of renal injury should be implemented. A sound understanding of current data on the efficacy of different preventive measures facilitates the use of an evidence-based approach to reduce risk.

Research on interventions for the prevention of CA-AKI has focused on four strategic approaches: (1) identification of contrast media that are less nephrotoxic; (2) utilization of renal replacement therapy to eliminate iodinated contrast from the vasculature prior to glomerular filtration; (3) administration of pharmacologic agents that neutralize the nephrotoxic actions of contrast; and (4) delivery of intravenous fluids to expand the intravascular space and diminish the adverse hemodynamic and direct tubular effects of contrast in the kidney.

6.5.2 Choice of Contrast Agent

Iodinated contrast media are commonly characterized by their osmolality relative to plasma. The first-generation contrast media, referred to as "high-osmolal" agents, were ionic compounds that had osmolalities of approximately 1500 mOsm/kg to over 2000 mOsm/kg and that were associated with relatively high rates of CA-AKI in at-risk patients. The development of a second generation of contrast media ("low-osmolal") with osmolalities of approximately 600–1000 mOsm/kg led to trials comparing these agents with the first-generation "high-osmolal" contrast media. The Iohexol Cooperative Study was a multi-center clinical trial that compared high-osmolal diatrizioate with low-osmolal iohexol in 1196 patients undergoing non-emergent coronary angiography [30]. Overall, CA-AKI was less common with iohexol than diatriazoate (3.2% vs. 7.1%, $p = 0.002$), and this difference was particularly notable among patients with both diabetes mellitus and renal impairment. Incorporating data from this and several other trials, Barrett and Carlisle conducted a meta-analysis demonstrating a lower risk of CA-AKI with low-osmolal contrast compared to high-osmolal contrast (OR = 0.61; 95% CI: 0.48–0.77) [44]. Among patients with underlying renal impairment, the risk of CA-AKI with low-osmolal contrast was even lower (OR = 0.5; 95% CI: 0.36–0.68); a finding that informed the preferential use of these agents in patients with impaired baseline kidney function.

More recently, clinical trials have compared the effects of low-osmolal contrast with iso-osmolal iodixanol. Although preliminary studies found lower rates of CA-AKI with iodixanol compared with certain low-osmolal agents (i.e., iohexol, ioxaglate), others reported comparable risk for CA-AKI [67–74]. The findings of meta-analyses comparing iodixanol to low-osmolal contrast agents reflect those of the clinical trials [75–79]. Clinical practice guidelines issued most recently by the American College of Cardiology/American Heart Association cite an absence of sufficient data to support the preferential use of iso-osmolal compared with low-osmolal contrast [80]. Similarly, the European Society of Urogenital Radiology recommends the use of either low- or iso-osmolal contrast in patients at elevated risk of CA-AKI [81].

6.5.3 Use of Renal Replacement Therapies to Prevent CA-AKI

Iodinated contrast media are highly water soluble, bind proteins to a very limited degree, and distribute in vivo to the extracellular space; properties that enable their efficient removal from the circulation by extracorporeal renal replacement therapy. Lee et al. reported that prophylactic hemodialysis at the time of coronary angiography resulted in a smaller decrement in creatinine clearance and lower likelihood of requring chronic hemodialysis among 82 patients with advanced CKD [82]. However, this trial had a very small sample size, used measured creatinine clearance as the primary endpoint despite the inherent limitations and inaccuracies of 24 h urine collection, and found that only a small number of patients developed dialysis-requring ESRD. Most other trials of prophylactic hemodialysis to date demonstrated no benefit, and in some instances noted a higher risk for AKI in patients who received prophylactic hemodialysis [83–88]. Thus, there is presently no role for this therapy for the prevention of CA-AKI.

Continuous renal replacement therapy (CRRT) also removes iodinated contrast from the vascular space. Marenzi and colleagues conducted two trials examining the effect of continuous venovenous hemofiltration (CVVH) on the prevention of CA-AKI, both of which found a lower risk for CA-AKI and death with this therapy [89, 90]. However, these trials used a surrogate primary study endpoint based on small increments in SCr, which is problematic given that CRRT lowers SCr independent of any effect it might have on the prevention of renal injury. CRRT is associated with significant costs and potential infectious and non-infectious complications and data drawn from clinical trials to date are insufficient to support the use of CRRT for the prevention of CA-AKI.

6.5.4 Pharmacological Agents to Prevent CA-AKI

Multiple pharmacological agents with different physiological actions have been evaluated for the prevention of CA-AKI. Some were found to be ineffective and in some cases potentially deleterious, whereas data on other agents are mixed, with some studies demonstrating benefit and others showing no effect (Table 6.5).

Loop diuretics inhibit active sodium transport in the ascending limb of the loop of Henle and by virtue of their potential to reduce tubular epithelial cell oxygen utilization were hypothesized to decrease the risk of renal injury from iodinated contrast. However, data from clinical trials fail to support the use of these agents for the prevention of CA-AKI [91]. A clinical trial by Solomon et al. reported a higher incidence of CA-AKI among patients who received peri-procedural furosemide and hypotonic saline compared with hypotonic saline alone (40% vs. 11%, $p = <0.02$) [91]. The lack of benefit with furosemide in this study mirrored the findings of an earlier study that found a higher risk for CA-AKI with the use of this agent [92].

Several studies have investigated the administration of dopamine as a potential treatment to reduce the risk for contrast-induced renal injury [93–95]. While small studies suggested a beneficial effect, larger clinical trials have failed to

Table 6.5 Pharmacological agents for CA-AKI prevention

Ineffective	Indeterminate effectiveness
Loop diuretics[a]	Atrial natriuretic peptide
Dopamine[a]	Theophylline/ aminophylline
Fenoldopam[a]	Statins
Calcium channel blockers	Prostaglandin analogs
N-acetylcysteine	Allopurinol
	Acetazolamide

[a]Associated with adverse effects

confirm these findings [93, 95, 96]. Weisberg et al. found no difference in the incidence of CA-AKI among patients who received dopamine and hypotonic saline compared to patients who received just hypotonic saline, yet observed higher rates of CA-AKI among diabetics who received dopamine [95]. Fenoldopam, a selective dopamine receptor agonist was reported in a series of small, mostly non-randomzied studies to be protective against the development of CA-AKI [97–102]. Subsequent studies, including a clinical trial by Stone et al. that enrolled 315 patients with CKD undergoing coronary angiography, failed to demonstrate a benefit of fenoldopam for the prevention of CA-AKI [103].

Atrial natriuretic peptide (ANP), which has renal vasodilatory properties, was studied in a multi-center randomized controlled trial by Kurnik et al. that enrolled 247 patients with baseline CKD. This trial reported no reduction in CA-AKI with the use of ANP compared to placebo [104]. Conversely, Morikawa and colleagues studied 254 patients with CKD undergoing coronary angiography and reported a lower incidence of CA-AKI among patients who received ANP and IV fluids compared to patients who received just IV fluids [105]. In light of the discordant findings on the benefit of ANP, and the potential side effects of this therapy, the use of ANP for the prevention of CA-AKI is not currently recommended.

Because of the role adenosine may play in the pathogenesis of CA-AKI, studies have examined the potential for adenosine antagonists such as theophylline to reduce the risk for renal injury from iodinated contrast [106, 107]. A clinical trial by Early et al. that enrolled 80 patients found no benefit to theophylline for the prevention of CA-AKI [106]. Conversely, Huber et al. reported a lower incidence of CA-AKI with the use of theophylline in a study of 100 patients with CKD. Subsequent meta-analyses reported inconsistent findings on the potential benefit of theophylline [108–110]. As theophylline has potential side effects, its use for the prevention of CA-AKI cannot be recommended based on currently available data.

Clinical trials on the role of statins for the prevention of CA-AKI have demonstrated conflicting findings although two recent trials demonstrated a benefit [111, 112]. However, the findings of these studies should be viewed with an understanding that the administration of rosuvastatin has been shown to be associated with an increase in estimated glomerular filtration rate [113]. Hence, the use of small increments in SCr as an endpoint in trials investigating statins for the prevention of CA-AKI is problematic due to the potential for these agents to affect renal function parameters independently of any potentially protective effect against contrast.

N-acetylcysteine (NAC) is an anti-oxidant with vasodilatory effects that has been the focus of substantial research as a preventive intervention for CA-AKI. The initial clinical trial of NAC by Tepel et al. randomized 83 patients and found a lower incidence of CA-AKI with NAC than with placebo (2% vs. 21%, $p = 0.01$) [114]. Since the publication of this study, a multitude of clinical trials evaluating NAC for the prevention of CA-AKI have been published, yielding highly conflicting results [50, 114–138]. The acetylcysteine for contrast nephropathy trial enrolled over 2300 patients undergoing angiography and found no reduction in the risk for CA-AKI with oral NAC compared with placebo. However, the large majority of participants in this trial were at low risk for CA-AKI, which significantly reduced the generalizability of the findings to those most likely to develop this condition. Multiple systematic reviews and meta-analyses sought to reconcile the discordant clinical trial findings, yet collectively documented similarly incongruous results [110, 139–148]. However, the recently published Prevention of Serious Adverse Events Following Angiography (PRESERVE) trial, which enrolled 4993 patients undergoing nonemergent angiography, has finally provided a definitive answer to the effectiveness of NAC [149]. As part of its 2 × 2 factorial design, PRESERVE randomized 2495 patients to receive oral NAC (1200 mg twice daily for 5 days beginning on the day of angiography), and 2498 patients to receive matching oral placebo [149].

The study demonstrated that compared with oral placebo, NAC was not associated with a reduction in 90-day death, need for dialysis, or persistent impairment in kidney function (OR = 1.02, 95% CI: 0.78–1.33), nor was it associated with a decrease in the incidence of CA-AKI (OR = 1.06, 95% CI: 0.87–1.28). Based on these findings in a very large and high-risk patient population, there is currently no role for oral NAC for the prevention of CA-AKI or associated serious, adverse outcomes.

While none of the aforementioned agents, or others including calcium channel blockers, prostaglandins, acetazolamide, or mannitol have been definitively shown to prevent CA-AKI, many of the trials of pharmacological thereapies were limited by small sample size, use of surrogate primary study endpoints based on nominal increments in SCr, and in some cases, inclusion of low-risk patients. Although current recommendations for the prevention of CA-AKI do not incorporate the administration of any of these pharmacological therapies, future research, other than with NAC, is needed to examine these and other novel agents in large, high-risk patient groups.

6.5.5 Intravenous Fluids for the Prevention of CA-AKI

The provision of intravenous (IV) fluid prior to and following contrast administration has been shown to reduce the risk for CA-AKI [91, 150–152]. Expanding the intravascular space with IV fluid is believed to counteract the vasoconstrictive effect of iodinated contrast and to decrease the concentration and viscosity of contrast media in the tubular lumen, reducing tubular damage [153].

Following a series of observational studies suggesting a benefit of IV fluid, Solomon et al. conducted a clinical trial that compared IV 0.45% saline alone to IV 0.45% saline with 25 g of IV mannitol or with 80 mg of IV furosemide [91]. CA-AKI occurred less frequently in patients who received IV fluid alone compared to IV fluids with either mannitol or furosemide. Subsequently, Trivedi et al. conducted a clinical trial that randomized patients undergoing coronary angiography to receive IV isotonic saline for 12 h prior to and 12 h following the procedure or unrestricted oral fluids [152]. The trial was stopped at a preliminary time point for safety reasons given a substantially lower incidence of CA-AKI in patients who received IV saline (3.7% vs. 34.6%; $p = 0.005$). Mueller et al. enrolled over 1600 patients undergoing coronary angiography into a trial that compared peri-procedural IV 0.45% saline to 0.9% saline [151]. Although the overall study population was at relatively low risk for renal injury, the administration of 0.9% saline was associated with a lower incidence of CA-AKI than 0.45% saline (0.7% v 2.0%, $p = 0.04$).

Recent research on IV fluid composition and the prevention of CA-AKI has focused on the comparative effects of isotonic sodium bicarbonate and isotonic sodium chloride. The underlying hypothesis for the benefit of sodium bicarbonate relates to enhanced urinary alkalinization with the filtration of $HCO3^-$ that decreases the generation of reactive oxygen species (ROS) and attenuates renal injury. This hypothesis was first tested by Merten et al. in a clinical trial that enrolled 119 patients and demonstrated a lower incidence of CA-AKI with IV isotonic bicarbonate compared with IV isotonic saline (1.6% vs. 13.6%, $p = 0.02$) [150]. These results resulted in a proliferation of clinical trials, some reporting a lower incidence of CA-AKI with IV sodium bicarbonate and others demonstrating no difference [51, 52, 154–160]. As occurred following the publications of clinical trials of NAC, these incongruent clinical trial results led to the performance of systematic reviews and meta-analyses, the results of which were as disparate as the component clinical trials [155, 161–169]. To definitively address the persistent clinical equipoise on the role of IV sodium bicarbonate, the PRESERVE trial randomized 4993 high-risk patients to receive IV isotonic sodium bicarbonate ($N = 2511$) or IV isotonic sodium chloride ($N = 2482$) prior to, during, and following angiography [149]. Compared with IV sodium chloride, sodium bicarbonate did not result in a decrease in 90-day death, need for dialysis, or persistent impairment in kidney function (OR = 0.93; 95% CI: 0.72–1.22) or in the incidence of CA-AKI (OR = 1.16, 95% CI: 0.96–1.41) [149]. Thus, at the present time, IV isotonic sodium chloride should be considered the standard of care with regard to the provision of IV fluid for the prevention of CA-AKI and associated adverse outcomes.

6.5.6 Limitations of Clinical Trials to Date

Notwithstanding the substantial effort to identify pharmacological and non-pharmacological interventions for the prevention of CA-AKI, many of the clinical trials to date had methodological limiations that precluded meaningful interpretation of potential benefit. First, most trials used small increments in SCr as the primary study endpoint based on observational data demonstrating an association of such biochemical perturbations with serious, adverse outcomes. However, the causal nature of such associations has not yet been proven, as it is plausible that small changes in kidney function are a marker of more hemodynamically tenuous patients who are at increased risk for adverse outcomes, rather than a mediator of such outcomes. Moreover, most patients who manifest small increments in SCr following contrast-enhanced procedures do not experience serious adverse outcomes (Fig. 6.2). The use of a surrogate primary endpoint defined by nominal increments in SCr, which occurs much more commonly after contrast-enhanced procedures than serious, adverse outcomes (e.g., death, need for dialysis), has facilitated the design of clinical trials with inflated event rates and relatively small sample sizes that are unable to effectively determine whether interventions reduce the development of clinical outcomes of greatest importance to patients and providers. Designing clinical trials based on the estimated effect of interventions on less common but far more serious patient-centered outcomes (e.g., death, need for dialysis) necessitates the enrollment of large numbers of patients as evidenced by the PRESERVE trial [149]. Unless and until the association of CA-AKI with serious, adverse short- and long-term events is confirmed to be causal, the conduct of clinical trials that utilize primary outcomes defined by small biochemically based short-term changes in kidney function to determine preventive efficacy will continue to generate disparate and inconclusive findings. Finally, some of the trials to date of preventive interventions for CA-AKI enrolled patients at low risk for CA-AKI. This can lead to

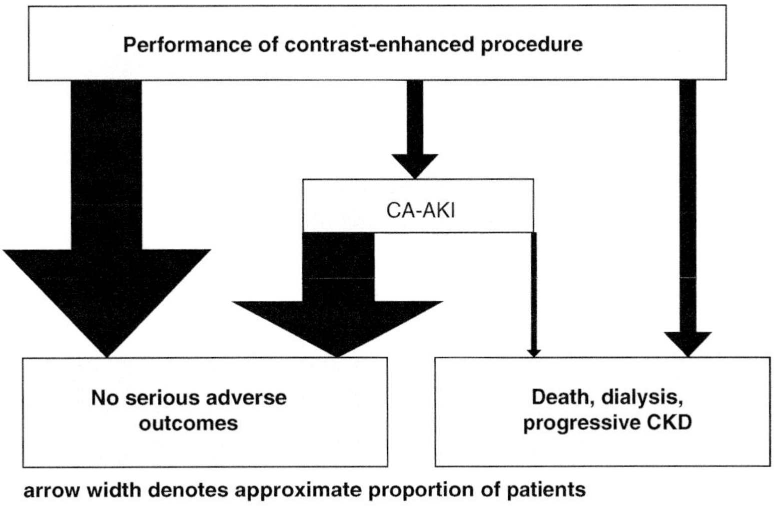

Fig. 6.2 Outcomes of contrast-enhanced procedures. Most patients undergoing contrast-enhanced procedures do not develop AKI (white arrow). Among patients with AKI defined by small increments in serum creatinine, most do not experience serious adverse outcomes (dark gray arrow)

lower-than-expected rates of CA-AKI, decreased statistical power, and reduced capacity to determine efficacy in patients truly at increased risk.

6.5.7 Current Recommendations for the Prevention of CA-AKI

The initial step in preventing the development of CA-AKI involves the identification of patients at increased risk. For such patients, consideration should be made to perform alternative imaging procedures that do not require iodinated contrast but that provide comparable diagnostic yield. Among those who require intravascular contrast, all modifiable risk factors should be addressed. Non-steroidal anti-inflammatory medications should be discontinued prior to contrast administration and held until CA-AKI has been ruled out. The lowest necessary volume of either low or iso-osmolal contrast should be used. Isotonic IV sodium chloride should be administered prior to, during, and after the procedure [149]. For hospitalized patients, particularly those undergoing non-emergent procedures, isotonic IV sodium chloride can be delivered at a rate of 1 ml/kg/h for 12 h preceding, during, and for 12 h following the procedure. For subjects undergoing outpatient or urgent inpatient procedures, IV sodium chloride can be administered at a rate of 3 ml/kg/h over 1 h prior to and 1–1.5 ml/kg/h during and for 4–6 h following contrast administration. The POSEIDON trial documented that the provision of isotonic IV fluid to patients undergoing coronary angiography with elevated left ventricular end-diastolic pressure is effective and safe [170]. Therefore, isotonic IV sodium chloride should be administered to patients with non-decompensated heart failure, albeit with careful monitoring for the development of pulmonary compromise. At present, there is no role for other pharmacological interventions for the prevention of CA-AKI. Similarly, available data do not support the discontinuation of diuretics or blockers of the renin-angiotensin aldosterone axis prior to contrast administration. In patients at-risk for CA-AKI, including those who receive appropriate preventive care, it is essential to assess SCr 48–96 h following contrast administration to determine whether CA-AKI has developed. This permits the timely implementation of supportive care to mitigate further renal injury.

Conclusion

The administration of intravascular iodinated contrast media is a common cause of acute kidney injury. Past research has elucidated the pathophysiology of and risk factors for CA-AKI. A series of studies, principally observational, have shown that CA-AKI is associated with serious adverse short- and long-term outcomes; findings that have likely contributed to the under-utilization of indicated diagnostic and therapeutic procedures in patients with kidney disease. However, the causal nature of these associations remains unproven. Therefore, contrast-enhanced procedures with clear clinical indications should be performed, albeit with appropriate preventive care. The cornerstone of prevention of CA-AKI is the provision of peri-procedural isotonic IV fluids, namely sodium chloride. Additional studies that enroll large numbers of high-risk patients and evaluate clinically relevant patient-centered outcomes are needed to determine if other pharmacological or non-pharmacological interventions have a role in the prevention of this iatrogenic condition.

References

1. Heyman SN, Brezis M, Epstein FH, Spokes K, Silva P, Rosen S. Early renal medullary hypoxic injury from radiocontrast and indomethacin. Kidney Int. 1991;40:632–42.
2. Heyman SN, Reichman J, Brezis M. Pathophysiology of radiocontrast nephropathy: a role for medullary hypoxia. Investig Radiol. 1999;34:685–91.
3. Nicot GS, Merle LJ, Charmes JP, et al. Transient glomerular proteinuria, enzymuria, and nephrotoxic reaction induced by radiocontrast media. JAMA. 1984;252:2432–4.
4. Haller C, Hizoh I. The cytotoxicity of iodinated radiocontrast agents on renal cells in vitro. Investig Radiol. 2004;39:149–54.
5. Hizoh I, Haller C. Radiocontrast-induced renal tubular cell apoptosis: hypertonic versus oxidative stress. Investig Radiol. 2002;37:428–34.

6. Hizoh I, Strater J, Schick CS, Kubler W, Haller C. Radiocontrast-induced DNA fragmentation of renal tubular cells in vitro: role of hypertonicity. Nephrol Dial Transplant. 1998;13:911–8.
7. Hardiek K, Katholi RE, Ramkumar V, Deitrick C. Proximal tubule cell response to radiographic contrast media. Am J Physiol Renal Physiol. 2001;280:F61–70.
8. Heyman SN, Rosen S, Khamaisi M, Idee JM, Rosenberger C. Reactive oxygen species and the pathogenesis of radiocontrast-induced nephropathy. Investig Radiol. 2010;45:188–95.
9. Moreau JF, Droz D, Noel LH, Leibowitch J, Jungers P, Michel JR. Tubular nephrotoxicity of water-soluble iodinated contrast media. Investig Radiol. 1980;15:S54–60.
10. Humes HD, Hunt DA, White MD. Direct toxic effect of the radiocontrast agent diatrizoate on renal proximal tubule cells. Am J Phys. 1987;252:F246–55.
11. Bakris GL, Lass N, Gaber AO, Jones JD, Burnett JC Jr. Radiocontrast medium-induced declines in renal function: a role for oxygen free radicals. Am J Phys. 1990;258:F115–20.
12. Bakris GL, Gaber AO, Jones JD. Oxygen free radical involvement in urinary Tamm-Horsfall protein excretion after intrarenal injection of contrast medium. Radiology. 1990;175:57–60.
13. Parvez Z, Rahman MA, Moncada R. Contrast media-induced lipid peroxidation in the rat kidney. Investig Radiol. 1989;24:697–702.
14. Yoshioka T, Fogo A, Beckman JK. Reduced activity of antioxidant enzymes underlies contrast media-induced renal injury in volume depletion. Kidney Int. 1992;41:1008–15.
15. Erley CM, Heyne N, Burgert K, Langanke J, Risler T, Osswald H. Prevention of radiocontrast-induced nephropathy by adenosine antagonists in rats with chronic nitric oxide deficiency. J Am Soc Nephrol. 1997;8:1125–32.
16. Schnackenberg CG. Physiological and pathophysiological roles of oxygen radicals in the renal microvasculature. Am J Physiol Regul Integr Comp Physiol. 2002;282:R335–42.
17. Szabo G, Bahrle S, Stumpf N, et al. Poly(ADP-Ribose) polymerase inhibition reduces reperfusion injury after heart transplantation. Circ Res. 2002;90:100–6.
18. Weisbord SD, Mor MK, Resnick AL, et al. Prevention, incidence, and outcomes of contrast-induced acute kidney injury. Arch Intern Med. 2008;168:1325–32.
19. Shema L, Ore L, Geron R, Kristal B. Contrast-induced nephropathy among Israeli hospitalized patients: incidence, risk factors, length of stay and mortality. Isr Med Assoc J. 2009;11:460–4.
20. D'Elia JA, Gleason RE, Alday M, et al. Nephrotoxicity from angiographic contrast material. A prospective study. Am J Med. 1982;72:719–25.
21. Bruce RJ, Djamali A, Shinki K, Michel SJ, Fine JP, Pozniak MA. Background fluctuation of kidney function versus contrast-induced nephrotoxicity. AJR Am J Roentgenol. 2009;192:711–8.
22. McDonald JS, McDonald RJ, Carter RE, Katzberg RW, Kallmes DF, Williamson EE. Risk of intravenous contrast material-mediated acute kidney injury: a propensity score-matched study stratified by baseline-estimated glomerular filtration rate. Radiology. 2014;271:65–73.
23. McDonald JS, McDonald RJ, Lieske JC, et al. Risk of acute kidney injury, dialysis, and mortality in patients with chronic kidney disease after intravenous contrast material exposure. Mayo Clin Proc. 2015;90:1046–53.
24. McDonald RJ, McDonald JS, Bida JP, et al. Intravenous contrast material-induced nephropathy: causal or coincident phenomenon? Radiology. 2013;267:106–18.
25. McDonald RJ, McDonald JS, Newhouse JH, Davenport MS. Controversies in contrast material-induced acute kidney injury: closing in on the truth? Radiology. 2015;277:627–32.
26. Wilhelm-Leen E, Montez-Rath ME, Chertow G. Estimating the risk of radiocontrast-associated nephropathy. J Am Soc Nephrol. 2017;28:653–9.
27. McDonald JS, McDonald RJ, Comin J, et al. Frequency of acute kidney injury following intravenous contrast medium administration: a systematic review and meta-analysis. Radiology. 2013;267:119–28.
28. McCullough PA, Adam A, Becker CR, et al. Risk prediction of contrast-induced nephropathy. Am J Cardiol. 2006;98:27K–36K.
29. McCullough PA, Wolyn R, Rocher LL, Levin RN, O'Neill WW. Acute renal failure after coronary intervention: incidence, risk factors, and relationship to mortality. Am J Med. 1997;103:368–75.
30. Rudnick MR, Goldfarb S, Wexler L, et al. Nephrotoxicity of ionic and nonionic contrast media in 1196 patients: a randomized trial. The Iohexol Cooperative Study. Kidney Int. 1995;47:254–61.
31. Cramer BC, Parfrey PS, Hutchinson TA, et al. Renal function following infusion of radiologic contrast material. A prospective controlled study. Arch Intern Med. 1985;145:87–9.
32. Weisberg LS, Kurnik PB, Kurnik BR. Risk of radiocontrast nephropathy in patients with and without diabetes mellitus. Kidney Int. 1994;45:259–65.
33. Stolker JM, McCullough PA, Rao S, et al. Pre-procedural glucose levels and the risk for contrast-induced acute kidney injury in patients undergoing coronary angiography. J Am Coll Cardiol. 2010;55:1433–40.
34. Taliercio CP, Vlietstra RE, Fisher LD, Burnett JC. Risks for renal dysfunction with cardiac angiography. Ann Intern Med. 1986;104:501–4.
35. Gomes AS, Baker JD, Martin-Paredero V, et al. Acute renal dysfunction after major arteriography. AJR Am J Roentgenol. 1985;145:1249–53.
36. Ahmad SR, Kortepeter C, Brinker A, Chen M, Beitz J. Renal failure associated with the use of celecoxib and rofecoxib. Drug Saf. 2002;25:537–44.

37. Nikolsky E, Mehran R, Lasic Z, et al. Low hematocrit predicts contrast-induced nephropathy after percutaneous coronary interventions. Kidney Int. 2005;67:706–13.
38. Mehran R, Aymong ED, Nikolsky E, et al. A simple risk score for prediction of contrast-induced nephropathy after percutaneous coronary intervention: development and initial validation. J Am Coll Cardiol. 2004;44:1393–9.
39. Hsu RK, Hsu CY. Proteinuria and reduced glomerular filtration rate as risk factors for acute kidney injury. Curr Opin Nephrol Hypertens. 2011;20:211–7.
40. He F, Zhang J, Lu ZQ, et al. Risk factors and outcomes of acute kidney injury after intracoronary stent implantation. World J Emerg Med. 2012;3:197–201.
41. Marenzi G, Assanelli E, Campodonico J, et al. Contrast volume during primary percutaneous coronary intervention and subsequent contrast-induced nephropathy and mortality. Ann Intern Med. 2009;150:170–7.
42. Nyman U, Almen T, Aspelin P, Hellstrom M, Kristiansson M, Sterner G. Contrast-medium-Induced nephropathy correlated to the ratio between dose in gram iodine and estimated GFR in ml/min. Acta Radiol. 2005;46:830–42.
43. Worasuwannarak S, Pornratanarangsi S. Prediction of contrast-induced nephropathy in diabetic patients undergoing elective cardiac catheterization or PCI: role of volume-to-creatinine clearance ratio and iodine dose-to-creatinine clearance ratio. J Med Assoc Thai. 2010;93 Suppl 1:S29–34.
44. Barrett BJ, Carlisle EJ. Metaanalysis of the relative nephrotoxicity of high- and low-osmolality iodinated contrast media. Radiology. 1993;188:171–8.
45. Levy EM, Viscoli CM, Horwitz RI. The effect of acute renal failure on mortality. A cohort analysis. JAMA. 1996;275:1489–94.
46. Bartholomew BA, Harjai KJ, Dukkipati S, et al. Impact of nephropathy after percutaneous coronary intervention and a method for risk stratification. Am J Cardiol. 2004;93:1515–9.
47. From AM, Bartholmai BJ, Williams AW, Cha SS, McDonald FS. Mortality associated with nephropathy after radiographic contrast exposure. Mayo Clin Proc. 2008;83:1095–100.
48. Weisbord SD, Chen H, Stone RA, et al. Associations of increases in serum creatinine with mortality and length of hospital stay after coronary angiography. J Am Soc Nephrol. 2006;17:2871–7.
49. Rihal CS, Textor SC, Grill DE, et al. Incidence and prognostic importance of acute renal failure after percutaneous coronary intervention. Circulation. 2002;105:2259–64.
50. Marenzi G, Assanelli E, Marana I, et al. N-acetylcysteine and contrast-induced nephropathy in primary angioplasty. N Engl J Med. 2006;354:2773–82.
51. Maioli M, Toso A, Leoncini M, et al. Sodium bicarbonate versus saline for the prevention of contrast-induced nephropathy in patients with renal dysfunction undergoing coronary angiography or intervention. J Am Coll Cardiol. 2008;52: 599–604.
52. Adolph E, Holdt-Lehmann B, Chatterjee T, et al. Renal Insufficiency Following Radiocontrast Exposure Trial (REINFORCE): a randomized comparison of sodium bicarbonate versus sodium chloride hydration for the prevention of contrast-induced nephropathy. Coron Artery Dis. 2008;19:413–9.
53. Subramanian S, Tumlin J, Bapat B, Zyczynski T. Economic burden of contrast-induced nephropathy: implications for prevention strategies. J Med Econ. 2007;10:119–34.
54. Goldenberg I, Chonchol M, Guetta V. Reversible acute kidney injury following contrast exposure and the risk of long-term mortality. Am J Nephrol. 2009;29:136–44.
55. Harjai KJ, Raizada A, Shenoy C, et al. A comparison of contemporary definitions of contrast nephropathy in patients undergoing percutaneous coronary intervention and a proposal for a novel nephropathy grading system. Am J Cardiol. 2008;101:812–9.
56. Roghi A, Savonitto S, Cavallini C, et al. Impact of acute renal failure following percutaneous coronary intervention on long-term mortality. J Cardiovasc Med (Hagerstown). 2008;9:375–81.
57. Solomon RJ, Mehran R, Natarajan MK, et al. Contrast-induced nephropathy and long-term adverse events: cause and effect? Clin J Am Soc Nephrol. 2009;4:1162–9.
58. Brown JR, Malenka DJ, DeVries JT, et al. Transient and persistent renal dysfunction are predictors of survival after percutaneous coronary intervention: insights from the Dartmouth Dynamic Registry. Catheter Cardiovasc Interv. 2008;72:347–54.
59. James MT, Ghali WA, Tonelli M, et al. Acute kidney injury following coronary angiography is associated with a long-term decline in kidney function. Kidney Int. 2010;78:803–9.
60. James MT, Ghali WA, Knudtson ML, et al. Associations between acute kidney injury and cardiovascular and renal outcomes after coronary angiography. Circulation. 2011;123:409–16.
61. Chertow GM, Normand SL, McNeil BJ. "Renalism": inappropriately low rates of coronary angiography in elderly individuals with renal insufficiency. J Am Soc Nephrol. 2004;15:2462–8.
62. Han JH, Chandra A, Mulgund J, et al. Chronic kidney disease in patients with non-ST-segment elevation acute coronary syndromes. Am J Med. 2006;119:248–54.
63. Szummer K, Lundman P, Jacobson SH, et al. Relation between renal function, presentation, use of therapies and in-hospital complications in acute coronary syndrome: data from the SWEDEHEART register. J Intern Med. 2010;268:40–9.
64. Goldenberg I, Subirana I, Boyko V, et al. Relation between renal function and outcomes in patients with non-ST-segment elevation acute coronary syndrome: real-world data from the European Public

Health Outcome Research and Indicators Collection Project. Arch Intern Med. 2010;170:888–95.
65. Nauta ST, van Domburg RT, Nuis RJ, Akkerhuis M, Deckers JW. Decline in 20-year mortality after myocardial infarction in patients with chronic kidney disease: evolution from the prethrombolysis to the percutaneous coronary intervention era. Kidney Int. 2013;84:353–8.
66. James MT, Tonelli M, Ghali WA, et al. Renal outcomes associated with invasive versus conservative management of acute coronary syndrome: propensity matched cohort study. BMJ. 2013;347:f4151.
67. Aspelin P, Aubry P, Fransson SG, Strasser R, Willenbrock R, Berg KJ. Nephrotoxic effects in high-risk patients undergoing angiography. N Engl J Med. 2003;348:491–9.
68. Jo SH, Youn TJ, Koo BK, et al. Renal toxicity evaluation and comparison between visipaque (iodixanol) and hexabrix (ioxaglate) in patients with renal insufficiency undergoing coronary angiography: the RECOVER study: a randomized controlled trial. J Am Coll Cardiol. 2006;48:924–30.
69. Carraro M, Malalan F, Antonione R, et al. Effects of a dimeric vs a monomeric nonionic contrast medium on renal function in patients with mild to moderate renal insufficiency: a double-blind, randomized clinical trial. Eur Radiol. 1998;8:144–7.
70. Chalmers N, Jackson RW. Comparison of iodixanol and iohexol in renal impairment. Br J Radiol. 1999;72:701–3.
71. Juergens CP, Winter JP, Nguyen-Do P, et al. Nephrotoxic effects of iodixanol and iopromide in patients with abnormal renal function receiving N-acetylcysteine and hydration before coronary angiography and intervention: a randomized trial. Intern Med J. 2009;39:25–31.
72. Laskey W, Aspelin P, Davidson C, et al. Nephrotoxicity of iodixanol versus iopamidol in patients with chronic kidney disease and diabetes mellitus undergoing coronary angiographic procedures. Am Heart J 2009;158:822–8 e3.
73. Nguyen SA, Suranyi P, Ravenel JG, et al. Iso-osmolality versus low-osmolality iodinated contrast medium at intravenous contrast-enhanced CT: effect on kidney function. Radiology. 2008;248:97–105.
74. Solomon RJ, Natarajan MK, Doucet S, et al. Cardiac Angiography in Renally Impaired Patients (CARE) study: a randomized double-blind trial of contrast-induced nephropathy in patients with chronic kidney disease. Circulation. 2007;115:3189–96.
75. McCullough PA, Bertrand ME, Brinker JA, Stacul F. A meta-analysis of the renal safety of isosmolar iodixanol compared with low-osmolar contrast media. J Am Coll Cardiol. 2006;48:692–9.
76. Sharma SK, Kini A. Effect of nonionic radiocontrast agents on the occurrence of contrast-induced nephropathy in patients with mild-moderate chronic renal insufficiency: pooled analysis of the randomized trials. Catheter Cardiovasc Interv. 2005;65:386–93.
77. Solomon R. The role of osmolality in the incidence of contrast-induced nephropathy: a systematic review of angiographic contrast media in high risk patients. Kidney Int. 2005;68:2256–63.
78. Reed M, Meier P, Tamhane UU, Welch KB, Moscucci M, Gurm HS. The relative renal safety of iodixanol compared with low-osmolar contrast media: a meta-analysis of randomized controlled trials. JACC Cardiovasc Interv. 2009;2:645–54.
79. Heinrich MC, Haberle L, Muller V, Bautz W, Uder M. Nephrotoxicity of iso-osmolar iodixanol compared with nonionic low-osmolar contrast media: meta-analysis of randomized controlled trials. Radiology. 2009;250:68–86.
80. Anderson JL, Adams CD, Antman EM, et al. 2012 ACCF/AHA focused update incorporated into the ACCF/AHA 2007 guidelines for the management of patients with unstable angina/non-ST-elevation myocardial infarction: a report of the American College of Cardiology Foundation/American Heart Association Task Force on Practice Guidelines. Circulation. 2013;127:e663–828.
81. ESUR Guidelines on Contrast Media; 2008.
82. Lee PT, Chou KJ, Liu CP, et al. Renal protection for coronary angiography in advanced renal failure patients by prophylactic hemodialysis. A randomized controlled trial. J Am Coll Cardiol. 2007;50:1015–20.
83. Reinecke H, Fobker M, Wellmann J, et al. A randomized controlled trial comparing hydration therapy to additional hemodialysis or N-acetylcysteine for the prevention of contrast medium-induced nephropathy: the Dialysis-versus-Diuresis (DVD) Trial. Clin Res Cardiol. 2007;96:130–9.
84. Holscher B, Heitmeyer C, Fobker M, Breithardt G, Schaefer RM, Reinecke H. Predictors for contrast media-induced nephropathy and long-term survival: prospectively assessed data from the randomized controlled Dialysis-Versus-Diuresis (DVD) trial. Can J Cardiol. 2008;24:845–50.
85. Hsieh YC, Ting CT, Liu TJ, Wang CL, Chen YT, Lee WL. Short- and long-term renal outcomes of immediate prophylactic hemodialysis after cardiovascular catheterizations in patients with severe renal insufficiency. Int J Cardiol. 2005;101:407–13.
86. Berger ED, Bader BD, Bosker J, Risler T, Erley CM. Contrast media-induced kidney failure cannot be prevented by hemodialysisDtsch Med Wochenschr. 2001;126:162–6.
87. Frank H, Werner D, Lorusso V, et al. Simultaneous hemodialysis during coronary angiography fails to prevent radiocontrast-induced nephropathy in chronic renal failure. Clin Nephrol. 2003;60:176–82.
88. Huber W, Jeschke B, Kreymann B, et al. Haemodialysis for the prevention of contrast-induced nephropathy: outcome of 31 patients with severely impaired renal function, comparison with patients at similar risk and review. Invest Radiol. 2002;37:471–81.
89. Marenzi G, Lauri G, Campodonico J, et al. Comparison of two hemofiltration protocols for

prevention of contrast-induced nephropathy in high-risk patients. Am J Med. 2006;119:155–62.
90. Marenzi G, Marana I, Lauri G, et al. The prevention of radiocontrast-agent-induced nephropathy by hemofiltration. N Engl J Med. 2003;349:1333–40.
91. Solomon R, Werner C, Mann D, D'Elia J, Silva P. Effects of saline, mannitol, and furosemide to prevent acute decreases in renal function induced by radiocontrast agents. [see comments.]. N Engl J Med. 1994;331:1416–20.
92. Weinstein JM, Heyman S, Brezis M. Potential deleterious effect of furosemide in radiocontrast nephropathy. Nephron. 1992;62:413–5.
93. Hall KA, Wong RW, Hunter GC, et al. Contrast-induced nephrotoxicity: the effects of vasodilator therapy. J Surg Res. 1992;53:317–20.
94. Kellum JA. The use of diuretics and dopamine in acute renal failure: a systematic review of the evidence. Crit Care (Lond). 1997;1:53–9.
95. Weisberg LS, Kurnik PB, Kurnik BR. Dopamine and renal blood flow in radiocontrast-induced nephropathy in humans. Ren Fail. 1993;15:61–8.
96. Kapoor A, Sinha N, Sharma RK, et al. Use of dopamine in prevention of contrast induced acute renal failure—a randomised study. Int J Cardiol. 1996;53:233–6.
97. Bakris GL, Lass NA, Glock D. Renal hemodynamics in radiocontrast medium-induced renal dysfunction: a role for dopamine-1 receptors. Kidney Int. 1999;56:206–10.
98. Madyoon H, Croushore L. Use of fenoldopam for prevention of radiocontrast nephropathy in the cardiac catheterization laboratory: a case series. J Interv Cardiol. 2001;14:179–85.
99. Madyoon H, Croushore L, Weaver D, Mathur V. Use of fenoldopam to prevent radiocontrast nephropathy in high-risk patients. Catheter Cardiovasc Interv. 2001;53:341–5.
100. Singer I, Epstein M. Potential of dopamine A-1 agonists in the management of acute renal failure. Am J Kidney Dis. 1998;31:743–55.
101. Madyoon H. Clinical experience with the use of fenoldopam for prevention of radiocontrast nephropathy in high-risk patients. Rev Cardiovasc Med. 2001;2 Suppl 1:S26–30.
102. Mathur VS. The role of the DA1 receptor agonist fenoldopam in the management of critically ill, transplant, and hypertensive patients. Rev Cardiovasc Med. 2003;4 Suppl 1:S35–40.
103. Stone GW, McCullough PA, Tumlin JA, et al. Fenoldopam mesylate for the prevention of contrast-induced nephropathy: a randomized controlled trial. JAMA. 2003;290:2284–91.
104. Kurnik BR, Allgren RL, Genter FC, Solomon RJ, Bates ER, Weisberg LS. Prospective study of atrial natriuretic peptide for the prevention of radiocontrast-induced nephropathy. Am J Kidney Dis. 1998;31:674–80.
105. Morikawa S, Sone T, Tsuboi H, et al. Renal protective effects and the prevention of contrast-induced nephropathy by atrial natriuretic peptide. J Am Coll Cardiol. 2009;53:1040–6.
106. Erley CM, Duda SH, Rehfuss D, et al. Prevention of radiocontrast-media-induced nephropathy in patients with pre-existing renal insufficiency by hydration in combination with the adenosine antagonist theophylline. Nephrol Dial Transplant. 1999;14:1146–9.
107. Katholi RE, Taylor GJ, McCann WP, et al. Nephrotoxicity from contrast media: attenuation with theophylline. Radiology. 1995;195:17–22.
108. Bagshaw SM, Ghali WA. Theophylline for prevention of contrast-induced nephropathy: a systematic review and meta-analysis. Arch Intern Med. 2005;165:1087–93.
109. Ix JH, McCulloch CE, Chertow GM. Theophylline for the prevention of radiocontrast nephropathy: a meta-analysis. Nephrol Dial Transplant. 2004;19:2747–53.
110. Kelly AM, Dwamena B, Cronin P, Bernstein SJ, Carlos RC. Meta-analysis: effectiveness of drugs for preventing contrast-induced nephropathy. Ann Intern Med. 2008;148:284–94.
111. Han Y, Zhu G, Han L, et al. Short-term rosuvastatin therapy for prevention of contrast-induced acute kidney injury in patients with diabetes and chronic kidney disease. J Am Coll Cardiol. 2014;63:62–70.
112. Leoncini M, Toso A, Maioli M, Tropeano F, Villani S, Bellandi F. Early high-dose rosuvastatin for contrast-induced nephropathy prevention in acute coronary syndrome: results from the PRATO-ACS Study (Protective Effect of Rosuvastatin and Antiplatelet Therapy On contrast-induced acute kidney injury and myocardial damage in patients with Acute Coronary Syndrome). J Am Coll Cardiol. 2014;63:71–9.
113. Vidt DG, Harris S, McTaggart F, Ditmarsch M, Sager PT, Sorof JM. Effect of short-term rosuvastatin treatment on estimated glomerular filtration rate. Am J Cardiol. 2006;97:1602–6.
114. Tepel M, van der Giet M, Schwarzfeld C, Laufer U, Liermann D, Zidek W. Prevention of radiographic-contrast-agent-induced reductions in renal function by acetylcysteine. N Engl J Med. 2000;343:180–4.
115. Baker CS, Baker LR. Prevention of contrast nephropathy after cardiac catheterisation. Heart. 2001:361–2.
116. Briguori C, Manganelli F, Scarpato P, et al. Acetylcysteine and contrast agent-associated nephrotoxicity. J Am Coll Cardiol. 2002;40:298–303.
117. Coyle LC, Rodriguez A, Jeschke RE, Simon-Lee A, Abbott KC, Taylor AJ. Acetylcysteine In Diabetes (AID): a randomized study of acetylcysteine for the prevention of contrast nephropathy in diabetics. Am Heart J. 2006;151:1032 e9–12.
118. Kay J, Chow WH, Chan TM, et al. Acetylcysteine for prevention of acute deterioration of renal function following elective coronary angiography and intervention: a randomized controlled trial. JAMA. 2003;289:553–8.

119. Gomes VO, Poli de Figueredo CE, Caramori P, et al. N-acetylcysteine does not prevent contrast induced nephropathy after cardiac catheterisation with an ionic low osmolality contrast medium: a multicentre clinical trial. Heart. 2005;91:774–8.
120. Fung JW, Szeto CC, Chan WW, et al. Effect of N-acetylcysteine for prevention of contrast nephropathy in patients with moderate to severe renal insufficiency: a randomized trial. Am J Kidney Dis. 2004;43:801–8.
121. Durham JD, Caputo C, Dokko J, et al. A randomized controlled trial of N-acetylcysteine to prevent contrast nephropathy in cardiac angiography. Kidney Int. 2002;62:2202–7.
122. Allaqaband S, Tumuluri R, Malik AM, et al. Prospective randomized study of N-acetylcysteine, fenoldopam, and saline for prevention of radiocontrast-induced nephropathy. Catheter Cardiovasc Interv. 2002;57:279–83.
123. Shyu KG, Cheng JJ, Kuan P. Acetylcysteine protects against acute renal damage in patients with abnormal renal function undergoing a coronary procedure. J Am Coll Cardiol. 2002;40:1383–8.
124. Sandhu C, Belli AM, Oliveira DB. The role of N-acetylcysteine in the prevention of contrast-induced nephrotoxicity. Cardiovasc Intervent Radiol. 2006;29:344–7.
125. Rashid ST, Salman M, Myint F, et al. Prevention of contrast-induced nephropathy in vascular patients undergoing angiography: a randomized controlled trial of intravenous N-acetylcysteine. J Vasc Surg. 2004;40:1136–41.
126. Oldemeyer JB, Biddle WP, Wurdeman RL, Mooss AN, Cichowski E, Hilleman DE. Acetylcysteine in the prevention of contrast-induced nephropathy after coronary angiography. Am Heart J. 2003;146:E23.
127. Ochoa A, Pellizzon G, Addala S, et al. Abbreviated dosing of N-acetylcysteine prevents contrast-induced nephropathy after elective and urgent coronary angiography and intervention. J Interv Cardiol. 2004;17:159–65.
128. MacNeill BD, Harding SA, Bazari H, et al. Prophylaxis of contrast-induced nephropathy in patients undergoing coronary angiography. Catheter Cardiovasc Interv. 2003;60:458–61.
129. Kefer JM, Hanet CE, Boitte S, Wilmotte L, De Kock M. Acetylcysteine, coronary procedure and prevention of contrast-induced worsening of renal function: which benefit for which patient? Acta Cardiol. 2003;58:555–60.
130. Goldenberg I, Shechter M, Matetzky S, et al. Oral acetylcysteine as an adjunct to saline hydration for the prevention of contrast-induced nephropathy following coronary angiography. A randomized controlled trial and review of the current literature. Eur Heart J. 2004;25:212–8.
131. Drager LF, Andrade L, Barros de Toledo JF, Laurindo FR, Machado Cesar LA, Seguro AC. Renal effects of N-acetylcysteine in patients at risk for contrast nephropathy: decrease in oxidant stress-mediated renal tubular injury. Nephrol Dial Transplant. 2004;19:1803–7.
132. Diaz-Sandoval LJ, Kosowsky BD, Losordo DW. Acetylcysteine to prevent angiography-related renal tissue injury (the APART trial). Am J Cardiol. 2002;89:356–8.
133. Azmus AD, Gottschall C, Manica A, et al. Effectiveness of acetylcysteine in prevention of contrast nephropathy. J Invasive Cardiol. 2005;17:80–4.
134. Webb JG, Pate GE, Humphries KH, et al. A randomized controlled trial of intravenous N-acetylcysteine for the prevention of contrast-induced nephropathy after cardiac catheterization: lack of effect. Am Heart J. 2004;148:422–9.
135. Balderramo DC, Verdu MB, Ramacciotti CF, et al. Renoprotective effect of high periprocedural doses of oral N-acetylcysteine in patients scheduled to undergo a same-day angiography. Rev Fac Cien Med Univ Nac Cordoba. 2004;61:13–9.
136. Carbonell N, Blasco M, Sanjuan R, et al. Intravenous N-acetylcysteine for preventing contrast-induced nephropathy: a randomised trial. Int J Cardiol. 2007;115:57–62.
137. Amini M, Salarifar M, Amirbaigloo A, Masoudkabir F, Esfahani F. N-acetylcysteine does not prevent contrast-induced nephropathy after cardiac catheterization in patients with diabetes mellitus and chronic kidney disease: a randomized clinical trial. Trials. 2009;10:45.
138. Miner SE, Dzavik V, Nguyen-Ho P, et al. N-acetylcysteine reduces contrast-associated nephropathy but not clinical events during long-term follow-up. Am Heart J. 2004;148:690–5.
139. Alonso A, Lau J, Jaber BL, Weintraub A, Sarnak MJ. Prevention of radiocontrast nephropathy with N-acetylcysteine in patients with chronic kidney disease: a meta-analysis of randomized, controlled trials. Am J Kidney Dis. 2004;43:1–9.
140. Bagshaw SM, Ghali WA. Acetylcysteine for prevention of contrast-induced nephropathy after intravascular angiography: a systematic review and meta-analysis. BMC Med. 2004;2:38.
141. Birck R, Krzossok S, Markowetz F, Schnulle P, van der Woude FJ, Braun C. Acetylcysteine for prevention of contrast nephropathy: meta-analysis. Lancet. 2003;362:598–603.
142. Duong MH, MacKenzie TA, Malenka DJ. N-acetylcysteine prophylaxis significantly reduces the risk of radiocontrast-induced nephropathy: comprehensive meta-analysis. Catheter Cardiovasc Interv. 2005;64:471–9.
143. Gonzales DA, Norsworthy KJ, Kern SJ, et al. A meta-analysis of N-acetylcysteine in contrast-induced nephrotoxicity: unsupervised clustering to resolve heterogeneity. BMC Med. 2007;5:32.
144. Isenbarger DW, Kent SM, O'Malley PG. Meta-analysis of randomized clinical trials on the usefulness of acetylcysteine for prevention of contrast nephropathy. Am J Cardiol. 2003;92:1454–8.

145. Kshirsagar AV, Poole C, Mottl A, et al. N-acetylcysteine for the prevention of radiocontrast induced nephropathy: a meta-analysis of prospective controlled trials. J Am Soc Nephrol. 2004;15:761–9.
146. Misra D, Leibowitz K, Gowda RM, Shapiro M, Khan IA. Role of N-acetylcysteine in prevention of contrast-induced nephropathy after cardiovascular procedures: a meta-analysis. Clin Cardiol. 2004;27:607–10.
147. Nallamothu BK, Shojania KG, Saint S, et al. Is acetylcysteine effective in preventing contrast-related nephropathy? A meta-analysis. Am J Med. 2004;117:938–47.
148. Pannu N, Manns B, Lee H, Tonelli M. Systematic review of the impact of N-acetylcysteine on contrast nephropathy. Kidney Int. 2004;65:1366–74.
149. Weisbord SD, Gallagher M, Jneid H, et al. Outcomes after angiography with sodium bicarbonate and acetylcysteine. N Engl J Med. 2017;
150. Merten GJ, Burgess WP, Gray LV, et al. Prevention of contrast-induced nephropathy with sodium bicarbonate: a randomized controlled trial. JAMA. 2004;291:2328–34.
151. Mueller C, Buerkle G, Buettner HJ, et al. Prevention of contrast media-associated nephropathy: randomized comparison of 2 hydration regimens in 1620 patients undergoing coronary angioplasty. [see comments.]. Arch Intern Med. 2002;162:329–36.
152. Trivedi HS, Moore H, Nasr S, et al. A randomized prospective trial to assess the role of saline hydration on the development of contrast nephrotoxicity. Nephron. 2003;93:C29–34.
153. Weisbord SD, Palevsky PM. Prevention of contrast-induced nephropathy with volume expansion. Clin J Am Soc Nephrol. 2008;3:273–80.
154. Brar SS, Shen AY, Jorgensen MB, et al. Sodium bicarbonate vs sodium chloride for the prevention of contrast medium-induced nephropathy in patients undergoing coronary angiography: a randomized trial. JAMA. 2008;300:1038–46.
155. Kanbay M, Covic A, Coca SG, Turgut F, Akcay A, Parikh CR. Sodium bicarbonate for the prevention of contrast-induced nephropathy: a meta-analysis of 17 randomized trials. Int Urol Nephrol. 2009;41:617–27.
156. Masuda M, Yamada T, Mine T, et al. Comparison of usefulness of sodium bicarbonate versus sodium chloride to prevent contrast-induced nephropathy in patients undergoing an emergent coronary procedure. Am J Cardiol. 2007;100:781–6.
157. Ozcan EE, Guneri S, Akdeniz B, et al. Sodium bicarbonate, N-acetylcysteine, and saline for prevention of radiocontrast-induced nephropathy. A comparison of 3 regimens for protecting contrast-induced nephropathy in patients undergoing coronary procedures. A single-center prospective controlled trial. Am Heart J. 2007;154:539–44.
158. Pakfetrat M, Nikoo MH, Malekmakan L, et al. A comparison of sodium bicarbonate infusion versus normal saline infusion and its combination with oral acetazolamide for prevention of contrast-induced nephropathy: a randomized, double-blind trial. Int Urol Nephrol. 2009;41:629–34.
159. Recio-Mayoral A, Chaparro M, Prado B, et al. The reno-protective effect of hydration with sodium bicarbonate plus N-acetylcysteine in patients undergoing emergency percutaneous coronary intervention: the RENO Study. J Am Coll Cardiol. 2007;49:1283–8.
160. Vasheghani-Farahani A, Sadigh G, Kassaian SE, et al. Sodium bicarbonate plus isotonic saline versus saline for prevention of contrast-induced nephropathy in patients undergoing coronary angiography: a randomized controlled trial. Am J Kidney Dis. 2009;54:610–8.
161. Zoungas S, Ninomiya T, Huxley R, et al. Systematic review: sodium bicarbonate treatment regimens for the prevention of contrast-induced nephropathy. Ann Intern Med. 2009;151:631–8.
162. Navaneethan SD, Singh S, Appasamy S, Wing RE, Sehgal AR. Sodium bicarbonate therapy for prevention of contrast-induced nephropathy: a systematic review and meta-analysis. Am J Kidney Dis. 2009;53:617–27.
163. Meier P, Ko DT, Tamura A, Tamhane U, Gurm HS. Sodium bicarbonate-based hydration prevents contrast-induced nephropathy: a meta-analysis. BMC Med. 2009;7:23.
164. Hoste EA, De Waele JJ, Gevaert SA, Uchino S, Kellum JA. Sodium bicarbonate for prevention of contrast-induced acute kidney injury: a systematic review and meta-analysis. Nephrol Dial Transplant. 2009;
165. Brown JR, Block CA, Malenka DJ, O'Connor GT, Schoolwerth AC, Thompson CA. Sodium bicarbonate plus N-acetylcysteine prophylaxis: a meta-analysis. JACC Cardiovasc Interv. 2009;2:1116–24.
166. Joannidis M, Schmid M, Wiedermann CJ. Prevention of contrast media-induced nephropathy by isotonic sodium bicarbonate: a meta-analysis. Wien Klin Wochenschr. 2008;120:742–8.
167. Hogan SE, L'Allier P, Chetcuti S, et al. Current role of sodium bicarbonate-based preprocedural hydration for the prevention of contrast-induced acute kidney injury: a meta-analysis. Am Heart J. 2008;156:414–21.
168. Ho KM, Morgan DJ. Use of isotonic sodium bicarbonate to prevent radiocontrast nephropathy in patients with mild pre-existing renal impairment: a meta-analysis. Anaesth Intensive Care. 2008;36:646–53.
169. Kunadian V, Zaman A, Spyridopoulos I, Qiu W. Sodium bicarbonate for the prevention of contrast induced nephropathy: a meta-analysis of published clinical trials. Eur J Radiol.
170. Brar SS, Aharonian V, Mansukhani P, et al. Haemodynamic-guided fluid administration for the prevention of contrast-induced acute kidney injury: the POSEIDON randomised controlled trial. Lancet. 2014;383:1814–23.

7 Acute Kidney Injury and Liver Disease: Incidence, Pathophysiology, Prevention/Treatment, and Outcomes

Justin M. Belcher and Chirag R. Parikh

Acute kidney injury (AKI) is a common and devastating complication in patients with cirrhosis, occurring in an estimated 19% of hospitalizations [1], and is associated with significant mortality, 55–91% [2–4]. The clinical impact of this grave confluence of illnesses will continue to worsen as the incidence of both AKI and cirrhosis is increasing [5]. Importantly, etiologies of AKI in patients with cirrhosis vary, and distinguishing between them is critical as distinct therapies exist. Approximately one third of such patients have acute tubular necrosis (ATN) [1]. Care in such patients is supportive, and, if clinically necessary, they are typically offered dialysis. Of the remaining patients, two thirds have prerenal azotemia, a functional AKI that is responsive to volume expansion. Such patients are managed by holding diuretics and providing albumin, typically dosed as 1 mg/kg/day. The remaining patients have kidneys that are primarily structurally intact but whose AKI is unresponsive to volume expansion. These patients are clinically diagnosed with hepatorenal syndrome (HRS), which can either be a rapidly progressive form (type 1) or a more indolent form, that more accurately can be thought of as an aggressive form of chronic kidney disease in patients with refractory cirrhosis (type 2). The management of type 1 HRS will be extensively discussed below but consists of attempting to shunt blood from the splanchnic to the systemic vasculature so as to improve renal perfusion.

J. M. Belcher · C. R. Parikh (✉)
Section of Nephrology, Department of Internal Medicine, Yale University School of Medicine, New Haven, CT, USA
e-mail: Justin.belcher@yale.edu; chirag.parikh@yale.edu

7.1 Pathogenesis of Hepatorenal Syndrome and Other Causes of AKI in Patients with Cirrhosis

Patients with cirrhosis have an increased propensity for renal failure secondary to the hemodynamic abnormalities associated with the progression of liver disease and the development of ascites. The initial precipitating factor is the onset of portal hypertension and portosystemic collaterals and consists of splanchnic vasodilatation. It is likely that much of this vasodilatation is driven by bacterial translocation, which has been demonstrated to be increased in both animals and patients with cirrhosis [6, 7]. Such translocation elicits an inflammatory response, with increased production of proinflammatory cytokines including tumor necrosis factor-α and interleukin-6 and vasodilator factors (nitric oxide) in the splanchnic area. In experimental cirrhosis, nitric oxide blockade increases systemic blood pressure and sodium excretion and decreases ascites [8, 9]. Indeed, patients with cirrhosis and increased levels of lipopolysaccharide-binding protein

S. S. Waikar et al. (eds.), *Core Concepts in Acute Kidney Injury*,
https://doi.org/10.1007/978-1-4939-8628-6_7

or circulating levels of bacterial DNA have increased serum levels of cytokines, reduced systemic vascular resistance, and increased cardiac output, as compared with those who have cirrhosis but are without these markers of bacterial translocation [10, 11]. More recent studies have indicated that increased angiogenic factors and endogenous cannabinoids also appear to contribute importantly to vasodilatation of the splanchnic arterial vessels [12].

This vasodilatation results in a decrease in effective arterial blood volume, resulting in the stimulation of neurohumoral systems, specifically the renin-angiotensin-aldosterone system (RAAS), sympathetic nervous system, and non-osmotic release of antidiuretic hormone. Activation of RAAS and the sympathetic nervous system induces sodium retention, increases intravascular volume, and results in a hyperdynamic circulatory state characterized by low systemic vascular resistance and increased cardiac output [13]. These compensatory mechanisms are initially able to maintain a reasonable arterial pressure and effective arterial blood volume. However, as cirrhosis progresses and vasodilatation worsens, such mechanisms are no longer sufficient, and patients experience a further decrease in effective blood volume with enhanced activation of vasoconstrictive systems [14]. This activation leads to preferential vasoconstriction in several vascular beds, most prominently the renal and central nervous systems [12, 15]. The predilection toward renal vasoconstriction cannot be countered by the usual intrarenal release of vasodilatory substances such as prostaglandins and prostacyclin owing to their decreased production in the renal vasculature in advanced cirrhosis, and vasoconstriction is exacerbated further by local release of vasoconstrictors such as endothelin and thromboxane [16]. The resulting progressive renal hypoperfusion perpetuates the increased sodium avidity and results in worsening of ascites and edema. While an increase in cardiac output initially acts as a compensatory mechanism, there is evidence that cardiac output decreases as cirrhosis progresses [17]. A relatively lower output (<6 L/min) with a lack of response to further arterial vasodilatation and physiological stressors can compound the deceased renal blood flow and has been shown to be a strong predictor of HRS [17–19]. The precipitants and physiologic derangements leading to AKI in patients with cirrhosis are shown in Fig. 7.1 [20].

In normal physiologic conditions, the renal vasculature is able to autoregulate renal perfusion in the setting of decreased flow via tubuloglomerular feedback and the myenteric stretch reflex. This autoregulation ensures an essentially constant blood flow to the kidneys irrespective of fluctuations in systemic blood pressure. However, when mean arterial pressure reaches a decisive threshold around 65 mmHg, autoregulatory mechanisms are overwhelmed, and renal blood flow begins to decrease in proportion to renal perfusion pressure [21]. That is, for any given perfusion pressure, the amount of blood the kidney actually receives will progressively decrease [22, 23]. With advancing cirrhosis it has been demonstrated that this ability to autoregulate renal perfusion is lost. Patients with advanced cirrhosis are therefore both predisposed to renal hypoperfusion and ill-equipped to respond to it. Strong evidence is lacking that such chronic hypoperfusion itself leads to ischemic injury. However, hypoperfusion clearly predisposes cirrhotic patients to structural kidney injury when coupled with a second hit. Such renal insults are common in cirrhosis and include hypovolemia secondary to gastrointestinal bleeding, diarrhea or excessive use of diuretics, use of nephrotoxic medications, and infections. Renal failure is particularly frequent and severe in patients with spontaneous bacterial peritonitis. Stemming from bacterial translocation, peritonitis is associated with an intense inflammatory response resulting in impairment of an already under functioning circulatory system [24, 25]. Nonsteroidal anti-inflammatory drugs may also cause renal failure in patients with cirrhosis as their renal perfusion is extremely dependent on renal prostaglandin synthesis [14]. Once structural injury is established in patients with cirrhosis, recovery may be retarded because of an inability to reconstitute optimal renal perfusion even after resolution of the precipitating insult.

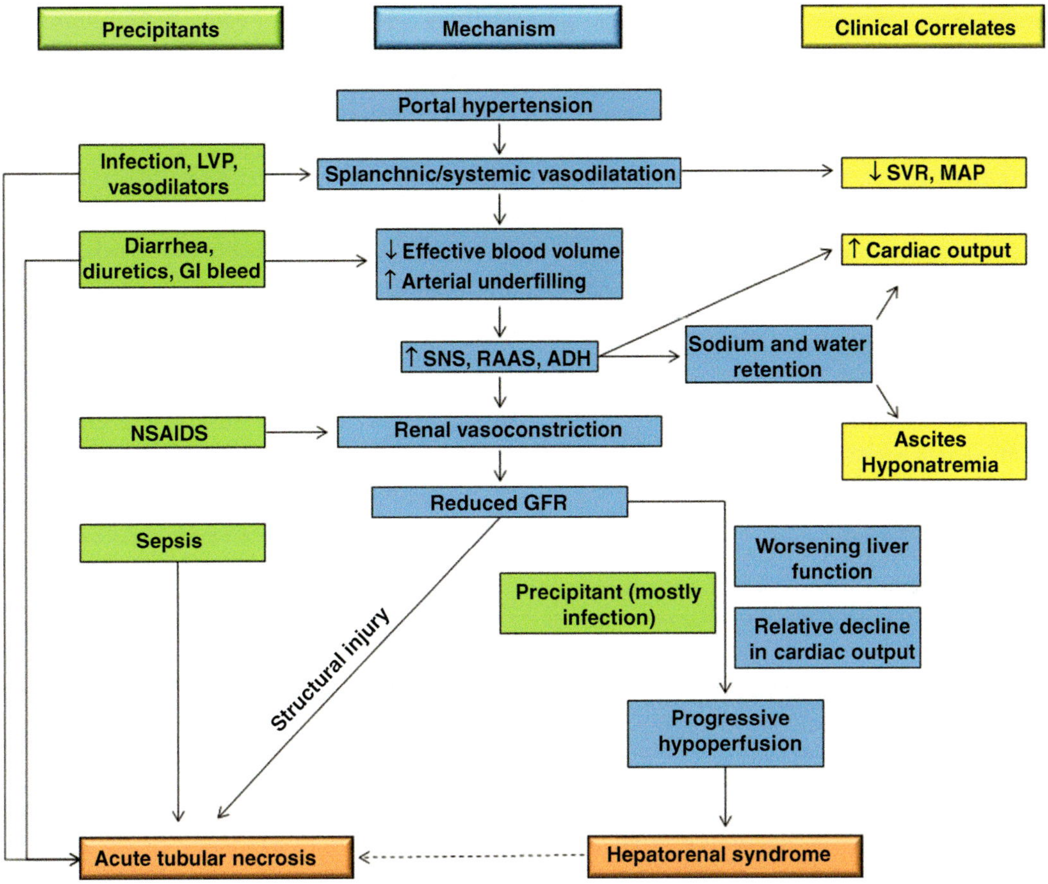

Fig. 7.1 Precipitants, mechanisms, and clinical correlates of HRS and ATN in cirrhosis. Portal hypertension leads to splanchnic and systemic vasodilatation, reducing effective arterial blood volume. This reduction stimulates activation of sympathetic nervous system (SNS), RAAS, and antidiuretic hormone (ADH) with ensuing retention of sodium and water, increasing cardiac output, ascites, and hyponatremia. The increased activity of vasoconstrictor systems results in renal vasoconstriction and consistently decreased renal perfusion. Any factor that worsens vasodilatation (infection, large-volume paracentesis [LVP], vasodilators) or decreases blood volume (diarrhea, over-diuresis, bleeding) will further decrease renal perfusion and lead to AKI. In advanced cirrhosis, splanchnic vasodilatation and renal vasoconstriction can become refractory to volume expansion and, compounded by decreased cardiac function, lead to severe renal hypoperfusion and development of HRS. Alternatively, precipitants may be severe enough to produce structural tubular injury (e.g., septic or hypovolemic shock) and AKI. The extent to which prolonged severe HRS can progress to ATN remains unclear and thus is depicted with a dashed line. Abbreviations: *GI* gastrointestinal, *MAP* mean arterial pressure, *NSAIDs* nonsteroidal anti-inflammatory drugs, *SVR* systemic vascular resistance. Reprinted from Belcher JM, Parikh CR, Garcia-Tsao G. Acute kidney injury in patients with cirrhosis: perils and promise. *Clin Gastroenterol Hepatol.* 2013;11(12):1550–1558; used with permission

7.2 Classification (Definition and Staging) of AKI in Cirrhosis

Despite improved understanding of the precipitants of and physiology underlying AKI in cirrhosis, considerable confusion continues to surround its diagnosis. One of the primary reasons for such struggles is that creatinine, the chief biomarker of glomerular filtration, is unsuited for this role in patients with cirrhosis. In this setting, low protein intake, loss of muscle mass, diminished hepatic synthesis of creatine, and an enlarged volume of distribution decrease serum creatinine level irrespective of renal function and thus lead to overestimation of glomerular filtration rate (GFR) [26]. Major extrarenal influences on serum creatinine level are shown in Fig. 7.2. The traditional definition of AKI in cirrhosis has involved an increase in creatinine to greater than 1.5 mg/dL [27]. However, with the above-described factors frequently resulting in a baseline creatinine level as low as 0.5 or 0.6 mg/dL, adherence to such an elevated threshold may result in delayed diagnosis for patients with severe AKI and likely fails to detect many cases of mild to moderate disease.

In 2010, a working group composed of members of the International Ascites Club (IAC) and the Acute Dialysis Quality Initiative (ADQI) published diagnostic criteria for what they term "hepatorenal disorders," covering AKI, chronic kidney disease (CKD), and HRS [28]. Recognizing that serum creatinine level is an especially poor biomarker of renal dysfunction in patients with cirrhosis [26], the group recommended the adaptation of a rise in serum creatinine of ≥0.3 mg/dL in <48 h as the threshold for AKI rather than a fixed cutoff greater than 1.5 mg/dL. However, the threshold of 2.5 mg/dL for the diagnosis of type 1 HRS (which was to be considered as special form of AKI) was left unchanged. The component of urine output included in the Acute Kidney Injury Network (AKIN); Risk, Injury, Failure, Loss, and End-Stage Renal Failure (RIFLE); and Kidney Disease: Improving Global Outcomes (KDIGO) sets of criteria was excluded from the new consensus guidelines as patients with decompensated cirrhosis frequently have reduced urine output as a result of their high renal sodium and water retention [29]. Such patients with refractory ascites unresponsive to diuretic therapy may have daily urine outputs below the threshold for the diagnosis of AKI but also have stable serum creatinine levels.

The IAC-ADQI diagnostic criteria were evaluated in a cohort of patients with decompensated cirrhosis and normal serum creatinine levels who were monitored regularly as outpatients. AKI was observed in 54% of patients, with many patients having repeated episodes of AKI over a 12-month period [30]. Despite peak serum

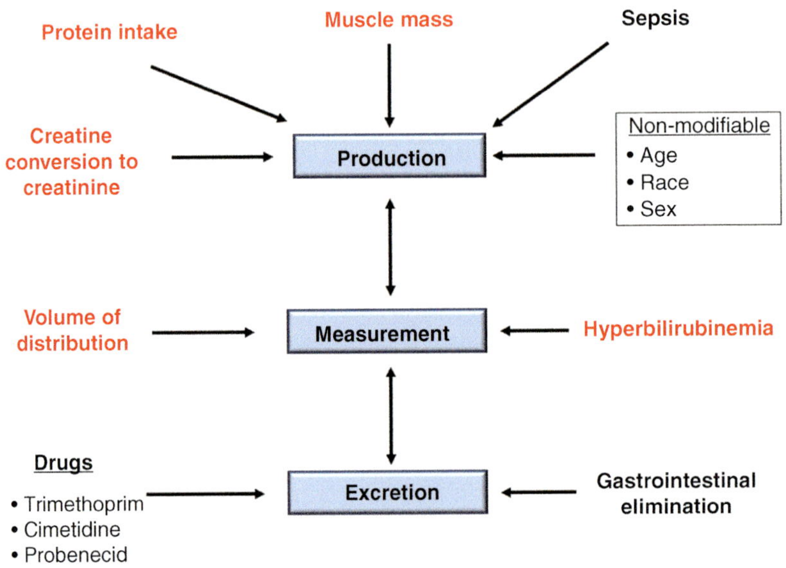

Fig. 7.2 Extrarenal influences on serum creatinine levels. Primary extrarenal influences on serum creatinine are depicted. In addition to the status of renal filtration, creatinine levels are affected by factors that influence its production and excretion as well as those that impact its measurement. Factors especially relevant to patients with cirrhosis are shown in *red*. Reprinted from Belcher JM, Parikh CR, Garcia-Tsao G. Acute kidney injury in patients with cirrhosis: perils and promise. *Clin Gastroenterol Hepatol*. 2013;11(12):1550–1558; used with permission

creatinine levels remaining within the normal laboratory range in the majority of episodes of AKI, there was a gradual and statistically significant ($P < 0.05$) rise in serum creatinine levels in the AKI group over the ensuing 12 months. This increase was associated with a significant reduction in survival in comparison with the non-AKI group ($P < 0.05$). Meeting the IAC-ADQI diagnostic criteria for AKI therefore has prognostic relevance even in the outpatient setting. When the same IAC-ADQI criteria were applied to a cohort of hospitalized patients with cirrhosis and a bacterial infection, those patients diagnosed with AKI using the new criteria had reduced 30-day survival compared with those who did not develop AKI [31]. Even in those patients whose creatinine returned to baseline, survival at 30 days was still substantially decreased in comparison with those patients who never developed AKI ($P < 0.05$).

Despite these findings, there has been considerable controversy on whether to adopt these new diagnostic criteria in lieu of the conventional standard of creatinine rising above 1.5 mg/dL out of concern that the increased sensitivity of the new criteria would ameliorate its predictive value [32, 33]. Two studies independently found that the short-term prognosis of hospitalized patients with cirrhosis and stage 1 AKI whose peak serum creatinine level was <1.5 mg/dL was excellent, similar to patients without AKI [34, 35]. Ferreira et al. evaluated the new definition in a study of 94 ICU patients with cirrhosis with a documented baseline creatinine level less than 1.5 mg/dL [36]. Forty-three patients (46%) had AKI by IAC-ADQI vs. 24 patients (26%) using the traditional definition. AKI by the traditional standard had a stronger association with mortality than AKI by IAC-ADQI, with an odds ratios (ORs) and 95% confidence intervals of 6.8 (2.4–18.8) and 3.1 (1.2–7.8), respectively. Similarly, patients meeting traditional criteria had higher mortality rates (58%) than those who only reached the IAC-ADQI threshold (40%). The authors concluded the new definition may not be better at defining in-hospital mortality risk. It is certainly true that adopting a more lenient definition of AKI will decrease specificity for predicting mortality. By labeling more patients as having AKI, cases on average will be less severe and on aggregate patients will have better outcomes, evidenced in the study by Ferreira et al. by IAC-ADQI's lower positive predictive value (40% vs. 58%).

The benefits of adopting the new, more sensitive definition, however, are twofold. First, although necessarily losing specificity, lowering the threshold for a diagnosis of AKI will increase sensitivity, and the association between even mild acute increases in creatinine and adverse outcomes has been well established [37]. In the study by Ferreira et al. [36], the AKIN definition identified 21% more patients who ultimately would die. Second, and perhaps more importantly, the lower threshold of AKIN will identify those more severe cases who ultimately would have qualified for the 1.5 mg/dL threshold as having AKI significantly earlier, thus facilitating earlier interventions and potentially improving outcomes [37]. Prospective validation of these potential benefits awaits definitive demonstration in further prospective trials.

7.2.1 Definition of Baseline Creatinine

With the adaptation of an AKI definition contingent upon changes in creatinine from a patient's baseline, the decision as to which creatinine value to consider as the baseline necessarily assumes tremendous import. Historically studies used ad hoc definitions of baseline serum creatinine levels, and the prevalence and mortality unsurprisingly differed considerably depending on which definition was used. The most commonly utilized value in the setting of cirrhosis was creatinine at hospital admission. However, when compared with the use of accurate outpatient baseline values, such an approach obscures the presence of nearly 40% of AKI cases [38]. At the recommendation of an expert consensus conference, the baseline serum creatinine level is now defined as a stable serum creatinine within the previous 3 months [39]. Only if none is available should the value obtained upon admission be considered the baseline.

7.2.2 Staging of AKI Severity in Cirrhosis

In addition to adopting new criteria for the diagnosis of AKI, the most recent IAC recommendations also endorse the breakdown of AKI into stages as per the AKIN guidelines. The applicability of the staging system in the assessment of AKI in cirrhosis was evaluated in a cohort of 192 patients admitted into hospital with AKI [38]. Patients were classified into different stages of AKI on admission according to the AKIN creatinine criterion. At enrollment, 91 patients were in AKIN stage 1, 56 in stage 2, and 42 in stage 3. A correlation between the in-hospital mortality with the initial stage at the time of diagnosis of AKI was found, with higher in-hospital mortality noted for higher stages of AKI. During their hospital stay, 85 of 192 (44%) patients' AKI progressed, and this worsening was associated with the development of significantly more medical- and cirrhosis-specific complications ($P < 0.05$) and an exponential increase in mortality (Fig. 7.3). Significantly more non-survivors had progression of AKI compared with survivors ($P < 0.0001$). Conversely, improvement of serum creatinine levels was more frequent among survivors than non-survivors ($P = 0.01$). A similar improvement in survival was observed after downstaging of AKI with terlipressin in a different cohort of patients with type 1 HRS [40].

The same findings were confirmed in the second study consisting of 110 prospectively enrolled patients with decompensated cirrhosis and AKI, and 52 retrospectively identified, but well-matched, controls who were cirrhotic inpatients admitted during the same period, but without AKI [41]. An overall mortality of 32% was observed in the AKI group, versus 4% in the control group ($P < 0.001$). In-hospital mortality increased significantly with ascending stages of AKI (14% stage 1, 38% stage 2, and 43% stage 3; $P < 0.001$).

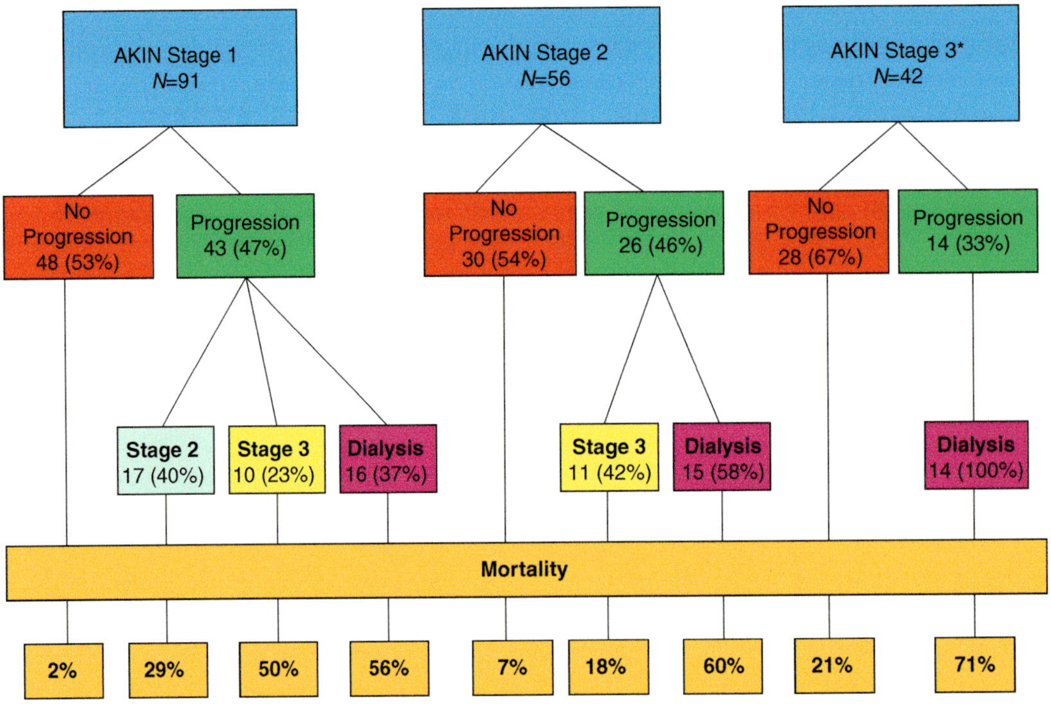

Fig. 7.3 Degree of AKI progression and mortality. Progression is defined by an increase in AKIN stage after initially fulfilling AKIN criteria. Progression to dialysis refers to any patient who presented as non-dialysis-dependent but subsequently developed the requirement for dialysis. Reprinted from Belcher JM, Garcia-Tsao G, Sanyal AJ, et al. Association of AKI with mortality and complications in hospitalized patients with cirrhosis. *Hepatology*. 2013;57(2):753–762; used with permission

7.3 Diagnostic Evaluation and Differential Diagnosis of AKI in Patients with Cirrhosis

The impact of AKI on mortality is not homogeneous but instead contingent on the etiology of AKI [42]. The primary causes of AKI in patients with cirrhosis are prerenal azotemia (PRA), acute tubular necrosis (ATN), and HRS. The prevalence of these diagnoses among patients with cirrhosis and AKI is shown in Fig. 7.4. HRS is one of the most common complications suffered by patients with advanced cirrhosis. In those with ascites, HRS will develop in 18% by 1 year and 40% after 5 years [43]. The functional nature of HRS has been convincingly demonstrated via the absence of significant morphologic damage on kidney biopsy, the restoration of renal function following liver transplant and subsequent restoration of renal perfusion, and the potential reversibility of the renal dysfunction following treatment with volume expansion and vasoconstrictors. The major diagnostic challenge (which is a critical one for prognosis and treatment strategies) is distinguishing structural (ATN) from functional (HRS) AKI. In spite of the severity of kidney dysfunction, kidneys in patients with HRS are primarily structurally intact. Kidney function in this setting, therefore, can be markedly improved if kidney blood flow is restored. In addition to treatment with vasoconstrictors (see below), liver transplantation in patients with advanced cirrhosis can restore systemic vascular resistance, mitigate systemic and kidney vasoconstriction, and restore normal kidney hemodynamics. Patients with HRS at the time of liver transplantation can, thus, experience rapid improvement in kidney function posttransplant [44]. Patients with ATN should be dialyzed if clinically indicated, but in such patients with frank structural injury, interventions to restore kidney perfusion do not result in resolution of AKI, and application of vasoconstrictors or liver transplantation is, therefore, inappropriate. Finally, patients with ATN must be differentiated from patients with HRS when considering a combined liver/kidney transplant.

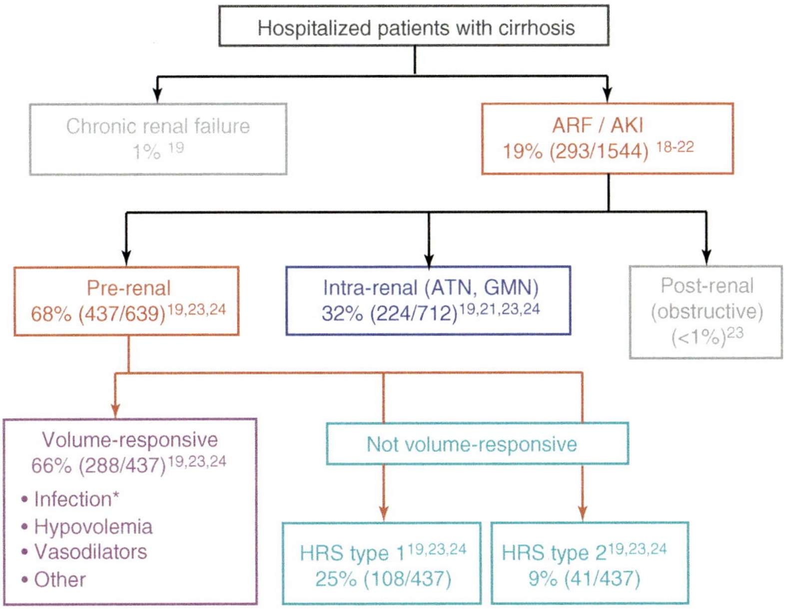

Fig. 7.4 Prevalence and types of acute kidney injury in hospitalized patients with cirrhosis. Abbreviations: *ARF* acute renal failure, *AKI* acute kidney injury, *ATN* acute tubular necrosis, *GN* glomerulonephritis, *HRS* hepatorenal syndrome. Reprinted from Garcia-Tsao G, Parikh CR, Viola A. Acute kidney injury in cirrhosis. *Hepatology*. 2008;48:2064–2077; used with permission

HRS is divided into two distinct clinical patterns based on intensity and rate of progression, type 1 and type 2. Type 1 HRS is the more severe and rapidly progressive and has been significantly more studied. It has traditionally been defined by a rapid loss of renal function with a doubling of creatinine to greater than 2.5 mg/dL in less than 2 weeks. Clinically patients with HRS are virtually always hypotensive with hyponatremia (serum sodium <130 mEq/L) and demonstrate extreme sodium avidity with urine sodium often <10 mEq/L. The mortality in type 1 HRS is severe, with untreated patients surviving an average of 2 weeks. Despite these characteristic clinical findings, it can frequently be very challenging to differentiate HRS from other causes of AKI in patients with cirrhosis, in particular ATN. In light of the cost, scarcity, and potential toxicity of HRS therapies, accurately making this distinction is critical.

Many of the tests typically used to identify ATN in the general population are ineffective in the setting of cirrhosis. The fractional excretion of sodium (FENa), so commonly used by nephrologists evaluating AKI, has historically been very challenging to interpret in patients with cirrhosis. While HRS is well recognized to be associated with very low urine sodium, such is the degree of renal sodium avidity in advanced cirrhosis that FENa is low even in the absence of AKI [45], and ATN can present with a FENa less than 1% despite the presence of tubular injury [46]. The traditional dichotomy where a FENa less than 1% indicates hypoperfusion and more than 1–2% signifies tubular dysfunction and ATN is, therefore, inapplicable. As a result, FENa has historically been thought of as less useful in the setting of cirrhosis. Similarly, urine microscopy is potentially helpful in the differential diagnosis of AKI but is complicated in patients with cirrhosis by biliary staining of sediment and has not been rigorously evaluated in this setting. The gold standard for diagnosing AKI, kidney biopsy, is rarely performed in patients with advanced cirrhosis for fear of bleeding complications.

In an attempt to standardize the diagnosis of HRS, the IAC established and then revised six clinical criteria [27]. Once prerenal azotemia is ruled out by failure to improve with withholding of diuretics and albumin resuscitation, those patients meeting all six IAC criteria were determined to have HRS, whereas those who do not were assumed to have ATN (barring signs consistent with a glomerulonephritis or interstitial nephritis). Unfortunately, these criteria lack specificity as patients with ATN often (1) present with ascites, (2) have creatinine more than 1.5 mg/dL, (3) do not respond to volume resuscitation, (4) lack significant proteinuria or hematuria, and (5) have no gross structural changes to the kidney. Although ATN can certainly be associated with shock, (6) ischemic ATN can develop in the absence of shock and, indeed, frequently occurs in the setting of ostensibly normal blood pressure [47]. In addition, the degree of creatinine elevation does not distinguish ATN from HRS [48]. In 2015, as part of adopting the IAC-ADQI diagnostic criteria, the IAC again revised the definition for type 1 HRS (Table 7.1) [39]. As long as they meet the criteria for AKI (an increase in creatinine of ≥0.3 mg/dL within 48 h or an increase of ≥50% from baseline within 7 days) and fulfill the other five traditional IAC criteria for HRS, there is no longer a fixed creatinine threshold that patients must cross before being diagnosed with HRS. In addition, as long as patients present with stage 2 or 3 AKI or progress from one stage to a higher stage, the creatinine no longer must be more than 2.5 mg/dL before treatment with vasoconstrictive agents is indicated.

Table 7.1 International Ascites Club diagnostic criteria for hepatorenal syndrome

Diagnosis of cirrhosis with ascites
Diagnosis of AKI according to IAC-ADQI criteria
No response after 2 consecutive days of diuretic withdrawal and plasma volume expansion with albumin 1 g/kg of body weight
Absence of shock
No current or recent use of nephrotoxic drugs
No macroscopic signs of structural kidney injury Absence of proteinuria (>500 mg/day) Absence of microscopic hematuria (>50 RBCs per high-power field) Normal finding of renal ultrasound

Abbreviations: *AKI* acute kidney injury, *IAC-ADQI* International Ascites Club-Acute Dialysis Quality Initiative, *RBC* red blood cell

7.3.1 Role of Biomarkers

While the updated HRS definition will lead to earlier initiation of therapy, it does not resolve the difficulty in distinguishing ATN from HRS. The critical diagnostic shortcoming is that serum creatinine is a marker of kidney filtration, not injury, and, thus, cannot distinguish functional from structural etiologies of AKI. Nearly 30 biomarkers of kidney tubular injury have recently been investigated for early detection, differential diagnosis, and prognosis of AKI [49]. Such biomarkers reflect frank structural injury and, thus, when appearing in consort with an acute drop in glomerular filtration rate (GFR), should indicate the drop is attributable to structural damage. Among the most promising are interleukin-18 (IL-18), kidney injury molecule-1 (KIM-1), liver-type fatty acid-binding protein (L-FABP), and neutrophil gelatinase-associated lipocalin (NGAL).

In one of the first studies investigating the potential of biomarkers for differential diagnosis in cirrhosis, Verna and colleagues assessed 118 cirrhotic patients with urine samples collected in the emergency room and evaluated the utility of NGAL for the differential diagnosis of their kidney status and risk stratification for mortality [48]. HRS was diagnosed via the IAC criteria, PRA as a rise in creatinine by at least 0.3 mg/dL to >1.5 mg/dL with a fall to either baseline or <1.5 mg/dL within 48 h and ATN as a rise in creatinine by at least 0.3 mg/dL to >1.5 mg/dL without a fall to <1.5 mg/dL in 48 h despite withdraw and diuretics and volume resuscitation in patients not meeting HRS criteria. Patients with HRS (n = 20) had urine NGAL levels intermediate between PRA (n = 17) (median [interquartile range] 105 ng/mL [27.5–387.5] vs. 20 ng/mL [15–45], P = 0.004) and ATN (n = 15) (325 ng/mL [100–700], P = 0.001). Serum creatinine, however, did not differ between ATN and HRS. Fifteen (13%) patients died. In adjusted analysis, NGAL at a cutoff of 110 ng/mL (odds ratio, 6.05; 95% confidence interval, 1.35–27.2) and diagnosis of HRS (odds ratio, 6.71; 95% confidence interval, 1.76–25.5) independently predicted mortality. Fagundes et al. studied urinary NGAL in 84 patients with kidney dysfunction, defined as creatinine greater than 1.5 mg/dL [50]. HRS was diagnosed via the IAC criteria. Prerenal azotemia was considered when patients had a history of fluid losses in the preceding days (due to either bleeding, diuretic overdose, or other causes), together with compatible findings, absence of other causes of impairment of kidney function, and reversibility of kidney impairment as indicated by decrease of serum creatinine below 1.5 mg/dL after fluid resuscitation. ATN was diagnosed in patients who had at least three of the following: hypovolemic and/or septic shock or treatment with potentially nephrotoxic agents, urine sodium greater than 40 mEq/L, urine osmolality lower than 400 mOsm/kg, and fractional excretion of sodium greater than 2% without diuretics. Patients with ATN (n = 11) had NGAL levels significantly higher than seen in PRA (n = 16), 417 ng/mL (239–2242) vs. 30 ng/mL (20–59). HRS (n = 33) was once again intermediate, 76 ng/mL (43–263), and differed significantly from both ATN and PRA. NGAL levels in patients with PRA were similar to cirrhotic patients without AKI, showing biomarker specificity for structural AKI. Qasem and colleagues evaluated the utility of both NGAL and IL-18 in 150 patients with cirrhosis admitted to ICU [51]. The diagnostic criteria utilized were identical to Fagundes. Values of both biomarkers in patients with HRS (n = 14) were found to be significantly higher than in those with PRA (n = 17) and significantly lower than in those with ATN (n = 22). NGAL and IL-18 demonstrated an excellent ability to discriminate ATN from HRS with area under the receiving operating characteristic curve (AUCs) of 0.91 and 0.98, respectively.

Belcher et al. used retrospective adjudication by a panel of nephrologists and hepatologists after the patients' death or discharge in a study of 102 patients with cirrhosis and AKI whose creatinine either returned to within 25% of baseline within 48 h of meeting Acute Kidney Injury Network (AKIN) criteria or whose AKI progressed to a higher stage after initially meeting the criteria [52]. Patients were adjudicated as PRA (n = 55), ATN (n = 19), and HRS (n = 16). Median values for NGAL, 565 (76–1000) vs. 59 ng/mL (22–203); IL-18, 124 (15–325) vs. 15 ng/mL (15–65); KIM-1, 8.4 (4.1–18.3) vs. 5.1 ng/mL (2.1–10.7); L-FABP, 27 (8–103) vs. 10 ng/mL (4–19); and albumin, 92 (44–253) vs. 21 mg/dL (4–70) were significantly higher in patients with ATN compared with those without ATN. Comparing the three distinct diagnoses, all biomarkers were significantly elevated in ATN relative to PRA, but only NGAL, IL-18, and albumin were statistically higher in ATN compared with HRS, and no injury markers distinguished PRA from HRS. Across the majority of studies, levels for NGAL, the most investigated biomarker, have been remarkably consistent in patients diagnosed with HRS, raising the tantalizing promise of NGAL as an objective test to distinguish primarily functional from structural AKI in patients with cirrhosis and guide decisions regarding vasoconstrictor therapy (see below). Ariza et al. investigated 55 patients with acutely decompensated cirrhosis [53]. Differential diagnosis was performed according to the criteria of Fagundes. In those patients who developed AKI, NGAL levels were once again lowest in PRA ($n = 12$), 36 μg/g creatinine (26–125); intermediate in HRS ($n = 15$), 104 (58–208); and highest in ATN ($n = 12$), 1807 (494–3716). Interestingly, in the study by Belcher et al., spot albuminuria was significantly higher in patients adjudicated with ATN, 92 mg/dL (44–254), than it was in either prerenal azotemia, 21 mg/dL (4–70), or HRS, 24 mg/dL (13–129), $P < 0.001$. The AUC identifying ATN at a cutoff of 44 mg/dL was 0.73 (0.64–0.83).

While NGAL and other biomarkers of structural injury hold great promise to distinguish HRS from ATN, the test is not clinically available in much of the world. Objective tests to make this distinction are therefore thought to be lacking, and the diagnosis of HRS is a clinical one and often one of exclusion. However, it is possible that a common, frequently utilized test in AKI, the fractional excretion of sodium (FENa), may hold unrecognized potential to assist with this differential diagnosis. In many settings of AKI, FENa is useful for distinguishing functional from structural disease. In functional, such as with prerenal azotemia, tubules are structurally intact, and sodium avid due to renal hypoperfusion and thus FENa is very low, below 1%. With structural etiologies such as ATN, tubular injury limits sodium resorption, and FENa increases, typically >2–3%. Due to the physiology of cirrhotic circulation, virtually patients with advanced cirrhosis have chronic renal hypoperfusion and have a FENa <1%, even in the absence of AKI. Such is the degree of sodium avidity in advanced cirrhosis that even patients with ATN typically have a FENa <1% and the test has thus historically been thought unhelpful in distinguishing HRS from ATN [46]. However, in the abovementioned studies by Verna, Fagundes, Qasem, Belcher, and Ariza et al., the FENa in patients diagnosed with HRS clustered tightly around 0.15% and in each case were significantly lower than those for patients with ATN. While the values for ATN varied across studies based on diagnostic definitions, it appears that FENa, after reconceptualizing how "low is low," may in fact be clinically useful for distinguishing HRS from ATN. Values for FENa in prerenal azotemia, HRS, and ATN are shown in Fig. 7.5.

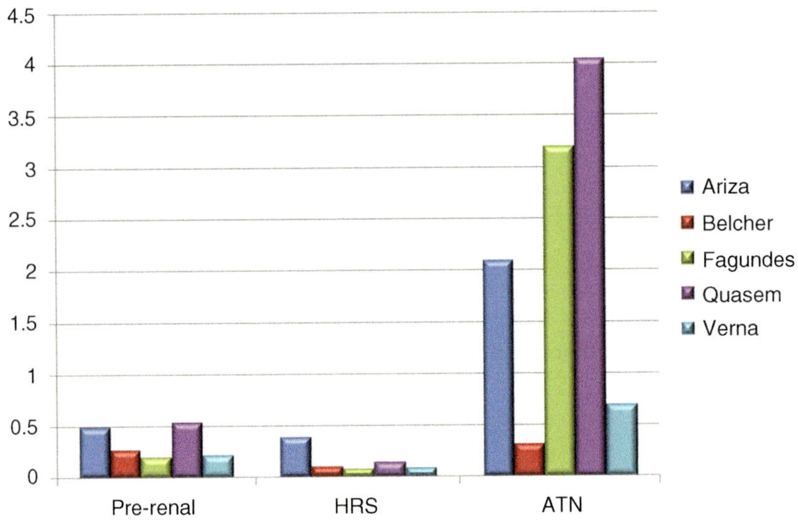

Fig. 7.5 Values for the fractional excretion of sodium (FENa) in patients with cirrhosis and acute kidney injury diagnosed with prerenal azotemia, hepatorenal syndrome, or acute tubular necrosis. Values given in percentage. Abbreviations: *HRS* hepatorenal syndrome, *ATN* acute tubular necrosis

7.4 Therapy

7.4.1 Vasoconstrictors

The current pharmacologic mainstay of treatment for HRS is the use of vasoconstrictors. While this may seems superficially paradoxical in a condition driven by renal artery vasoconstriction, the physiologic rationale is that they improve circulatory function by causing constriction of the dilated splanchnic vasculature, shunting the blood back to the systemic circulation, and subsequently de-escalating the endogenous vasoconstrictor systems with a resulting improvement in renal perfusion. The most commonly used and extensively studied vasoconstrictors in the management of HRS include vasopressin analogues (terlipressin) and alpha-adrenergic agonists (midodrine and norepinephrine). Studies have shown that renal response to vasoconstrictors is enhanced when paired with albumin in order to further improve systemic underfilling and this is thus the standard of care. Despite not being approved for clinical use in the United States, the majority of studies have focused on the use of terlipressin in the treatment of type 1 HRS.

Terlipressin (paired with albumin) is typically started intravenously at 1 mg every 4–6 h and increased up to a maximum of 2 mg every 4–6 h after 3 days if there has not been response to therapy as defined by a fall in creatinine of at least 25% from pretreatment values. If the patient has not responded in 10–14 days, the treatment is discontinued. A full response has traditionally been considered a fall in creatinine to below 1.5 mg/dL. Meta-analysis has shown response rates to be approximately 40–50% [54]. More recently, Boyer et al. studied 196 patients randomized to either terlipressin administered as 1 mg every 6 h or placebo, with both groups receiving concomitant albumin. While patients in the terlipressin arm had a significantly greater fall in creatinine, there was no difference between the groups in HRS reversal or in survival. Those receiving terlipressin who did have reversal had significantly improved survival versus those who did not, while in the placebo arm, there was no difference in survival between patients who did and did not have HRD reversal [55]. However, when this study was analyzed together with another similar large trial by the same authors, resulting in a total of 153 patients receiving terlipressin and 155 placebo, HRS reversal was more common with terlipressin than placebo, 27% vs. 14%; $P = 0.004$ [56]. The effect was more profound in male patients, those with creatinine <3 mg/dL at treatment initiation, Model for End-Stage Liver Disease (MELD) <34, and baseline mean arterial pressure (MAP) ≥70 mmHg. Despite the improved renal recovery, there was no difference in transplant-free or overall survival at 90 days. Interestingly, a very recent randomized controlled trial demonstrated that continuous infusion of terlipressin rather than intermittent boluses produced a trend toward improved response rates and was associated with significantly fewer adverse events and lower cumulative dose [57].

7.4.2 Predictors of Nonresponse

Several studies have looked to established predictors of response to vasoconstrictor therapy. Nazar et al. found bilirubin levels at the initiation of treatment and an increase in mean arterial pressure (MAP) by ≥5 mmHg by day 3 of treatment as independent predictors of renal recovery [58]. Response rates in patients with serum bilirubin <10 or ≥10 mg/dL were 67% and 13%, respectively ($P = 0.001$). Corresponding values in patients with an increase in mean arterial pressure ≥5 or <5 mmHg at day 3 were 73% and 36%, respectively ($P = 0.037$). In a trial by Sharma et al. [59], creatinine level, MAP, and plasma renin activity at the initiation of treatment were associated with renal response on multivariate analysis, while Boyer et al. found only creatinine level at the initiation of therapy to be independently associated [60]. Given these findings that creatinine at the initiation of treatment is predictive of response, it was realized that it is likely imprudent to wait until it rises to 2.5 mg/dL to initiate therapy. According to the newly proposed IAC algorithm, HRS can now be diagnosed when patients have stage 1 AKI and meet the other five criteria and vasoconstrictor therapy

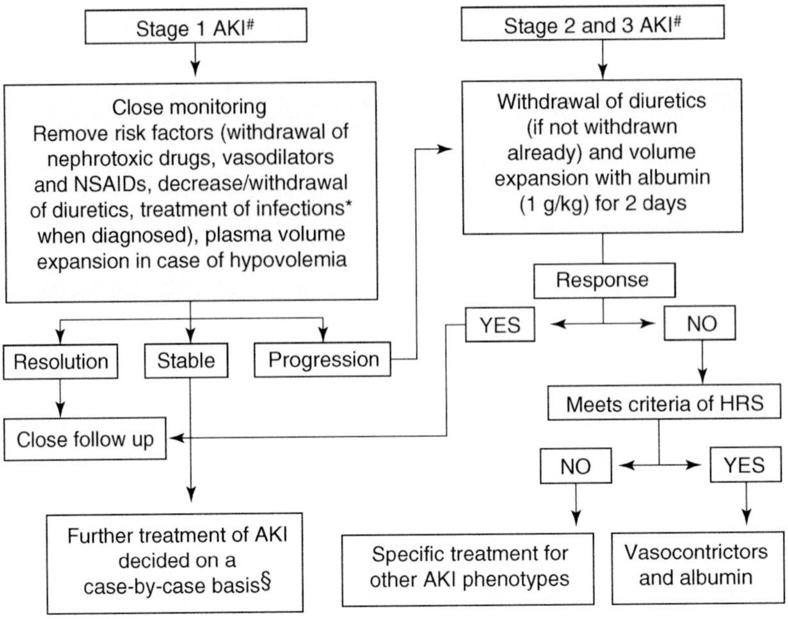

Fig. 7.6 Proposed algorithm for the management of acute kidney injury (AKI) according to the International Ascites Club-Acute Dialysis Quality Initiative (IAC-ADQI) consensus criteria for patients with cirrhosis and ascites. There was considerable concern during the formulation of the algorithm regarding the use of vasoconstrictors in patients with AKI stage 1 and sCr <1.5 mg/dL. Their utility in this setting remains to be established. #Initial AKI stage is defined as AKI stage at the time of first fulfilment of the AKI criteria. §No global consensus was reached on this point. Abbreviations: *HRS* hepatorenal syndrome, *NSAIDs* nonsteroidal anti-inflammatory drugs, *sCr* serum creatinine. Reprinted from Angeli P, Gines P, Wong F, et al. Diagnosis and management of acute kidney injury in patients with cirrhosis: revised consensus recommendations of the International Club of Ascites. *Gut*. 2015;64(4):531–537; used with permission

can be initiated when AKI presents in stage 2 or 3 or if there is progression of the initial stage despite general therapeutic measures [39]. An algorithm for HRS treatment is shown in Fig. 7.6.

7.4.3 Alternatives to Terlipressin

With terlipressin unavailable, the tradition alternative utilized in the United States has been a combination of midodrine and octreotide along with albumin. However, this regimen is inferior to intravenous vasopressor agents. Cavallin et al. randomized 27 patients with type 1 HRS to receive terlipressin and albumin, while 22 received midodrine, octreotide, and albumin [61]. Both groups could receive escalating doses if there was no response to a maximum of 12 mg/24 h of terlipressin and 12.5 mg and 200 μg thrice daily of midodrine and octreotide, respectively. They found a dramatically higher rate of recovery of renal function in the terlipressin group (19/27, 70.4%) compared to the midodrine/octreotide group (6/21, 28.6%), $P = 0.01$. Few prospective trials have compared terlipressin and norepinephrine. However, a meta-analysis of four small randomized trials (totaling 78 patients treated with terlipressin and 76 with norepinephrine, all treated with albumin) found no difference in either HRS response rate or 30-day mortality between the two vasopressors [62]. Therefore, in situations where terlipressin is not available, norepinephrine is likely a superior alternative to midodrine and octreotide.

Srivastava and colleagues compared terlipressin versus a combination of dopamine, furosemide, and Lasix over 5 days in patients with both type 1 and type 2 HRS [63]. In both groups, the two treatment arms resulted in similar increase in urine output and urine sodium along with similar falls in plasma renin activity. Thirty-day mortality was also similar between the two groups. Interestingly though, neither arm in the type 1 HRS patients had a significant decreased in serum creatinine.

7.4.4 Transjugular Intrahepatic Portosystemic Shunts

The use of transjugular intrahepatic portosystemic shunts (TIPS) for the treatment of HRS has long held physiologic promise. By shunting blood for the splanchnic to the systemic circulation, TIPS alleviates systemic underfilling and should therefore lead to a reduction in the activation of RAAS and the SNS. However, the setting where HRS is typically encountered (advanced cirrhosis) is also one in which TIPS is often contraindicated for fear of provoking or worsening hepatic encephalopathy. Therefore, few studies have prospectively investigated TIPS in the treatment of HRS. In two small studies, the use of TIPS in patients with type 1 HRS significantly improved GFR and reduced plasma renin activity, serum aldosterone, and norepinephrine levels in approximately 60% of patients [64, 65]. However, both studies excluded patients with advanced cirrhosis as defined by Child-Pugh score ≥12 or serum bilirubin >5 mg/dL as well as those with hepatic encephalopathy.

Type 2 HRS develops in patients with ascites refractory to treatment with diuretics. In such patients both therapeutic paracentesis and TIPS have been shown to be effective in reducing ascites. Randomized trials suggest that TIPS may improve survival compared to paracentesis [66]. In such patients, the MELD score has been shown to predict survival in patients treated with elective TIPS and should be included in the process of selecting patients who would benefit from TIPS placement.

7.4.5 Renal Replacement Therapy

The role of renal replacement therapy in patients with HRS is controversial. Most clinicians agree that its use is appropriate when intended as a bridge to transplant but there are no randomized trials comparing its efficacy for this to other forms of therapy such as vasoconstrictors. More problematic are instances when patients are not transplant candidates. There is scant data on outcomes for patients with cirrhosis and AKI requiring dialysis as such patients are routinely excluded from trials and, when included, are typically not distinguished as having HRS or ATN. Those studies that have specifically investigated dialysis in patients with HRS have either had extremely small numbers [67] or utilized outdated HRS definitions [67, 68]. Wong et al. studied 102 liver transplant candidates receiving RRT for AKI [69]. A total of 32 (31%) survived to transplant, with 1-year postoperative survival of 70% versus 90% for patients not requiring RRT. Mortality in those not receiving a transplant was near universal, 64/69 (94%); 50% of patients died within 8 days of initiating RRT, and the survival curve did not begin leveling off until 15–20 days. Little is known about the relative outcomes with continuous versus intermittent dialysis. Given the near universal hypotension in patients with decompensated cirrhosis, continuous renal replacement therapy (CRRT) is frequently employed as a matter of necessity. In the study by Wong et al., patients receiving CRRT had a significantly higher mortality than those receiving intermittent hemodialysis, 48/66 (73%) versus 18/36 (50%), OR 2.67 (1.14–6.23). However, as CRRT patients had significantly higher APACHE II scores, lower mean arterial pressure, increased rates of intubation, and higher rates of infection, this finding is clearly influenced by selection bias. Zhang retrospectively studied 80 patients who received vasoconstrictors and albumin for HRS, 37 of whom received dialysis and 43 of whom did not [70]. Baseline serum creatinine was similar between the groups though it is not clear what time-point was considered as the baseline in the non-dialysis group. There was no difference in 30 and 180 days mortality between the two groups, even after censoring for liver transplantation.

While the development of any successful treatment for AKI is to be celebrated, there is considerable cause for skepticism as to whether the results of trials of vasoconstrictors are applicable to patients requiring dialysis. Patients already on dialysis have been excluded from randomized trials to date. Critically, across multiple studies looking at both terlipressin and norepinephrine, serum creatinine at initiation of treatment is one of the strongest independent predictors of renal response [60]. It is very unlikely that, either not having started vasoconstrictor therapy before dialysis is required or having progressed to RRT despite being on vasoconstrictors, patients would respond at this advanced stage. In addition, the majority of trials excluded patients in shock or with uncontrolled infections, complications frequently present in ICU patients with HRS. In light of this, dialysis of HRS patients ineligible for transplant is unlikely to prolong length or quality of life and should typically not be performed.

7.5 Acute-On-Chronic Liver Failure

Historically the study of AKI in cirrhosis was understood to revolve around the setting of decompensated cirrhosis. Recently an appreciation has developed for the unique entity of acute-on-chronic liver failure (ACLF) and its relation to AKI. ACLF combines an acute deterioration in liver function in an individual with pre-existing chronic liver disease with hepatic and extrahepatic organ failures and is associated with substantial short-term mortality. Common precipitants include bacterial and viral infections, alcoholic hepatitis, and surgery, but in more than 40% of patients, no precipitating event is identified. Although clinicians have recognized acute decompensation and acute-on-chronic liver failure as separate clinical entities for many years, no universally accepted diagnostic criteria were available [71, 72]. Recently, two definitions have been proposed, by the Asian Pacific Association for the Study of the Liver (APASL) [73] and the European and American associations for the study of liver disease [74]. The definitions were merged under the auspices of the World Congress of Gastroenterology, affirming that acute-on-chronic liver failure is distinct from both acute liver failure and decompensated cirrhosis, with clear clinical, laboratory, and pathophysiological features [75]. Subsequently investigators in two large, prospective, observational studies, one in Europe (Chronic Liver Failure [CLIF] Consortium Acute-on-Chronic [CANONIC]) [76] and one in Canada and the United States (North American Consortium for the Study of End-Stage Liver Disease [NACSELD]) [77], have attempted to define groups of patients with cirrhosis at high risk for ACLF and associated increased short-term mortality [78].

ACLF develops in approximately 30% of hospitalized patients with cirrhosis who have an acute complication of their liver disease [79]. In the CANONIC study which prospectively enrolled 1343 hospitalized patients with cirrhosis and an acute complication, kidney dysfunction (defined as serum creatinine 1.5–1.9 mg/dL) was reported in 13% and kidney failure (defined as serum creatinine ≥2 mg/dL or requirement of renal replacement therapy) in 56% of ACLF patients [76]. Studies based on APASL criteria have reported kidney dysfunction in 23–51% of patients [80–82] with ACLF as compared to the reported prevalence of 20% in overall hospitalized patients with cirrhosis [1]. Few studies have assessed the prevalence of AKI in ACLF employing the new definitions of AKI. As reported in one abstract, utilizing the AKIN criteria and APASL ACLF definition, a significantly higher incidence of AKI was noted in patients with ACLF (51%) as compared to 32% in patients with decompensated cirrhosis not meeting ACLF criteria [82].

Angeli et al. studied 510 patients prospectively enrolled in the CANONIC study and assessed for the development of AKI at 48 h [83]. Two hundred and forty patients (47%) met the criteria for ACLF, while 98 (19%) developed AKI. The development of both ACLF and AKI was strongly associated with mortality. 28-day transplant-free mortality and 90-day transplant-free mortality of patients with ACLF (32% and 50%, respectively) were significantly higher with respect to those of patients without ACLF (6% and 16%, respectively; both $P < 0.001$). Corresponding values in patients with and without AKI were 46% and 59% and 12% and 26%, respectively (both

$P < 0.0001$). ACLF classification was more accurate than AKI classification in predicting 90-day mortality (AUC 0.72 vs. 0.62; $P < 0.0001$) in the whole series of patients. Moreover, assessment of ACLF classification at 48 h had significantly better prognostic accuracy compared with that of both AKI classification and ACLF classification at enrollment.

Ariza et al. noted that *LCN2*, the gene responsible for NGAL production, is upregulated in experimental models of liver injury and cultured hepatocytes as a result of injury by toxins or pro-inflammatory cytokines, particularly interleukin-6 [84]. To investigate whether NGAL could be a biomarker of ACLF and whether the *LCN2* gene may be upregulated in the liver in ACLF, they measured both urinary and plasma NGAL levels in 716 patients from the CANONIC study hospitalized for complications of cirrhosis, 148 of whom developed ACLF. *LCN2* expression was assessed in liver biopsies from 29 additional patients with decompensated cirrhosis with and without ACLF. The authors found urine NGAL (uNGAL) was markedly increased in ACLF vs. no ACLF (108 (35–400) vs. 29 (12–73) μg/g creatinine; $P < 0.001$) and was an independent predictive factor of ACLF. The independent association persisted after adjustment for kidney function and exclusion of variables present in ACLF definition. uNGAL was also an independent predictive factor of 28-day transplant-free mortality together with MELD score and leukocyte count (AUC 0.88). uNGAL significantly improved the accuracy of MELD in predicting prognosis. For example, for a MELD score of 30, the probability of death at 28 days was only 5% in patients with uNGAL below 15 μg/g of creatinine compared to 41% in those with uNGAL above 105 μg/g of creatinine. *LCN2* gene expression was markedly upregulated in the liver of patients with ACLF. Conversely, expression did not differ between patients with acute decompensation but no ACLF and those with compensated cirrhosis.

While structural injury accounts for only approximately one third of AKI generally occurring in cirrhosis, this percentage increases in the setting of ACLF due to increased prevalence of inflammation and infection [82, 85]. In nearly 500 patients in hospital with cirrhosis and clinically significant renal dysfunction, 3-month survival was only 15% in those developing hepatorenal syndrome; however these patients accounted for only 13% of all cases [42]. Patients with cirrhosis whose renal failure had other causes were more than twice as likely to survive. Studies are needed to determine if biomarkers can assist with AKI differential diagnosis in ACLF as well as to evaluate the efficacy of vasoconstrictor therapy in those patients who do develop HRS.

Little data exists regarding the prevention of ACLF or of mitigating the risk of AKI in those who do suffer it. Administration of albumin for the prevention of HRS [86] in patients with SBP and also use of prophylactic antibiotics have shown reduction in the incidence of kidney failure by modulation of NFkB and cytokines and by a TLR-4-based mechanism [87]. Use of norfloxacin for primary prophylaxis of SBP also holds promise in the prevention of AKI [86]. While some trials in patients with severe alcoholic hepatitis have shown reductions in HRS and/or mortality with treatment with pentoxifylline and *N*-acetylcysteine [88–90] with or without steroids, others have found no effect [91, 92]. Administration of granulocyte colony-stimulating factor (G-CSF) in patients with ACLF diagnosed as per APASL criteria has also been shown to reduce the development of HRS as well as decreasing the incidence of sepsis [93, 94].

Conclusions

AKI is a common complication in patients with cirrhosis and remains associated with significant mortality. Advances in understanding its pathogenesis and better delineating its etiologies have however provided hope for improved outcomes. The critical issue remains establishing an accurate and timely distinction between functional (HRS or prerenal azotemia) and structural (ATN) causes. Prerenal azotemia can often be ruled out by holding diuretics and challenging the patient with 2 days of albumin dosed at 1 mg/kg/day. While distinguishing between HRS and ATN in the remaining patients is clinically very challenging, new tools and a reappraisal of some nephrology old standbys hold the promise of illuminating a path through the diagnostic fog. Urinary biomarkers reflecting frank structural injury to the tubules such as NGAL are significantly elevated in ATN compared with HRS, while FENa, reflecting tubular integrity and sodium avidity, is significantly lower in HRS. Moving forward, a panel of structural and functional markers will likely provide significant clarity to this clinically vexing differential diagnosis. Once HRS is identified, new therapies hold promise to improve outcomes in what was once, outside of receiving a transplant, an essentially universally fatal condition. The vasoconstrictor terlipressin, in conjunction with albumin, has been shown to lower serum creatinine and lead to an increased rate of durable HRS reversal, though data demonstrating improved mortality remain scant. Importantly, norepinephrine appears to be as effective as terlipressin and is an acceptable clinical alternative in areas of the world where terlipressin is not available. In patients with ATN, dialysis should be offered when clinically indicated, and, if renal failure is persistent, patients should be evaluated for a combined liver-kidney transplant.

References

1. Garcia-Tsao G, Parikh CR, Viola A. Acute kidney injury in cirrhosis. Hepatology. 2008;48:2064–77.
2. Du Cheyron D, Bouchet B, Parienti JJ, et al. The attributable mortality of acute renal failure in critically ill patients with liver cirrhosis. Intensive Care Med. 2005;31(12):1693–9.
3. Fang JT, Tsai MH, Tian YC, et al. Outcome predictors and new score of critically ill cirrhotic patients with acute renal failure. Nephrol Dial Transplant. 2008;23(6):1961–9.
4. Cholongitas E, Senzolo M, Patch D, et al. Cirrhotics admitted to intensive care unit: the impact of acute renal failure on mortality. Eur J Gastroenterol Hepatol. 2009;21(7):744–50.
5. Hsu CY, McCulloch CE, Fan D, et al. Community-based incidence of acute renal failure. Kidney Int. 2007;72(2):208–12.
6. Wiest R, Das S, Cadelina G, et al. Bacterial translocation in cirrhotic rats stimulates eNOS-derived NO production and impairs mesenteric vascular contractility. J Clin Invest. 1999;104:1223–33.
7. Wiest R, Garcia-Tsao G. Bacterial translocation (BT) in cirrhosis. Hepatology. 2005;41:422–33.
8. Martin PY, Ohara M, Gines P, et al. Nitric oxide synthase (NOS) inhibition for one week improves renal sodium and water excretion in cirrhotic rats with ascites. J Clin Invest. 1998;101:235–42.
9. Lee FY, Colombato LA, Albillos A, et al. N omega-nitro-L-arginine administration corrects peripheral vasodilation and systemic capillary hypotension, and ameliorates plasma volume expansion and sodium retention in portal hypertensive rats. Hepatology. 1993;17:84–90.
10. Albillos A, de la Hera A, González M, et al. Increased lipopolysaccharide binding protein in cirrhotic patients with marked immune and hemodynamic derangement. Hepatology. 2003;37:208–17.
11. Francés R, Zapater P, González Navajas JM, et al. Bacterial DNA in patients with cirrhosis and noninfected ascites mimics the soluble immune response established in patients with spontaneous bacterial peritonitis. Hepatology. 2008;47:978–85.
12. Mejias M, Garcia-Pras E, Tiani C, et al. Beneficial effects of sorafenib on splanchnic, intrahepatic, and portocollateral circulations in portal hypertensive and cirrhotic rats. Hepatology. 2009;49:1245–56.
13. Schrier RW, Arroyo V, Bernardi M, et al. Peripheral arterial vasodilation hypothesis: a proposal for the initiation of renal sodium and water retention in cirrhosis. Hepatology. 1988;8:1151–7.
14. Arroyo V, Ginès P, Gerbes AL, et al. Definition and diagnostic criteria of refractory ascites and hepatorenal syndrome in cirrhosis. Hepatology. 1996;23:164–76.
15. Guevara M, Bru C, Ginès P, et al. Increased cerebrovascular resistance in cirrhotic patients with ascites. Hepatology. 1998;28:39–44.
16. Laffi G, La Villa G, Pinzani M, et al. Arachidonic acid derivatives and renal function in liver cirrhosis. Semin Nephrol. 1997;17:530–48.
17. Ruiz-del-Arbol L, Monescillo A, Arocena C, et al. Circulatory function and hepatorenal syndrome in cirrhosis. Hepatology. 2005;42:439–47.
18. Krag A, Bendtsen F, Henriksen JH, et al. Low cardiac output predicts development of hepatorenal syndrome and survival in patients with cirrhosis and ascites. Gut. 2010;59:105–10.
19. Nazar A, Guevara M, Sitges M, et al. Left ventricular function assessed by echocardiography in cirrhosis: relationship to systemic hemodynamics and renal dysfunction. J Hepatol. 2013;58:51–7.
20. Belcher JM, Parikh CR, Garcia-Tsao G. Acute kidney injury in patients with cirrhosis: perils and promise. Clin Gastroenterol Hepatol. 2013;11(12):1550–8.
21. Cupples WA, Braam B. Assessment of renal autoregulation. Am J Physiol Ren Physiol. 2007;292:F1105–23.
22. Sansoé E, Silvano S, Mengozzi G, et al. Loss of tubuloglomerular feedback in decompensated liver cirrhosis: physiopathological implications. Dig Dis Sci. 2005;50:955–63.

23. Stadlbauer VP, Wright GAK, Banaji M, et al. Relationship between activation of the sympathetic nervous system and renal blood flow autoregulation in cirrhosis. Gastroenterology. 2008;134:111–9.
24. Bories PN, Campillo B, Azaou L, et al. Long-lasting NO overproduction in cirrhotic patients with spontaneous bacterial peritonitis. Hepatology. 1997;25:1328–33.
25. Grangé JD, Amiot X. Nitric oxide and renal function in cirrhotic patients with ascites: from pathophysiology to practice. Eur J Gastroenterol Hepatol. 2004;16:567–70.
26. Davenport A. Difficulties in assessing renal function in patients with cirrhosis: potential impact on patient treatment. Intensive Care Med. 2011;37:930–2.
27. Salerno F, Gines A, Ginès P, et al. Diagnosis, prevention and treatment of hepatorenal syndrome in cirrhosis. Gut. 2007;56:1310–8.
28. Wong F, Nadim MK, Kellum JA, et al. Working Party proposal for a revised classification system of renal dysfunction in patients with cirrhosis. Gut. 2011;60:702–9.
29. Angeli P, Gatta A, Caregaro L, et al. Tubular site of renal sodium retention in ascitic liver cirrhosis evaluated by lithium clearance. Eur J Clin Investig. 1990;20:111–7.
30. Tsien CD, Rabie R, Wong F. Acute kidney injury in decompensated cirrhosis. Gut. 2013;62:131–7.
31. Wong F, O'Leary JG, Reddy KR, et al. New consensus definition of acute kidney injury accurately predicts 30-day mortality in patients with cirrhosis and infection. Gastroenterology. 2013;145(6):1280–8.
32. Arroyo V. Acute kidney injury (AKI) in cirrhosis: should we change current definition and diagnostic criteria of renal failure in cirrhosis? J Hepatol. 2013;59:415–7.
33. Cardenas A. Defining renal failure in cirrhosis—acute kidney injury classification or traditional criteria? Ann Hepatol. 2013;12:984–5.
34. Piano S, Rosi S, Maresio G, et al. Evaluation of the Acute Kidney Injury Network criteria in hospitalized patients with cirrhosis and ascites. J Hepatol. 2013;59:482–9.
35. Fagundes C, Barreto R, Guevara M, et al. A modified acute kidney injury classification for diagnosis and risk stratification of impairment of kidney function in cirrhosis. J Hepatol. 2013;59:474–81.
36. Ferreira CN, Rodrigues T, Cortez-Pinto H, et al. The new definition of acute kidney injury in patients with cirrhosis: a critical look. Gut. 2012;61:1513.
37. Newsome BB, Warnock DG, McClellan WM, et al. Long-term risk of mortality and end-stage renal disease among the elderly after small increases in serum creatinine level during hospitalization for acute myocardial infarction. Arch Intern Med. 2008;168:609–16.
38. Belcher JM, Garcia-Tsao G, Sanyal AJ, et al. Association of AKI with mortality and complications in hospitalized patients with cirrhosis. Hepatology. 2013;57(2):753–62.
39. Angeli P, Gines P, Wong F, et al. Diagnosis and management of acute kidney injury in patients with cirrhosis: revised consensus recommendations of the International Club of Ascites. Gut. 2015;64(4):531–7.
40. Wong F, et al. Reduction in acute kidney injury (AKI) is a strong predictor of survival in patients with hepatorenal syndrome type-1 (HRS-1) treated with terlipressin plus albumin or albumin alone. Nephrol Dial Transplant. 2015;30:Siii451.
41. Scott RA, Austin AS, Kolhe NV, et al. Acute kidney injury is independently associated with death in patients with cirrhosis. Frontline Gastroenterol. 2013;4:191–7.
42. Martin-Llahi M, Guevara M, Torre A, et al. Prognostic importance of the cause of renal failure in patients with cirrhosis. Gastroenterology. 2011;140:488–96.
43. Gines A, Escorsell A, Gines P, et al. Incidence, predictive factors, and prognosis of the hepatorenal syndrome in cirrhosis with ascites. Gastroenterology. 1993;105:229–36.
44. Wong F, Leung W, Beshir M, et al. Outcomes of patients with cirrhosis and hepatorenal syndrome type 1 treated with liver transplantation. Liver Transpl. 2015;21(3):300–7.
45. Magri P, Auletta M, Andreucci M, et al. Sodium retention in preascitic stage of cirrhosis. Semin Nephrol. 2001;21(3):317–22.
46. Diamond JR, Yoburn DC. Nonoligouric acute renal failure associated with a low fractional excretion of sodium. Ann Intern Med. 1982;96(5):597–600.
47. Abuelo JG. Normotensive ischemic acute renal failure. N Engl J Med. 2007;357(8):797–805.
48. Verna EC, Brown RS, Farrand E, et al. Urinary neutrophil gelatinase-associated lipocalin predicts mortality and identifies acute kidney injury in cirrhosis. Dig Dis Sci. 2012;57(9):2362–70.
49. Belcher JM, Edelstein CL, Parikh CR. Clinical applications of biomarkers for acute kidney injury. Am J Kidney Dis. 2011;57(6):930–40.
50. Fagundes C, Pepin MN, Guevara M, et al. Urinary neutrophil gelatinase-associated lipocalin as biomarker in the differential diagnosis of impairment of kidney function in cirrhosis. J Hepatol. 2012;57(2):267–73.
51. Qasem AA, Farag SE, Hamed E, et al. Urinary biomarkers of acute kidney injury in patients with cirrhosis. ISRN Nephrol. 2014:376795. https://doi.org/10.1155/2014/376795.
52. Belcher JM, Sanyal AJ, Peixoto AJ, et al. Kidney biomarkers and differential diagnosis of patients with cirrhosis and acute kidney injury. Hepatology. 2014;60(2):622–32.
53. Ariza X, Solà E, Elia C, et al. Analysis of a urinary biomarker panel for clinical outcomes assessment in cirrhosis. PLoS One. 2015;10(6):e0128145.
54. Cavallin M, Fasolato S, Marenco S, et al. The treatment of hepatorenal syndrome. Dig Dis. 2015;33(4):548–54.
55. Boyer TD, Sanyal AJ, Wong F, et al. Terlipressin plus albumin is more effective than albumin alone in improving renal function in patients with cirrhosis

and hepatorenal syndrome type 1. Gastroenterology. 2016;150(7):1579–89.
56. Sanyal AJ, Boyer TD, Frederick RT, et al. Reversal of hepatorenal syndrome type 1 with terlipressin plus albumin vs. placebo plus albumin in a pooled analysis of the OT-0401 and REVERSE randomized clinical studies. Aliment Pharmacol Ther. 2017;45(11):1390–401.
57. Cavallin M, Piano S, Romano A, et al. Terlipressin given by continuous intravenous infusion verses intravenous boluses in the treatment of hepatorenal syndrome: a randomized controlled study. Hepatology. 2016;63:983–92.
58. Nazar A, Pereira GH, Guevara M, et al. Predictors of response to therapy with terlipressin and albumin in patients with cirrhosis and type 1 hepatorenal syndrome. Hepatology. 2010;51(1):219–26.
59. Sharma P, Kumar A, Sharma BC, et al. An open label, pilot, randomized controlled trial of noradrenaline versus terlipressin in the treatment of type 1 hepatorenal syndrome and predictors of response. Am J Gastroenterol. 2008;103(7):1689–97.
60. Boyer TD, Sanyal AJ, Garcia-Tsao G, et al. Predictors of response to terlipressin plus albumin in hepatorenal syndrome (HRS) type 1: relationship of serum creatinine to hemodynamics. J Hepatol. 2011;55(2):315–21.
61. Cavallin M, Kamath PS, Merli M, et al. Terlipressin plus albumin versus midodrine and octreotide plus albumin in the treatment of hepatorenal syndrome: a randomized trial. Hepatology. 2015;62(2):567–74.
62. de Mattos AZ, de Mattos AA, Ribeiro RA. Terlipressin versus noradrenaline in the treatment of hepatorenal syndrome: systematic review with meta-analysis and full economic evaluation. Eur J Gastroenterol Hepatol. 2016;28:345–51.
63. Srivastava S, Shalimar, Vishnubhatla S, et al. Randomized controlled trial comparing the efficacy of Terlipressin and albumin with a combination of concurrent dopamine, furosemide, and albumin in hepatorenal syndrome. J Clin Exp Hepatol. 2015;5(4):276–85.
64. Guevara M, Ginès P, Bandi JC, et al. Transjugular intrahepatic portosystemic shunt in hepatorenal syndrome: effects on renal function and vasoactive systems. J Hepatol. 1998;28(2):416–22.
65. Brensing KA, Textor J, Perz J, et al. Long term outcome after transjugular intrahepatic portosystemic stent-shunt in non-transplant cirrhotics with hepatorenal syndrome: a phase II study. Gut. 2000;47:288–95.
66. Bai M, Qi XS, Yang ZP, et al. TIPS improves liver transplantation-free survival in cirrhotic patients with refractory ascites: an updated meta-analysis. World J Gastroenterol. 2014;20(10):2704–14.
67. Capling RK, Bastani B. The clinical course of patients with type 1 hepatorenal syndrome maintained on hemodialysis. Ren Fail. 2004;26:563–8.
68. Keller F, Heinze H, Jochimsen F, et al. Risk factors and outcomes of 107 patients with decompensated liver disease and acute renal failure (including 26 patients with hepatorenal syndrome): the role of hemodialysis. Ren Fail. 1995;17:135–46.
69. Wong LP, Blackley MP, Andreoni KA, et al. Survival of liver transplant candidates with acute renal failure receiving renal replacement therapy. Kidney Int. 2005;68:362–70.
70. Zhang Z, Maddukuri G, Jaipail N, et al. Role of renal replacement therapy in patients with type 1 hepatorenal syndrome receiving combination treatment of vasoconstrictor therapy and albumin. J Crit Care. 2015;30(5):969–74.
71. Wlodzimirow KA, Eslami S, Abu-Hanna A, et al. A systematic review on prognostic indicators of acute on chronic liver failure and their predictive value for mortality. Liver Int. 2013;33:40–52.
72. Jalan R, Williams R. Acute-on-chronic liver failure: pathophysiological basis of therapeutic options. Blood Purif. 2002;20:252–61.
73. Sarin S, Kumar A, Almeida JA, et al. Acute-on-chronic-liver failure: consensus recommendations of the Asian Pacific Association for the study of the liver (APASL). Hepatol Int. 2009;3(1):269–82.
74. Moreau R, Jalan R, Gines P, et al. Acute-on-chronic liver failure is a distinct syndrome that develops in patients with acute decompensation of cirrhosis. Gastroenterology. 2013;144(7):1426–37.
75. Jalan R, Yurdaydin C, Bajaj JS, et al. Toward an improved definition of acute-on-chronic liver failure. Gastroenterology. 2014;147:4–10.
76. Jalan R, Saliba F, Pavesi M, et al. Development and validation of a prognostic score to predict mortality in patients with acute-on-chronic liver failure. J Hepatol. 2014;61(5):1038–47.
77. Bajaj JS, O'Learey JG, Reddy KR, et al. Survival in infection-related acute-on-chronic liver failure is defined by extrahepatic organ failures. Hepatology. 2014;60(1):250–6.
78. Bernal W, Jalan R, Quaglia A, et al. Acute-on-chronic liver failure. Lancet. 2015;386(10003):1576–87.
79. Moreau R, Arroyo A. Acute-on-chronic liver failure: a new clinical entity. Clin Gastroenterol Hepatol. 2015;13(5):836–41.
80. Garg H, Kumar A, Garg V, et al. Clinical profile and predictors of mortality in patients of acute-on-chronic liver failure. Dig Liver Dis. 2012;44(2):166–71.
81. Jindal A, Sarin SK, et al. Acute kidney injury (AKI) at admission and its response to terlipressin as a predictor of mortality in patients with acute-on-chronic liver failure (ACLF). J Hepatol. 2013;58(Suppl 1):S89.
82. Maiwall R, Kumar S, Vashishtha C, et al. Acute kidney injury (AKI) in patients with acute on chronic liver failure (ACLF) is different from patients with cirrhosis. Hepatology. 2012;58(4 Suppl):36A–91A.
83. Angeli P, Rodríguez E, Piano S, et al. Acute kidney injury and acute-on-chronic liver failure classifications in prognosis assessment of patients with acute decompensation of cirrhosis. Gut. 2015;64(10):1616–22.
84. Ariza X, Graupera I, Coll M, et al. Neutrophil gelatinase-associated lipocalin is a biomarker of acute-on-chronic liver failure and prognosis in cirrho-

sis. J Hepatol. 2016;65:57. https://doi.org/10.1016/j.jhep.2016.03.002
85. Jalan R, Gines P, Olson JC, et al. Acute-on chronic liver failure. J Hepatol. 2012;57(6):1336–48.
86. Fernandez J, Navasa M, Planas R, et al. Primary prophylaxis of spontaneous bacterial peritonitis delays hepatorenal syndrome and improves survival in cirrhosis. Gastroenterology. 2007;133:818–24.
87. Shah N, El Zahraa Dhar D, Mohammed F, et al. Prevention of acute kidney injury in a rodent model of cirrhosis following selective gut decontamination is associated with reduced renal TLR4 expression. J Hepatol. 2012;56:1047–53.
88. Parker R, Armstrong MJ, Corbett C, et al. Systematic review: pentoxifylline for the treatment of severe alcoholic hepatitis. Aliment Pharmacol Ther. 2013;37(9):845–54.
89. Sidhu SS, Goyal O, Singla M, et al. Pentoxifylline in severe alcoholic hepatitis: a prospective, randomized trial. J Assoc Physicians India. 2012;60:20–2.
90. Nguyen-Khac E, Thevenot T, Piquet MA, et al. Glucocorticoids plus N-acetylcysteine in severe alcoholic hepatitis. N Engl J Med. 2011;365(19):1781–9.
91. Lebrec D, Thabut D, Oberti F, et al. Pentoxifylline does not decrease short-term mortality but does reduce complications in patients with advanced cirrhosis. Gastroenterology. 2010;138:1755–62.
92. Thursz MR, Richardson P, Allison M, et al. Prednisolone or pentoxifylline for alcoholic hepatitis. N Engl J Med. 2015;372:1619–28.
93. Duan XZ, Liu FF, Tong JJ, et al. Granulocyte-colony stimulating factor therapy improves survival in patients with hepatitis B virus-associated acute-on-chronic liver failure. World J Gastroenterol. 2013;19(7):1104–10.
94. Garg V, Garg H, Khan A, et al. Granulocyte colony-stimulating factor mobilizes CD34(+) cells and improves survival of patients with acute-on-chronic liver failure. Gastroenterology. 2012;142(3):505–12.

Acute Kidney Injury and Cancer: Incidence, Pathophysiology, Prevention/Treatment, and Outcomes

8

Colm C. Magee

8.1 Introduction

Acute kidney injury (AKI) is an important complication of cancer and its treatment [1] [1–3].

Although AKI in the cancer patient is often multifactorial, it is useful to consider the causes of AKI in the traditional categories of prerenal, intrarenal, and postrenal [1]. These are summarized in Table 8.1. Risk factors which predispose to AKI in the cancer patient include advanced age, pre-existing renal disease, hypovolemia, intrinsic nephrotoxicity of a given chemotherapy drug, the cumulative dose received of that drug, and exposure to other nephrotoxins such as nonsteroidal anti-inflammatory drugs (NSAIDs). Not only does AKI complicate the general management of the cancer patient, but it can delay or prevent administration of optimal anticancer therapy. As in many areas of medical practice, the development of AKI is generally associated with a poorer overall prognosis.

C. C. Magee
Department of Nephrology, Beaumont Hospital, Dublin, Ireland
e-mail: colmmagee@beaumont.ie

8.2 Prerenal AKI

Hypovolemia is a common complication of cancer. Fluid intake may be inadequate due to anorexia from the underlying disease or from the chemotherapy. Cancers involving the abdomen and pelvis—particularly when advanced—can cause small bowel obstruction (an example being ovarian cancer with peritoneal metastases). The chemotherapy may directly cause vomiting and diarrhea. Hypercalcemia of malignancy can exacerbate volume depletion.

Anticancer drugs can cause renal hypoperfusion and prerenal AKI by other mechanisms. High-dose interleukin-2 can cause a capillary leak syndrome (and nausea + vomiting), leading to reduced effective circulatory volume. Cancer patients are at increased risk of NSAID-induced prerenal syndromes because (a) NSAIDs are often prescribed to treat cancer pain and (b) hypovolemia is common in these patients. The topic of NSAID-induced AKI is discussed in more detail in Chap. 9.

8.2.1 Hepatorenal Syndrome

Hepatorenal syndrome can be a rare complication of massive liver infiltration by tumor cells. Occasional cases occur because of severe drug-induced hepatitis, e.g., with erlotinib, a tyrosine kinase inhibitor. Hepatorenal syndrome is most

S. S. Waikar et al. (eds.), *Core Concepts in Acute Kidney Injury*,
https://doi.org/10.1007/978-1-4939-8628-6_8

Table 8.1 Causes of AKI in the cancer patient

Prerenal
Hypovolemia (poor fluid intake, vomiting, diarrhea, capillary leak syndrome with IL2)
NSAIDs
Hypercalcemia
Hepatorenal syndrome (after HCT, massive infiltration by cancer cells)
Intrarenal
Glomerular
Rapidly progressive glomerulonephritis syndromes (rare)
Collapsing glomerulopathy (IV bisphosphonates, interferon)
Tubulointerstitial
ATN due to septic or hypovolemic shock
ATN due to IV contrast
ATN due to drugs (cisplatin, ifosfamide, zoledronate)
Acute cast nephropathy (myeloma)[a]
Tumor lysis syndrome (uric acid and calcium-phosphate deposition)[a]
High-dose methotrexate[a]
Interstitial nephritis (immune checkpoint inhibitors such as ipilimumab, nivolumab, and pembrolizumab)
Lysozymuria
Vascular
HUS (gemcitabine, mitomycin C, and other drugs; conditioning regimen for allogeneic HCT)
Anti-VEGF inhibitors and tyrosine kinase inhibitors
Postrenal
Obstruction of both urinary tracts by urological and non-urological cancers
Retroperitoneal fibrosis
Other
Bilateral nephrectomy (renal cancer)
Massive infiltration of kidneys by lymphoma
Partial or total nephrectomy for renal cell carcinoma

This list is not exhaustive
ATN acute tubular necrosis, *HCT* hematopoietic cell transplantation
[a]Associated with both tubular injury and tubular obstruction

commonly seen after myeloablative hematopoietic cell transplantation.

8.2.2 Hypercalcemia

Hypercalcemia is a relatively common complication of malignancy and indeed may be its presenting feature [2, 4]. Most cases of cancer-associated hypercalcemia are due to release of parathyroid hormone-related peptide (PTHrp) or local bone breakdown (mediated by cytokines)—see Table 8.2. Rarely, hypercalcemia is due to ectopic production of 1,25-dihydroxyvitamin D (calcitriol) in patients with lymphoma. AKI associated with hypercalcemia is predominantly due to renal vasoconstriction and hypovolemia. Treatment typically involves large volumes of normal saline (followed later by loop diuretics), high-dose bisphosphonates, steroids (where the tumor is presumed to be steroid sensitive, e.g., myeloma or lymphoma), and treatment of the underlying disease. Occasionally, oliguric AKI associated with severe hypercalcemia is treated with hemodialysis with a low calcium dialysate. In general, the renal prognosis is good because the hypercalcemia is usually reversible. The overall prognosis is frequently poor, however.

Table 8.2 Causes of hypercalcemia in the cancer patient

Type	Approximate % of total cases	Typical cancers	Bone metastases	Mediators
Humoral hypercalcemia of malignancy	80	Squamous cell cancers (of the lung, head + neck, uterine cervix), ovarian cancer, renal cancer	Minimal	PTH-related protein (PTHrP)
Local bone breakdown	20	Multiple myeloma, breast cancer, lymphoma	Extensive	Cytokines, chemokines
Excess 1,25 vitamin D3	<1	Lymphomas	Variable	1,25 vitamin D3
Ectopic PTH	<1	Various	Variable	PTH

8.3 Intrarenal AKI

Cancer and its treatment are associated with multiple intrarenal causes of AKI which can be subdivided into glomerular, tubulointerstitial, and vascular—see Table 8.1.

8.3.1 Glomerular Diseases

In general, cancer-associated glomerular disease tends to present with proteinuric syndromes and/or subacute deterioration in renal function (rather than AKI; see "angiogenesis inhibitors" below). Well-described—but rare—examples of such presentations are tumor-associated membranous nephropathy and minimal change disease. Light chain deposition disease and amyloidosis are well-known complications of myeloma and other forms of monoclonal gammopathy. Again, "pure" AKI with these conditions is rare.

Other glomerular diseases (membranoproliferative glomerulonephritis, ANCA-associated vasculitis) have been reported in patients with cancer, although the association overall is not strong. In patients with membranoproliferative glomerulonephritis, however, an underlying monoclonal gammopathy should always be excluded.

One glomerular disease that has been described almost exclusively in cancer patients is bisphosphonate-induced collapsing focal segmental glomerulosclerosis (FSGS). This form of FSGS is thought to be a direct toxic effect of high doses of intravenous bisphosphonates, particularly pamidronate (historically, cancer patients tended to receive higher doses of bisphosphonates than other non-cancer patients). Patients with this form of kidney damage typically present with nephrotic syndrome and renal failure [3, 5]. Stopping the bisphosphonate may improve renal function somewhat, but many patients have residual CKD. This complication can be minimized by avoiding very high-dose bisphosphonate regimens (especially in patients with pre-existing renal disease), administering the drug slowly and with IV fluids, and monitoring the patient's plasma creatinine and urinalysis. Another clue to bisphosphonate "overdose" is the development of hypocalcemia. Fortunately, bisphosphonate nephrotoxicity appears to be less common because of greater awareness of this significant adverse effect.

8.3.2 Tubulointerstitial Diseases

Acute tubular necrosis may occur (just as in any patient) after inadequate renal perfusion associated with the shock syndromes (hypovolemic, septic, or cardiogenic shock). Again, cancer patients are more at risk of hypovolemic and septic shock due to their underlying diagnosis and the toxic effects of chemotherapy (neutropenia, mucositis, etc.). The management of AKI from ATN in this setting is broadly similar to that of the non-cancer patient. Acute tubular injury/necrosis may also have more "cancer-specific" causes—typically nephrotoxic effects of a chemotherapy drug or of a toxic substance released by the tumor cells. General measures to prevent chemotherapy nephrotoxicity are summarized in Table 8.3.

Table 8.3 General strategies to minimize the nephrotoxicity of chemotherapy

Avoid supra-therapeutic doses
Adjust dose for lower GFR
Administer high volumes of NS or other solution to maintain high urine output before/during/after infusion of drug
Monitor patient for rising creatinine and proteinuria; consider switching or postponing therapy if these occur
Avoid other nephrotoxins such as NSAIDs

NS normal saline

AKI due to acute interstitial nephritis has recently been associated with a new class of drug called immune checkpoint inhibitors. These drugs function—at least in part—by unblocking checkpoints in the patient's immune response. Not surprisingly, severe inflammatory reactions have been reported in a number of organs including the kidneys, lungs, and GI tract [3, 6].

8.3.3 Cisplatin

Cisplatin, commonly used in the treatment of solid organ cancer, is associated with dose-related nephrotoxicity [4, 7]. Its nephrotoxic effects include AKI, CKD, Fanconi-like syndrome, and magnesium wasting. Hemolytic uremic syndrome (HUS) has been reported when cisplatin is combined with gemcitabine or bleomycin.

Typically, the patient presents with non-oliguric AKI after repeated exposure to cisplatin. Hypomagnesemia is common. There may be other evidence of tubular injury such as glycosuria and hypophosphatemia. Prevention involves adequate hydration at the time of administration and monitoring plasma creatinine. Worsening renal function may prompt a switch to a less nephrotoxic alternative such as carboplatin. Some degree of renal dysfunction and electrolyte wasting may persist for years, even after stopping the offending agent.

8.3.4 Ifosfamide

Ifosfamide can also cause severe tubular injury again resulting in AKI, CKD, and electrolyte wasting [4–8]. Nephrotoxicity is associated with higher cumulative doses. Preventive strategies are as described above for cisplatin.

8.3.5 Bisphosphonates

High doses of intravenous bisphosphonates, particularly zoledronate, can cause acute tubular necrosis, as opposed to the collapsing glomerulopathy described above [6, 9]. Prevention of this form of AKI is similar to that proposed for the glomerular lesion.

8.3.6 Acute (Myeloma) Cast Nephropathy

The term "cast nephropathy" is preferable to the less specific "myeloma kidney." The AKI in acute cast nephropathy is due to a combination of tubular injury and tubular obstruction (by casts containing light chains) [2].

In the healthy person, small amounts of light chains are filtered across the glomerular barrier and resorbed in the proximal tubule. In the setting of massive production of a pathological light chain (i.e., multiple myeloma), the normal kidney resorptive mechanisms are overwhelmed, and the light chains cause direct tubular injury and—when combined with Tamm-Horsfall protein—intratubular obstruction. Risk factors for acute cast nephropathy (in addition to production of a nephrotoxic light chain) include hypovolemia, hypercalcemia, and NSAIDs.

AKI in the setting of myeloma (or presumed myeloma) is a medical emergency. A high index of suspicion for acute cast nephropathy should be entertained in any elderly patient presenting with AKI especially if bone pain, hypercalcemia, anemia, or high plasma globulins are present. Urgent serum electrophoresis, urine electrophoresis (or serum free light chain assay), and bone marrow biopsy should be performed. Immediate treatment includes large volumes of intravenous fluids and treatment of exacerbating factors (hypercalcemia, sepsis, etc.). Where the index of suspicion for acute cast nephropathy is high and results are pending, dexamethasone therapy should be started immediately. Renal biopsy is sometimes useful in making the diagnosis of cast nephropathy but may not be required where the diagnosis of myeloma is very likely or already known.

Once the diagnosis is established, definitive chemotherapy can be given. The goal of such chemotherapy is *to reduce light chain production as quickly as possible*. Current regimens in this setting usually incorporate the proteasome inhibitor, bortezomib, plus dexamethasone. In theory, extracorporeal removal of light chains might hasten renal recovery. Early small trials of plasmapheresis were somewhat encouraging in this regard, but the most recent randomized controlled trial showed little benefit [7, 10]. Similarly, high cutoff dialysis showed promise in preliminary studies, but a benefit has not yet been shown in larger randomized controlled trials. It should be noted that plasmapheresis *is* useful in the rare cases of AKI due to hyperviscosity syndrome.

In summary, the management of presumed or confirmed acute cast nephropathy involves a high index of suspicion, rapid diagnosis, IV fluids, and early aggressive chemotherapy to rapidly reduce light chain production. Other causes of AKI in the myeloma patient are summarized in Table 8.4.

8.3.7 Tumor Lysis Syndrome

TLS is a metabolic syndrome that can complicate cancer treatment but can occasionally arise de novo, in the setting of rapid cell turnover [2].

It is most commonly associated with lymphomas and leukemias but can complicate any rapidly proliferating malignancy, particularly if highly sensitive to chemotherapy. The metabolic abnormalities that occur in TLS result from massive cell death with the release of intracellular contents—see Fig. 8.1. The pathogenesis of the AKI is twofold. Firstly, uric acid crystals are deposited within the renal tubules, causing direct tubular toxicity and intratubular obstruction. Such deposition will be favored by a low ambient pH. Secondly, calcium-phosphate crystals precipitate in the renal parenchyma—this is exacerbated by a high ambient pH.

Table 8.4 Causes of AKI in the myeloma patient

Hypercalcemia
NSAIDs
Hyperviscosity syndrome
Acute cast nephropathy
ATN
High-dose bisphosphonates

The typical onset of TLS is within 24–72 h of starting cancer treatment. TLS is characterized by hyperkalemia, hyperphosphatemia, hyperuricemia, hypocalcemia, and AKI. Plasma lactate dehydrogenase (LDH) is also elevated. With appropriate measures TLS is preventable—see also Table 8.5:

(a) Identify those at high risk of developing TLS, e.g., patients with pre-existing renal impairment or hypovolemia and high tumor load with a rapid cell turnover.
(b) Administer large volumes of IV fluids to ensure a high urine output. Typically, normal saline is used because of concerns that sodium bicarbonate solutions might worsen calcium-phosphate deposition (see above). Overuse of bicarbonate solutions might also cause significant hypocalcemia. Intravenous normal saline at >200 mL/h should commence *prior* to starting cancer treatment.
(c) Allopurinol or rasburicase (recombinant uricase) should be started prior to chemotherapy to treat or prevent hyperuricemia. Allopurinol is the less costly option. Note that these drugs do not prevent calcium-phosphate deposition.

Established TLS is a medical emergency. Treatment involves high-volume normal saline to maintain a high urine output and high-dose allopurinol or rasburicase (usually the latter). The metabolic derangements, such as hyperkalemia, should be aggressively treated. In advanced or severe cases, renal replacement therapy should be started early. *High-dose* hemodialysis or CRRT (preferably the former) is required to remove the large amounts of potassium being liberated; high-dose dialysis will also tend to rapidly normalize uric acid, calcium, and phosphate concentrations, thus treating the underlying

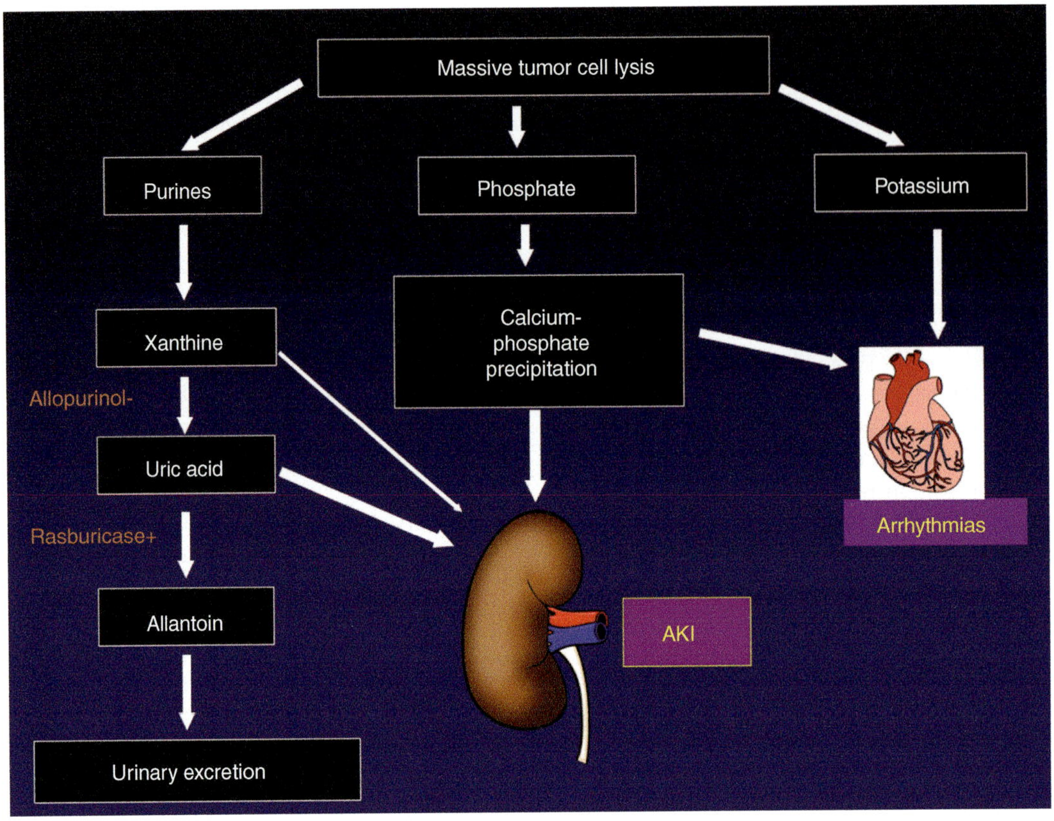

Fig. 8.1 Pathophysiology of tumor lysis syndrome. The mechanisms by which allopurinol and rasburicase prevent uric acid deposition in the kidneys are also illustrated

Table 8.5 Prevention of tumor lysis syndrome in the high-risk patient

Therapy	Comment
Large volumes of IV fluids	Aim to keep urine output >150 mL/h
Allopurinol	High doses needed. Safe and moderately effective; not expensive
Rasburicase	Recombinant form of uricase. Rapid acting, safe, and very effective but expensive. Can be used to treat established cases

causes of AKI and hastening renal recovery. In general, the renal prognosis with TLS is good, assuming the patient survives the acute event.

8.3.8 Methotrexate

High-dose IV methotrexate followed by folinic acid rescue is used in the treatment of certain leukemias, lymphomas, and solid organ cancers. High-dose protocols can cause severe AKI [3].

Nephrotoxicity is not a concern with low or standard dose methotrexate, but at high doses the drug and its metabolites can crystallize in the tubular lumina (causing obstruction and direct tubular damage). Precipitation of the drug is exacerbated by a lower urine pH. The resultant fall in GFR reduces the elimination of methotrexate—potentially exposing the patient to severe toxic effects such as myelosuppression and hepatitis.

Risk factors for methotrexate nephrotoxicity include pre-existing renal impairment, hypovolemia, and a high drug concentration at 72 h post-infusion. As urinary alkalinization reduces the intrarenal precipitation of methotrexate, a bicarbonate-based hydration regimen is recommended for the prevention of nephrotoxicity. This solution should be commenced *prior* to therapy and continued for 24–48 h after the infusion, aiming to achieve a urinary pH of >7.0.

An acute rise in plasma creatinine during or immediately after methotrexate infusion is usually the first marker of AKI. Established cases are treated with ongoing urinary alkalinization and additional folinic acid. Glucarpidase (a rescue agent, which cleaves methotrexate into nontoxic metabolites) is used in severe cases [8, 11]. Although methotrexate is not readily dialyzable and a rebound in levels occurs after cessation of dialysis, dialysis is sometimes prescribed in severe, established cases of MTX-induced AKI, pending administration of glucarpidase. Early recognition and treatment of this complication is essential.

8.3.9 Vascular Diseases

The most common vascular cause of AKI in patients with cancer is hemolytic uremic syndrome (HUS). HUS is a well-described complication of both cancer and its treatment. In some cases, an underlying adenocarcinoma of the stomach, pancreas, or prostate is directly responsible. However, most cases arise in the setting of cancer *plus* chemotherapy. The most frequently implicated chemotherapy drugs are gemcitabine, mitomycin C, and the combination of cisplatin + bleomycin. HUS can also complicate hematopoietic cell transplantation (HCT), particularly if the conditioning regimen includes irradiation and high-dose cyclophosphamide. Other causes of AKI in the patient with HCT are summarized in Table 8.6.

The renal dysfunction in cancer-associated HUS may be acute or subacute and is often associated with severe hypertension. Other clues to the diagnosis are the laboratory features of thrombotic microangiopathy (raised plasma LDH, schistocytes on blood film, falling hemoglobin, falling platelets, low haptoglobin), but these abnormalities can be subtle. The AKI may not manifest until several months after initial exposure to the offending drug (median time to diagnosis in our gemcitabine series was 8 months) [9, 12]. Patients who are receiving the above drugs should have regular monitoring of blood pressure, platelet count, renal function, and LDH. New or exacerbated hypertension is often the first sign of an evolving HUS. Further tests such as serum haptoglobin and blood films can be done when clinical suspicion for HUS is high. Urinalysis typically shows blood and protein. Renal biopsy is occasionally performed when the diagnosis is not apparent. Management involves cessation of the offending agent, control of hypertension, and supportive care. Data to support the use of plasma exchange is lacking, but some centers use it in severe cases. The overall prognosis in cancer patients who develop HUS is often guarded.

Table 8.6 Types of hematopoietic cell transplant (HCT) and associated AKI

	Allogeneic myeloablative	Autologous myeloablative	Allogeneic nonmyeloablative
Cancers treated	Many leukemias, lymphomas, myelodysplastic syndromes	Lymphomas, multiple myeloma	As for allogeneic myeloablative
Intensity of conditioning regimen	High	High	Low
AKI after HCT	Common; sometimes severe	Rare	Common; rarely severe
Causes of AKI (usually first 3 months)	HRS, shock syndromes, nephrotoxic drugs[a], CNIs, sirolimus	Shock syndromes, nephrotoxic drugs, occasionally HRS	CNIs

This list is not exhaustive
HRS hepatorenal syndrome, *CNI* calcineurin inhibitor
[a]Aminoglycosides, amphotericin

8.3.10 Angiogenesis Inhibitors

Both vascular endothelial growth factor (VEGF) inhibitors (bevacizumab, aflibercept) and tyrosine kinase inhibitors (imatinib and dasatinib) have been reported to cause proteinuria and hypertension. Less commonly, AKI may occur. The predominant histological findings have been renal thrombotic microangiopathy [4] [2, 7].

8.4 Postrenal AKI

Postrenal causes of AKI are common and should always be considered in the differential diagnosis of causes of AKI in the cancer patient. Conversely, malignancy should be considered in any patient who presents with bilateral urinary tract obstruction. Obstruction can be intrarenal (intratubular) or extrarenal—only the latter will be associated with hydronephrosis on imaging.

Intratubular obstruction can be caused by light chain casts, uric acid crystals (in tumor lysis syndrome), or crystallization of certain drugs (such as high-dose methotrexate). Acute cast nephropathy, tumor lysis syndrome, and methotrexate nephrotoxicity are discussed above. Maintaining a high urine output in "at-risk" patients is the best way to avoid intratubular precipitation and AKI.

Extrarenal obstruction typically occurs at the level of the ureters or bladder (urethral obstruction is rare). Of course, both urinary tracts must be obstructed for severe AKI to occur, unless the patient has, at baseline, a solitary functioning kidney. Bilateral ureteric obstruction can be caused by a wide range of cancers, most commonly gynecological, gastrointestinal, or urological; its presence usually indicates metastatic (and advanced) disease. Pelvic irradiation and certain malignancies such as lymphomas and sarcoma can cause retroperitoneal fibrosis and ureteric obstruction; here there may be minimal or no hydronephrosis/hydroureter.

The clinical presentation of postrenal failure depends to some extent on the degree, the acuity, and the site of the obstruction. Severe, acute cases may present with oliguria and suprapubic or flank pain. Examination may show an enlarged bladder and/or flank tenderness. There may be other symptoms and signs (such as bone pain) suggesting a diagnosis of cancer. Ultrasound is the initial imaging modality of choice because it is inexpensive, is readily available, involves no IV contrast, and is a sensitive test for hydronephrosis—see Fig. 8.2. It does not, however, provide good visualization of the distal ureters. CT or MRI are often used to define the level of obstruction and to stage the underlying malignancy. Initial treatment involves relief of the obstruction (see Fig. 8.2) and treatment of the underlying malignancy. Nephrostomies and ureteric stenting often result in reasonable recovery of renal function—assuming renal parenchyma is reasonably well preserved at the time of presentation. Unfortunately, the overall prognosis is often guarded because the obstruction is usually due to extensive tumor. The prognosis can be better, however, with lymphoma-induced obstruction; indeed effective treatment of the lymphoma can dramatically reduce tumor and lymph node bulk in the retroperitoneum, allowing safe removal of nephrostomies/stents.

In summary, the general management of postrenal AKI involves:

(a) Making the diagnosis based on history, examination, and basic tests (e.g., ultrasound showing bilateral hydronephrosis)
(b) Where appropriate, excluding prerenal and intrarenal causes
(c) Rapid relief of the obstruction and treatment of its underlying cause

8.4.1 Miscellaneous Conditions

8.4.1.1 Bilateral or Unilateral Nephrectomy

Von Hippel-Lindau (VHL) disease is an autosomal dominant condition manifested by a variety of benign and malignant tumors, including clear cell carcinoma of the kidney. Renal cancers may be bilateral—see Fig. 8.3. Bilateral renal call cancers may also occur in the absence of VHL. Although partial nephrectomy and other nephron-sparing treatments are now widely used in such cases, some patients ultimately require

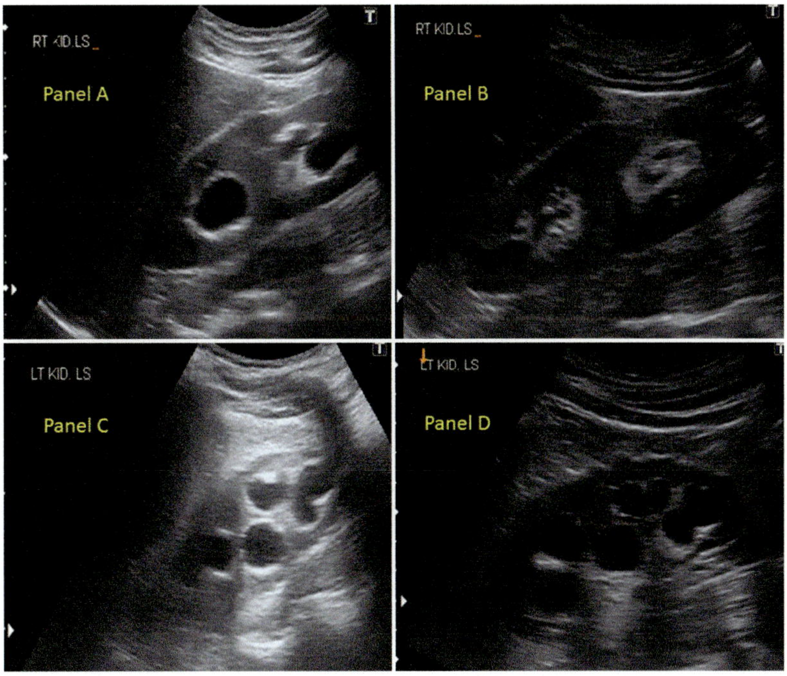

Fig. 8.2 Ultrasound images of a 70-year-old male who presented with suprapubic discomfort and oliguria and was ultimately diagnosed with prostate adenocarcinoma. Examination showed a palpable suprapubic mass (bladder). Plasma creatinine was 4.3 mg/dL. Insertion of a bladder catheter improved urine output, and creatinine fell, but not to normal. Panels (**a**) and (**b**) show the right kidney before and after insertion of a bladder catheter (resolution of the hydronephrosis). Panels (**c**) and (**d**) show the left kidney before and after insertion of the bladder catheter (persistent hydronephrosis). Further imaging showed obstruction of the left ureter by enlarged lymph nodes. Note the left kidney is also somewhat atrophic

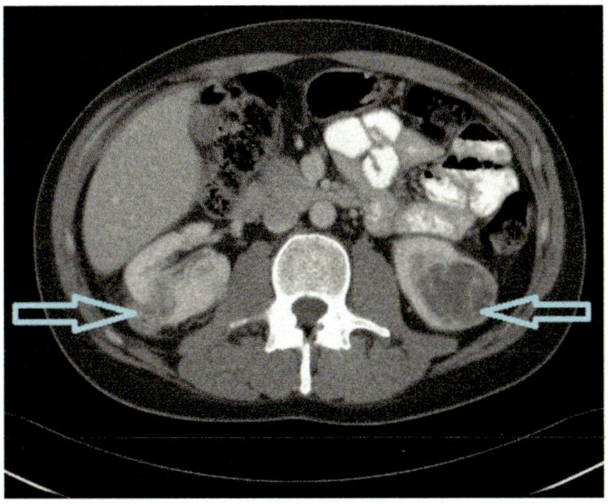

Fig. 8.3 CT of a 27-year-old male recently diagnosed with intracranial hemangioblastoma. Arrows show complex cysts/masses in both kidneys. The patient ultimately needed bilateral nephrectomy

single and then double nephrectomy. This obviously precipitates the need for dialysis.

Unilateral or partial nephrectomy is often required for the optimal treatment of renal cell carcinoma. Such surgery can precipitate AKI, particularly in the patient with risk factors for renal disease [2, 13].

8.4.1.2 Tumor Infiltration

Metastases to the kidney are not uncommon, particularly on autopsy. However, involvement severe enough to cause AKI requires that both kidneys are extensively involved—this happens occasionally with rapidly growing hematologic malignancies, such as lymphoma or acute leukemia. Affected patients usually present with AKI, a bland urinalysis, and enlarged kidneys. The presence of large kidneys on imaging in a patient with known lymphoma or leukemia is suggestive of tumor infiltration. When large kidneys and AKI are observed in a patient with no known malignancy, the diagnosis can be established by renal biopsy. The renal prognosis depends on the responsiveness of the tumor to therapy. A rapid reduction in kidney size and improvement in renal function may be seen within days if the tumor responds rapidly to therapy. Appropriate prophylaxis to prevent tumor lysis syndrome is important.

8.4.2 AKI after Hematopoietic Cell Transplantation

The general purpose of HCT is to allow administration of otherwise lethal (and ideally curative) doses of chemoradiotherapy, followed by engraftment of stem or progenitor cells for marrow recovery. Most commonly, HCT is used to treat hematologic cancers, but other indications now include certain nonhematologic cancers, severe genetic disorders (such as immunodeficiencies), and severe autoimmune diseases. The three main types of HCT are summarized in Table 8.6. Of note, calcineurin inhibitors are commonly prescribed after forms of allogeneic HCT, to prevent graft-versus-host disease.

AKI is common after HCT, but its incidence and severity depend on the type of HCT (and on the definition of AKI used in reported series) [10, 14]. It is most common after myeloablative allogeneic HCT, reflecting the propensity of this regimen to cause profound immunosuppression (with associated risk of severe sepsis) and liver damage (with associated risk of hepatorenal syndrome); furthermore, CNIs are routinely prescribed for the first 100 days after transplantation. Severe AKI is least common after nonmyeloablative HCT—even though patients are older and sometimes sicker—reflecting the shorter period of pancytopenia and the rarity of severe posttransplant liver disease [10, 14]. The principal cause of AKI in this setting is probably CNI toxicity; severe AKI necessitating dialysis is relatively rare. Myeloablative autologous HCT has an intermediate incidence of AKI. If dialysis is required for severe AKI, the overall prognosis is usually very poor, whatever the type of HCT. Fortunately, rates of AKI appear to be decreasing—probably related to multiple improvements in peritransplant care [11, 15].

Hepatic sinusoidal obstructive syndrome (SOS), also known as veno-occlusive disease of the liver, is one of the most common causes of severe AKI after myeloablative HCT, particularly allogeneic myeloablative HCT. The pathophysiology is thought to involve radiotherapy—and chemotherapy-induced damage to the hepatic venules. Clinically, SOS is manifested as a form of hepatorenal syndrome and usually appears in the first 30 days. In mild to moderate cases, sodium and fluid restriction, diuresis, and analgesia may be required, and the syndrome eventually resolves. Severe SOS complicated by liver and renal failure (and frequently respiratory failure) carries a very high mortality >80% [12, 16]. Treatment involves supportive care (sodium and fluid restriction, avoidance of all hepatotoxins, etc.) and, in severe cases, defibrotide [13, 17]. Hemodialysis or CRRT may be required; the latter has the potential advantages of minimizing changes in intracranial pressure and more easily controlling the large daily obligate fluid intake.

Conclusion

AKI is an important complication of cancer and its treatment. As new therapies are constantly being introduced into oncology, physicians need to be aware of the possibility of new nephrotoxic drugs and "new" renal syndromes. Common sense strategies such as identifying the high-risk patient in advance (allowing close monitoring of renal function), minimizing unnecessary exposure to nephrotoxins, and avoiding hypovolemia can prevent some cases of AKI. Early diagnosis and treatment of AKI is important—this is most likely to happen when there is close collaboration between oncologists and nephrologists.

References

1. Humphreys BD, Soiffer RJ, Magee CC. Renal failure associated with cancer and its treatment: an update. J Am Soc Nephrol [Internet]. 2005 Jan [cited 2012 Sep 17];16(1):151–61. Available from: http://www.ncbi.nlm.nih.gov/pubmed/15574506.
2. Rosner MH, Perazella MA. Acute kidney injury in patients with cancer. N Engl J Med. 2017;377(5):500–1.
3. Malyszko J, Kozlowska K, Kozlowski L, Malyszko J. Nephrotoxicity of anticancer treatment. Nephrol Dial Transplant. 2017;32(6):924–36.

4. Stewart AF. Clinical practice. Hypercalcemia associated with cancer. N Engl J Med [Internet]. 2005 Jan 27 [cited 2016 Sep 10];352(4):373–9. Available from: http://www.ncbi.nlm.nih.gov/pubmed/15673803.
5. Markowitz GS, Appel GB, Fine PL, Fenves AZ, Loon NR, Jagannath S, et al. Collapsing focal segmental glomerulosclerosis following treatment with high-dose pamidronate. J Am Soc Nephrol [Internet]. 2001 Jun [cited 2016 Sep 9];12(6):1164–72. Available from: http://www.ncbi.nlm.nih.gov/pubmed/11373339.
6. Belliere J, Meyer N, Mazieres J, Ollier S, Boulinguez S, Delas A, Ribes D, Faguer S. Acute interstitial nephritis related to immune checkpoint inhibitors. Br J Cancer. 2016;115(12):1457–61.
7. Perazella MA. Onco-nephrology: renal toxicities of chemotherapeutic agents. Clin J Am Soc Nephrol [Internet]. 2012 Oct [cited 2016 Sep 10];7(10):1713–21. Available from: http://www.ncbi.nlm.nih.gov/pubmed/22879440.
8. Schlondorff JS, Mendez GP, Rennke HG, Magee CC. Electrolyte abnormalities and progressive renal failure in a cancer patient. Kidney Int [Internet]. 2007 Jun [cited 2012 Sep 17];71(11):1181–4. Available from: http://www.ncbi.nlm.nih.gov/pubmed/17332730.
9. Markowitz GS, Fine PL, Stack JI, Kunis CL, Radhakrishnan J, Palecki W, et al. Toxic acute tubular necrosis following treatment with zoledronate (Zometa). Kidney Int [Internet]. 2003 Jul [cited 2016 Sep 9];64(1):281–9. Available from: http://www.ncbi.nlm.nih.gov/pubmed/12787420.
10. Clark WF, Stewart AK, Rock GA, Sternbach M, Sutton DM, Barrett BJ, et al. Plasma exchange when myeloma presents as acute renal failure: a randomized, controlled trial. Ann Intern Med [Internet]. 2005 Dec 6 [cited 2016 Sep 9];143(11):777–84. Available from: http://www.ncbi.nlm.nih.gov/pubmed/16330788.
11. Widemann BC, Balis FM, Kim A, Boron M, Jayaprakash N, Shalabi A, et al. Glucarpidase, leucovorin, and thymidine for high-dose methotrexate-induced renal dysfunction: clinical and pharmacologic factors affecting outcome. J Clin Oncol [Internet]. 2010 Sep 1 [cited 2016 Sep 9];28(25):3979–86. Available from: http://www.ncbi.nlm.nih.gov/pubmed/20679598.
12. Humphreys BD, Sharman JP, Henderson JM, Clark JW, Marks PW, Rennke HG, et al. Gemcitabine-associated thrombotic microangiopathy. Cancer [Internet]. 2004 Jun 15 [cited 2012 Aug 22];100(12):2664–70. Available from: http://www.ncbi.nlm.nih.gov/pubmed/15197810.
13. Cho A, Lee JE, Kwon GY, Huh W, Lee HM, Kim YG, Kim DJ, Oh HY, Choi HY. Post-operative acute kidney injury in patients with renal cell carcinoma is a potent risk factor for new-onset chronic kidney disease after radical nephrectomy. Nephrol Dial Transplant. 2011;26(11):3496–501.
14. Parikh CR, Schrier RW, Storer B, Diaconescu R, Sorror ML, Maris MB, et al. Comparison of ARF after myeloablative and nonmyeloablative hematopoietic cell transplantation. Am J Kidney Dis [Internet]. 2005 Mar [cited 2016 Sep 10];45(3):502–9. Available from: http://www.ncbi.nlm.nih.gov/pubmed/15754272.
15. Gooley TA, Chien JW, Pergam SA, Hingorani S, Sorror ML, Boeckh M, et al. Reduced mortality after allogeneic hematopoietic-cell transplantation. N Engl J Med [Internet]. 2010 Nov 25 [cited 2016 Sep 10];363(22):2091–101. Available from: http://www.ncbi.nlm.nih.gov/pubmed/21105791.
16. Coppell JA, Richardson PG, Soiffer R, Martin PL, Kernan NA, Chen A, et al. Hepatic veno-occlusive disease following stem cell transplantation: incidence, clinical course, and outcome. Biol Blood Marrow Transplant [Internet]. 2010 Feb [cited 2016 Sep 10];16(2):157–68. Available from: http://www.ncbi.nlm.nih.gov/pubmed/19766729.
17. Richardson PG, Riches ML, Kernan NA, Brochstein JA, Mineishi S, Termuhlen AM, et al. Phase 3 trial of defibrotide for the treatment of severe veno-occlusive disease and multi-organ failure. Blood [Internet]. 2016 Mar 31 [cited 2016 Sep 10];127(13):1656–65. Available from: http://www.ncbi.nlm.nih.gov/pubmed/26825712.

9 Drug-Induced Acute Kidney Injury

Randy L. Luciano and Mark A. Perazella

9.1 Introduction

Therapeutic and diagnostic agents have long been noted to alter kidney function. The kidney is a common site of drug toxicity since many drugs are filtered, secreted, reabsorbed, biotransformed, and excreted by the kidney. The resulting enhanced and prolonged renal exposure to various drugs and drug metabolites can lead to injury within all compartments of the kidney: the interstitium, tubules, glomeruli, and renal blood vessels. Recognizing acute kidney injury (AKI) syndromes that are associated with various agents can lead to early identification in the treatment course of potentially harmful drugs and therapeutic agents. Once identified, the medication or agent can be withheld or dose-reduced, thereby significantly impacting and potentially reducing the duration and severity of kidney injury. This chapter focuses on diagnosis and recognition of patterns of AKI associated with certain drugs. While not all encompassing, it highlights major drugs.

R. L. Luciano
Section of Nephrology, Department of Internal Medicine, Yale University School of Medicine, New Haven, CT, USA
e-mail: randy.luciano@yale.edu

M. A. Perazella (✉)
Section of Nephrology, Yale University School of Medicine, New Haven, CT, USA

Department of Medicine, Yale University, New Haven, CT, USA
e-mail: mark.perazella@yale.edu

9.2 Epidemiology of Drug-Induced Kidney Injury

The incidence and prevalence of drug-induced acute kidney injury (DI-AKI) are problematic and difficult to determine for several reasons. While therapeutic agents have been implicated in up to 60% of all hospital-acquired acute kidney injury (AKI) [1], the incidence is actually quite variable. In-hospital administration of medications has contributed to approximately 17–27% of all AKI, based on various studies [2–6]. The wide variability of estimating AKI prevalence in these studies is multifactorial. First, the prevalence variability of AKI may be related to the definition of AKI employed in certain studies. Second, most studies capture data on ICU patients yet miss the data on non-ICU patients, and very few studies examine AKI in non-hospitalized patients. Third, the inclusion of diagnostic agents, such as radiocontrast, can significantly alter the percentages of drug-induced versus other causes of AKI in hospitalized patients. Fourth, the effect of therapeutic agents on patients with chronic kidney disease (CKD) is often overlooked or actively excluded. Despite the variability, drug-induced AKI does have a high incidence and

S. S. Waikar et al. (eds.), *Core Concepts in Acute Kidney Injury*,
https://doi.org/10.1007/978-1-4939-8628-6_9

prevalence and is associated with an increased morbidity and mortality.

9.3 Risk Factors for Drug-Induced Kidney Injury

Risk factors for drug-induced AKI can be divided into risks specific to the drug or diagnostic agent, factors specific to the kidney's drug handling, or characteristics specific to the patient (Table 9.1) Distinguishing these various risks is critical to assess whether any modifiable factors exist that can facilitate the use of measures that prevent or alleviate injury. While medications or therapeutic agents themselves are directly toxic or injurious to the kidney, development of AKI is significantly influenced by the presence of concurrent patient risk factors for nephrotoxicity.

Table 9.1 Risk factors for drug-induced acute kidney injury

Kidney-specific factors
High blood flow rate (up to 25% if cardiac output)
Differential sensitivity based on metabolic activity with kidney (cells in loop of Henle are more sensitive)
Increased accumulation and concentration of drugs or metabolites
Transport properties of renal tubular epithelial cells
Enzymes specific for biotransformation that can lead to generation of reactive oxygen species
Patient-specific factors
Older ager (>65 years)
Female gender
Acute kidney injury
Chronic kidney disease
Nephrotic syndrome
Acute and chronic heart failure
Cirrhosis
True or effective volume depletion
Metabolic derangements
Hypercalcemia, hypokalemia, hypomagnesemia
Alkaline or acidic urine pH
Host genetic factors
Gene mutations in hepatic or renal CYP450 enzymes
Gene mutations in renal transport channels
Drug-specific factors
Prolonged exposure
Direct nephrotoxic effects of a compound
Combinations of medications leading to or enhancing nephrotoxicity
Insolubility leading to crystal precipitation

9.3.1 Renal Risk Factors

The kidney itself is more prone to injury based on several factors. First, the kidney has significant exposure to potentially nephrotoxic medications and therapeutic agents by virtue of its high blood flow rate, which averages approximately 20–25% of cardiac output. As a result, therapeutic and diagnostic agents are delivered at a high rate to the kidney, allowing for greater exposure of potentially toxic substance to the kidney, thereby contributing to the burden of kidney injury [7].

On a cellular level, certain areas of the kidney are more prone to injury. Renal tubular epithelial cells (RTECs) that exist deep in the renal medullary regions are highly metabolically active, resulting in increased oxygen consumption. This demand creates a relatively hypoxic environment that makes cells exquisitely sensitive to toxic injury. As a result, these RTECs, through localized hypoxia, have a decreased ability to adequately respond to nephrotoxic substances that are encountered. In addition to this inherent hypoxic property of the cellular environment, the medullary region also has a significant concentrating ability, which can lead to the accumulation of drugs or drug metabolites at high concentrations. Ultimately, this concentrating effect on drug levels may promote toxic renal injury [7].

The unique transport properties of proximal RTECs make this region more prone to injury. These cells have extensive apical and basolateral cellular uptake mechanisms. Apical uptake of compounds occurs through endocytosis and other uptake mechanisms [8–10]. Upon uptake via the megalin/cubilin receptor, compounds enter lysosomes, accumulate and form myeloid bodies and/or rupture, and spill toxic substances into the cytoplasm. This results in the accumulation and concentration of potentially nephrotoxic substances within cells that can result in signaling pathways and cascades that ultimately lead to cell injury and death. Basolateral delivery also leads to proximal tubular exposure of compounds. Delivery occurs via peritubular capillaries, with uptake occurring through transporters called human organic anion/cation transporters (HOAT/HOCT) [9, 11]. This movement of potentially toxic substances into the intracellular space, and subsequent shuttling and apical excretion, increases the exposure of the proximal tubular cells to these substances, thereby contributing to AKI.

On a biochemical level, the kidney has several enzymes responsible for the biotransformation of drugs. These include CYP450 and flavin-containing monooxygenases. The breakdown of compounds in the kidney results in the generation of potentially nephrotoxic metabolites and reactive oxygen species that can promote injury (apoptosis and/or necrosis). Reactive oxygen species generation leads to oxidative stress and the generation of free radicals. Through nucleic acid oxidation and alkylation causing DNA breaks, direct protein damage, and lipid peroxidation, kidney injury can occur [7].

9.3.2 Patient Risk Factors

Various patient-specific factors also contribute to drug-induced kidney injury. Certain factors are not modifiable including age and sex. Both older age (>65 years old) and female sex increase the risk of drug-induced AKI. This effect is generally multifactorial. First, reductions in total body water are common in the elderly due to decreased lean body mass, leading to a decrease in total body water that affects drug distribution and plasma concentrations of water-soluble drugs. Second, lower muscle mass may impair the ability to detect abnormal GFRs masked by apparently normal serum creatinine concentrations. GFR estimating equations that are based on age attempt to ameliorate this concern, but oftentimes serum creatinine concentration, and not estimated GFR is assessed when clinicians are dosing drugs. Lastly, the elderly also tend to be more prone to increased renal arteriolar vasoconstriction secondary to angiotensin II or endothelin excess. This renal effect may expose the patient to increased drug concentrations [12–14].

Additional risk factors for drug-related injury unique to patients include the presence of acute or chronic kidney disease. Underlying kidney injury, either current AKI or CKD, makes a patient more susceptible to drug nephrotoxicity. Acutely injured kidneys may have ischemia preconditioned tubules that generate a more pronounced renal oxidative injury response to toxins. In both AKI and CKD, there may be an increased exposure of a decreased number of functioning nephrons to toxins, which will exacerbate pre-existing kidney dysfunction. Employing GFR estimating equations during AKI may also result in an overestimation of the GFR, especially with rapidly declining renal function. This can potentially lead to mis-dosing of medications leading to the accumulation of toxic doses of medications or metabolites [7]. More severe and prolonged AKI often develops, which risks development of CKD.

Apart from underlying kidney disease, other systemic diseases that are known to impair renal perfusion can increase susceptibility to drug injury. These include edematous states such as acute and chronic heart failure, nephrotic syndrome, and cirrhosis, which create a state of effective circulating volume depletion and renal underperfusion. This effectively volume-depleted state will lead to the activation of neurohormonal cascades that reduce renal perfusion. Patients with nephrotic syndrome and cirrhosis, and to a minor degree in malnourished heart failure patients, will develop hypoalbuminemia. As a result of reduced protein binding of drugs, low serum albumin can lead to increased free drug concentrations, thereby increasing exposure of certain potentially toxic drugs to the kidney [13, 14].

Certain host genetic differences can explain the heterogenous response that patients have to drug-induced kidney injury. For example, differences in innate host immune response genes can predispose certain patients to allergic drug reactions with acute interstitial nephritis (AIN) developing. In addition, the kidney has CYP450 enzymes, and polymorphisms in these genes may lead to altered metabolism with the potential for increased nephrotoxicity [15, 16]. Also, specific polymorphisms in transport channels may lead to altered metabolism with associated drug nephrotoxicity.

9.4 Diagnosis of Drug-Induced Acute Kidney Injury

Diagnosis of DI-AKI is similar to that of other forms of AKI and utilizes a combination of clinical, laboratory, and imaging findings (Table 9.2).

Table 9.2 Tests use to diagnose drug-induced acute kidney injury

Test	Findings	Advantages	Disadvantages
Physical exam			
Volume assessment	Peripheral or pulmonary edema	Relatively easy to assess	May not be an accurate representation of intravascular volume status
Rash	Multiple rashes	Superficial and easy to assess or biopsy	Non-specific and non-sensitive
Fever	Elevated temperature vs. hyperpyrexia	Objective	Non-specific and non-sensitive
Flank pain	Associated flank swelling or tenderness	Easy to obtain history	Non-specific and non-sensitive
Serum laboratories			
BUN or creatinine	Elevated BUN or creatinine	Easy to measure	Need to know baseline creatinine
Electrolytes	Decreased phosphorous or potassium in tubular disorders	Easy to measure	May be due to non-kidney causes
CBC	Elevated eosinophils could suggest allergic reaction	Easy to assess	Non-specific and non-sensitive
Urine evaluations			
FeNa, FeUrea	Alterations around a predetermined value	Easy to obtain and calculate	Non-specific and non-sensitive
Urinalysis	Evaluate for specific gravity, protein, glucose, heme, leukocyte esterase, red and white blood cells, bacteria, yeast, and casts	Easy to obtain	False negatives exist, inaccuracy with cast and crystal interpretation
Urine eosinophils	Presence of eosinophils in urine with Hansel stain	Should not be used	Low sensitivity and specificity
Urine sediment analysis	Identify abnormal cells, casts, crystals	Direct correlation with kidney injury that can be localized to the site of injury	Requires a trained nephrologist and the presence of a microscope and centrifuge
Imaging			
Ultrasound	Kidney size, echogenicity, hydronephrosis	Evaluation of obstruction in noninvasive safe way	Technologist dependent, limited in diagnostic capabilities
Computed tomography	Kidney size, echogenicity, hydronephrosis	Noninvasive	Requires radiation exposure, contrast not often used, but is a nephrotoxin
Gallium scintigraphy	Enhancement of kidneys with active inflammatory cells	Noninvasive	Low sensitivity and specificity, may be difficult to order
FDG-PET scan	Enhancement of kidneys with active inflammatory cells	Noninvasive	Only small studies have looked at this
Biopsy	Identifies kidney injury based on light, immunofluorescence, and electron microscopy	Direct look at site of kidney injury	Invasive with risks of bleeding and infection

Kidney injury may lead to various physical exam abnormalities. If allergic in nature, drug-induced injury may lead to a fever or rash; however these findings are relatively uncommon. The rash can present as a morbilliform, maculopapular, toxic epidermal necrolysis or a purpuric rash depending on the underlying renal lesion [17]. In addition to these findings, the patient may experience flank pain if there is swelling in the renal parenchyma and stretching of the renal capsule.

Laboratory evaluations can provide insight into the type of kidney injury. Elevations in blood urea nitrogen (BUN) and serum creatinine concentrations are often the first clinical manifestation of drug-induced kidney injury. As shown in animal (and some human) studies, novel serum and urinary biomarkers of kidney injury may provide an earlier diagnosis of acute kidney injury but are currently not available in the USA. Serum potassium and phosphorous are usually elevated in AKI; however hypophosphatemia and hypokalemia can also be important findings in the setting of certain forms of drug-induced tubular injury. Low serum phosphorus and potassium, in the correct context, can indicate adequate or modestly reduced GFR, yet impaired tubular reabsorption, suggesting proximal RTEC dysfunction. This injury pattern is often seen in a Fanconi syndrome, which occurs with several drugs.

A complete blood count can also provide clues into the type of kidney injury. Increased serum eosinophils may be seen with allergic or hypersensitivity-related renal disorders, both of which are common forms of drug-induced kidney injury. The combination of anemia and thrombocytopenia is very suggestive of a microangiopathic hemolytic anemic disease, such as drug-induced thrombotic microangiopathy, which is associated with AKI.

When evaluating drug-induced kidney injury, a thorough examination of the urine, through both automated laboratory analysis and direct sediment analysis, is critical in classifying the various types of renal injury and predicting the severity of injury. Automated urinalysis provides information that is complimentary to clinical labs and the urine sediment findings. Normoglycemic glucosuria suggests decreased proximal tubular glucose reabsorption, indicative of tubular dysfunction. Positive leukocyte esterase indicates the presence of leukocytes in the urine suggesting infection when accompanied by bacteria or yeast in the urine or, in the absence of microorganisms, inflammation along the genitourinary tract. Urinary eosinophils have been used in the past to suggest the possibility of AIN. However, the sensitivity and specificity of this test are quite low, and therefore, it is not recommended in the diagnostic workup [18].

Protein present on automated urinalysis indicates urinary albumin and not other proteins. Protein positive on a urinalysis is qualitative and should prompt protein quantification by the direct measurement of urinary albumin and total protein. Kidney injury that is predominantly glomerular in nature will generally have a large amount of albuminuria relative to total urinary protein. In contrast, low urinary albumin levels relative to total protein suggest either the presence of excess filtered non-albumin serum proteins or tubular dysfunction with tubular proteinuria [19, 20].

Urine sediment examination is an extremely useful diagnostic tool. The presence of RTECs, white blood cells (WBCs), or red blood cells (RBCs) can be suggestive of kidney injury. While RTECs may exist in low numbers in a patient without kidney injury, an abundance of RTECs often indicates underlying tubular injury. The presence of isomorphic RBCs can suggest an injury anywhere along the genitourinary tract, from the kidney to the urethra. However, dysmorphic RBCs is highly specific for glomerular injury, although they can be seen with certain inflammatory tubular disorders. The presence of urinary WBCs suggests inflammation anywhere along the genitourinary tract. The presence of bacteria or yeast alongside WBCs should raise the suspicion for an infection, whereas sterile pyuria raises suspicion for a renal inflammatory process [21].

Apart from cells, the urinary sediment is also useful in the identification of casts (cellular and noncellular) and crystals. Casts are composed of Tamm Horsfall protein, or uromodulin, a protein secreted by loop of Henle renal tubular cells. Hyaline casts are made of this protein and form in the setting of sluggish urinary flow rates. Cellular casts, whether RBC, WBC, RTEC, or a mix of these cells, is indicative of intrinsic kidney injury [22]. Muddy brown granular casts are also indicative of kidney injury and generally reflect ischemic or nephrotoxic acute tubular injury. Crystals may also be present in the urinary sediment [23]. Crystal-induced kidney disease will be discussed in detail in subsequent sections.

Imaging may be a useful tool in the diagnosis of acute and chronic kidney disease. Ultrasound demonstrates kidney size and echogenicity, which may indicate the possibility of chronic kidney disease or congenital or acquired unilateral kidney. Ultrasound is also helpful in evaluating for obstruction, manifested by hydronephrosis and/or hydroureter. Gallium scintigraphy and FDG-PET scans have also been used to diagnose AKI due to kidney inflammation such as AIN but are insensitive and non-specific findings [17].

Kidney biopsy is the gold standard in the diagnosis of drug-induced kidney injury. With examination of renal histology, the vasculature, glomeruli, tubules, and interstitium should be evaluated for injury patterns that can differentiate between the different etiologies of drug-induced kidney injury. Examples include drug-induced thrombotic microangiopathy and vasculitis as indicative of drug-associated vascular injury and immune-complex deposition and podocytopathies from a large number of drugs causing glomerular injury. Numerous medications promote acute tubular injury and necrosis through direct toxic effects, ischemic injury, osmotic effects, and crystal deposition within tubular lumens. An inflammatory infiltrate within the renal interstitium along with tubulitis and sometimes granulomas are histologic manifestations of drug-induced acute interstitial nephritis observed on kidney biopsy.

9.5 Drug-Induced Acute Kidney Injury

Many drugs can affect kidney function. The following sections describe drug-induced kidney injury patterns based on the underlying location in the kidney. Common drugs or drug classes are included, with more in-depth listings of drugs included in associated tables.

9.5.1 Prerenal (Hemodynamic) Acute Kidney Injury

Glomerular filtration is modulated by a number of local and systemic hormones which include the prostaglandins (PG), angiotensin, endothelin, catecholamines, and atrial natriuretic peptide, to name a few. Afferent vasodilation and efferent vasoconstriction allow maintenance of glomerular filtration, especially when renal perfusion is compromised by hypotension and true or effective volume depletion. Perturbations of these vascular forces can lead to prerenal physiology or hemodynamic reductions in GFR. Several drugs may reduce GFR by altering afferent or efferent vascular tone (Fig. 9.1).

9.5.1.1 Afferent Vasoconstriction

Nonsteroidal anti-inflammatory drugs Nonsteroidal anti-inflammatory drugs (NSAIDs) are commonly employed as analgesics, antipyretics, and anti-inflammatory medications. NSAIDs are implicated in many forms of drug-related injury including hemodynamic AKI from dysregulation of glomerular blood flow [24, 25]. NSAIDs inhibit cyclooxygenase (COX) enzymes, which convert arachidonic acid (AA) to various PGs. Inhibition of the COX enzymes leads to a decrease in prostaglandin synthesis, thereby severely curtailing prostaglandin function to modulate afferent arteriolar tone. As PGs potentiate afferent arteriolar dilatation, inhibition of their synthesis through NSAID use can lead afferent vasoconstriction, thereby impairing renal blood flow leading to a decreased GFR and hemodynamic AKI. Normally the effects of prostaglandins on arteriolar tone are minimal; however in severe acute volume depletion, in effective volume depletion (cirrhosis, heart failure, nephrotic syndrome), or in CKD, patients are prostaglandin dependent for maintenance of GFR. In these settings, PG inhibition can tip the afferent arteriole to vasoconstriction, thus leading to decreased GFR. COX

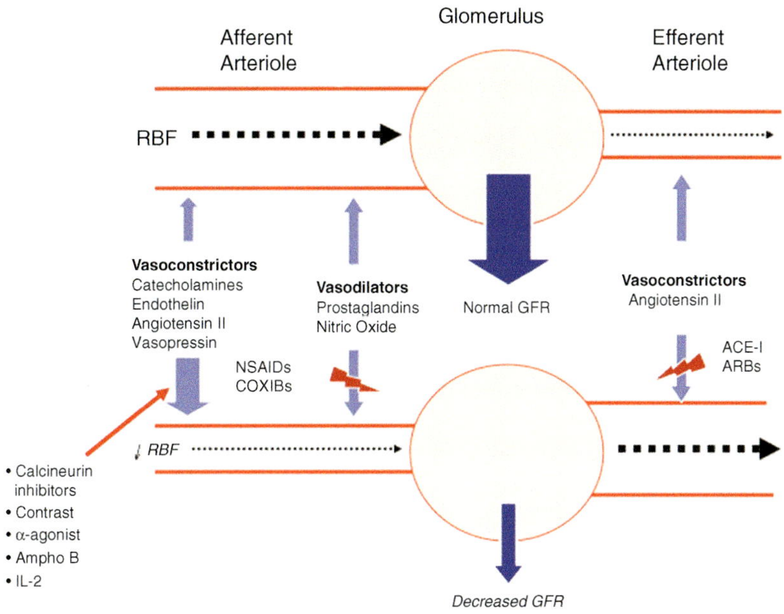

Fig. 9.1 Glomerular filtration is determined in part by afferent arteriolar and efferent arteriolar vascular tone. In states of reduced blood flow and low blood pressure, the afferent arteriole is dilated, and the efferent arteriole is constricted. The medications noted in the figure disturb this response and reduce GFR

enzymes can exist as either a COX-1 or COX-2 subtypes, both of which are important to maintain GFR and inhibition of either can hemodynamic AKI [26–28].

Calcineurin inhibitors Cyclosporine and tacrolimus belong to a class of medications known as the calcineurin inhibitors (CNI). These medications function by binding cytoplasmic proteins (cyclophilins and FK-binding protein, respectively), which leads to the inhibition of calcineurin, which in turn prevents the transcription of certain immune cytokines. These medications are widely used as immunosuppressants for solid organ transplantation and a variety of autoimmune disorders. One side effect of these drugs, especially at higher doses with supratherapeutic levels, is afferent and efferent arteriolar vasoconstriction caused primarily by endothelial dysfunction. This leads to the decreased production of vasodilators, such as PGs and nitric oxide, and the release of vasoconstrictors, such as thromboxane A2 and endothelin, which reduce renal perfusion and GFR [29, 30]. As with the NSAIDs, true or effective volume depletion and CKD predispose to reductions in GFR and AKI. In addition, the use of these agents in the setting of graft ischemia can prolong primary graft dysfunction and failure. In addition to CNI dose reduction, discontinuation of certain drugs (NSAIDs, ACE/ARBs), calcium channel blocker therapy, and administration of intravenous volume can mitigate the effects of CNI nephrotoxicity.

Angiotensin converting enzyme inhibition/angiotensin receptor blockade Activation of the angiotensin type I receptor (AT-I) of the efferent arteriole causes arteriolar vasoconstriction that leads to an increase in intraglomerular capillary pressure and thereby maintains GFR in the setting of mild to moderate renal underperfusion. In normal states, angiotensin antagonism by angiotensin converting enzyme inhibitors (ACEI) or angiotensin receptor blockers (ARBs) has little effect on renal hemodynamics. However, ACEI or ARBS are administered in settings of reduced RBF, as with severe renal artery stenosis, states of true or effective volume depletion, with CKD, or NSAID or CNI therapy, intraglomerular capillary pressure decreases and GFR declines [31, 32]. A decline in GFR that stabilizes is typically beneficial in patients with proteinuric CKD. However, in severe RAS and volume-depleted states, AKI with rising serum creatinine develops and warrants investigation with temporary drug discontinuation (and correction of the underlying disease state).

9.5.2 Intrinsic Kidney Disease

9.5.2.1 Vascular Disease

Several medications have been implicated in drug-induced AKI as a result of vascular injury. As the kidney is extremely vascular organ, local and systemic disease causing renal vascular injury is often associated with AKI. Below are three forms of vascular injury that have been associated with drug-induced AKI.

Cholesterol embolization is a syndrome that can be induced by anticoagulant and thrombolytic therapy. While this complication more often occurs following arteriography and certain vascular procedures, the diagnosis is sometimes difficult to differentiate from radiocontrast-induced AKI. Upon administration of the thrombolytic agents, which dissolve thrombus covering atherosclerotic plaques, cholesterol fragments embolize to vessels in various end organs including the kidneys. Most often the skin, as manifested by acute distal cyanosis in the form of infarcted digits or livedo reticularis, or the kidney, as manifested by AKI and acute hypertension, is involved. Recognition of the syndrome can be tricky as AKI usually manifests upward to 1–2 weeks, and it mimics other syndromes including vasculitis [33, 34]. Therapy is supportive although cases of steroid therapy responsiveness have been reported. Outcomes are quite poor, with one study showing greater than 25% of patients requiring chronic hemodialysis and a large percentage of patients developing nondialysis-dependent CKD.

Drug-induced thrombotic microangiopathy (TMA) has also been reported with numerous medications (Fig. 9.2). TMA following drug administration can either be caused by drug-related induction of antibody production (targeting ADAMTS-13, inhibitory complement factors, or platelets) or direct toxicity of the drug leading to vascular injury and platelet-rich thrombus formation in small blood vessels. A list of drugs implicated in both forms of TMA is listed in Table 9.3. Anticancer agents such as the anti-angiogenesis drugs, gemcitabine, and mitomycin C are associated with TMA. Proteinuria and hypertension are the most common renal effects of the ADs; however AKI often signal

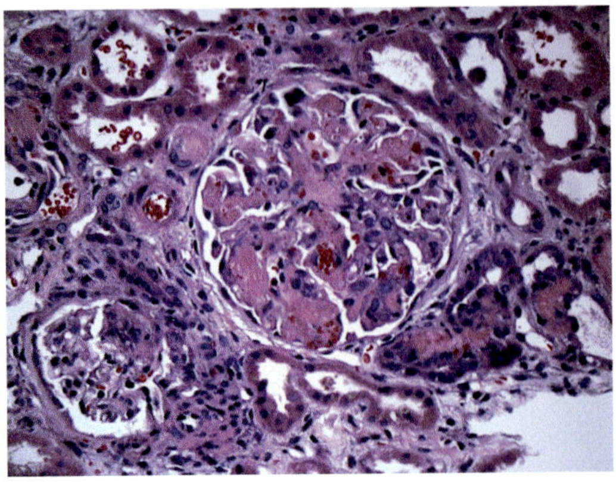

Fig. 9.2 Thrombotic microangiopathy (TMA) is seen in the glomerulus of a patient treated with gemcitabine. As seen in this image, the glomeruli containing multiple intracapillary fibrin thrombi, mesangiolysis, and numerous red blood cell fragments within the injured subendothelial and mesangial areas of the glomerular tuft. These findings characterize TMA

severe TMA. This class of drugs is now the most common cause of drug-induced TMA. Systemic evidence of TMA is absent in 50% of patients, and a renal limited form of TMA must be entertained in patients with AKI. Although relatively rare, a cumulative TMA incidence of 0.31% has been noted in patients exposed to gemcitabine. Gemcitabine use has been noted to have both immune-mediated and direct toxicity leading to its nephrotoxicity profile [35, 36]. Interferon when used in high dose and for prolonged periods is associated with TMA, especially in patients with chronic myelogenous leukemia. The antiplatelet agents (ticlopidine, clopidogrel, and prasugrel) are all associated with TMA, while quinine exposure through prescription, beverages, and health food stores is associated with TMA via formation of quinine-dependent IgG antibodies to platelets.

Kidney-specific ANCA-associated vasculitis (AAV) has been associated with certain drugs, including hydralazine, minocycline, phenytoin, penicillamine, allopurinol, sulfasalazine, antitumor necrosis factor agents, and propylthiouracil (PTU) (Table 9.4). Cocaine cut with levamisole is another cause of AAV. ANCA-associated vasculitides refer to a disease that results in the production of anti-neutrophil cytoplasmic antibodies (ANCA) that can either have a cytoplasmic

Table 9.3 Drugs associated with thrombotic microangiopathy

Antiplatelet agents
Ticlopidine, clopidogrel, prasugrel
Dipyridamole
Defibrotide
Antineoplastic agents
Anti-angiogenesis drugs
Mitomycin C
Gemcitabine
Cisplatin/carboplatin
Estramustine/lomustine
Cytarabine
Tamoxifen
Bleomycin
Daunorubicin
Hydroxyurea
Interferon
IFN-α
IFN-β
Immunosuppressive agents
Calcineurin inhibitors
Anti-CD33
Antimicrobial agents
Valacyclovir
Penicillins
Rifampin
Metronidazole
Tetracycline
Sulfisoxazole
Albendazole
Nonsteroidal anti-inflammatory agents
Diclofenac
Piroxicam
Ketorolac
Hormones
Conjugated estrogens ± progestins
Others
Quinine
Simvastatin
Iodine
Cocaine

(C-ANCA) or perinuclear (P-ANCA) pattern. The C-ANCA pattern is almost exclusively caused by antibodies directed against proteinase 3 (PRC), while P-ANCA is usually due to antibodies directed against myeloperoxidase (MPO) but also can be seen with antibodies against lactoferrin and human leukocyte esterase (HLE) [37, 38]. Presence of these antibodies leads to small vessel injury and when present in the kidney is manifested as a necrotizing glomerulonephritis (Fig. 9.3). Induction of vasculitis is quite rare in these medications. PTU is the drug that is most commonly associated with an AAV. PTU-associated ANCA conversion has been reported in 20–64% of patients, with only a very small fraction of patients (4–6%) having clinical evidence of vasculitis. Although vasculitis is not common, it should be recognized early, as consequences can be fatal if the medication is not withheld and immunosuppressive therapy not administered.

Table 9.4 Drugs associated with immune-mediated glomerular injury

ANCA-associated vasculitis
Hydralazine
Antithyroid medications
Propylthiouracil, methimazole
Minocycline
Allopurinol
Penicillamine
Sulfasalazine
Cocaine (levamisole)
Drug-induced lupus
Anti-arrhythmics
Procainamide, quinidine, amiodarone
Antihypertensives
Hydralazine, methyldopa, captopril
Antipsychotics
Chlorpromazine, lithium
Antibiotics
Isoniazid, minocycline, sulfamethoxazole
Anticonvulsants
Carbamazepine, phenytoin, valproic acid
Antithyroids
Propylthiouracil
Diuretics
Chlorthalidone, hydrochlorothiazide
Biologics
TNF-α inhibitors, IFN-α
Miscellaneous
Statins, levodopa

9.5.2.2 Glomerular Disease

Several forms of drug-induced glomerular disease (Table 9.5) have been reported, and these agents target all glomerular cell types (podocyte, endothelial cell, and mesangial cell). Classic

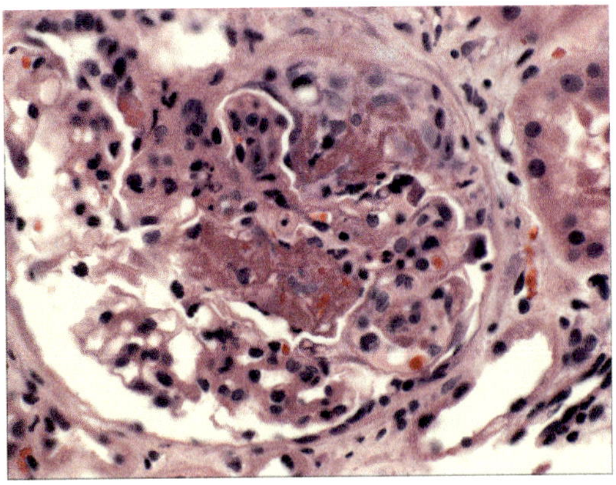

Fig. 9.3 The glomerulus reveals fibrinoid necrosis and early crescent formation in a patient with an ANCA-associated vasculitis (AAV) due to cocaine contaminated with levamisole

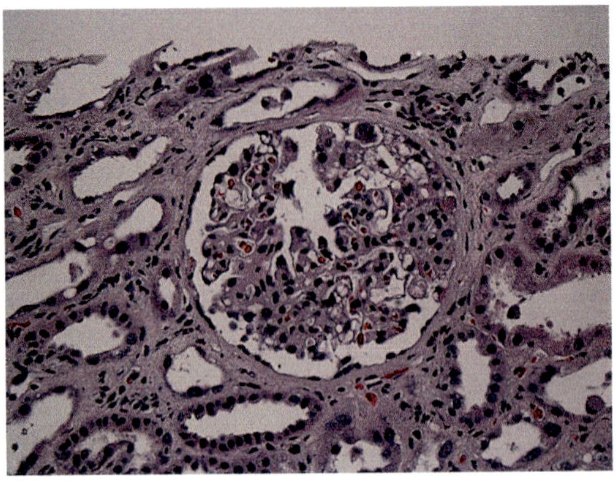

Fig. 9.4 Focal segmental glomerulosclerosis (FSGS) is a glomerular lesion due to a number of drugs including pamidronate, anabolic androgenic steroids, and interferon. There is sclerosis in a segment of the glomerular tuft (arrow), which is diagnostic for the FSGS lesion

Table 9.5 Drugs associated with glomerular injury

Minimal change disease
IFN-α, IFN-β
Pamidronate
Lithium
Nonsteroidal anti-inflammatory drugs
FSGS
IFN-α, IFN-γ
Pamidronate
Lithium
Sirolimus
Anabolic steroids

lesions include minimal change disease (MCD), membranous nephropathy (MGN), and focal and segmental glomerulosclerosis (FSGS). These are secondary forms of glomerulopathy which, while relatively uncommon, must be recognized to facilitate drug discontinuation and therapy to limit kidney injury. In these cases, drug-induced glomerular disease presents similarly to idiopathic or primary forms of glomerular diseases, although the effects, often proteinuria, may not be as severe. In general, one can demonstrate a temporal association between offending agent exposure and development of the glomerulopathy.

Drug-induced podocyte (glomerular epithelial cell) injury leading to either MCD or FSGS is well described. As with the idiopathic or primary counterparts, patients will usually have nephrotic-range proteinuria and peripheral edema; however, it can be less severe. Drugs that have been implicated in MCD include interferon, pamidronate, lithium, and NSAIDs. Another podocytopathy associated with glomerular scarring is FSGS. Drugs implicated in causing FSGS (Fig. 9.4) include interferon, pamidronate, sirolimus, lithium, and anabolic steroids. These patients tend to have more severe AKI and may not fully recover kidney function following discontinuation. As with other forms of drug-induced injury, care is largely supportive with removal of the offending agent and sometimes a course of steroids [39].

Membranous nephropathy (Fig. 9.5) is a form of glomerular disease characterized by nephrotic syndrome and varying severities of AKI. Biopsy, unlike the two previously mentioned nephropathies, will demonstrate with thick capillary loops on light microscopy, granular immunofluorescence (IF) pattern, and glomerular subepithelial membrane immune complexes on electron microscopy. In contrast to primary MGN, immunofluorescence is often negative for anti-PLAR2 antibodies with absent IgG4 subtype staining on IF [40]. MGN is described with penicillamine/bucillamine and gold salts, three antiquated agents that were used to treat rheumatoid arthritis. Now, however, MGN is reported, albeit rarely, with NSAIDs and selective COX inhibitors, the antitumor necrosis factor agent adalimumab,

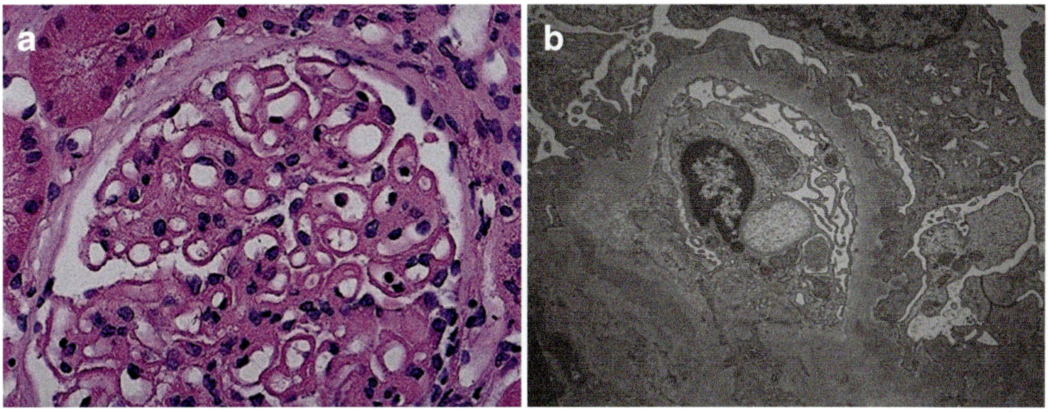

Fig. 9.5 (**a**) Membranous glomerulonephritis is seen on light microscopy in a patient treated with a nonsteroidal anti-inflammatory drug. The capillary loops are thickened and appear rigid. (**b**) On electron microscopy, electron dense deposits are seen in the subepithelial space. These findings are diagnostic for membranous glomerulonephritis

captopril, and certain organic mercurials contained in skin-lightening creams. As NSAIDs are widely used, recognition that MGN can occur is important for clinicians, although it is less common than MCD. Drug discontinuation may reverse the lesion, but immunosuppressive therapy may also be employed.

Drug-induced lupus (DIL) is relatively uncommon, occurring more commonly in older patients (Table 9.4). Major organ involvement is rare but has been reported with glomerular involvement associated with hydralazine, sulfasalazine, penicillamine, and anti-TNF-a therapy [41]. Serologies in drug-induced lupus nephritis are slightly different than idiopathic lupus, with antihistone antibodies more prevalent, yet anti-dsDNA antibodies still present in hydralazine-induced lupus nephritis. Complement levels are variably reduced, and other abnormalities may be reported, such as the presence of p-ANCA antibodies. Treatment of drug-induced lupus nephritis includes removing the offending agent, with manifestations of disease resolving within days to weeks of this intervention. Major organ involvement including AKI can require the use of immunosuppressive agents.

9.5.2.3 Acute Interstitial Nephritis

Drugs are the most predominant cause of acute interstitial nephritis (AIN), ahead of autoimmune disorders and infections. In developed countries, studies have shown upward of 70% of AIN attributed to medications, especially hospital-acquired AIN. AIN typically presents as a steady, not abrupt, rise in serum creatinine approximately 2 weeks after introduction of a medications. This is not always the case, as repeat exposure may lead to a more abrupt rise in serum creatinine. Along this line, drugs such as the NSAIDs and proton-pump inhibitors may present with a gradual and prolonged rise in serum creatinine. Except for methicillin, AIN rarely presents with a systemic hypersensitivity reaction, with triad of fever, skin rash, and eosinophilia <5–10% and clearly much less common than kidney involvement. In contrast, AKI, as evidenced by a rise in serum creatinine, sterile pyuria with the presence of leukocyturia and white blood cell casts, and low-grade proteinuria are more commonly present [17].

AIN is an allergic response that is mediated predominantly by T cells in concert with plasma cells, eosinophils, neutrophils, and mast cells. The end result is an inflammatory cell-rich interstitial infiltrate accompanied by tubulitis and sometimes granuloma (Fig. 9.6). Certain factors can play a role in the development of AIN, including drugs acting as haptens, molecular mimicry, and an individual's underlying immune response genes. However at times, although rarely, a humoral

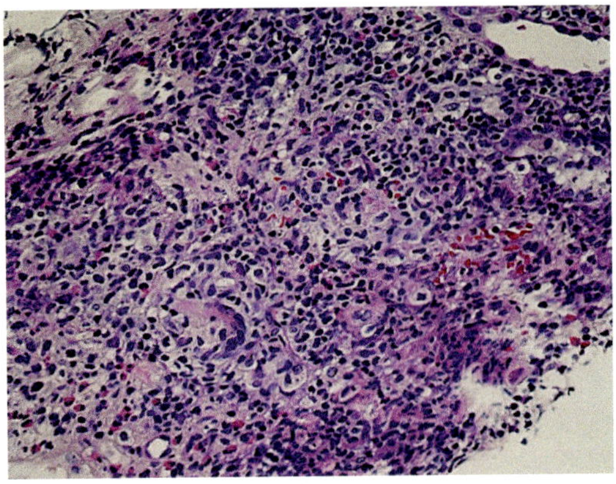

Fig. 9.6 An inflammatory infiltrate within the renal interstitium along with separation and injury to the tubules is seen. This is diagnostic of acute interstitial nephritis, which can be due to any number of medications

response may lead to the inflammatory response, whereby portion of the drug, which acts as a hapten, binds to the tubular basement membrane and evokes an antibody response with formation of tubulointerstitial immune complexes [17].

All drugs are suspect when AIN has been diagnosed, but certain medications, perhaps based on usage patterns, are more common. When discovered, the first and foremost therapy is to remove the offending agent. If AKI is severe enough, time of recognition is recent, minimal interstitial fibrosis is present on histology, and the resulting AIN is from a more acute rather than chronic exposure, a course of steroids may be warranted with the hopes of preserving kidney function. Table 9.6 lists drugs that are commonly associated with AIN. Three classes of medications that have been commonly implicated in acute interstitial nephritis are discussed.

Antimicrobials have a high potential to cause AIN [42]. Beta-lactams (penicillin derivatives and cephalosporins) are more common inducers of AIN than other antibiotics. Methicillin frequently caused AIN with an associated hypersensitivity syndrome and for this reason is no longer routinely used. Other beta-lactams remain a common cause of AIN along with the sulfonamides. As with methicillin, these drugs more tend to cause more hypersensitivity reactions, with fever, rash, and eosinophilia than other drugs. Fluoroquinolones have also been implicated in AIN, with ciprofloxacin being more common than the others. Several antiviral agents can also cause AIN and must be considered when AKI develops. Discontinuation of the culprit drug is the mainstay of therapy. However, it may be difficult identifying the causative agent when several are employed. In addition, it may also be difficult to discontinue the antibiotic that is being used for a documented infection unless other good options are available. Avoidance of the particular antibiotic and possibly similar antibiotics of the same class is advised. Steroid therapy may also be warranted in cases of severe AKI, especially when AIN is documented within 2–3 weeks of drug initiation and histology has limited interstitial fibrosis. This can be tricky when patient has severe underlying infection although steroids have been employed in sepsis and septic shock. Discussion with the infectious disease consultant is often warranted.

Table 9.6 Drugs associated with interstitial nephritis

Antibiotics
β-lactams
Fluoroquinolones
Rifampin
Sulfa-based drugs
Vancomycin
Minocycline
Ethambutol
Antivirals
Acyclovir
Abacavir
Indinavir
Atazanavir
GI medications
Proton-pump inhibitors
Histamine-2 receptor blockers
Analgesics
Nonsteroidal anti-inflammatory drugs (including COX-2 inhibitors)
Anticonvulsants
Phenytoin
Carbamazepine
Phenobarbital
Miscellaneous
Allopurinol
Captopril
Tyrosine kinase inhibitors
Thiazide diuretics
Loop diuretics
Immune Checkpoint Inhibitors

NSAIDs are another important cause of AIN [43]. Clinical presentation tends to be more subacute or chronic and usually falls well outside the classical range of the medication initiation within 1–2 weeks. Hypersensitivity symptoms and signs are extremely rare with these drugs. Unlike other forms of AIN, NSAIDs may be accompanied by nephrotic-range proteinuria due to associated MCD. The interstitial infiltrate typically shows a mononuclear infiltrate with few or no eosinophils. NSAID-induced AIN may develop due to inhibition of COX enzyme, which leads to leukotriene overproduction through the activity of lipoxygenases on arachidonic acid. These proinflammatory cytokines can be responsible for the interstitial inflammatory lesion observed with NSAID therapy. All NSAIDs, including topical preparations and the selective COX-2 inhibitor celecoxib, can cause AIN [44].

Proton-pump inhibitors (PPIs), which are a mainstay of therapy for acid-related gastrointestinal (GI) disease, are a well-described cause of AIN [45–47]. AIN was first described with omeprazole and subsequently with several other PPIs. Unlike other forms of drug-induced AIN, PPIs develop the lesion at a mean time of approximately 11 weeks. Like NSAIDs, patients often do not develop a typical hypersensitivity reaction. Early recognition of PPI-induced AIN and drug discontinuation is generally associated with a good prognosis. Importantly, AIN with the PPIs is a class affect, and switching to H2 antagonists is required for further treatment of acid-related GI disorders. While kidney function usually recovers, many patients may develop CKD.

9.5.2.4 Acute Tubular Injury/Necrosis

One of the most common renal lesions associated with drug therapy is acute tubular injury/necrosis (ATI/ATN), which often develops from direct tubular toxicity [48]. As mentioned, most patients have underlying risk factors for drug-induced tubular injury (Fig. 9.7). Tubular injury usually occurs in a dose-dependent fashion with increased exposure producing progressively worse injury moving from subclinical damage to advanced stage 3 AKI from severe ATN. The proximal tubule is particularly prone to injury as it is the site of drug reabsorption through multiple pathways. Medications may injure cells through promoting mitochondrial dysfunction, disrupting lysosomal or cell membranes, enhancing cellular entry of calcium and other ions, and directly promoting the formation of free radicals. Indirect tubular injury by drugs can occur through induction of rhabdomyolysis with associated myoglobinuria and direct tubular pigment toxicity, as seen with the statin drugs. Table 9.7 lists various drugs associated with acute tubular injury/necrosis. Selected drugs or drug classes that have been commonly associated with acute tubular injury/necrosis are reviewed.

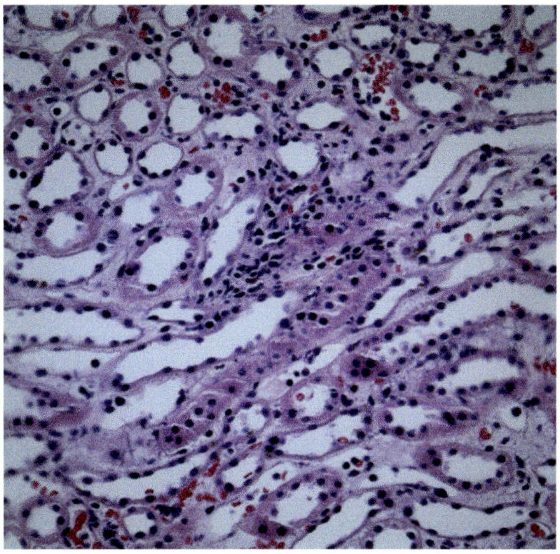

Fig. 9.7 Acute tubular injury/acute tubular necrosis (ATI/ATN) is seen with a number of medications. This lesion is characterized by tubular dilatation, tubular cell flattening with simplification, and dropout of cells into the tubular space

Aminoglycosides are bactericidal agents that have been employed for many years to treat gram-negative infections. Kidney injury with select aminoglycosides has been reported as high as 25% [49]. Aminoglycosides are freely filtered and due to cationic charge are attracted by apical phospholipids and reabsorbed in proximal tubules via megalin/cubilin receptor binding. Toxicity is associated with cationic charge with neomycin (most cationic) demonstrating a high degree of nephrotoxicity, followed by gentamicin, tobramycin, amikacin, and streptomycin. Tubular injury usually occurs 5–7 days

Table 9.7 Drugs associated with acute tubular necrosis

Antibiotics
Aminoglycosides
Gentamicin > amikacin > tobramycin
Cephalosporins
Cefazolin > cephalexin > ceftazidime
Vancomycin
Amphotericin B
Osmotically active agents
Contrast
Hydroxyethyl starch
Intravenous sucrose
Intravenous cyclodextrin
Mannitol
Antineoplastic agents
Platin-based chemotherapy agents
Cisplatin > carboplatin
Ifosfamide
Nucleotide analogues
Tenofovir
Cidofovir
Adefovir

after administration, with nephrotoxicity being dose dependent. Risks for AKI include volume depletion, underlying AKI or CKD, and patient age. AKI is generally nonoliguric and may be associated with electrolyte and acid-base disturbances due to aminoglycoside-related Fanconi or Bartter-like syndromes. Prevention or reductions in AKI are based on volume repletion and careful calculation of loading and maintenance doses based on eGFR. While monitoring peak and trough serum aminoglycoside levels can reduce risk of nephrotoxicity, single daily versus multiple doses per day reduced tubular injury and maintains drug efficacy. Dialysis is sometimes required for severe ATI/ATN. Dialysis does effectively remove aminoglycosides.

Several osmotically active agents that are excreted by the kidney can cause AKI from tubular injury [50]. These agents, which include intravenous sucrose (a carrier in some forms of intravenous immunoglobulin), radiocontrast dye, hydroxyethylstarch, mannitol, and intravenous cyclodextrin, are filtered macromolecules that are not metabolized by the kidney due to a lack of enzymes. These substances undergo proximal tubular uptake via pinocytosis, are internalized, and taken up by lysosomes. Lysosomes are packed with these substances and due to inefficient removal cause severe cell swelling. Cellular swelling leads to disturbed cell function and tubular luminal occlusion, a process termed osmotic nephrosis or nephropathy. Risks for AKI include volume depletion, excessive drug concentrations, and underlying AKI or CKD. Patients may develop oliguric AKI and may require dialysis until renal recovery occurs within 5–7 days. Several large trials demonstrate increased AKI and dialysis requirement in critical care patients treated with hydroxyethyl starch [51, 52]. Treatment is largely supportive with avoidance of further nephrotoxin exposure and dialysis when indicated, which may also reduce drug levels and facilitate renal recovery.

Cisplatin is a member of the platinum-based chemotherapeutic agents utilized to effectively treat various malignancies. Tumor killing results from the ability of cisplatin to bind to and crosslink DNA, thereby leading to tumor cell apoptosis. AKI has long been recognized as a complication of cisplatin and is due primarily to direct tubular toxicity with some contribution from glomerular and vascular injury [11, 53]. Drug uptake into proximal tubular cells occurs primarily via OCT2. Once inside of cells, it can cause injury and apoptosis via inflammation, oxidative stress, and activation of cell death pathways (caspase, cyclin-dependent kinases, etc.). Chloride at the cis position of the molecule is thought to promote much of the injury. Risks for toxicity include volume depletion and underlying CKD. Forced diuresis with normal saline and 3% saline may reduce tubular injury. Intravenous magnesium, amifostine, and other agents may also reduce AKI. Other platin agents such as carboplatin and oxaliplatin are less nephrotoxic in part due to absent OCT2 transport and replacement of chloride at the cis position with carboxylate and cyclobutane. Therapy is mainly supportive and dialysis initiated for the usual indication, but it will not remove the drug. Other anticancer agents associated with various degrees of tubular injury include ifosfamide, pemetrexed, zoledronate, pentostatin, imatinib, and the BRAF inhibitors among others.

Tenofovir is a reverse transcriptase inhibitor that is used as part of combination anti-retroviral therapy (cART) in patients with HIV infection. The drug is structurally similar to naturally occurring oligonucleotides and the known nephrotoxins adefovir and cidofovir. This structure, along with its pathway of excretion through proximal tubular cells via OAT1, promotes cellular injury. While initial clinical trials suggested renal safety, subsequent case reports/series, systematic reviews, VHA database study, and more recent phase 3 trials have shown clear-cut AKI and proximal tubulopathy (Fanconi syndrome) associated with tenofovir [54, 55]. Animal studies and patient biopsies demonstrate ATI/ATN with associated mitochondrial disturbance/disruption [55]. Risks for tenofovir-associated kidney injury include underlying CKD, coadministration of medications that increase tenofovir levels, and endogenous apical efflux transport mutations (MRP2 gene) [56]. AKI typically resolves with drug discontinuation, and patients may rarely require dialysis. Up to 50% of patient may be left with some level of CKD [55].

9.5.2.5 Crystalline Nephropathy

Certain drugs and/or their metabolites can precipitate within tubular lumens to form crystals (Fig. 9.8). This process usually occurs in distal tubular lumens leading to both a tubular obstruction and an interstitial cellular activation and inflammation [57]. Crystals generally form due to inherent insoluble properties, sluggish urine flow rates, urine pH effects on drug solubility, and underlying kidney disease. Risks that can therefore lead to intratubular crystal formation include true or effective volume depletion as seen in cirrhosis, CHF, renal salt wasting or chronic diarrhea, underlying AKI or CKD, and excessive drug dosing. Table 9.8 lists drugs that have been reported to cause crystalline nephropathy. A couple of illustrative examples are discussed.

Acyclovir is an antiviral agent that is used to treat herpes simplex virus infection and when employed intravenously can cause crystalluria and AKI. Rapid high-dose acyclovir bolus employed for viral meningoencephalitis leads to high concentrations of drug within tubular lumens. In fact, upward of 90% of the drug is eliminated through the kidney. Due to high urinary concentrations and the relative insolubility of acyclovir, drug crystals precipitate within the tubular lumens. As a result, AKI has been described in between 12 and 48% of patients receiving high-dose intravenous acyclovir, a number that increases with concomitant volume depletion and underlying CKD

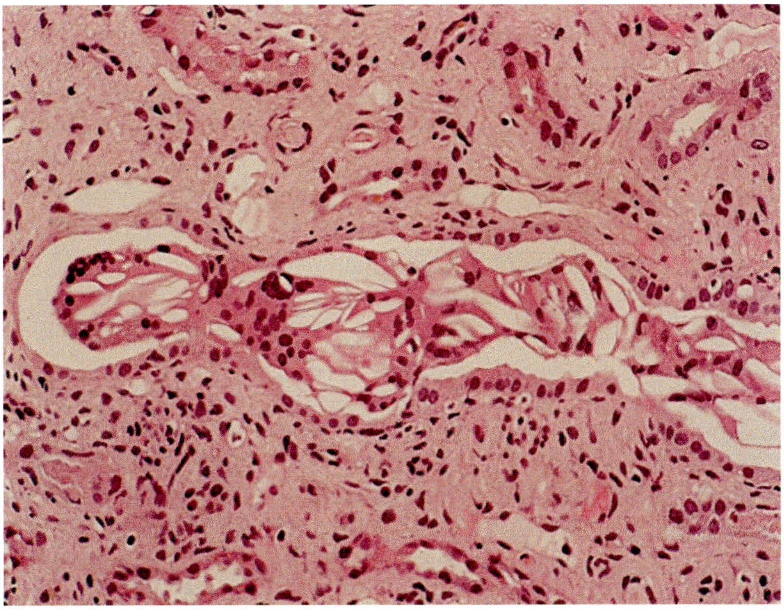

Fig. 9.8 Crystalline nephropathy is seen with a number of medications that are insoluble in the urine and precipitate within the tubular lumens. Classic medications include acyclovir, sulfadiazine, methotrexate, and certain protease inhibitors (like indinavir seen in this biopsy specimen)

Table 9.8 Drugs associated with crystal nephropathy

Sulfadiazine
Acyclovir
Indinavir
Atazanavir
Triamterene
Methotrexate
Orlistat
Ciprofloxacin

[58, 59]. Acyclovir crystals can be identified on urine sediment exam where they are usually needle shaped and positively birefringent with polarization. Prevention or reduction of AKI can be achieved with appropriate drug dosing adjusted to GFR, volume repletion prior to drug administration, and slower infusion of drug (versus bolus). When AKI occurs and is associated with neurotoxicity, dialysis can effectively remove the drug. Most patients recover kidney function with supportive therapy.

Orlistat, an inhibitor of gastric and pancreatic lipase, is approved as a prescription and an over-the-counter medication for weight loss. It functions by promoting fat malabsorption, which can promote enteric hyperoxaluria. Fat within the bowel lumen saponifies calcium, which allows unbound oxalate to be absorbed and increase serum oxalate levels. The resulting hyperoxaluria promotes calcium oxalate precipitation with tubular lumens. This results in acute/subacute oxalate nephropathy and AKI, which stems from both tubulointerstitial inflammation and luminal obstruction. Several case reports of AKI in the setting of orlistat therapy have demonstrated biopsy-proven calcium oxalate nephropathy [60, 61]. All patients in these cases had underlying diabetes mellitus and CKD. A population-based study of 953 patients also documented increased AKI in patient-administered orlistat. CKD, hypertension, and CHF were AKI risks for those taking orlistat. Drug avoidance in patients with known CKD and careful monitoring in high-risk patients prone to volume depletion can help reduce the risk. Using lower doses may also decrease AKI risk as well. In general, AKI recovers with drug discontinuation and supportive care.

Methotrexate is dihydrofolate reductase inhibitor that is used in high intravenous doses to treat certain malignancies. The drug and its metabolite (7-OH methotrexate) are filtered and secreted by the tubules into the urine. Nephrotoxicity develops predominantly in patients treated with doses ranging from 1 to 12 grams/m^2, and AKI incidence ranges from 1.8 to 12% depending on the population studied [58, 62]. Methotrexate crystal precipitation within tubular lumens is associated with kidney injury (plus interstitial inflammation), although direct tubular injury from oxidative stress associated with reduced adenosine deaminase activity may contribute. The poor solubility of methotrexate/7-OH methotrexate in acidic urine as well as reduced urine flow rates enhances crystal precipitation. Prevention of or reduction in AKI involves urinary alkalinization (pH > 7.1) and induction of high urinary flow rates. Treatment of AKI revolves around leucovorin rescue and in some instances the use of high-flux hemodialysis or carboxypeptidase G2 administration (to convert the drug to a harmless metabolite) [63].

Atazanavir is a protease inhibitor that is used as a once daily medication to treat HIV. IT has a rather favorable side effect profile. However, case reports of atazanavir crystal nephropathy have been reported. Early reports have shown stones with birefringent atazanavir crystals [64, 65]. About 7% of the medication is excreted non-metabolized in the urine [66]. It is poorly soluble and more likely to precipitate in alkaline urine. A large retrospective study has demonstrated nephrolithiasis in approximately 1% of patients on atazanavir with a median time of onset of 23 months [67].

9.5.3 Postrenal AKI

AKI can also present as the result of post-kidney obstruction promoted by a medication [48]. Obstruction occurring downstream of the kidney can be the result of injury or obstruction to the ureters, bladder, prostate, or urethra. This can either be the result of direct injury to these organs, luminal or outflow obstruction, or

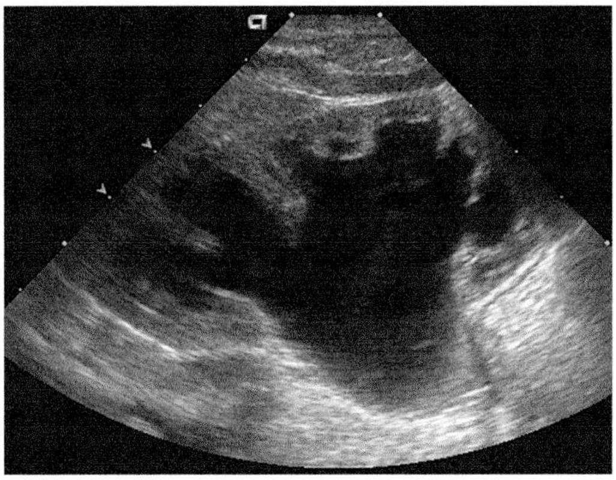

Fig. 9.9 Hydronephrosis is seen in this ultrasound image. Severe dilatation of the pelvis and calyces is demonstrated. Obstruction anywhere along the renal collecting system can cause acute kidney injury if both kidneys are involved (or a single functioning kidney is obstructed)

extrinsic compression of these organs impeding urinary flow. Ultrasonography reveals dilatation of the pelvis and calyces of the kidneys (Fig. 9.9).

Medications that increase the risk of nephrolithiasis should be suspected in patients who present with stone-related obstruction. Approximately 1–2% of kidney stones are caused by drugs with lithogenic potential [48]. Either the drug or its metabolite may form all or part of the stone, or the drug or metabolite may impair calcium oxalate or purine metabolism, thereby leading to the formation of these stones [68]. Coadministration of medications that alter drug metabolism can also enhance stone formation. Lastly, chronic drug use or high medication dose can increase the risk of stone formation. Patient-specific factors increase the risk of nephrolithiasis including either a personal or family history of lithogenesis, abnormal urine pH, current or frequent genitourinary tract infections, low urine volume, acute or chronic states of volume depletion, and underlying AKI or CKD. Table 9.9 lists drugs commonly associated with nephrolithiasis.

Aside from the formation of kidney stones, medications that cause retroperitoneal fibrosis (RPF) can also lead to ureteral encasement thereby creating a significant urinary obstruction and AKI. Ergot derivatives, beta-blockers, and dopaminergic agents have all been reported as causing RPF. Finally agents that promote urinary retention, including anticholinergics, antihistamines, anesthetic agents, opiates, ecstasy, and alcohol, can also lead to AKI from impaired bladder emptying.

Table 9.9 Drugs associated with postrenal kidney injury

Nephrolithiasis
Antibacterials
Sulfonamides
Aminopenicillins
Quinolones
Nitrofurantoin
Protease inhibitors
Indinavir
Nelfinavir
Atazanavir
Diuretics
Acetazolamide
Triamterene
Miscellaneous
Guaifenesin
Aluminum derivatives
Silicum derivatives
Calcium-vitamin D supplements
Retroperitoneal fibrosis
β-blockers
Ergot derivatives
Dopaminergic agonists
Urinary retention
Anticholinergic agents
Antihistamines
Anesthetic agents
Opiates

9.5.4 Summary

All parts of the kidney are vulnerable to effects of medication. Certain patient- and kidney-specific factors are not modifiable and may make some patients more susceptible to injury. Medications themselves or metabolites can have varied nephrotoxic potential. Injury can take the form of hemodynamic, tubular, interstitial, or glomerular injury. Recognizing signs of kidney injury early and identifying potential medications that can cause injury can help to decrease the burden and impact of medication-induced acute kidney injury.

References

1. Schetz M, Dasta J, Goldstein S, Golper T. Drug-induced acute kidney injury. Curr Opin Crit Care. 2005;11:555–65.
2. Choudhury D, Ahmed Z. Drug-induced nephrotoxicity. Med Clin North Am. 1997;81:705–17.
3. Leape LL, Brennan TA, Laird N, et al. The nature of adverse events in hospitalized patients. Results of the Harvard Medical Practice Study II. N Engl J Med. 1991;324:377–84.
4. Mehta RL, Pascual MT, Soroko S, et al. Spectrum of acute renal failure in the intensive care unit: the PICARD experience. Kidney Int. 2004;66:1613–21.
5. Nash K, Hafeez A, Hou S. Hospital-acquired renal insufficiency. Am J Kidney Dis. 2002;39:930–6.
6. Uchino S, Kellum JA, Bellomo R, et al. Acute renal failure in critically ill patients: a multinational, multicenter study. JAMA. 2005;294:813–8.
7. Perazella MA. Renal vulnerability to drug toxicity. Clin J Am Soc Nephrol. 2009;4:1275–83.
8. Fanos V, Cataldi L. Renal transport of antibiotics and nephrotoxicity: a review. J Chemother. 2001;13:461–72.
9. Enomoto A, Endou H. Roles of organic anion transporters (OATs) and a urate transporter (URAT1) in the pathophysiology of human disease. Clin Exp Nephrol. 2005;9:195–205.
10. Nagai J, Takano M. Molecular aspects of renal handling of aminoglycosides and strategies for preventing the nephrotoxicity. Drug Metab Pharmacokinet. 2004;19:159–70.
11. Ciarimboli G, Ludwig T, Lang D, et al. Cisplatin nephrotoxicity is critically mediated via the human organic cation transporter 2. Am J Pathol. 2005;167:1477–84.
12. Jerkic M, Vojvodic S, Lopez-Novoa JM. The mechanism of increased renal susceptibility to toxic substances in the elderly. Part I. The role of increased vasoconstriction. Int Urol Nephrol. 2001;32:539–47.
13. Singh NP, Ganguli A, Prakash A. Drug-induced kidney diseases. J Assoc Physicians India. 2003;51:970–9.
14. Guo X, Nzerue C. How to prevent, recognize, and treat drug-induced nephrotoxicity. Cleveland Clin J Med. 2002;69:289–90, 293–284, 296–287 passim.
15. Ciarimboli G, Koepsell H, Iordanova M, et al. Individual PKC-phosphorylation sites in organic cation transporter 1 determine substrate selectivity and transport regulation. J Am Soc Nephrol. 2005;16:1562–70.
16. Harty L, Johnson K, Power A. Race and ethnicity in the era of emerging pharmacogenomics. J Clin Pharmacol. 2006;46:405–7.
17. Perazella MA. Diagnosing drug-induced AIN in the hospitalized patient: a challenge for the clinician. Clin Nephrol. 2014;81:381–8.
18. Muriithi AK, Nasr SH, Leung N. Utility of urine eosinophils in the diagnosis of acute interstitial nephritis. Clin J Am Soc Nephrol. 2013;8:1857–62.
19. Smith ER, Cai MM, McMahon LP, Wright DA, Holt SG. The value of simultaneous measurements of urinary albumin and total protein in proteinuric patients. Nephrol Dial Transplant. 2012;27:1534–41.
20. Samarawickrama A, Cai M, Smith ER, et al. Simultaneous measurement of urinary albumin and total protein may facilitate decision-making in HIV-infected patients with proteinuria. HIV Med. 2012;13:526–32.
21. Fogazzi GB, Verdesca S, Garigali G. Urinalysis: core curriculum 2008. Am J Kidney Dis. 2008;51:1052–67.
22. Perazella MA. The urine sediment as a biomarker of kidney disease. Am J Kidney Dis. 2015;66:748.
23. Fogazzi GB. Crystalluria: a neglected aspect of urinary sediment analysis. Nephrol Dial Transplant. 1996;11:379–87.
24. Clive DM, Stoff JS. Renal syndromes associated with nonsteroidal antiinflammatory drugs. N Engl J Med. 1984;310:563–72.
25. Schlondorff D. Renal complications of nonsteroidal anti-inflammatory drugs. Kidney Int. 1993;44:643–53.
26. Perazella MA. COX-2 selective inhibitors: analysis of the renal effects. Expert Opin Drug Saf. 2002;1:53–64.
27. Perazella MA, Tray K. Selective cyclooxygenase-2 inhibitors: a pattern of nephrotoxicity similar to traditional nonsteroidal anti-inflammatory drugs. Am J Med. 2001;111:64–7.
28. Eras J, Perazella MA. NSAIDs and the kidney revisited: are selective cyclooxygenase-2 inhibitors safe? Am J Med Sci. 2001;321:181–90.
29. Nankivell BJ, Borrows RJ, Fung CL, O'Connell PJ, Chapman JR, Allen RD. Calcineurin inhibitor nephrotoxicity: longitudinal assessment by protocol histology. Transplantation. 2004;78:557–65.
30. Fellstrom B. Cyclosporine nephrotoxicity. Transplant Proc. 2004;36:220S–3S.
31. Navar LG, Harrison-Bernard LM, Imig JD, Wang CT, Cervenka L, Mitchell KD. Intrarenal angiotensin II generation and renal effects of AT1 receptor blockade. J Am Soc Nephrol. 1999;10(Suppl 12):S266–72.
32. Brewster UC, Perazella MA. The renin-angiotensin-aldosterone system and the kidney: effects on kidney disease. Am J Med. 2004;116:263–72.
33. Lee KG, Loh HL, Tan CS. Spontaneous cholesterol crystal embolism—a rare cause of renal failure. Ann Acad Med Singapore. 2012;41:176–7.
34. Hitti WA, Wali RK, Weinman EJ, Drachenberg C, Briglia A. Cholesterol embolization syndrome induced by thrombolytic therapy. Am J Cardiovasc Drugs. 2008;8:27–34.
35. Walter RB, Joerger M, Pestalozzi BC. Gemcitabine-associated hemolytic-uremic syndrome. Am J Kidney Dis. 2002;40:E16.
36. Fung MC, Storniolo AM, Nguyen B, Arning M, Brookfield W, Vigil J. A review of hemolytic uremic syndrome in patients treated with gemcitabine therapy. Cancer. 1999;85:2023–32.
37. Harper L, Savage CO. Pathogenesis of ANCA-associated systemic vasculitis. J Pathol. 2000;190:349–59.

38. Gao Y, Zhao MH. Review article: drug-induced anti-neutrophil cytoplasmic antibody-associated vasculitis. Nephrology. 2009;14:33–41.
39. Markowitz GS, Bomback AS, Perazella MA. Drug-induced glomerular disease: direct cellular injury. Clin J Am Soc Nephrol. 2015;10:1291–9.
40. Hofstra JM, Debiec H, Short CD, et al. Antiphospholipase A2 receptor antibody titer and subclass in idiopathic membranous nephropathy. J Am Soc Nephrol. 2012;23:1735–43.
41. Hogan JJ, Markowitz GS, Radhakrishnan J. Drug-induced glomerular disease: immune-mediated injury. Clin J Am Soc Nephrol. 2015;10:1300–10.
42. Perazella MA, Markowitz GS. Drug-induced acute interstitial nephritis. Nat Rev Nephrol. 2010;6:461–70.
43. Pirani CL, Valeri A, D'Agati V, Appel GB. Renal toxicity of nonsteroidal anti-inflammatory drugs. Contrib Nephrol. 1987;55:159–75.
44. Alper AB Jr, Meleg-Smith S, Krane NK. Nephrotic syndrome and interstitial nephritis associated with celecoxib. Am J Kidney dis. 2002;40:1086–90.
45. Brewster UC, Perazella MA. Proton pump inhibitors and the kidney: critical review. Clin Nephrol. 2007;68:65–72.
46. Brewster UC, Perazella MA. Acute kidney injury following proton pump inhibitor therapy. Kidney Int. 2007;71:589–93.
47. Geevasinga N, Coleman PL, Webster AC, Roger SD. Proton pump inhibitors and acute interstitial nephritis. Clin Gastroenterol Hepatol. 2006;4:597–604.
48. Perazella MA. Drug-induced nephropathy: an update. Expert Opin Drug Saf. 2005;4:689–706.
49. Lopez-Novoa JM, Quiros Y, Vicente L, Morales AI, Lopez-Hernandez FJ. New insights into the mechanism of aminoglycoside nephrotoxicity: an integrative point of view. Kidney Int. 2011;79:33–45.
50. Dickenmann M, Oettl T, Mihatsch MJ. Osmotic nephrosis: acute kidney injury with accumulation of proximal tubular lysosomes due to administration of exogenous solutes. Am J Kidney Dis. 2008;51:491–503.
51. Perner A, Haase N, Guttormsen AB, et al. Hydroxyethyl starch 130/0.42 versus Ringer's acetate in severe sepsis. N Engl J Med. 2012;367:124–34.
52. Myburgh JA, Finfer S, Bellomo R, et al. Hydroxyethyl starch or saline for fluid resuscitation in intensive care. N Engl J Med. 2012;367:1901–11.
53. Miller RP, Tadagavadi RK, Ramesh G, Reeves WB. Mechanisms of cisplatin nephrotoxicity. Toxins. 2010;2:2490–518.
54. Zaidan M, Lescure FX, Brocheriou I, et al. Tubulointerstitial nephropathies in HIV-infected patients over the past 15 years: a clinico-pathological study. Clin J Am Soc Nephrol. 2013;8:930–8.
55. Herlitz LC, Mohan S, Stokes MB, Radhakrishnan J, D'Agati VD, Markowitz GS. Tenofovir nephrotoxicity: acute tubular necrosis with distinctive clinical, pathological, and mitochondrial abnormalities. Kidney Int. 2010;78:1171–7.
56. Perazella MA. Tenofovir-induced kidney disease: an acquired renal tubular mitochondriopathy. Kidney Int. 2010;78:1060–3.
57. Luciano RL, Perazella MA. Crystalline-induced kidney disease: a case for urine microscopy. Clin Kidney J. 2015;8:131–6.
58. Yarlagadda SG, Perazella MA. Drug-induced crystal nephropathy: an update. Expert Opin Drug Saf. 2008;7:147–58.
59. Fleischer R, Johnson M. Acyclovir nephrotoxicity: a case report highlighting the importance of prevention, detection, and treatment of acyclovir-induced nephropathy. Case Rep Med. 2010;2010:1.
60. Chaudhari D, Crisostomo C, Ganote C, Youngberg G. Acute oxalate nephropathy associated with orlistat: a case report with a review of the literature. Case Rep Nephrol. 2013;2013:124604.
61. Singh A, Sarkar SR, Gaber LW, Perazella MA. Acute oxalate nephropathy associated with orlistat, a gastrointestinal lipase inhibitor. Am J Kidney Dis. 2007;49:153–7.
62. Perazella MA, Moeckel GW. Nephrotoxicity from chemotherapeutic agents: clinical manifestations, pathobiology, and prevention/therapy. Semin Nephrol. 2010;30:570–81.
63. Widemann BC, Balis FM, Kim A, et al. Glucarpidase, leucovorin, and thymidine for high-dose methotrexate-induced renal dysfunction: clinical and pharmacologic factors affecting outcome. J Clin Oncol. 2010;28:3979–86.
64. Chang HR, Pella PM. Atazanavir urolithiasis. N Engl J Med. 2006;355:2158–9.
65. Pacanowski J, Poirier JM, Petit I, Meynard JL, Girard PM. Atazanavir urinary stones in an HIV-infected patient. AIDS. 2006;20:2131.
66. Jao J, Wyatt CM. Antiretroviral medications: adverse effects on the kidney. Adv Chronic Kidney Dis. 2010;17:72–82.
67. Couzigou C, Daudon M, Meynard JL, et al. Urolithiasis in HIV-positive patients treated with atazanavir. Clin Infect Dis. 2007;45:e105–8.
68. Daudon M, Jungers P. Drug-induced renal calculi: epidemiology, prevention and management. Drugs. 2004;64:245–75.

Sepsis and Acute Kidney Injury: Epidemiology, Pathophysiology, Diagnosis, and Management

10

Rashid Alobaidi and Sean M. Bagshaw

10.1 Introduction

Acute kidney injury (AKI) is increasingly encountered, particularly in critically ill patients, with sepsis consistently identified as a leading contributing factor. The short- and long-term consequences of an episode of AKI complicating critical illness are considerable, predisposing to increased risk of death and major morbidity. Importantly, not only does sepsis predispose to AKI, but the development of AKI increases patient susceptibility to de novo infection and sepsis, likely through an array of effects on humoral and cell-mediated immune function. The distinction between septic and non-septic AKI may have particular clinical relevance considering evolving evidence to suggest that sepsis-associated AKI (SA-AKI) is characterized by a unique pathophysiology. SA-AKI has distinct complex and dynamic mechanisms that include systemic and intrarenal hemodynamic mechanisms, renal microcirculatory dysfunction, and activation of immune and inflammatory pathways resulting in direct kidney damage and dysfunction. Presently, there is a paucity of treatment options specific for SA-AKI, making this a challenging problem for clinicians. However, rigorous attention to basic medical care, risk identification, early diagnosis, harm avoidance, and planning for renal replacement therapy support when complications are anticipated or ensue are of critical importance to improve outcomes for those at risk of or with early evidence of SA-AKI.

R. Alobaidi
Division of Critical Care, Department of Pediatrics, Faculty of Medicine and Dentistry, University of Alberta, Edmonton, AB, Canada

S. M. Bagshaw (✉)
Department of Critical Care Medicine, Faculty of Medicine and Dentistry, University of Alberta, Edmonton, AB, Canada
e-mail: bagshaw@ualberta.ca

10.2 SA-AKI Epidemiology

AKI is common in critically ill patients with accumulating evidence to suggest increasing incidence. A recent systematic review of worldwide incidence of AKI, synthesizing 312 studies that included over 49 million patients, found that AKI affects 1 in 5 adults and 1 in 3 children hospitalized with acute illness [1]. A large 10-year cohort that included more than 90,000 patients from 20 intensive care units reported that AKI incidence increased by 2.8% per year [2]. Overall, recent estimates of AKI incidence in ICU has been reported to range between 39 and 65% [3–6]. Similar to AKI, secular trends of growing sepsis incidence have been described. A 22-year retrospective analysis of hospitalization records in the United States found an 8.7% annual increase for a primary diagnosis of sepsis [7]. The incidence of

S. S. Waikar et al. (eds.), *Core Concepts in Acute Kidney Injury*,
https://doi.org/10.1007/978-1-4939-8628-6_10

severe sepsis between 2004 and 2009 showed an average annual increase of 13% [8]. A recent meta-analysis of 27 sepsis studies reported a population incidence rate of 288 cases per 100,000 person-years. When the results were restricted to the last decade, the incidence rate increased to 437 cases per 100,000 person-years [9].

Numerous observational studies have found sepsis to be a foremost contributing factor for AKI (Table 10.1). A large study from 57 adult ICUs in Australia and New Zealand identified AKI in 36.1% of 120,123 patients, with 32.4% of them having SA-AKI (11.7% of the total cohort) [10]. The Beginning and Ending Supportive Therapy (BEST) for the Kidney, a large prospective observational study of more than 29,000 patients, reported an AKI incidence of 5.7%, with sepsis being described as the most common contributing factor (47.5%) [11]. Analysis of 276,731 admissions to 170 adult critical care units of the UK Intensive Care National Audit and Research Center identified AKI in 17,326 ICU admissions in the first 24 h, of those 47.3% were associated with sepsis [12]. Recent AKI cohorts reported similar high incidence of SA-AKI ranging between 30 and 49% [3, 4, 6]. Studies in primarily sepsis cohorts have also reported high occurrence of SA-AKI (Table 10.2). More than 60% of 4532 adult patients with septic shock from 1989 to 2005 suffered AKI [13]. Another multicenter

Table 10.1 Selected observational studies of SA-AKI in cohorts with AKI

Study	Year	Cohort (*n*)	AKI (%)	SA-AKI (%)	AKI definition
BEST kidney [11]	2007	29,269	5.7	47.5	Any of: BUN >84 mg/dL[a], UOP <200 mL/12 h, RRT
Cruz [99]	2007	2164	10.8	25.6	RIFLE
Bagshaw [100]	2008	120,123	36.1	32.4	RIFLE
Kolhe [12]	2008	276,326	6.3	47.3	SCr >3.4 mg/dL[b] and/or BUN >112 mg/dL[a] during the first 24 h
Andrikos [101]	2009	1062	16	45	RIFLE
Piccinni [3]	2011	576	65	30.6	RIFLE
Nisula [4]	2013	2901	39.3	32.2	AKIN
Shum [6]	2016	3687	54.7	49.2	KDIGO

Abbreviations: *SCr* serum creatinine, *SA-AKI* sepsis-associated acute kidney injury, *BUN* blood urea nitrogen, *UOP* urine output

[a]BUN: 1.0 mg/dL = 0.357 mmol/L

[b]SCr: 1.0 mg/dL = 88.4 mcmol/L

Table 10.2 Selected observational studies of SA-AKI in cohorts with sepsis

Study	Year	Cohort (*n*)	SA-AKI (%)	AKI definition
Hoste [21]	2003	185	16.2	SCr >2 mg/dL[a]
Yegenaga [22]	2004	257	11	SCr >2 mg/dL[a] or urine output <400 mL/24 h
Lopes [102]	2007	182	37.4	RIFLE
Oppert [103]	2008	401	41.4	SCr twice normal Or urine output <0.5 mL/kg
Daher [104]	2008	722	17.7	RIFLE
Bagshaw [10]	2008	33,375	42.1	RIFLE
Bagshaw [13]	2009	4532	64.4	RIFLE
Lopes [20]	2009	315	31.4	AKIN
Poukkanen [105]	2013	918	53.2	KDIGO
Suh [23]	2013	992	57.7	RIFLE
Sood [14]	2014	5443	77.6	RIFLE

Abbreviations: *SCr* serum creatinine, *SA-AKI* sepsis-associated acute kidney injury

[a]SCr: 1 mg/dL = 88.4 mcmol/L

cohort reported that SA-AKI affected 77.6% of 5443 septic shock patients [14]. Likewise, sepsis carries a strong association with the development of AKI in critically ill children. Infection was identified as an independent predictor of AKI in a large pediatric cohort of 2106 critically ill children (AKI incidence, 18%) [15]. Similarly, sepsis was a primary risk factor for the development of AKI in 18–58% of pediatric patients [16–19]. The incidence of SA-AKI appears to closely correlate with severity of sepsis. In a cohort of 315 patients, AKI incidence increased significantly from 4.2% for sepsis, 22.7% for severe sepsis, and 52.8% for septic shock, respectively [20].

10.3 SA-AKI Risk Factors

The risk of developing SA-AKI is higher in the elderly. Patients with a greater burden of baseline comorbid disease are also at greater risk. In particular, these comorbidities include chronic kidney disease, diabetes mellitus, heart failure, liver disease, and malignancy [10, 11, 13, 21–24]. Selected sources of infection have shown association with greater likelihood of developing AKI; specifically sources include bloodstream, chest, abdominal, and genitourinary infections [11, 13]. A recent large retrospective multicenter analysis showed that non-pulmonary infections have higher risk of developing AKI compared with other sources. The specific pathogen has not shown clear association with modified risk for SA-AKI [24]. However, in another small cohort study, bloodstream infection, in particular gram-negative bacilli and fungi, has shown modest increased risk for SA-AKI [23].

AKI alone likely increases the short- and longer-term susceptibility to infection and sepsis through a variety of mechanisms (Fig. 10.1). Uremia is known to induce immune system dysfunction including abnormal phagocytic function, depletion in B-cell and T-cell functions, and impaired leukocyte trafficking [25]. Critically ill patients with AKI were found to have reduced monocyte cytokine production and high plasma cytokine levels [26]. Additionally, AKI is associated with fluid accumulation which can potentially disrupt normally protective cellular and tissue barriers. Multicenter analysis of 618 patients with AKI found that 56% developed sepsis after AKI diagnosis. Risk factors for sepsis development included higher severity of illness scores, oliguria, fluid overload, and receipt of RRT [27].

10.4 SA-AKI Clinical Characteristics and Outcomes

Observational data suggest that kidney injury associated with SA-AKI occurs early in the course of critical illness. Several studies report that AKI occurred within 24 h of ICU admission for adult patients with sepsis [13, 28]. In a large

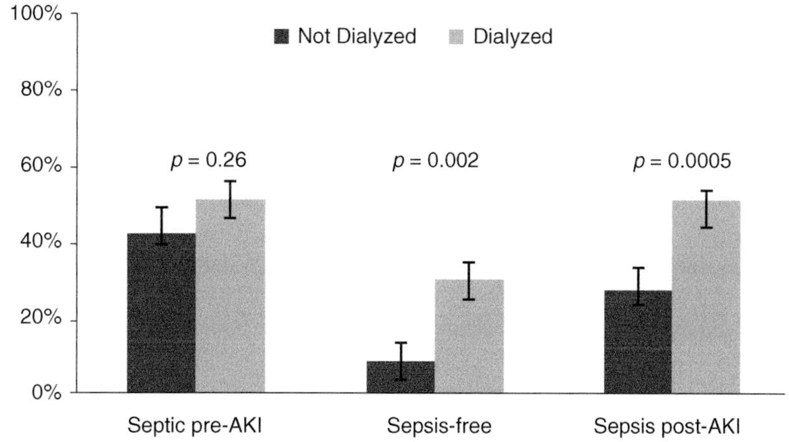

Fig. 10.1 In-hospital mortality stratified by AKI severity (received RRT or not) and timing of sepsis (pre- or post-AKI) (Reproduced with permission from Mehta R et al. Intensive Care Med. 2011 Feb; 37(2): 241–248)

recent cohort, 68% of 5443 patients with septic shock had evidence of AKI within 6 h after presentation [14]. Compared with non-septic AKI, SA-AKI has generally been associated higher acuity of illness. Observational studies showed that SA-AKI patients have higher Acute Physiology and Chronic Health Evaluation II (APACHE II) and Sequential Organ Failure Assessment (SOFA) scores. Similarly, SA-AKI patients received larger volumes of fluid resuscitation and had higher vasopressor needs, worse pulmonary function, higher central venous pressure, and more abnormalities in blood chemistry. Additionally, SA-AKI patients often have more pronounced oliguria and achieve greater degrees of positive fluid balance and overload [10, 11, 21]. Finally, SA-AKI patients have greater relative and absolute changes to serum creatinine from baseline, and more SA-AKI patients fulfill severe AKI criteria (RIFLE-Failure or KDIGO stage 3) [10].

Accumulating data suggest that SA-AKI portends a worse prognosis. Lengths of ICU stay are generally longer in patients with SA-AKI versus AKI without sepsis or sepsis alone. This is likely driven by underlying illness severity and the alternative contributing factors for AKI among non-septic patients. Septic patients developing AKI were found to have twice the duration of ICU stay compared with septic patients without AKI [21]. Similar findings from a larger cohort found SA-AKI patients to have longer ICU and hospital stays compared with non-septic AKI or sepsis alone. Moreover, there was a stepwise increase in length of stay according to AKI severity. The median ICU length of stay increased from 3.1 to 4.8 days as SA-AKI patients had worsening AKI, progressing from RIFLE-Injury to RIFLE-Failure [10].

Recovery of renal function was similar for patients with SA-AKI versus AKI without sepsis. Complete renal function recovery occurred in 95.7% of 315 SA-AKI patients, with a mean time for complete recovery of 10.1 ± 8 days. Interestingly, the BEST Kidney study showed similar rates of progression to ESKD and RRT dependence for septic AKI (5.7%) versus non-septic AKI (7.8%) survivors [11].

Both ICU and in-hospital mortality rates have consistently been described as higher for SA-AKI compared with non-septic AKI (ICU mortality, 19.8% vs. 13.4%; in-hospital mortality, 29.7% vs. 21.6%) [10]. In addition, there was a stepwise increase for ICU, in-hospital, and 90-day mortality rates in septic AKI patients reported when patients were stratified by increasing severity of AKI [13]. Mortality was significantly higher in patients with SA-AKI for AKI-AKIN stage 3 (64.1%) compared with AKI-AKIN stage 1 (34.6%) after adjustment for illness severity [20].

10.5 SA-AKI Pathophysiology

Our evolving understanding of SA-AKI suggests that septic AKI is precipitated by unique and complex mechanisms. Previously, sepsis-mediated kidney hypoperfusion leading to ischemic injury was often cited as the primary pathophysiological mechanism contributing to SA-AKI. Acute tubular necrosis (ATN) has been classically used to describe the cellular effects of sepsis-driven ischemia-reperfusion injury. However, this terminology is dated and likely should be supplanted by modern clinical descriptions of AKI. Autopsy studies have shown that only 22% of 184 patients with clinically defined SA-AKI had classic histopathologic features suggestive of tubular necrosis on biopsy [29]. Accumulating evidence suggests that AKI in sepsis may occur in settings of preserved or increased global renal blood flow (RBF). This provides clues to why early restoration of renal hemodynamics does not necessarily reverse AKI in a significant proportion of patients with SA-AKI. Experimental data are beginning to unravel the scope of additional drivers of kidney damage and dysfunction in sepsis, including the simultaneous and amplifying effects of renal microcirculatory dysfunction (i.e., endothelial dysfunction, inflammation, coagulation disruption), systemic and kidney-derived inflammation, tubular epithelial cell adaptation to injurious stimuli, and the often multiple baseline susceptibilities and discrete insults experienced by patients (Fig. 10.2).

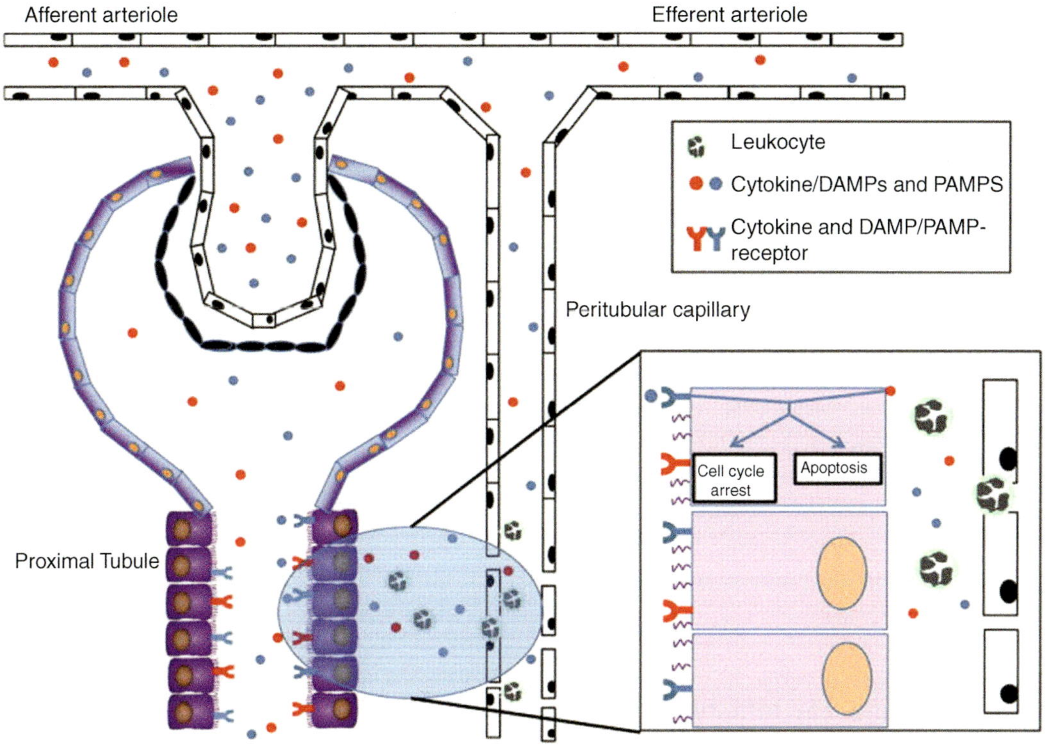

Fig. 10.2 During sepsis, DAMPs, PAMPs, and additional inflammatory mediators can injure renal tubular epithelial cells from both the tubular lumen and interstitial side. Inflammatory mediators derived from bacteria (PAMPs) or immune cells (DAMPs) are filtered through the glomerulus, where they enter the tubular lumen and can contribute to tubular cell injury by binding to specific receptors (e.g., TLR). Similarly, cytokines, DAMPs, and PAMPs are also released from extravasated leukocytes, where they amplify damage by binding to receptors on the interstitial side of tubular cells. The activation of cytokine or DAMP/PAMP receptors may induce apoptosis or cell-cycle arrest, depending on the pattern and severity of the signaling. Reproduced with permission from Zarbock A et al. Curr Opin Crit Care 2014;20(6):588–95

10.5.1 Alteration in Renal Hemodynamics and Microcirculatory Dysfunction

Experimental studies in animal models suggest that sepsis leads to aberrations in global and regional microvascular RBF. In an ovine model, *Escherichia coli*-induced sepsis conferred a period of hyperdynamic RBF associated with 50% reduction in glomerular filtration rate (GFR) [30]. Similar findings were reported in another experimental model where sepsis induced significant increases in RBF associated with reductions in creatinine clearance [31]. In humans, renal vein thermodilution measurement of renal blood flow (RBF) in eight septic critically ill patients showed preservation of renal plasma flow. In these patients, decreases in GFR did not correlate with changes in RBF and vice versa [32]. A systematic review of 159 animal studies of experimental sepsis found that majority (62%) reported diminished RBF; however, this was predominantly related to sepsis-induced low cardiac output states [33]. Overall, RBF seems to be less contributory to renal perfusion during hyperdynamic sepsis unless cardiac output is impaired. A randomized trial in an ovine model of hyperdynamic sepsis evaluated the impact of angiotensin II infusion (ATII) on renal hemodynamics. AT II infusion resulted in a further reduction of RBF; however, it contributed to a significant increase in creatinine clearance (70%) and urine output (sevenfold increase) compared with placebo [34]. These findings suggest that an early primary irregularity occurring in sepsis may be the loss of glomerular perfusion pressure and relative shunting, coupled with the maldistribution of regional blood flow and deranged microcirculatory perfusion. Indeed, grossly impaired microcirculatory flow can occur in regional tissues beds, such as the renal cortex or medulla, despite preserved or even increased global RBF [35]. Numerous factors coalesce to disrupt the microcirculation. Loss of the endothelial glycocalyx contributes to altered vascular permeability, excess fluid extravasation, and renal tissue edema. Cellular debris, including leukocytes and platelets, and coagulation activation further contribute to endothelial disruption and occlusion [36]. These factors contribute to impaired microcirculatory perfusion and may be further exacerbated by intrarenal pressure (encapsulated organ) and macro-hemodynamic factors such as elevated renal venous pressure and/or excessive intra-abdominal pressure.

10.5.2 Immune- and Inflammatory-Mediated Injury

Sepsis is known to release a vast array of inflammatory mediators, commonly referred to as damage-associated molecular proteins (DAMPs—derived from the host response [e.g., DNA, RNA, HMGBP1]) and pathogen-associated molecular proteins (PAMPs—derived from pathogens) [37] (Fig. 10.2). Elevated circulating levels of selected inflammatory mediators in sepsis are known to be associated with development of SA-AKI. Renal tubular apoptosis, cell-cycle arrest, and overt necrosis are adaptive responses to DAMPs/PAMPs and cytokine signaling pathways from the luminal and interstitial (i.e., peritubular capillary) surfaces of the epithelial cells and may be a potent contributing mechanism of kidney damage and dysfunction in SA-AKI. Indeed, in a side-by-side experimental comparison of murine models of SA-AKI versus ischemia-reperfusion (using cecal-ligation puncture model), renal cell apoptosis was more prominent on histology in the SA-AKI mice with minimal tubular injury or inflammation. In addition, the SA-AKI mice showed increased renal interleukin-10 expression and proliferation of regulatory T cells. Inhibition of caspase-3 modulated the severity of AKI, supporting a mechanistic role for apoptosis in propagating injury [38]. In a porcine model of fecal peritonitis, renal tubular cells showed vacuolization and injury to cellular brush borders but no evidence of necrosis [39]. A comparison of postmortem kidney biopsy specimens from 19 patients with septic shock versus trauma and non-septic patients showed an increase in renal tubular cell apoptosis and leukocyte infiltration in the septic group, while apoptosis was not observed in the non-septic group [40].

10.5.3 Adaptive Response to Cellular Stress

Oxidative stress, bioenergetic failure, and cellular hypoxia are molecular drivers of injury during SA-AKI. Tissue hypoxia in the kidney during sepsis may be defined by inflammation, changes in intrarenal nitric oxide, nitrosative stress or oxygen radical homeostasis, and dysregulation [41, 42]. Downregulation of mediators of oxidative phosphorylation occurs during sepsis, and protection of mitochondrial respiration as an adaptive response may mitigate kidney damage during sepsis [43]. In a model of lipopolysaccharide-induced endotoxemic AKI, reactive nitrogen species and reactive oxygen species (ROS) were overexpressed in the renal cytosolic dysfunction during sepsis. This study suggests that injury occurs during SA-AKI from dysregulation of transcriptional events, ROS signaling, mitochondrial activity, and metabolic orientation such as apoptosis [44]. However, recent data have shown renal epithelial cells may adapt to local milieu to limit apoptosis and/or necrosis in SA-AKI. These data imply epithelial cells may adapt to limit cellular damage by altering metabolic processes and entering a state of cell-cycle arrest [45]. This adaptive response phenotypically manifests as reduced kidney function; however, the cellular level provides opportunity for renal epithelial cell repair and recovery.

10.6 SA-AKI Diagnosis and Risk Recognition

The risk of poor outcomes associated with SA-AKI worsens with delays in recognition of injury. Because no singular effective therapy has been discovered, early initiation of supportive care targeting the drivers of injury is the mainstay of therapy. The activation of such support relies on risk identification, early recognition, and timely diagnosis of injury. The recent diagnostic and staging criteria by the Kidney Disease: Improving Global Outcomes (KDIGO) utilizes absolute and relative changes in serum creatinine level and urine output to define and assess the severity of kidney injury [46]. While the KDIGO classification is an important advance in the field of AKI, use of creatinine and urine output come with well recognized limitations. Serum creatinine is insensitive and can vary widely by age, sex, diet, muscle mass, and the volume status of the patient. Changes to serum creatinine are often delayed, usually requiring >24 h to increase significantly, and several days to reach a new steady state after acute changes to glomerular filtration rate (GFR). Due to the nonlinear relationship between GFR and serum creatinine, GFR may decrease by more than 50% prior to significant increments in serum creatinine occurring. Septic patients typically receive aggressive fluid resuscitation, which can have a dilutional effect on serum creatinine. Similarly, sepsis has been shown to reduce the muscular production and/or release of creatinine, even in the absence of any changes in weight, hematocrit, or extracellular fluid volume [47]. These pitfalls impair the sensitivity of serum creatinine and limit its efficacy in the early detection of SA-AKI.

The role of classic urine biochemistry and derived indices in the diagnosis and discrimination of AKI remains controversial. Data from observational studies have found many of these parameters, in particular urine sodium (UNa), and fractional excretion of sodium and urea (FeNa, FeU) has relatively poor operative characteristics to inform about diagnosis and provide clinical decision support [48]. In a study of 83 critically ill adults, fractional excretion of sodium and urea (FeNa and FeU) was not significantly different in patients with SA-AKI versus AKI without sepsis. In addition, they were not predictive of worsening AKI severity, renal replacement therapy, or mortality [49]. On the other hand, the evaluation of the urinary sediment for renal epithelial cells and casts can provide diagnostic and prognostic information about the risk for worsening AKI. A prospective evaluation of a urine microscopy score derived from renal tubular cells and casts correlated with urinary neutrophil gelatinase-associated lipocalin (NGAL) levels and with severity of AKI [50].

The precise role of novel kidney damage biomarkers, such as cystatin C; neutrophil gelatinase-associated lipocalin (NGAL); insulin-like growth factor-binding protein 7 (IGFBP7) and tissue inhibitor of metalloproteinases-2 (TIMP-2); kidney injury molecule-1; interleukin-18; and L-type fatty acid-binding protein, detectable in the blood and urine for the diagnosis of AKI and for clinical decision support, while very promising, is still undergoing investigation. Novel biomarkers have shown an ability to identify SA-AKI before changes in serum creatinine levels. Plasma and urine NGAL levels were significantly higher at 0, 12, and 24 h in 83 patients with SA-AKI compared with patients with non-septic AKI [51]. While other studies showed inconsistent findings, a recent systematic review that included 15 studies evaluating plasma and urine NGAL in septic patients suggested that they have good precision in diagnosing SA-AKI and predicting outcome including receipt of RRT and mortality [52]. Other markers specific for sepsis-induced cellular injury may carry high predictive precision for SA-AKI. An increase of E-selectin, typical of inflammatory and endothelial activation, is associated with future risk of AKI in septic patients [53]. In a large multicenter study of critically ill adults, cell-cycle arrest markers TIMP-2 and IGFB7 showed superior discrimination for AKI compared with other novel biomarkers such as NGAL, interleukin-18, liver-type fatty acid-binding protein, and kidney injury molecule-1 (AUC, 0.80 for TIMP-2/IGFBP7 versus <0.72 for the others). In this study, the predictive performance of TIMP-2/IGFBP7 for AKI was increased further in patients with sepsis (AUC, 0.82) [54]. The use of Doppler-based renal resistance index has shown potential utility in the diagnosis of SA-AKI. However, its use remains limited by inter-operator variability and the influence of age, other hemodynamic variables, and intra-abdominal pressure [55–57]. Newer modalities such as contrast-enhanced ultrasound might have promising role in early detection of AKI in the future [58].

Table 10.3 The renal angina index (RAI) to predict risk of AKI among critically ill children [59]

Risk				Injury		
Demographics	Class	Score		↓eCCl	↑%FO	Score
ICU admission	Moderate	1	×	0	<5%	1
Transplantation	High	3		1–24%	≥5–10%	2
Ventilation + inotropic support	Very high	5		25–49%	≥10–15%	4
				≥50%	≥15%	8

Abbreviations: *eCCl* estimated creatinine clearance by the Schwartz formula; *%FO* percentage of fluid overload normalized for ICU admission weight
The RAI is calculated by multiplying the patient risk score by the injury score. The higher score for either of the injury criteria (eCCl or FO) is used. A RAI product of ≥8 fulfills the renal angina classification. Transplantation refers to solid organ or stem cell transplantation

Risk prediction tools can be utilized to identify patients at greater risk of developing overt or worsening AKI. The concept of renal angina index (RAI), a composite based on risk factors and early signs of kidney injury, has shown good predictive performance in severe AKI in critically ill children with sepsis (Table 10.3) [59]. The use of automated electronic alerting (e-alert) from electronic medical records and clinical information systems has been suggested to improve the recognition of AKI in hospitalized patients at risk. Electronic alerting has shown promise in triggering earlier interventions and improving AKI outcomes [60].

10.7 SA-AKI Management

The general principles in the evaluation and management of SA-AKI are aimed at early resuscitation targets to physiological endpoints, source control, and antimicrobial administration, followed by strategy of limiting injury, avoiding life-threatening complications, and eliminating any potential contributors to worsening kidney function to facilitate recovery (Fig. 10.2). While numerous novel therapies have been evaluated for the prevention and management of SA-AKI, no specific intervention has been shown to contribute to improved patient outcomes.

10.7.1 Fluid Resuscitation

When shock is identified, resuscitation and optimization of intravascular volume should be performed promptly by the administration of fluid and vasoactive therapy titrated to physiological endpoints. Optimizing systemic and kidney hemodynamics should always be a priority, as reestablishment of adequate intravascular volume and perfusion pressure using early aggressive fluid administration and vasoactive support can be lifesaving [61, 62]. Of the numerous strategies evaluated for the prevention of AKI, only fluid therapy has been shown to be effective. However, following the acute resuscitation phase, patients who are no longer "fluid responsive" should be carefully monitored for complications of fluid accumulation and overload. Fluid overload is associated with less favorable outcomes including higher mortality, higher utilization of RRT, and reduced probability of renal recovery [63–66]. A recent meta-analysis of three large randomized trials that evaluated protocolized early goal directed therapy (EGDT) resuscitation compared to standard care found no difference in 90-day mortality (OR 0.97; 95% CI, 0.82–1.14, $p = 0.68$) [67]. In addition, the use and duration of RRT were similar between the two groups.

Recent data have provided additional insights into the type of fluid to be used for acute resuscitation in patients with sepsis. In randomized trials of fluid resuscitation in septic patients, the use of synthetic colloid hydroxyethyl starch (HES) compared with crystalloids was associated with increased risk of AKI, greater RRT utilization, and increased mortality [68–70]. Based on these data, the use of HES fluids for resuscitation in sepsis should be discouraged. Evidence for albumin use in acute resuscitation in sepsis has suggested some benefit; however, it remains controversial. A secondary analysis of the SAFE study and a recent systematic review have shown use of albumin solutions is associated with reduced mortality; however, there is no significant difference in the incidence of AKI [71, 72]. Although the ALBIOS trial showed that albumin replacement in sepsis was not associated with survival benefit, a post hoc analysis suggested albumin-containing solutions may improve the hemodynamic profile and reduce fluid volumes, organ dysfunction, and survival in patients with septic shock [73]. However, there remain a number of uncertainties regarding the routine use of albumin for resuscitation in septic shock (i.e., cost-effectiveness). Recent data have also focused on the composition of crystalloid solutions and the risk of adverse kidney sequelae. The preferential use of balanced crystalloid solutions (such as Ringer's lactate and PlasmaLyte) has been shown in observational studies to reduce the risk of iatrogenic metabolic acidosis, AKI, and mortality [74, 75]. A recent large randomized crossover trial enrolling 2278 predominantly non-septic, low-risk, postoperative patients from 4 ICUs did not show significant differences in the occurrence of AKI or mortality; however, AKI occurred in relatively few patients [76]. The issue of the ideal crystalloid solution for acute resuscitation to optimize kidney and patient survival remains to be definitively proven.

10.7.2 Antimicrobial Therapy

Early antibiotic administration has been shown to improve outcome in sepsis [62]. Similarly, delayed administration of appropriate antimicrobial therapy was found to be an independent predictor of the development of SA-AKI [13]. Incremental delays in antimicrobial delivery after the onset of hypotension showed a direct relationship with increased SA-AKI incidence and severity. In that cohort, the mean time to receive antimicrobials in SA-AKI patients was 6.0 h versus 4.2 h in patients with no AKI ($p < 0.001$). For every 1-h delay in administering antibiotics, the odds of AKI increased by >40% (OR 1.41; 95% CI, 1.10–1.20, $p < 0.001$). In another recent study, early administration of antimicrobials was associated with greater likelihood of recovery of SA-AKI within 24 h from admission [14].

10.7.3 Vasoactive Support

The optimal perfusion pressure to target vasoactive support in sepsis and septic shock remains to be determined. The SEPSISPAM trial suggested a lower MAP target (MAP 65–70 mmHg compared with 80–85 mmHg) was as effective as a higher MAP target for survival and occurrence of adverse events in septic shock; however, in the subgroup of patients with chronic hypertension, the higher MAP target was associated with lower utilization of RRT [77]. Whether a greater MAP target reduces risk for AKI and RRT utilization remains uncertain. The Surviving Sepsis Campaign recommends the preferential use of norepinephrine as first vasopressor agent in treating adult septic shock patients who remain hypotensive following fluid resuscitation [62]. This recommendation is supported by evidence showing superiority of norepinephrine over dopamine [78]. Specific to AKI, the use of "renal-dose" dopamine has not proven effective for preventing the development of AKI [79]. Fenoldopam (selective dopamine receptor-1 agonist) was found to have protective effect against the development of SA-AKI in a small RCT; however, that did not show survival benefit, suggesting the need for further verification in high-quality trials [80]. In the VASST trial, low-dose vasopressin plus norepinephrine was not associated with reduced mortality compared to norepinephrine alone in patients with septic shock [80]. A post hoc analysis suggested that vasopressin may reduce the progression of SA-AKI (from RIFLE-Risk to Failure or Loss) and reduce the utilization of RRT [81]. Recently, the VANISH trial showed that vasopressin was not associated with decreased mortality or significant differences in kidney failure-free days compared to norepinephrine-treated in patients with septic shock (difference −2.3 days; 95% CI: −13.0 to 8.5 days); however, the vasopressin-treated patients had lower use of RRT (difference −9.9%; 95% CI: −19.3 to −0.6%) [82]. Use of recombinant angiotensin II (ANGII) infusion as a novel vasopressor has shown kidney-specific benefits in experimental sepsis models, and a recent phase 3 RCT showed use of ANGII showed significant improvements in mean arterial pressure in patients with catecholamine-resistant vasodilatory shock compared to placebo [83]. Further trials are anticipated to evaluate whether these findings can further translate to survival and kidney benefits.

10.7.4 Renal Replacement Therapy (RRT)

Renal support therapy is the cornerstone for treatment of established, persistent, or complicated AKI following acute resuscitation. The decision to start RRT is often complex and shows considerable variability. RRT should be initiated when confronted with life-threatening complications attributed to AKI, such as medically refractory metabolic acidosis, hyperkalemia, azotemia, or fluid overload. Starting RRT in the absence of these criteria remains controversial, with selected data from observational studies suggesting early or preemptive RRT initiation before the onset of overt complications of AKI may be associated with improved survival. A systematic review that included 15 studies comparing early versus late initiation of RRT therapy found improved mortality with early RRT use (odds ratio 0.45; 95% CI, 0.28–0.72). However, the studies included in the meta-analysis were generally small and heterogeneous, suffered low methodological quality, and had considerable risk of bias, limiting their applicability [84]. Recently, two large RCTs evaluated the question of when to optimally start RRT in AKI [85, 86]. The single-center Early Versus Late Initiation of Renal Replacement Therapy in Critically Ill Patients with Acute Kidney Injury (ELAIN) trial showed decreased in 90-day mortality in the early RRT group (39.3% vs. 53.6%; $p = 0.03$). In addition, early RRT was associated with improved kidney recovery, decreased duration of RRT, and reduction in selected plasma pro-inflammatory mediators. On the other hand, the multicenter Artificial Kidney Initiation in Kidney Injury (AKIKI) trial showed no difference in 60-day mortality between early and delayed RRT initiation strategies (48.5% vs. 49.7%, $p = 0.79$). RRT-free days were greater, and the occurrence of catheter-related bloodstream infection was lower in the delayed RRT strategy group. These conflicting findings will hopefully be further clarified with the completion of two ongoing large multicenter RCTs [87, 88].

The ideal modality to support critically ill septic patients with AKI remains unresolved. Continuous renal replacement therapy (CRRT) is used most commonly early in the course for hemodynamically unstable patients because of its adaptability to the patient condition, achievement of more consistent hemodynamic tolerance, and metabolic and fluid homeostasis. Although no definitive evidence has shown a survival advantage with one particular modality, recent data have suggested that initial support with CRRT may better facilitate recovery of kidney function to RRT independence and reduce the long-term risk of incident chronic kidney disease [89, 90].

Despite early data by Ronco et al. [91] suggesting a potential benefit from higher-intensity dose RRT (CRRT effluent 35–45 mL/kg/h), subsequent evidence from two large multicenter RCTs (Randomized Evaluation of Normal Versus Augmented Level Renal Replacement Therapy [RENAL] and Veterans Affairs/National Institutes of Health Acute Renal Failure Trial Network [ATN] study) showed no incremental benefit of higher-intensity compared to lower-intensity RRT, with fewer metabolic complications occurring in those receiving lower-intensity support [92, 93]. In addition, in both the RENAL and ATN studies, there was no significant difference in the odds ratios (ORs) for mortality in the subgroups with sepsis who received higher- vs. lower-intensity RRT.

Experimental and preliminary clinical data had suggested that high-volume CRRT may confer survival benefit by exerting a nonspecific immunomodulatory effect in sepsis. The hIgh VOlume in Intensive caRE (IVOIRE) study investigated high-volume hemofiltration (HVHF) in septic shock patients with AKI and found no survival or clinical benefits [94]. A recent systematic review evaluating high-volume hemofiltration (CRRT effluent >50 mL/kg/h) for SA-AKI found no outcome benefits and more metabolic abnormalities using higher effluent rates compared to standard doses [78]. A number of additional extracorporeal blood purification techniques are being actively investigated as potential adjuvant therapies in sepsis, including novel membranes and hemofilters, plasma exchange, sorbent technologies (i.e., polymyxin B hemoperfusion); however, definitive evidence of patient and kidney survival benefit are pending.

10.7.5 Targeted Molecular- and Cell-Based Therapy

The pathogenesis of SA-AKI is as a multifactorial process involving apoptotic, immune, and inflammatory processes. Novel perspective medical therapies directed at these pathways have emerged and could be of potential therapeutic value.

Recent preclinical and clinical studies of alkaline phosphatase (ALP) have shown promise for improving outcome in SA-AKI. The precise mechanism for ALP remains uncertain; however, it may exert its anti-inflammatory activity by direct dephosphorylation of bacterial endotoxins and through conversion of adenosine triphosphate into adenosine [95]. In a phase 2 clinical trial of 36 patients with sepsis, recombinant ALP infusion was associated with improved creatinine clearance and reduction in inflammatory markers; however, there is no evidence for reduced utilization of RRT [96]. Targeting the apoptotic pathway with caspase inhibitors and suppressing inflammatory cascades have shown some promising results in experimental models. In a septic mouse model, caspase-3 and interleukin-10 inhibitors had some protective effect against the development of SA-AKI [38]. Similar findings were observed in an earlier rat model with glycerol-induced AKI, where early caspase inhibition attenuated apoptosis and inflammation processes, and reduced kidney injury [97]. Modulation of mitochondrial oxidative phosphorylation through antioxidants also may be of benefit in SA-AKI by mediating hypoxia-induced reactive oxygen species (ROS) and nitric oxide synthase renal epithelial tubular cell injury during sepsis [98]. Other therapeutic agents have shown some kidney anti-inflammatory and apoptosis-suppressing qualities (Table 10.4). Further evidence assessing their beneficial effect in SA-AKI patients is needed.

Table 10.4 Selected novel therapeutic agents with potential in the prevention and treatment of SA-AKI

Agent	Proposed mechanism of action	Study design (*n*)
Fenoldopam [80]	Dopamine-1 receptor agonist Increase renal blood flow	RCT (300)
Low-dose vasopressin [81]	Glomerular efferent arteriolar vasoconstriction Catecholamine sparing	Post hoc analysis of VASST trial (778)
Alkaline phosphatase [96]	Anti-inflammatory activity Dephosphorylation of endotoxins Conversion of adenosine triphosphate to adenosine	RCT [36]
Caspase-3 inhibitors [38, 97]	Suppressing apoptotic pathways	Experimental
Ghrelin [106, 107]	Anti-inflammatory activity Reduce cytokine levels Decrease serum nitric oxide levels	Experimental
Soluble thrombomodulin [108]	Anti-inflammatory and anticoagulant effects Reduce microvascular endothelial injury Improve microvascular perfusion	Experimental
Resveratrol [109, 110]	Anti-inflammatory activity Reduce cytokine levels Minimize endothelial injury Suppress macrophage activity Decrease reactive nitrogen species	Experimental
Adenosine receptor agonists [111]	Anti-inflammatory activity	Experimental
Erythropoietin [112]	Anti-apoptotic and antioxidant activity	Experimental
Temsirolimus [113]	Promote autophagy and kidney recovery	Experimental

Conclusion

SA-AKI is a major clinical challenge for the clinicians. SA-AKI can be a catastrophic complication that exacerbates an already less than favorable outcome in patients with sepsis and septic shock. Identification of those at greatest risk or with early signs of injury is critical. Clinical risk scores, electronic alerting systems, enhanced monitoring, and novel damage-specific markers can aid in risk identification, early diagnosis, and implementation of bundled interventions aimed at mitigating the course of SA-AKI. Our understanding of SA-AKI pathophysiology suggests a redundant and multifactorial process that remains incompletely understood. Early aggressive fluid resuscitation and vasoactive support to restore hemodynamics and perfusion, coupled with harm avoidance, are the cornerstones of treatment. Crystalloid solutions are generally preferred over colloids solutions. HES solutions should be avoided. Balanced crystalloids have theoretical advantages over 0.9% saline for preventing iatrogenic acidosis and AKI during large volume resuscitations; however, definitive evidence is pending. Unnecessary fluid accumulation with excessive central venous pressures and/or intra-abdominal hypertension should be avoided. Norepinephrine remains the first-line vasopressor in septic shock. While sparing high catecholamine exposure by the additional of vasopressin may reduce AKI progression, more evidence is needed. The optional timing of RRT initiation in the absence of life-threatening complications of AKI remains unknown. CRRT is generally first-line renal support in septic shock; however, it may be adapted to intermittent therapies as resuscitation evolves. Less intensive RRT is preferable and current evidence would not support an adjuvant role for high-volume hemofiltration. As our understanding of the pathobiology of SA-AKI expands, additional rigorous investigation is needed to develop novel and effective preventative and therapeutic interventions.

Acknowledgment Dr. Bagshaw is supported by a Canada Research Chair in Critical Care Nephrology.

References

1. Susantitaphong P, Cruz DN, Cerda J, Abulfaraj M, Alqahtani F, Koulouridis I, et al. World incidence of AKI: a meta-analysis. Clin J Am Soc Nephrol. 2013;8(9):1482–93.
2. Bagshaw SM, George C, Bellomo R, Committee ADM. Changes in the incidence and outcome for early acute kidney injury in a cohort of Australian intensive care units. Crit Care. 2007;11(3):R68.
3. Piccinni P, Cruz DN, Gramaticopolo S, Garzotto F, Dal Santo M, Aneloni G, et al. Prospective multicenter study on epidemiology of acute kidney injury in the ICU: a critical care nephrology Italian collaborative effort (NEFROINT). Minerva Anestesiol. 2011;77(11):1072–83.
4. Nisula S, Kaukonen KM, Vaara ST, Korhonen AM, Poukkanen M, Karlsson S, et al. Incidence, risk factors and 90-day mortality of patients with acute kidney injury in Finnish intensive care units: the FINNAKI study. Intensive Care Med. 2013;39(3):420–8.
5. Hoste EA, Bagshaw SM, Bellomo R, Cely CM, Colman R, Cruz DN, et al. Epidemiology of acute kidney injury in critically ill patients: the multinational AKI-EPI study. Intensive Care Med. 2015;41(8):1411–23.
6. Shum HP, Kong HH, Chan KC, Yan WW, Chan TM. Septic acute kidney injury in critically ill patients—a single-center study on its incidence, clinical characteristics, and outcome predictors. Ren Fail. 2016;38(5):706–16.
7. Martin GS, Mannino DM, Eaton S, Moss M. The epidemiology of sepsis in the United States from 1979 through 2000. N Engl J Med. 2003;348(16):1546–54.
8. Gaieski DF, Edwards JM, Kallan MJ, Carr BG. Benchmarking the incidence and mortality of severe sepsis in the United States. Crit Care Med. 2013;41(5):1167–74.
9. Fleischmann C, Scherag A, Adhikari NK, Hartog CS, Tsaganos T, Schlattmann P, et al. Assessment of global incidence and mortality of hospital-treated sepsis. Current estimates and limitations. Am J Respir Crit Care Med. 2016;193(3):259–72.
10. Bagshaw SM, George C, Bellomo R, Committee ADM. Early acute kidney injury and sepsis: a multicentre evaluation. Crit Care. 2008;12(2):R47.
11. Bagshaw SM, Uchino S, Bellomo R, Morimatsu H, Morgera S, Schetz M, et al. Septic acute kidney injury in critically ill patients: clinical characteristics and outcomes. Clin J Am Soc Nephrol. 2007;2(3):431–9.
12. Kolhe NV, Stevens PE, Crowe AV, Lipkin GW, Harrison DA. Case mix, outcome and activity for patients with severe acute kidney injury during the first 24 hours after admission to an adult, general critical care unit: application of predictive models from a secondary analysis of the ICNARC Case Mix Programme database. Crit Care. 2008;12(Suppl 1):S2.
13. Bagshaw SM, Lapinsky S, Dial S, Arabi Y, Dodek P, Wood G, et al. Acute kidney injury in septic shock:

clinical outcomes and impact of duration of hypotension prior to initiation of antimicrobial therapy. Intensive Care Med. 2009;35(5):871–81.
14. Sood MM, Shafer LA, Ho J, Reslerova M, Martinka G, Keenan S, et al. Early reversible acute kidney injury is associated with improved survival in septic shock. J Crit Care. 2014;29(5):711–7.
15. Alkandari O, Eddington KA, Hyder A, Gauvin F, Ducruet T, Gottesman R, et al. Acute kidney injury is an independent risk factor for pediatric intensive care unit mortality, longer length of stay and prolonged mechanical ventilation in critically ill children: a two-center retrospective cohort study. Crit Care. 2011;15(3):R146.
16. Bailey D, Phan V, Litalien C, Ducruet T, Merouani A, Lacroix J, et al. Risk factors of acute renal failure in critically ill children: a prospective descriptive epidemiological study. Pediatr Crit Care Med. 2007;8(1):29–35.
17. Plotz FB, Bouma AB, van Wijk JA, Kneyber MC, Bokenkamp A. Pediatric acute kidney injury in the ICU: an independent evaluation of pRIFLE criteria. Intensive Care Med. 2008;34(9):1713–7.
18. Duzova A, Bakkaloglu A, Kalyoncu M, Poyrazoglu H, Delibas A, Ozkaya O, et al. Etiology and outcome of acute kidney injury in children. Pediatr Nephrol. 2010;25(8):1453–61.
19. Mehta P, Sinha A, Sami A, Hari P, Kalaivani M, Gulati A, et al. Incidence of acute kidney injury in hospitalized children. Indian Pediatr. 2012;49(7):537–42.
20. Lopes JA, Jorge S, Resina C, Santos C, Pereira A, Neves J, et al. Acute kidney injury in patients with sepsis: a contemporary analysis. Int J Infect Dis. 2009;13(2):176–81.
21. Hoste EA, Lameire NH, Vanholder RC, Benoit DD, Decruyenaere JM, Colardyn FA. Acute renal failure in patients with sepsis in a surgical ICU: predictive factors, incidence, comorbidity, and outcome. J Am Soc Nephrol. 2003;14(4):1022–30.
22. Yegenaga I, Hoste E, Van Biesen W, Vanholder R, Benoit D, Kantarci G, et al. Clinical characteristics of patients developing ARF due to sepsis/systemic inflammatory response syndrome: results of a prospective study. Am J Kidney Dis. 2004;43(5):817–24.
23. Suh SH, Kim CS, Choi JS, Bae EH, Ma SK, Kim SW. Acute kidney injury in patients with sepsis and septic shock: risk factors and clinical outcomes. Yonsei Med J. 2013;54(4):965–72.
24. Sood M, Mandelzweig K, Rigatto C, Tangri N, Komenda P, Martinka G, et al. Non-pulmonary infections but not specific pathogens are associated with increased risk of AKI in septic shock. Intensive Care Med. 2014;40(8):1080–8.
25. Vaziri ND, Pahl MV, Crum A, Norris K. Effect of uremia on structure and function of immune system. J Ren Nutr. 2012;22(1):149–56.
26. Himmelfarb J, Le P, Klenzak J, Freedman S, McMenamin ME, Ikizler TA, et al. Impaired monocyte cytokine production in critically ill patients with acute renal failure. Kidney Int. 2004;66(6):2354–60.
27. Mehta RL, Bouchard J, Soroko SB, Ikizler TA, Paganini EP, Chertow GM, et al. Sepsis as a cause and consequence of acute kidney injury: program to improve care in acute renal disease. Intensive Care Med. 2011;37(2):241–8.
28. Lima RS, Marques CN, Silva Junior GB, Barbosa AS, Barbosa ES, Mota RM, et al. Comparison between early and delayed acute kidney injury secondary to infectious disease in the intensive care unit. Int Urol Nephrol. 2008;40(3):731–9.
29. Langenberg C, Bagshaw SM, May CN, Bellomo R. The histopathology of septic acute kidney injury: a systematic review. Crit Care. 2008;12(2):R38.
30. Langenberg C, Wan L, Egi M, May CN, Bellomo R. Renal blood flow in experimental septic acute renal failure. Kidney Int. 2006;69(11):1996–2002.
31. Langenberg C, Wan L, Bagshaw SM, Egi M, May CN, Bellomo R. Urinary biochemistry in experimental septic acute renal failure. Nephrol Dial Transplant. 2006;21(12):3389–97.
32. Brenner M, Schaer GL, Mallory DL, Suffredini AF, Parrillo JE. Detection of renal blood flow abnormalities in septic and critically ill patients using a newly designed indwelling thermodilution renal vein catheter. Chest. 1990;98(1):170–9.
33. Langenberg C, Bellomo R, May C, Wan L, Egi M, Morgera S. Renal blood flow in sepsis. Crit Care. 2005;9(4):R363–74.
34. Wan L, Langenberg C, Bellomo R, May CN. Angiotensin II in experimental hyperdynamic sepsis. Crit Care. 2009;13(6):R190.
35. Bezemer R, Legrand M, Klijn E, Heger M, Post IC, van Gulik TM, et al. Real-time assessment of renal cortical microvascular perfusion heterogeneities using near-infrared laser speckle imaging. Opt Express. 2010;18(14):15054–61.
36. De Backer D, Donadello K, Taccone FS, Ospina-Tascon G, Salgado D, Vincent JL. Microcirculatory alterations: potential mechanisms and implications for therapy. Ann Intensive Care. 2011;1(1):27.
37. Gustot T. Multiple organ failure in sepsis: prognosis and role of systemic inflammatory response. Curr Opin Crit Care. 2011;17(2):153–9.
38. Lee SY, Lee YS, Choi HM, Ko YS, Lee HY, Jo SK, et al. Distinct pathophysiologic mechanisms of septic acute kidney injury: role of immune suppression and renal tubular cell apoptosis in murine model of septic acute kidney injury. Crit Care Med. 2012;40(11):2997–3006.
39. Chvojka J, Sykora R, Krouzecky A, Radej J, Varnerova V, Karvunidis T, et al. Renal haemodynamic, microcirculatory, metabolic and histopathological responses to peritonitis-induced septic shock in pigs. Crit Care. 2008;12(6):R164.
40. Lerolle N, Nochy D, Guerot E, Bruneval P, Fagon JY, Diehl JL, et al. Histopathology of septic shock induced acute kidney injury: apoptosis and leukocytic infiltration. Intensive Care Med. 2010;36(3):471–8.
41. Evans RG, Ince C, Joles JA, Smith DW, May CN, O'Connor PM, et al. Haemodynamic influences on

kidney oxygenation: clinical implications of integrative physiology. Clin Exp Pharmacol Physiol. 2013;40(2):106–22.
42. Heyman SN, Rosen S, Rosenberger C. A role for oxidative stress. Contrib Nephrol. 2011;174:138–48.
43. Heyman SN, Evans RG, Rosen S, Rosenberger C. Cellular adaptive changes in AKI: mitigating renal hypoxic injury. Nephrol Dial Transplant. 2012;27(5):1721–8.
44. Quoilin C, Mouithys-Mickalad A, Lecart S, Fontaine-Aupart MP, Hoebeke M. Evidence of oxidative stress and mitochondrial respiratory chain dysfunction in an in vitro model of sepsis-induced kidney injury. Biochim Biophys Acta. 2014;1837(10):1790–800.
45. Takasu O, Gaut JP, Watanabe E, To K, Fagley RE, Sato B, et al. Mechanisms of cardiac and renal dysfunction in patients dying of sepsis. Am J Respir Crit Care Med. 2013;187(5):509–17.
46. Outcomes KDIG. KDIGO clinical practice guidelines on acute kidney injury. Kidney Int. 2012;2(1):8–12.
47. Doi K, Yuen PS, Eisner C, Hu X, Leelahavanichkul A, Schnermann J, et al. Reduced production of creatinine limits its use as marker of kidney injury in sepsis. J Am Soc Nephrol. 2009;20(6):1217–21.
48. Carvounis CP, Nisar S, Guro-Razuman S. Significance of the fractional excretion of urea in the differential diagnosis of acute renal failure. Kidney Int. 2002;62(6):2223–9.
49. Bagshaw SM, Bennett M, Devarajan P, Bellomo R. Urine biochemistry in septic and non-septic acute kidney injury: a prospective observational study. J Crit Care. 2013;28(4):371–8.
50. Bagshaw SM, Haase M, Haase-Fielitz A, Bennett M, Devarajan P, Bellomo R. A prospective evaluation of urine microscopy in septic and non-septic acute kidney injury. Nephrol Dial Transplant. 2012;27(2):582–8.
51. Bagshaw SM, Bennett M, Haase M, Haase-Fielitz A, Egi M, Morimatsu H, et al. Plasma and urine neutrophil gelatinase-associated lipocalin in septic versus non-septic acute kidney injury in critical illness. Intensive Care Med. 2010;36(3):452–61.
52. Zhang A, Cai Y, Wang PF, Qu JN, Luo ZC, Chen XD, et al. Diagnosis and prognosis of neutrophil gelatinase-associated lipocalin for acute kidney injury with sepsis: a systematic review and meta-analysis. Crit Care. 2016;20(1):41.
53. Powell TC, Powell SL, Allen BK, Griffin RL, Warnock DG, Wang HE. Association of inflammatory and endothelial cell activation biomarkers with acute kidney injury after sepsis. Springerplus. 2014;3:207.
54. Kashani K, Al-Khafaji A, Ardiles T, Artigas A, Bagshaw SM, Bell M, et al. Discovery and validation of cell cycle arrest biomarkers in human acute kidney injury. Crit Care. 2013;17(1):R25.
55. Lerolle N, Guerot E, Faisy C, Bornstain C, Diehl JL, Fagon JY. Renal failure in septic shock: predictive value of Doppler-based renal arterial resistive index. Intensive Care Med. 2006;32(10):1553–9.
56. Dewitte A, Coquin J, Meyssignac B, Joannes-Boyau O, Fleureau C, Roze H, et al. Doppler resistive index to reflect regulation of renal vascular tone during sepsis and acute kidney injury. Crit Care. 2012;16(5):R165.
57. Ninet S, Schnell D, Dewitte A, Zeni F, Meziani F, Darmon M. Doppler-based renal resistive index for prediction of renal dysfunction reversibility: a systematic review and meta-analysis. J Crit Care. 2015;30(3):629–35.
58. Schneider AG, Goodwin MD, Schelleman A, Bailey M, Johnson L, Bellomo R. Contrast-enhanced ultrasound to evaluate changes in renal cortical perfusion around cardiac surgery: a pilot study. Crit Care. 2013;17(4):R138.
59. Basu RK, Zappitelli M, Brunner L, Wang Y, Wong HR, Chawla LS, et al. Derivation and validation of the renal angina index to improve the prediction of acute kidney injury in critically ill children. Kidney Int. 2014;85(3):659–67.
60. Hoste EA, Kashani K, Gibney N, Wilson FP, Ronco C, Goldstein SL, et al. Impact of electronic-alerting of acute kidney injury: workgroup statements from the 15(th) ADQI Consensus Conference. Can J Kidney Health Dis. 2016;3:10.
61. Rivers E, Nguyen B, Havstad S, Ressler J, Muzzin A, Knoblich B, et al. Early goal-directed therapy in the treatment of severe sepsis and septic shock. N Engl J Med. 2001;345(19):1368–77.
62. Dellinger RP, Levy MM, Rhodes A, Annane D, Gerlach H, Opal SM, et al. Surviving sepsis campaign: international guidelines for management of severe sepsis and septic shock: 2012. Crit Care Med. 2013;41(2):580–637.
63. Boyd JH, Forbes J, Nakada TA, Walley KR, Russell JA. Fluid resuscitation in septic shock: a positive fluid balance and elevated central venous pressure are associated with increased mortality. Crit Care Med. 2011;39(2):259–65.
64. Sadaka F, Juarez M, Naydenov S, O'Brien J. Fluid resuscitation in septic shock: the effect of increasing fluid balance on mortality. J Intensive Care Med. 2014;29(4):213–7.
65. Payen D, de Pont AC, Sakr Y, Spies C, Reinhart K, Vincent JL, et al. A positive fluid balance is associated with a worse outcome in patients with acute renal failure. Crit Care. 2008;12(3):R74.
66. Bouchard J, Soroko SB, Chertow GM, Himmelfarb J, Ikizler TA, Paganini EP, et al. Fluid accumulation, survival and recovery of kidney function in critically ill patients with acute kidney injury. Kidney Int. 2009;76(4):422–7.
67. Investigators P, Rowan KM, Angus DC, Bailey M, Barnato AE, Bellomo R, et al. Early, goal-directed therapy for septic shock—a patient-level meta-analysis. N Engl J Med. 2017;376(23):2223–34.
68. Perner A, Haase N, Guttormsen AB, Tenhunen J, Klemenzson G, Aneman A, et al. Hydroxyethyl starch 130/0.42 versus Ringer's acetate in severe sepsis. N Engl J Med. 2012;367(2):124–34.
69. Myburgh JA, Finfer S, Bellomo R, Billot L, Cass A, Gattas D, et al. Hydroxyethyl starch or saline for

fluid resuscitation in intensive care. N Engl J Med. 2012;367(20):1901–11.
70. Zarychanski R, Abou-Setta AM, Turgeon AF, Houston BL, McIntyre L, Marshall JC, et al. Association of hydroxyethyl starch administration with mortality and acute kidney injury in critically ill patients requiring volume resuscitation: a systematic review and meta-analysis. JAMA. 2013;309(7):678–88.
71. Investigators SS, Finfer S, McEvoy S, Bellomo R, McArthur C, Myburgh J, et al. Impact of albumin compared to saline on organ function and mortality of patients with severe sepsis. Intensive Care Med. 2011;37(1):86–96.
72. Delaney AP, Dan A, McCaffrey J, Finfer S. The role of albumin as a resuscitation fluid for patients with sepsis: a systematic review and meta-analysis. Crit Care Med. 2011;39(2):386–91.
73. Caironi P, Tognoni G, Masson S, Fumagalli R, Pesenti A, Romero M, et al. Albumin replacement in patients with severe sepsis or septic shock. N Engl J Med. 2014;370(15):1412–21.
74. Yunos NM, Bellomo R, Hegarty C, Story D, Ho L, Bailey M. Association between a chloride-liberal vs chloride-restrictive intravenous fluid administration strategy and kidney injury in critically ill adults. JAMA. 2012;308(15):1566–72.
75. Raghunathan K, Shaw A, Nathanson B, Sturmer T, Brookhart A, Stefan MS, et al. Association between the choice of IV crystalloid and in-hospital mortality among critically ill adults with sepsis*. Crit Care Med. 2014;42(7):1585–91.
76. Young P, Bailey M, Beasley R, Henderson S, Mackle D, McArthur C, et al. Effect of a buffered crystalloid solution vs saline on acute kidney injury among patients in the intensive care unit: the SPLIT randomized clinical trial. JAMA. 2015;314(16):1701–10.
77. Asfar P, Meziani F, Hamel JF, Grelon F, Megarbane B, Anguel N, et al. High versus low blood-pressure target in patients with septic shock. N Engl J Med. 2014;370(17):1583–93.
78. De Backer D, Aldecoa C, Njimi H, Vincent JL. Dopamine versus norepinephrine in the treatment of septic shock: a meta-analysis*. Crit Care Med. 2012;40(3):725–30.
79. Bellomo R, Chapman M, Finfer S, Hickling K, Myburgh J. Low-dose dopamine in patients with early renal dysfunction: a placebo-controlled randomised trial. Australian and New Zealand Intensive Care Society (ANZICS) Clinical Trials Group. Lancet. 2000;356(9248):2139–43.
80. Morelli A, Ricci Z, Bellomo R, Ronco C, Rocco M, Conti G, et al. Prophylactic fenoldopam for renal protection in sepsis: a randomized, double-blind, placebo-controlled pilot trial. Crit Care Med. 2005;33(11):2451–6.
81. Gordon AC, Russell JA, Walley KR, Singer J, Ayers D, Storms MM, et al. The effects of vasopressin on acute kidney injury in septic shock. Intensive Care Med. 2010;36(1):83–91.
82. Gordon AC, Mason AJ, Thirunavukkarasu N, Perkins GD, Cecconi M, Cepkova M, et al. Effect of early vasopressin vs norepinephrine on kidney failure in patients with septic shock: the VANISH randomized clinical trial. JAMA. 2016;316(5):509–18.
83. Khanna A, English SW, Wang XS, Ham K, Tumlin J, Szerlip H, et al. Angiotensin II for the treatment of vasodilatory shock. N Engl J Med. 2017;377(5):419–30.
84. Karvellas CJ, Farhat MR, Sajjad I, Mogensen SS, Leung AA, Wald R, et al. A comparison of early versus late initiation of renal replacement therapy in critically ill patients with acute kidney injury: a systematic review and meta-analysis. Crit Care. 2011;15(1):R72.
85. Zarbock A, Kellum JA, Schmidt C, Van Aken H, Wempe C, Pavenstadt H, et al. Effect of early vs delayed initiation of renal replacement therapy on mortality in critically ill patients with acute kidney injury: the ELAIN randomized clinical trial. JAMA. 2016;315(20):2190–9.
86. Gaudry S, Hajage D, Schortgen F, Martin-Lefevre L, Pons B, Boulet E, et al. Initiation strategies for renal-replacement therapy in the intensive care unit. N Engl J Med. 2016;375(2):122–33.
87. Smith OM, Wald R, Adhikari NK, Pope K, Weir MA, Bagshaw SM, et al. Standard versus accelerated initiation of renal replacement therapy in acute kidney injury (STARRT-AKI): study protocol for a randomized controlled trial. Trials. 2013;14:320.
88. Barbar SD, Binquet C, Monchi M, Bruyere R, Quenot JP. Impact on mortality of the timing of renal replacement therapy in patients with severe acute kidney injury in septic shock: the IDEAL-ICU study (initiation of dialysis early versus delayed in the intensive care unit): study protocol for a randomized controlled trial. Trials. 2014;15:270.
89. Schneider AG, Bellomo R, Bagshaw SM, Glassford NJ, Lo S, Jun M, et al. Choice of renal replacement therapy modality and dialysis dependence after acute kidney injury: a systematic review and meta-analysis. Intensive Care Med. 2013;39(6):987–97.
90. Bonnassieux M, Duclos A, Schneider AG, Schmidt A, Benard S, Cancalon C, et al. Renal replacement therapy modality in the ICU and renal recovery at hospital discharge. Crit Care Med. 2018;46(2):e102–10.
91. Ronco C, Bellomo R, Homel P, Brendolan A, Dan M, Piccinni P, et al. Effects of different doses in continuous veno-venous haemofiltration on outcomes of acute renal failure: a prospective randomised trial. Lancet. 2000;356(9223):26–30.
92. VA/NIH Acute Renal Failure Trial Network, Palevsky PM, Zhang JH, O'Connor TZ, Chertow GM, Crowley ST, et al. Intensity of renal support in critically ill patients with acute kidney injury. N Engl J Med. 2008;359(1):7–20.
93. RENAL Replacement Therapy Study Investigators, Bellomo R, Cass A, Cole L, Finfer S, Gallagher M, et al. Intensity of continuous renal-replacement therapy in critically ill patients. N Engl J Med. 2009;361(17):1627–38.

94. Joannes-Boyau O, Honore PM, Perez P, Bagshaw SM, Grand H, Canivet JL, et al. High-volume versus standard-volume haemofiltration for septic shock patients with acute kidney injury (IVOIRE study): a multicentre randomized controlled trial. Intensive Care Med. 2013;39(9):1535–46.
95. Peters E, Heemskerk S, Masereeuw R, Pickkers P. Alkaline phosphatase: a possible treatment for sepsis-associated acute kidney injury in critically ill patients. Am J Kidney Dis. 2014;63(6):1038–48.
96. Pickkers P, Heemskerk S, Schouten J, Laterre PF, Vincent JL, Beishuizen A, et al. Alkaline phosphatase for treatment of sepsis-induced acute kidney injury: a prospective randomized double-blind placebo-controlled trial. Crit Care. 2012;16(1):R14.
97. Homsi E, Janino P, de Faria JB. Role of caspases on cell death, inflammation, and cell cycle in glycerol-induced acute renal failure. Kidney Int. 2006;69(8):1385–92.
98. Pathak E, MacMillan-Crow LA, Mayeux PR. Role of mitochondrial oxidants in an in vitro model of sepsis-induced renal injury. J Pharmacol Exp Ther. 2012;340(1):192–201.
99. Cruz DN, Bolgan I, Perazella MA, Bonello M, de Cal M, Corradi V, et al. North East Italian Prospective Hospital Renal Outcome Survey on Acute Kidney Injury (NEiPHROS-AKI): targeting the problem with the RIFLE Criteria. Clin J Am Soc Nephrol. 2007;2(3):418–25.
100. Bagshaw SM, George C, Dinu I, Bellomo R. A multi-centre evaluation of the RIFLE criteria for early acute kidney injury in critically ill patients. Nephrol Dial Transplant. 2008;23(4):1203–10.
101. Andrikos E, Tseke P, Balafa O, Cruz DN, Tsinta A, Androulaki M, et al. Epidemiology of acute renal failure in ICUs: a multi-center prospective study. Blood Purif. 2009;28(3):239–44.
102. Lopes JA, Jorge S, Resina C, Santos C, Pereira A, Neves J, et al. Acute renal failure in patients with sepsis. Crit Care. 2007;11(2):411.
103. Oppert M, Engel C, Brunkhorst FM, Bogatsch H, Reinhart K, Frei U, et al. Acute renal failure in patients with severe sepsis and septic shock—a significant independent risk factor for mortality: results from the German Prevalence Study. Nephrol Dial Transplant. 2008;23(3):904–9.
104. Daher EF, Marques CN, Lima RS, Silva Junior GB, Barbosa AS, Barbosa ES, et al. Acute kidney injury in an infectious disease intensive care unit - an assessment of prognostic factors. Swiss Med Wkly. 2008;138(9–10):128–33.
105. Poukkanen M, Vaara ST, Pettila V, Kaukonen KM, Korhonen AM, Hovilehto S, et al. Acute kidney injury in patients with severe sepsis in Finnish Intensive Care Units. Acta Anaesthesiol Scand. 2013;57(7):863–72.
106. Wang W, Bansal S, Falk S, Ljubanovic D, Schrier R. Ghrelin protects mice against endotoxemia-induced acute kidney injury. Am J Physiol Renal Physiol. 2009;297(4):F1032–7.
107. Khowailed A, Younan SM, Ashour H, Kamel AE, Sharawy N. Effects of ghrelin on sepsis-induced acute kidney injury: one step forward. Clin Exp Nephrol. 2015;19(3):419–26.
108. Sharfuddin AA, Sandoval RM, Berg DT, McDougal GE, Campos SB, Phillips CL, et al. Soluble thrombomodulin protects ischemic kidneys. J Am Soc Nephrol. 2009;20(3):524–34.
109. Holthoff JH, Wang Z, Seely KA, Gokden N, Mayeux PR. Resveratrol improves renal microcirculation, protects the tubular epithelium, and prolongs survival in a mouse model of sepsis-induced acute kidney injury. Kidney Int. 2012;81(4):370–8.
110. Chen L, Yang S, Zumbrun EE, Guan H, Nagarkatti PS, Nagarkatti M. Resveratrol attenuates lipopolysaccharide-induced acute kidney injury by suppressing inflammation driven by macrophages. Mol Nutr Food Res. 2015;59(5):853–64.
111. Lee HT, Kim M, Joo JD, Gallos G, Chen JF, Emala CW. A3 adenosine receptor activation decreases mortality and renal and hepatic injury in murine septic peritonitis. Am J Physiol Regul Integr Comp Physiol. 2006;291(4):R959–69.
112. Coldewey SM, Khan AI, Kapoor A, Collino M, Rogazzo M, Brines M, et al. Erythropoietin attenuates acute kidney dysfunction in murine experimental sepsis by activation of the beta-common receptor. Kidney Int. 2013;84(3):482–90.
113. Howell GM, Gomez H, Collage RD, Loughran P, Zhang X, Escobar DA, et al. Augmenting autophagy to treat acute kidney injury during endotoxemia in mice. PLoS One. 2013;8(7):e69520.

Acute Kidney Failure and Minimal Change Disease

11

Alain Meyrier and Patrick Niaudet

11.1 Introduction

Minimal change disease (MCD), a subset of "idiopathic nephrotic syndrome" (INS), defines a glomerulopathy with a normal appearance of glomeruli by light microscopy, negative immunofluorescence, and foot process flattening (or effacement) and fusion by electron microscopy. This definition excludes other variants of INS, such as focal segmental glomerulosclerosis and membranous glomerulopathy. Minimal change disease is the main cause of nephrotic syndrome in children—"childhood nephrosis"—representing about 95% of all cases before adolescence. It accounts for 70–90% of the NS in children who are younger than 10 years and 50% in older children.

Minimal change disease is also an important cause of INS in adults of all ages, accounting for 10–20% of cases, and is also observed in patients older than 60 years, especially in association with acute kidney injury (AKI) [1–5].

The functional expression of MCD is characterized by a profound change in the permselectivity of the glomerular capillary barrier to serum albumin. Proteinuria is greater than 40 mg/m^2 body surface area/h (>3.5 g/24 h in a 70 kg adult). This results in hypoalbuminemia, with serum albumin concentration lower than 30 g/L. Proteinuria can be massive, greater than 20 g daily with serum albumin levels below 10 g/L. Profuse proteinuria and severe hypoalbuminemia are associated with widespread pitting edema. Pleural and peritoneal serosal exudates can be abundant. Conversely, at variance with the nephritic syndrome, severe hypertension and visceral edema involving the brain or the lung (at least clinically significant [6]) are not features of nephrotic edema, a first clinical indication that sodium and water retention is mostly restricted to the extravascular compartment. Contrary to other causes of extracellular sodium and fluid retention, edema involves the face, especially in children and young adults. This and the fact that blood pressure is usually normal give the clinical impression that MCD is a particular form of nephrotic syndrome in which a vascular permeability factor is at work [7].

The pathogenesis of nephrotic edema is not entirely understood. The issue at stake is to determine why as soon as profuse proteinuria appears the renal tubules start reabsorbing massive amounts of sodium filtered at the glomerulus. Two pathophysiologic mechanisms have been proposed. One hypothesis, prevalent until the 1970s, maintained that low plasma colloid osmotic (or "oncotic") pressure (COP) is the cause of capillary leakage of extracellular fluid

A. Meyrier (✉)
Service de Néphrologie, Hôpital Georges Pompidou, Université Paris-Descartes Medical School, Paris, France

P. Niaudet
Department of Pediatric Nephrology, Hôpital Necker-Enfants Malades, Université Paris-Descartes, Paris, France

S. S. Waikar et al. (eds.), *Core Concepts in Acute Kidney Injury*,
https://doi.org/10.1007/978-1-4939-8628-6_11

into the interstitium, reduced plasma volume, and intense hormonal stimulation of renal sodium reabsorption. Since, this “underfill” explanation was refuted by a number of studies demonstrating that in nephrotic MCD the blood volume is not diminished and that sodium retention proceeds from changes of the intrinsic properties of the capillary endothelial filtration barrier [8].

In a majority of cases of MCD, renal function, defined by the glomerular filtration rate (GFR), is normal or moderately impaired. However, over the past 50 years, a number of reports of acute, oliguric, and in most cases reversible kidney insufficiency (AKI) in the course of idiopathic nephrotic syndrome with minimal glomerular changes have stimulated interest on this complication of a form of glomerular disease considered in most cases as entailing little risk of renal failure and a high rate of corticosteroid-induced remission.

The subject of this chapter requires to recalling the acquired knowledge regarding nephrotic edema in patients with minimal histopathologic glomerular changes.

11.2 Background

11.2.1 Nephrotic Edema: Movements of Blood Extracellular Fluid to the Interstitium, Lymphatic Uptake and Return to Plasma

In a normal physiological state (for a comprehensive review, see [9]), the extracellular compartment of total body water (ECF) is made up of plasma water and interstitial fluid. The movements of water and albumin along an interstitial capillary, from the arterial to the venous ends, are the result of a balance between filtration (*F*) and reabsorption (*R*). *F* and *R* are a function of capillary (*c*) and interstitial tissue (*i*) hydraulic (*P*) and oncotic (π) pressure and of capillary permeability (Kf: the ultrafiltration coefficient). These factors are integrated in the Starling equation where fluid movement (Jv) = Kf × *S* × EFP. EFP is the effective filtration pressure, *S* the capillary surface area, and Kf the ultrafiltration coefficient. EFP = (Pc − Pi) minus (πc − πi) [for figures in mmHg, see [10]].

To simplify these basic physiological data, it suffices to indicate that in nephrotic edema a new equilibrium is achieved between a decrease of albumin concentration in the plasma and in the interstitial fluid and a higher tissue pressure. In this setting interstitial fluid is taken up by lymphatics, and the increased lymph flow contributes to maintain a near normal blood volume. In order to explain why in most patients with the nephrotic syndrome blood volume is not low despite a reduced plasma colloid osmotic pressure (COP), Koomans et al. measured the transcapillary oncotic pressure difference in 12 patients with the nephrotic syndrome and in 6 patients during complete ($n = 3$) and partial ($n = 3$) remission [11]. Subcutaneous nylon wicks were used to collect tissue fluid and measure the albumin content. The albumin content and COP were low in both plasma and tissue fluid in the nephrotic phase and rose gradually during recovery. During these changes the transcapillary COP difference only rose slightly: from 6.2 ± 1.7 mmHg when the plasma COP was below 10 mmHg ($n = 11$) to 8.7 ± 1.5 mmHg when the plasma COP exceeded 20 mmHg ($n = 12$). These observations indicated that in hypoalbuminemia preservation of the intravascular volume is strongly dependent on maintenance of the difference in oncotic pressure across the capillary wall.

The same group, using a similar experimental protocol (subcutaneous wicks), studied the role of adjustments of tissue-fluid COP in the maintenance of the blood volume in ten patients with the nephrotic syndrome before and after diuretic treatment until dry weight [12]. A mean weight reduction of 13.5 ± 6.4 kg was attended by a fall in blood volume in three patients and no change in six, but the final blood volume was within the normal range. Albumin content and COP of tissue fluid were low before edema removal and rose slightly after it, parallel to changes in the plasma. Thus, the transcapillary gradient in COP did not change before and after diuretic treatment. Considering the low COP (8.6 ± 1.6 mmHg in edematous and

11.7 ± 3.7 mmHg in dry conditions), this gradient was only slightly below the value of about 10 mmHg normally found with this technique. The authors concluded that a lowered tissue-fluid COP is important for preserving the blood volume in non-edematous proteinuric and hypoalbuminemic patients. They suggested that this adaptation can explain why the blood volume is often normal and not expanded despite massive overhydration in these patients. However, these findings apply to nephrotic adults in a steady state of hypoalbuminemia. This is not the case when the onset of the nephrotic syndrome is explosive, a situation mostly observed in children [13–16].

On the same line, factors that abruptly diminish blood volume, such as vigorous loop diuretic treatment, tip the balance between interstitial and plasma volume toward hypovolemia and severe impairment of the glomerular filtration rate.

11.2.2 Nephrotic Patients with MCD in Steady-State Conditions Are Not Hypovolemic

As stated by Dorhout Mees, "The notion that fluid retention in the nephrotic syndrome is caused by a decreased circulating blood volume (hypovolemic concept) has dominated medical thinking and practice for decades. During recent years evidence has accumulated that this concept, logical as it may seem, does not reflect reality in most patients" [17, 18].

In fact these studies conducted by nephrologists from Utrecht in the Netherlands confirmed initial observations made by Eisenberg in 1968 that demonstrated that the blood volume is normal in nephrotic syndrome, observations confirmed in numerous subsequent studies [19]. These studies were based on blood and plasma volume measurements [12, 20–28] and/or on demonstrating that sodium retention and edema formation in the nephrotic syndrome was not the consequence of a hormonal response to hypovolemia but, rather, to an intrarenal defect, the nature of which is still not perfectly clear [29–36].

A remarkable experiment of unilateral proteinuria was performed by Ichikawa et al. [37]. This group produced a unilateral model of puromycin aminonucleoside (PAN)-induced albuminuria in Munich-Wistar rats to examine the mechanisms responsible for renal salt retention. Two weeks after selective perfusion of left kidneys with PAN or isotonic saline, increases in albumin excretion and decreases in sodium excretion were demonstrated in PAN-perfused but not in non-perfused kidneys of PAN-treated rats, although systemic plasma protein concentration remained at control level. Total kidney GFR and superficial single-nephron GFR were also reduced selectively in PAN-perfused kidneys, on average by approximately 30%, due primarily to a marked decline in the glomerular capillary ultrafiltration coefficient (Kf), which was also confined to PAN-perfused kidneys.

In vitro microperfusion experiments showed an increased rate of sodium reabsorption in the cortical collecting ducts from PAN nephrotic rats. The increased sodium reabsorption is associated with the stimulation of two selective sodium channels, Na,K-ATPase and ENaC [38–40].

11.2.3 Renal Function Is Moderately Altered in Nephrotic Syndrome with Minimal Glomerular Changes

Mild to moderate reduction in GFR has been observed in approximately 30% of children and adults. This reduction of the GFR is reversible with remission of proteinuria. The International Study of Kidney Disease in Children (ISKDC) reported that among 345 children with MCD, one third had serum creatinine levels greater than the 95th percentile of age-matched controls [41]. Similar observations were made in children by White et al. and by Habib and Kleinknecht [42, 43]. Bohlin reported on 13 unselected children with MCD who were followed up to 7.5 years. GFR determined as clearance of inulin was decreased at the first episode in six patients, but none of them had a decreased GFR later during the course of the disease [44]. The same trend to depressed GFR measured by creatinine clearance was observed in nephrotic adults with minimal change disease by Hopper et al. in a series of 31 patients studied by light, electron, and immunofluorescence microscopy [45].

However creatinine clearance is a poor marker of GFR in glomerular proteinuric diseases, in which the tubular secretion of creatinine is greatly increased, overestimating the glomerular filtration by about 40% [46]. More reliable clearance measurements with inulin confirmed depression of the GFR in the active, proteinuric phase of MCD, a depression in the order of 25%, followed by a return to normal GFR when treatment has induced a remission [44, 47–49].

Several studies analyzed the relationship between proteinuria, effective blood volume, and glomerular function. Considering the wealth of observations that rule out a state of hypovolemia that would ascribe reduced GFR to functional renal insufficiency, investigators sought other explanations.

Lowenstein et al. proposed a theory of "nephrosarca," that is, interstitial edema of the kidney, which would physically cause vascular and/or tubular occlusion and consequent filtration failure [50].

In fact, although some kidney biopsies demonstrate severe interstitial edema in grossly enlarged kidneys [51, 52], this is far from being a constant finding, and renal pathologists rarely mention conspicuous interstitial edema with tubular compression and collapse in their laboratory reports.

In severe forms of nephrotic syndrome, urinary albumin may reach extremely high concentrations with excretion of viscous urine, as in one case of AKI reported by Koomans whose patient voided small amounts of gel-like urine, which contained >120 g/L albumin and virtually no sodium [53].

Increased tubular urine viscosity might explain GFR reduction in less severe forms of INS, even in the absence of tubular protein casts.

In fact a simple explanation stems from the histological changes observed by electron microscopy in MCD, changes made of flattening and fusion of the podocyte foot processes along the outer aspect of the GBM [54].

Bohman et al. also analyzed the role of podocyte foot process flattening and fusion on the glomerular capillary permeability to small molecules, such as creatinine or inulin [55]. The authors studied a group of children with minimal change nephrotic syndrome to investigate the possible relationship between the fusion of glomerular epithelial foot processes and the reduction in GFR. The degree of foot process fusion was estimated as the harmonic true mean of foot process width and the length density of epithelial slit pores as determined by quantitative electron microscopic stereology. In the patients the GFR ranged between 40 and 127 mL/min/1.73 m^2 body surface area, the filtration fraction between 6.9 and 22.5%, and the serum albumin concentration between 14 and 46 g/L. The mean foot process width, which varied between 330 and 870 nm, showed a close correlation with the GFR and the filtration fraction, as well as with the serum albumin concentration. As expected, a reduction of epithelial slit pore length occurred concomitant with the broadening of the foot processes. These observations agree with the hypothesis that the reduction in the total length of glomerular epithelial slit pores, due to the fusion of foot processes, results in a reduced glomerular capillary permeability to water and small solutes.

Other studies by renal physiologists confirmed that in MCD the filtration coefficient (Kf) of the glomerular basement membrane (GBM) to small molecules is impaired, with a decrease in filtration slit frequency that causes the average path length for the filtrate to increase, thereby explaining the decreased hydraulic permeability [56].

To summarize these findings, it appears that the poorly identified factor that reversibly affects the glomerular capillary framework in patients with MCD leads to a lesion that increases the permeability of the GBM to serum albumin and reduces its permeability to small molecules, such as water, urea, creatinine, and inulin [57].

11.3 Acute Kidney Injury Complicating Minimal Change Disease

11.3.1 Historical Period: 1966–1992

The first report of oliguric acute renal failure in the course of nephrotic syndrome dates back to 1966 with a remarkable paper by Chamberlain et al. [58] but presented at a time when immunofluorescence was not available for studying kidney biopsies. There were nine cases that had been observed between 1961 and 1964. Four patients (all four were women aged 42–49 years) had initially minimal glomerular changes by light and electron microscopy. In fact the third case exhibited glomerular hypercellularity and most probably suffered from acute GN following vaccination, and the fourth case who died with bilateral renal vein thrombosis exhibited membranous glomerulopathy (MGN) at autopsy. Three other patients had MGN and two a proliferative GN. Thus two patients only were without doubt cases of MCD, while the others were cases of nephritic rather than nephrotic syndrome. These two patients were oliguric (<500 mL/day). The period of oliguria lasted, respectively, 48 and 114 days. They were grossly edematous and one was hypertensive with distended cervical veins. They were treated with dialysis and survived. In their discussion the authors considered, according to the prevalent belief, that their patients' oliguria was explained by hypovolemia. In fact the clinical reports show that the blood volume was most probably increased and the main factor of recovery consisted of corticosteroid therapy inducing remission of proteinuria.

Since the time when this seminal paper was published, several reports appeared in the English literature on AKI complicating nephrotic syndrome [45, 49, 50, 52, 59–68]. This literature was the subject of a comprehensive in-depth review by Smith and Hayslett in 1992 [69]. They analyzed 84 cases and excluded 9 of these (including 2 of Chamberlain et al.) whose kidney histology was not compatible with MCD and 3 cases in which the precipitating event was an allergic interstitial nephritis [52]. This selection yielded 75 cases with the following clinical attributes. There were 49 males and 26 females, with a mean age of 58 ± (SEM) 2 years (range 15–83). In 38 (84%) edema was described as massive. Forty-nine were hypertensive (systolic blood pressure 161 ± 4 mmHg, diastolic BP 91 ± 2 mmHg). The majority demonstrated a rather severe form of nephrotic syndrome with 11.6 ± 0.6 g/day of proteinuria (range 3.5–25) and hypoalbuminemia (19 ± 01 g/L, range 4–34). Most were oliguric at the time of referral, which made the concentration of urinary albumin per liter unusually high. The time between onset of nephrotic syndrome and AKI was 29 ± 5 days (range 7–90) and the time between onset of AKI and recovery 47 ± 11 days (range 3–180 days), although the two latter pieces of information were often lacking in the analyzed reports (21 and 19 cases, respectively). In any event the time to recovery was on average much longer than in cases of acute ischemic tubular necrosis, in which the average duration is in the order of 2 weeks.

In these 75 cases, a kidney biopsy was performed, in most but not all cases at the time of AKI. In fact the histopathologic diagnosis was one of minimal changes in 64, but in 11 cases, the kidney biopsy disclosed other lesions: focal segmental glomerulosclerosis in 6, mesangial proliferation in 4, and focal proliferation in 1. We have indicated above that kidney histology cannot be considered fully reliable when immunofluorescence along with electron microscopy was not done. As an example, careful reading of the paper by Chamberlain et al. reveals that two cases out of four were wrongly interpreted as being "MCD," including one in which different glomerular lesions strongly suggest MGN were found at autopsy [58].

With regard to lesions affecting the tubulointerstitium in cases where a kidney biopsy was done during the renal failure, about two thirds comprised a sufficient description of this compartment. In 65 biopsies the tubular lesions were compatible with a diagnosis of acute tubular necrosis with frank interstitial edema and in some scattered interstitial infiltrates. In the other 26 cases, tubular necrosis was specifically denied. Despite these uncertainties regarding the tubulointerstitial lesions, on the whole it seemed that in cases without tubular necrosis, the degree of renal insufficiency was relatively moderate with serum creatinine levels averaging 460 moles per liter and no necessity to treat AKI with dialysis.

In these reports little attention was directed to the vascular lesions. However Jennette and Falk, in a report of 21 cases of MCD and renal failure, noted vascular lesions that are common in hypertensive persons [64]. Their study included a control group and revealed that systolic blood pressure was significantly higher in nephrotic patients with AKI than in those without. Esparza et al. also noted in their relatively old patients lesions of arterial and arteriolar sclerosis [52]. We shall comment below on the issue of idiopathic nephrotic syndrome in older patients with so-called lesions of "nephrosclerosis."

More disquieting were some observations of patients whose kidney biopsy did not reveal unusually severe lesions and in whom AKI was irreversible. Raij et al. reported five such cases in adults aged 44–74 years in whom irreversible acute renal failure developed [65]. Prior to renal disease, associated systemic illness or occlusion of major renal vasculature was not present. All patients continued to excrete large amounts of proteins (8.6–15 g/24 h) despite a minimal glomerular filtration rate and severe oliguria. One patient died after 5 months without recovering renal function. Four patients required hemodialysis for a period of 12–58 months. The failure to recover renal function could not be explained by the light microscopic findings. The authors suggested that the irreversibility of the renal failure might be related to either permanent alterations in renal blood flow or ultrastructural changes or to both. They stressed the fact that some adult patients in whom acute renal failure develops during the course of idiopathic nephrotic syndrome seem to have a grave prognosis and that protracted oliguria or irreversible renal failure can be expected to occur.

Despite some drawbacks the review by Smith and Hayslett remains usefully informative. In particular their commentary illustrates the variability of treatments and outcomes in this compilation of 75 cases scattered over a period of 25 years. Treatments variably comprised volume expansion, or diuretics and/or ultrafiltration, or glucocorticoids alone. The overall impression is that recovery of renal function was achieved in about two thirds of the cases (58/75) within an average of 7 weeks but with wide variations in this length of time. However 14 patients died of various complications, and as mentioned above, some remained indefinitely on dialysis. These patients who did not recover were older than their fellow sufferers and more hypertensive.

Following this "historical" period that covers 25 years (1966–1991), the matter of AKI complicating minimal change nephrotic syndrome continued to stimulate the interest of nephrologists. The following section analyzes the publications that appeared over the subsequent quarter of a century.

11.3.2 Experience Acquired Between 1992 and 2014

11.3.2.1 Acute Kidney Injury in Adults with Minimal Glomerular Changes

By comparison with the "historical" period analyzed above, a Medline search covering the two following decades does not yield many publications specifically dealing with AKI complicating adult MCD. Large series of histopathologic studies indeed mention that MCD is not rare among patients undergoing a kidney biopsy in the setting of acute renal failure, especially in older patients [1–5], but few articles add useful information to the pre-existing literature. Some papers reporting large numbers of patients with MCD do not even mention cases of AKI in their experience [70]. Others mix up various forms of nephrotic glomerulopathies without specifically focusing on MCD [71].

We analyze below the main articles comprising sufficient information for the renal clinician, information based on well-documented cases of AKI and MCD.

Waldman et al. performed a retrospective review of 95 adults who had MCD and were observed in the same referral center between 1990 and 2005 [72]. Most patients (84%) were referred for a second opinion regarding treatment. The majority of them were white (80.6%) with more women (61%) than men, and mean age was 45.1 ± 1.6 year. Hypertension was present in 42.9%, and microscopic hematuria in 28.9%. Mean serum creatinine was 1.39 ± 0.13 mg/dL and mean GFR was 71.7 ± 4.0 mL/min per 1.73 m^2. Mean serum albumin was 2.21 ± 0.08 g/dL and urinary protein excretion was 9.93 ± 0.71 g/day. Mean duration of follow-up for the cohort as a whole was 132 weeks. AKI associated with the NS occurred in 24 patients. In 17 patients, it was concurrent with the initial presentation of MCD, and in 7 it occurred during a relapse. Patients with AKI, compared with 75 patients without AKI, were more likely to be male (63.2% vs. 33.3%), older (54.5 ± 3.4 vs. 41.7 ± 1.7 years), and hypertensive (68.8 vs. 36.8 years) with lower serum albumin (18.3 g/L vs. 23.1 g/L) and greater protein excretion (13.14 ± 2.03 vs. 9.1 ± 0.7 g/day) than those without AKI. There were no differences in the use of medications, including diuretics, angiotensin-converting enzyme inhibitors, angiotensin receptor blockers, and nonsteroidal anti-inflammatory agents between patients with or without AKI. Mean time to recovery of renal function was 6.4 ± 2.0 weeks. Four patients required hemodialysis that ranged from 5 to 24 weeks. Serum creatinine at last follow-up was significantly higher in patients with AKI (2.11 ± 0.44 vs. 1.15 ± 0.17 mg/dL in those without AKI). It was not possible to define treatments that best correlated with recovery of renal function. Kidney biopsies that were performed in 22 patients during an episode of AKI were reviewed. Features of acute tubular injury, evident in 14 biopsies, were mild in 9, moderate in 2, and severe in 3. Patchy interstitial inflammation, seen in 13 biopsies, was mild in 11, moderate in 1, and severe in 1. Interstitial edema was mild in six biopsies, moderate in two, and severe in one. Mild tubular atrophy and interstitial fibrosis were seen in 13 biopsies. Arteriosclerosis was mild in 13 and moderate in 2 biopsies. Six biopsies did not have any evidence of acute tubular injury, interstitial edema, or interstitial inflammation. At mean follow-up of 223 weeks, patients with an episode of AKI had a significantly higher mean serum creatinine compared with those without ARF (2.11 ± 0.44 versus 1.15 ± 0.17 mg/dL; $P < 0.001$). Four had developed lesions of FSGS.

Chen et al. presented data on 25 patients with MCD and AKI and focused their study on an interesting pathophysiologic hypothesis dealing with endothelin-1 (ET-1) expression in vessels, tubules, and glomeruli [73]. Their patient population consisted of 53 patients consecutively diagnosed with adult-onset MCN during a 10-year period. Based on creatinine clearance, 25 patients were assigned to the AKI group and 28 patients to the non-AKI group. The AKI group had a higher blood pressure, higher serum cholesterol level, and lower serum albumin level than the non-AKI group. Pathological data showed more severe foot process effacement, interstitial edema, and flattened tubular epithelium in the same group. Greater ET-1 expression was detected in vessels, tubules, and glomeruli of the AKI compared with non-AKI group. The AKI group experienced a lower steroid response rate. However, there was no significant difference in stability of remission to steroid treatment in patients who achieved a remission. The authors hypothesized that AKI associated with enhanced kidney ET-1 expression is a reversible complication of MCN that occurs frequently in patients with apparently expanded extracellular fluid. They presumed that AKI may develop as an amplification of the underlying pathogenesis of MCN involved in enhanced ET-1 expression, which may be superimposed by a transient episode of circulatory insufficiency during diuretic treatment.

11.3.2.2 Acute Kidney Injury in Children with Minimal Change Nephrosis

Acute kidney injury is much less frequent in children with MCD compared to adults. In a study including 1006 patients observed between 1990 and 1999, the incidence of acute kidney injury was 0.8% [74]. However, the frequency of AKI is higher if we consider those children with minimal change disease who are hospitalized. A recent publication from the Midwest Pediatric

Nephrology Consortium in the USA reports that AKI occurred in 58.6% of 336 children and 50.9% of 615 hospitalizations of children with nephrotic syndrome [75]. In this study, risk factors for AKI were steroid-resistant nephrotic syndrome, infection, and nephrotoxic medication exposure.

In children with MCD, AKI may be secondary to severe volume depletion, infection, acute tubular necrosis, allergic interstitial nephritis (due to antibiotics or nonsteroidal anti-inflammatory drugs), or drug toxicity such as calcineurin inhibitors (cyclosporine and tacrolimus which are often used in children with steroid-dependent nephrotic syndrome) or ACE inhibitors [76, 77]. ACE inhibitors or angiotensin receptor blockers are often prescribed to reduce proteinuria in steroid-resistant children and may be responsible for AKI. Volume depletion may be exacerbated by the use of diuretics or diarrhea. Peritonitis is a well-known complication of idiopathic nephrotic syndrome and may occur at presentation or at onset of a relapse. This serious infection may be associated with AKI [78, 79]. Sakarcan et al. reported AKI in four children, three of them in association with peritonitis [79]. Renal biopsy showed acute tubular ischemia. All children required dialysis, and renal function recovered in all of them within 12 days and in some of them up to 1 year.

These factors, which are associated with a risk of AKI, may be absent, and changes in renal perfusion and glomerular permeability are suspected. Vande Walle et al. studied 11 children with biopsy-proven MCD and oliguric acute renal failure [80]. They measured inulin and para-aminohippurate clearances before and after the intravenous administration of an albumin solution. Prior to albumin infusion, the GFR was significantly decreased in all patients, but renal plasma flow (RPF) values were in the normal range in most patients. This indicated a significant decrease of the filtration fraction. The response to albumin infusion was a slight but not significant increase of the RPF. The GFR increased in some patients and decreased in others. The authors concluded that although volume depletion may contribute to a reduced renal function in some patients, changes in glomerular permeability probably have a major role in AKI that occurs in the absence of precipitating factors. These data are in accordance with those reported by Bohman et al. [55], analyzed above in Sect. 11.2.3.

11.4 Pathophysiology of AKI in Minimal Change Nephrotic Syndrome

The foregoing commentary reveals several points of interest with regard to idiopathic nephrotic syndrome with minimal glomerular changes. First, it appears that in this form of nephrotic syndrome, the blood volume is normal, but can be abruptly diminished by a reckless use of loop diuretics for treating edema in a patient whose foot process flattening moderately decreases the GFR. Second, that AKI with tubular cell injury is more frequent in older patients with pre-existing hypertension and arterial/arteriolar lesions. Other factors that may cause AKI in MCD include drugs, contrast media, infection, and renal vein thrombosis.

11.4.1 Vascular Lesions

Vascular lesions are common in aged and/or hypertensive patients with MCD. They are interpreted as "nephrosclerosis," an umbrella term that covers microvascular lesions that do not uniformly reduce the afferent arteriolar blood supply to the glomerular tuft [81–83]. However these microvascular lesions along with inflammatory interstitial fibrosis and tubular atrophy undoubtedly contribute to compromise the viability of renal tubules, tubules that already suffer from reabsorption of proteins filtered at the glomerulus with droplets of athrocytosis.

Other vascular factors may contribute to jeopardize the kidney blood supply, in particular atherosclerotic stenosis of the renal arteries [84]. The common factor among these vascular lesions is ischemia. This explains the frequent finding of tubular necrosis on kidney biopsies in nephrotic patients with AKI, a form of postischemic injury with delayed improvement of renal function, irrespective of corticosteroid treatment.

11.4.2 Diuretics

Loop diuretics are widely used for treating nephrotic edema, and overtreatment resulting in hypovolemia is cited in most of the analyzed publications as having induced an acute rise in serum creatinine levels. Hypovolemic shock may occur, especially in elderly patients with a background of compromised cardiac function.

In fact, as indicated above extracellular salt and water retention in MCD can be rather crippling but not life threatening, as it would be in some cases of nephritic syndrome. As long as remission of proteinuria has not been achieved, essentially with corticosteroids, the patient remains edematous.

11.4.3 Iodinated Contrast Media

Iodinated contrast media are nephrotoxic and may induce AKI in a nephrotic patient older than ≈60 years [85]. The risk of AKI is greater when a high-osmolality ionic contrast medium is used in a nephrotic patient with an eGFR <60 mL/min/1.73 m^2.

11.4.4 Nonsteroidal Anti-inflammatory Drugs (NSAIDs)

11.4.4.1 NSAID-Induced MCD with or Without Acute Interstitial Nephritis

Since the late 1970s, NSAIDs have been identified among the causes of "secondary minimal change disease" [86]. NSAIDs can produce nephrotic syndrome associated with glomerular lesions identical to that seen in primary MCD. In most, but not all, cases there is a concomitant acute interstitial nephritis characterized by the influx of polyclonal T and B cells [87–93]. The association of NSAID with MCD is characterized by an abrupt decline in renal function, usually eventuating in AKI. Skin rashes and fever are uncommon.

Recrudescence may occur upon reexposure to the drug, implying that a cell-mediated hypersensitivity reaction is operative. Withdrawal of the agent is usually associated with full recovery, but glucocorticoids may hasten the rate of return of renal function and disappearance of proteinuria. Nevertheless, a clear beneficial effect of steroids on the course of NSAID-induced MCD is not clearly established.

11.4.4.2 NSAID-Induced AKI in Preexisting Minimal Change Disease

Nonsteroidal anti-inflammatory drugs diminish renal function in patients with minimal change disease by decreasing the synthesis of vasodilator prostaglandins, thereby inducing renal vasoconstriction [94].

Selective NSAIDs (COX-2 inhibitors) are credited with fewer symptomatic gastric and duodenal ulcers than nonselective ones. However they have a renal toxicity.

In a large cohort study, Lafrance and Miller found a higher risk of AKI, defined by a creatinine increase of greater than 50% in new users of any single NSAID compared to nonusers without recent use [95]. The risk of AKI varied among different NSAIDs with risk generally increasing with decrease in selectivity. The higher risk was observed with the selective NSAIDs and was lower with selective NSAIDs (COX-2 inhibitors).

Almansori et al. reported one case of AKI in a patient with biopsy-proven MCD plus acute tubular necrosis, without interstitial nephritis, which was attributed to celecoxib, a selective COX-2 inhibitor [96]. Proteinuria resolved after the agent was discontinued, although impaired renal function did not completely improve.

Chen and Tarng presented a case of celecoxib-associated minimal change disease with profound urinary protein loss and AKI [97]. Renal function and nephrotic syndrome in this patient resolved completely after discontinuation of celecoxib and treatment with methylprednisolone.

These observations demonstrate that a high index of suspicion exists in patients developing nephrotic syndrome and acute renal failure after taking COX-2 inhibitors. This cause of secondary MCD responds well to timely cessation of COX-2 inhibitors and administration of steroid therapy.

11.4.4.3 Other Causes of AKI in Minimal Change Disease

Renal vein thrombosis Renal vein thrombosis is occasionally cited among the causes of AKI complicating MCD [98]. In fact thromboembolism is a well-known complication of any etiology of nephrotic syndrome, a hazard that justifies preventive anticoagulation when serum albumin concentration is durably lower than 20 g/L. However renal vein thrombosis which is unusually frequent in membranous glomerulopathy rarely leads to AKI as a vicarious circulation relieves the pressure in the renal venous circulation [99]. Bilateral massive thrombosis of the whole renal venous circulation is a cause of AKI in dehydrated and febrile newborns, but it is not specifically cited in papers dealing with adult [72] or childhood MCD [75].

Folk medicines Traditional medicines are widely used in Eastern countries [100]. These folk remedies that may contain heavy metals, including mercury, can be a cause of AKI in Asian patients with the nephrotic syndrome. These patients should be questioned about their intake of such medications.

11.5 Treatment Recommendations

While there are many published reports describing MCD and AKI, there are no firm treatment recommendations. In adults with MCD and AKI, one cannot rely on publications that appeared before the 1970s, at a time when—as an example—mercurial diuretics were still occasionally used, and the "underfill" hypothesis led to advocating blood volume replenishment with albumin solutions and macromolecules along with loop diuretics. The acquired experience shows that infused albumin is rapidly wasted the next day in the urine, and neither improves serum albumin levels nor renal function. In the same line, treatment with loop diuretics may help reduce massive edema, but edema and renal failure are independent variables, and overtreatment with diuretics was for decades cited among the main causes of hypovolemia and AKI in nephrotic adults. In any event AKI complicating minimal change disease often requires performing a kidney biopsy in order to determine the nature and the degree of tubular injury, the involvement of the interstitium, and the appearance of arteries and arterioles. In a patient with hypertension and atherosclerosis, the main renal arteries must be examined by pulsed Doppler ultrasonography. Management of AKI is based on supportive treatment, including dialysis when necessary, in order to buy time until remission is—hopefully—achieved with glucocorticoids. In steroid-resistant cases with persistent massive proteinuria, regression of AKI is unlikely. In some of such cases, a repeat kidney biopsy may reveal lesions of FSGS [72].

In children with MCD, the occurrence of AKI requires a careful investigation of precipitating factors, such as severe intravascular volume depletion aggravated by the use of diuretics, infection, or nephrotoxic drugs. In the absence of precipitating factors, changes in glomerular permeability may explain AKI which most often resolve when corticosteroid therapy induces a remission. The management of AKI is supportive. It rarely requires dialysis.

Conflict of Interest Statement The authors deny any conflict of interest with regard to this chapter.

References

1. Cameron JS. Nephrotic syndrome in the elderly. Semin Nephrol. 1996;16:319–29.
2. Haas M, Spargo BH, Wit EJ, Meehan SM. Etiologies and outcome of acute renal insufficiency in older adults: a renal biopsy study of 259 cases. Am J Kidney Dis. 2000;35:433–47.
3. Moutzouris DA, Herlitz L, Appel GB, Markowitz GS, Freudenthal B, Radhakrishnan J, D'Agati VD. Renal biopsy in the very elderly. Clin J Am Soc Nephrol. 2009;4:1073–82.

4. Uezono S, Hara S, Sato Y, Komatsu H, Ikeda N, Shimao Y, Hayashi T, Asada Y, Fujimoto S, Eto T. Renal biopsy in elderly patients: a clinicopathological analysis. Ren Fail. 2006;28:549–55.
5. Zech P, Colon S, Pointet P, Deteix P, Labeeuw M, Leitienne P. The nephrotic syndrome in adults aged over 60: etiology, evolution and treatment of 76 cases. Clin Nephrol. 1982;17:232–6.
6. Marino F, Martorano C, Tripepi R, Bellantoni M, Tripepi G, Mallamaci F, Zoccali C. Subclinical pulmonary congestion is prevalent in nephrotic syndrome. Kidney Int. 2016;89(2):421–8.
7. Rostoker G, Behar A, Lagrue G. Vascular hyperpermeability in nephrotic edema. Nephron. 2000;85:194–200.
8. Doucet A, Favre G, Deschenes G. Molecular mechanism of edema formation in nephrotic syndrome: therapeutic implications. Pediatr Nephrol. 2007;22:1983–90.
9. Bhave G, Neilson EG. Body fluid dynamics: back to the future. J Am Soc Nephrol. 2011;22:2166–81.
10. Vande Walle JG, Donckerwolcke RA. Pathogenesis of edema formation in the nephrotic syndrome. Pediatr Nephrol. 2001;16:283–93.
11. Koomans HA, Kortlandt W, Geers AB, Dorhout Mees EJ. Lowered protein content of tissue fluid in patients with the nephrotic syndrome: observations during disease and recovery. Nephron. 1985;40:391–5.
12. Koomans HA, Geers AB, Dorhout Mees EJ, Kortlandt W. Lowered tissue-fluid oncotic pressure protects the blood volume in the nephrotic syndrome. Nephron. 1986;42:317–22.
13. Reimold EW, Marks JF. Hypovolemic shock complicating the nephrotic syndrome in children. J Pediatr. 1966;69:658–60.
14. Theuns-Valks SD, van Wijk JA, van Heerde M, Dolman KM, Bokenkamp A. Abdominal pain and vomiting in a boy with nephrotic syndrome. Clin Pediatr (Phila). 2011;50:470–3.
15. Van de Walle JG, Donckerwolcke RA, Greidanus TB, Joles JA, Koomans HA. Renal sodium handling in children with nephrotic relapse: relation to hypovolaemic symptoms. Nephrol Dial Transplant. 1996;11:2202–8.
16. Wang SJ, Tsau YK, Lu FL, Chen CH. Hypovolemia and hypovolemic shock in children with nephrotic syndrome. Acta Paediatr Taiwan. 2000;41:179–83.
17. Dorhout Mees EJ. Does it make sense to administer albumin to the patient with nephrotic oedema? Nephrol Dial Transplant. 1996;11:1224–6.
18. Dorhout Mees EJ, Koomans HA. Understanding the nephrotic syndrome: what's new in a decade? Nephron. 1995;70:1–10.
19. Eisenberg S. Blood volume in persons with the nephrotic syndrome. Am J Med Sci. 1968;255:320–6.
20. Dorhout EJ, Roos JC, Boer P, Yoe OH, Simatupang TA. Observations on edema formation in the nephrotic syndrome in adults with minimal lesions. Am J Med. 1979;67:378–84.
21. Dorhout Mees EJ, Geers AB, Koomans HA. Blood volume and sodium retention in the nephrotic syndrome: a controversial pathophysiological concept. Nephron. 1984;36:201–11.
22. Fauchald P, Noddeland H, Norseth J. Interstitial fluid volume, plasma volume and colloid osmotic pressure in patients with nephrotic syndrome. Scand J Clin Lab Invest. 1984;44:661–7.
23. Fauchald P, Noddeland H, Norseth J. An evaluation of ultrafiltration as treatment of diuretic-resistant oedema in nephrotic syndrome. Acta Med Scand. 1985;217:127–31.
24. Geers AB, Koomans HA, Boer P, Dorhout Mees EJ. Plasma and blood volumes in patients with the nephrotic syndrome. Nephron. 1984;38:170–3.
25. Geers AB, Koomans HA, Roos JC, Dorhout Mees EJ. Preservation of blood volume during edema removal in nephrotic subjects. Kidney Int. 1985;28:652–7.
26. Koomans HA, Braam B, Geers AB, Roos JC, Dorhout Mees EJ. The importance of plasma protein for blood volume and blood pressure homeostasis. Kidney Int. 1986;30:730–5.
27. Koomans HA, Geers AB, vd Meiracker AH, Roos JC, Boer P, Dorhout Mees EJ. Effects of plasma volume expansion on renal salt handling in patients with the nephrotic syndrome. Am J Nephrol. 1984;4:227–34.
28. Meltzer JI, Keim HJ, Laragh JH, Sealey JE, Jan KM, Chien S. Nephrotic syndrome: vasoconstriction and hypervolemic types indicated by renin-sodium profiling. Ann Intern Med. 1979;91:688–96.
29. Brown EA, Markandu N, Sagnella GA, Jones BE, MacGregor GA. Sodium retention in nephrotic syndrome is due to an intrarenal defect: evidence from steroid-induced remission. Nephron. 1985;39:290–5.
30. Brown EA, Markandu ND, Roulston JE, Jones BE, Squires M, MacGregor GA. Is the renin-angiotensin-aldosterone system involved in the sodium retention in the nephrotic syndrome? Nephron. 1982;32:102–7.
31. Brown EA, Markandu ND, Sagnella GA, Squires M, Jones BE, MacGregor GA. Evidence that some mechanism other than the renin system causes sodium retention in nephrotic syndrome. Lancet. 1982;2:1237–40.
32. Fadnes HO, Pape JF, Sundsfjord JA. A study on oedema mechanism in nephrotic syndrome. Scand J Clin Lab Invest. 1986;46:533–8.
33. Geers AB, Koomans HA, Roos JC, Boer P, Dorhout Mees EJ. Functional relationships in the nephrotic syndrome. Kidney Int. 1984;26:324–30.
34. Hammond TG, Whitworth JA, Saines D, Thatcher R, Andrews J, Kincaid-Smith P. Renin-angiotensin-aldo sterone system in nephrotic syndrome. Am J Kidney Dis. 1984;4:18–23.
35. Shapiro MD, Nicholls KM, Groves BM, Schrier RW. Role of glomerular filtration rate in the impaired sodium and water excretion of patients with the nephrotic syndrome. Am J Kidney Dis. 1986;8:81–7.
36. Usberti M, Federico S, Meccariello S, Cianciaruso B, Balletta M, Pecoraro C, Sacca L, Ungaro B, Pisanti

N, Andreucci VE. Role of plasma vasopressin in the impairment of water excretion in nephrotic syndrome. Kidney Int. 1984;25:422–9.
37. Ichikawa I, Rennke HG, Hoyer JR, Badr KF, Schor N, Troy JL, Lechene CP, Brenner BM. Role for intrarenal mechanisms in the impaired salt excretion of experimental nephrotic syndrome. J Clin Invest. 1983;71:91–103.
38. Deschenes G, Doucet A. Collecting duct (Na+/K+)-ATPase activity is correlated with urinary sodium excretion in rat nephrotic syndromes. J Am Soc Nephrol. 2000;11:604–15.
39. Feraille E, Vogt B, Rousselot M, Barlet-Bas C, Cheval L, Doucet A, Favre H. Mechanism of enhanced Na-K-ATPase activity in cortical collecting duct from rats with nephrotic syndrome. J Clin Invest. 1993;91:1295–300.
40. Kim SW, de Seigneux S, Sassen MC, Lee J, Kim J, Knepper MA, Frokiaer J, Nielsen S. Increased apical targeting of renal ENaC subunits and decreased expression of 11betaHSD2 in HgCl2-induced nephrotic syndrome in rats. Am J Physiol Renal Physiol. 2006;290:F674–87.
41. Nephrotic syndrome in children: prediction of histopathology from clinical and laboratory characteristics at time of diagnosis. A report of the International Study of Kidney Disease in Children. Kidney Int. 1978;13:159–65.
42. Habib R, Kleinknecht C. The primary nephrotic syndrome of childhood. Classification and clinicopathologic study of 406 cases. Pathol Annu. 1971;6: 417–74.
43. White RH, Glasgow EF, Mills RJ. Clinicopathological study of nephrotic syndrome in childhood. Lancet. 1970;1:1353–9.
44. Bohlin AB. Clinical course and renal function in minimal change nephrotic syndrome. Acta Paediatr Scand. 1984;73:631–6.
45. Hopper J Jr, Ryan P, Lee JC, Rosenau W. Lipoid nephrosis in 31 adult patients: renal biopsy study by light, electron, and fluorescence microscopy with experience in treatment. Medicine (Baltimore). 1970;49:321–41.
46. Carrie BJ, Golbetz HV, Michaels AS, Myers BD. Creatinine: an inadequate filtration marker in glomerular diseases. Am J Med. 1980;69:177–82.
47. Gur A, Adefuin PY, Siegel NJ, Hayslett JP. A study of the renal handling of water in lipoid nephrosis. Pediatr Res. 1976;10:197–201.
48. Koomans HA, Boer WH, Dorhout Mees EJ. Renal function during recovery from minimal lesions nephrotic syndrome. Nephron. 1987;47:173–8.
49. Nolasco F, Cameron JS, Heywood EF, Hicks J, Ogg C, Williams DG. Adult-onset minimal change nephrotic syndrome: a long-term follow-up. Kidney Int. 1986;29:1215–23.
50. Lowenstein J, Schacht RG, Baldwin DS. Renal failure in minimal change nephrotic syndrome. Am J Med. 1981;70:227–33.
51. Cameron MA, Peri U, Rogers TE, Moe OW. Minimal change disease with acute renal failure: a case against the nephrosarca hypothesis. Nephrol Dial Transplant. 2004;19:2642–6.
52. Esparza AR, Kahn SI, Garella S, Abuelo JG. Spectrum of acute renal failure in nephrotic syndrome with minimal (or minor) glomerular lesions. Role of hemodynamic factors. Lab Investig. 1981;45:510–21.
53. Koomans HA. Pathophysiology of acute renal failure in idiopatic nephrotic syndrome. Nephrol Dial Transplant. 2001;16:221–4.
54. Robson AM, Giangiacomo J, Kienstra RA, Naqvi ST, Ingelfinger JR. Normal glomerular permeability and its modification by minimal change nephrotic syndrmone. J Clin Invest. 1974;54:1190–9.
55. Bohman SO, Jaremko G, Bohlin AB, Berg U. Foot process fusion and glomerular filtration rate in minimal change nephrotic syndrome. Kidney Int. 1984;25:696–700.
56. Drumond MC, Kristal B, Myers BD, Deen WM. Structural basis for reduced glomerular filtration capacity in nephrotic humans. J Clin Invest. 1994;94:1187–95.
57. Maas RJ, Deegens JK, Wetzels JF. Permeability factors in idiopathic nephrotic syndrome: historical perspectives and lessons for the future. Nephrol Dial Transplant. 2014;29:2207–16.
58. Chamberlain MJ, Pringle A, Wrong OM. Oliguric renal failure in the nephrotic syndrome. Q J Med. 1966;35:215–35.
59. Conolly ME, Wrong OM, Jones NF. Reversible renal failure in idiopathic nephrotic syndrome with minimal glomerular changes. Lancet. 1968;1:665–8.
60. Harats D, Friedlander M, Koplovic Y, Friedman G. Prolonged reversible acute renal failure in focal glomerulonephritis with severe nephrotic syndrome in an elderly patient. Klin Wochenschr. 1989;67: 502–5.
61. Holdsworth DR, Stephenson P, Dowling JP, Atkins RC. Reversible acute renal failure in the nephrotic syndrome with minimal glomerular pathology. Med J Aust. 1977;2:532–3.
62. Hulter HN, Bonner EL Jr. Lipoid nephrosis appearing as acute oliguric renal failure. Arch Intern Med. 1980;140:403–5.
63. Imbasciati E, Ponticelli C, Case N, Altieri P, Bolasco F, Mihatsch MJ, Zollinger HU. Acute renal failure in idiopathic nephrotic syndrome. Nephron. 1981;28:186–91.
64. Jennette JC, Falk RJ. Adult minimal change glomerulopathy with acute renal failure. Am J Kidney Dis. 1990;16:432–7.
65. Raij L, Keane WF, Leonard A, Shapiro FL. Irreversible acute renal failure in idiopathic nephrotic syndrome. Am J Med. 1976;61:207–14.
66. Scully RE, Galdabini JJ, McNeely BU. Case records of the Massachusetts General Hospital. Weekly clinicopathological exercises. Case 17–1978. N Engl J Med. 1978;298:1014–21.
67. Searle M, Cooper C, Elliman J, Dathan R, Maciver A. Reversibility of acute renal failure in elderly patients with the nephrotic syndrome. Postgrad Med J. 1985;61:741–4.

68. Stephens VJ, Yates AP, Lechler RI, Baker LR. Reversible uraemia in normotensive nephrotic syndrome. Br Med J. 1979;2:705–6.
69. Smith JD, Hayslett JP. Reversible renal failure in the nephrotic syndrome. Am J Kidney Dis. 1992;19:201–13.
70. Mak SK, Short CD, Mallick NP. Long-term outcome of adult-onset minimal-change nephropathy. Nephrol Dial Transplant. 1996;11:2192–201.
71. Chen T, Lv Y, Lin F, Zhu J. Acute kidney injury in adult idiopathic nephrotic syndrome. Ren Fail. 2011;33:144–9.
72. Waldman M, Crew RJ, Valeri A, Busch J, Stokes B, Markowitz G, D'Agati V, Appel G. Adult minimal-change disease: clinical characteristics, treatment, and outcomes. Clin J Am Soc Nephrol. 2007;2:445–53.
73. Chen CL, Fang HC, Chou KJ, Lee JC, Lee PT, Chung HM, Wang JS. Increased endothelin 1 expression in adult-onset minimal change nephropathy with acute renal failure. Am J Kidney Dis. 2005;45:818–25.
74. Kilis-Pstrusinska K, Zwolinska D, Musial K. [Acute renal failure in children with idiopathic nephrotic syndrome]. Pol Merkur Lekarski. 2000;8:462–4.
75. Rheault MN, Zhang L, Selewski DT, Kallash M, Tran CL, Seamon M, Katsoufis C, Ashoor I, Hernandez J, Supe-Markovina K, D'Alessandri-Silva C, DeJesus-Gonzalez N, Vasylyeva TL, Formeck C, Woll C, Gbadegesin R, Geier P, Devarajan P, Carpenter SL, Kerlin BA, Smoyer WE, Midwest Pediatric Nephrology C. AKI in children hospitalized with nephrotic syndrome. Clin J Am Soc Nephrol. 2015;10:2110.
76. Rheault MN, Wei CC, Hains DS, Wang W, Kerlin BA, Smoyer WE. Increasing frequency of acute kidney injury amongst children hospitalized with nephrotic syndrome. Pediatr Nephrol. 2014;29:139–47.
77. Agarwal N, Phadke KD, Garg I, Alexander P. Acute renal failure in children with idiopathic nephrotic syndrome. Pediatr Nephrol. 2003;18:1289–92.
78. Cavagnaro F, Lagomarsino E. Peritonitis as a risk factor of acute renal failure in nephrotic children. Pediatr Nephrol. 2000;15:248–51.
79. Sakarcan A, Timmons C, Seikaly MG. Reversible idiopathic acute renal failure in children with primary nephrotic syndrome. J Pediatr. 1994;125:723–7.
80. Vande Walle J, Mauel R, Raes A, Vandekerckhove K, Donckerwolcke R. ARF in children with minimal change nephrotic syndrome may be related to functional changes of the glomerular basal membrane. Am J Kidney Dis. 2004;43:399–404.
81. Hill GS. Hypertensive nephrosclerosis. Curr Opin Nephrol Hypertens. 2008;17:266–70.
82. Meyrier A. Nephrosclerosis: update on a centenarian. Nephrol Dial Transplant. 2014.
83. Meyrier A. Nephrosclerosis: a term in quest of a disease. Nephron. 2015;129:276–82.
84. Textor SC. Atherosclerotic renal artery stenosis: flaws in estimated glomerular filtration rate and the problem of progressive kidney injury. Circ Cardiovasc Interv. 2011;4:213–5.
85. Aspelin P, Aubry P, Fransson SG, Strasser R, Willenbrock R, Berg KJ, Nephrotoxicity in High-Risk Patients Study of Iso-Osmolar, Low-Osmolar Non-Ionic Contrast Media Study Investigators. Nephrotoxic effects in high-risk patients undergoing angiography. N Engl J Med. 2003;348:491–9.
86. Glassock RJ. Secondary minimal change disease. Nephrol Dial Transplant. 2003;18 Suppl 6:vi52–8.
87. Brezin JH, Katz SM, Schwartz AB, Chinitz JL. Reversible renal failure and nephrotic syndrome associated with nonsteroidal anti-inflammatory drugs. N Engl J Med. 1979;301:1271–3.
88. Curt GA, Kaldany A, Whitley LG, Crosson AW, Rolla A, Merino MJ, D'Elia JA. Reversible rapidly progressive renal failure with nephrotic syndrome due to fenoprofen calcium. Ann Intern Med. 1980;92:72–3.
89. Feinfeld DA, Olesnicky L, Pirani CL, Appel GB. Nephrotic syndrome associated with use of the nonsteroidal anti-inflammatory drugs. Case report and review of the literature. Nephron. 1984;37:174–9.
90. Kleinknecht C, Broyer M, Gubler MC, Palcoux JB. Irreversible renal failure after indomethacin in steroid-resistant nephrosis. N Engl J Med. 1980;302:691.
91. Kleinknecht D. Interstitial nephritis, the nephrotic syndrome, and chronic renal failure secondary to nonsteroidal anti-inflammatory drugs. Semin Nephrol. 1995;15:228–35.
92. Lomvardias S, Pinn VW, Wadhwa ML, Koshy KM, Heller M. Nephrotic syndrome associated with sulindac. N Engl J Med. 1981;304:424.
93. Morgenstern SJ, Bruns FJ, Fraley DS, Kirsch M, Borochovitz D. Ibuprofen-associated lipoid nephrosis without interstitial nephritis. Am J Kidney Dis. 1989;14:50–2.
94. Clive DM, Stoff JS. Renal syndromes associated with nonsteroidal antiinflammatory drugs. N Engl J Med. 1984;310:563–72.
95. Lafrance JP, Miller DR. Selective and non-selective non-steroidal anti-inflammatory drugs and the risk of acute kidney injury. Pharmacoepidemiol Drug Saf. 2009;18:923–31.
96. Almansori M, Kovithavongs T, Qarni MU. Cyclooxygenase-2 inhibitor-associated minimal-change disease. Clin Nephrol. 2005;63:381–4.
97. Chen YH, Tarng DC. Profound urinary protein loss and acute renal failure caused by cyclooxygenase-2 inhibitor. Chin J Physiol. 2011;54:264–8.
98. Singhal R, Brimble KS. Thromboembolic complications in the nephrotic syndrome: pathophysiology and clinical management. Thromb Res. 2006;118:397–407.
99. Llach F, Papper S, Massry SG. The clinical spectrum of renal vein thrombosis: acute and chronic. Am J Med. 1980;69:819–27.
100. Luyckx VA, Naicker S. Acute kidney injury associated with the use of traditional medicines. Nat Clin Pract Nephrol. 2008;4:664–71.

12 Core Concepts: Post-cardiac Surgery Acute Kidney Injury

Jason B. O'Neal, Frederic T. Billings IV, and Andrew D. Shaw

12.1 Diagnosis and Epidemiology

Acute kidney injury (AKI) following cardiac surgery occurs in up to 30% of patients, and the incidence is highest in patients with known risk factors [1, 2]. Patients undergoing cardiac surgery typically have several risk factors (Table 12.1) [3]. Many of these risk factors including hypertension, advanced age, hyperlipidemia, and peripheral vascular disease are not modifiable, which makes the prevention of AKI in their presence more challenging [4]. Certain characteristics unique to cardiac surgery also contribute to an increased risk of AKI postoperatively, including cardiopulmonary bypass (CPB), the use of ventricular assist devices (VAD), use of extracorporeal membrane oxygenation (ECMO), and aortic cross-clamping. These interventions may lead to end-organ hypoperfusion and the initiation of a systemic inflammatory response, which both may play roles in the development of AKI [5].

J. B. O'Neal
Department of Anesthesiology, Vanderbilt University Medical Center, Nashville, TN, USA
e-mail: jason.b.oneal@vanderbilt.edu

F. T. Billings IV
Department of Anesthesiology, Vanderbilt University, Nashville, TN, USA
e-mail: frederic.t.billings@vanderbilt.edu

A. D. Shaw (✉)
Department of Anesthesiology and Pain Medicine, University of Alberta, Edmonton, AB, Canada
e-mail: andrew.shaw@vanderbilt.edu

The development of AKI may contribute to several complications, while also increasing mortality in this patient population. Complications of AKI after cardiac surgery include the need for dialysis, a prolonged length of stay in the intensive care unit, a prolonged hospital stay, and an increased risk for stroke [6]. Given the known high risk associated with cardiac surgery, increasing the risk for these complications has major implications on this patient population.

The incidence of AKI after cardiac surgery in the pediatric population is similar to that in adults, with rates up to 42% in the published literature [7]. The short-term outcomes in these patients are already suboptimal, but the development of AKI also places these patients at risk for the development of chronic kidney disease [8]. While certain risk factors such as atherosclerosis, hypertension, and diabetes are not typically present in this population, several other characteristics can place them at high risk. Some of the known risk factors for AKI in the pediatric patient undergoing cardiac surgery include elevated preoperative creatinine, age less than 1 year old, lesions associated with cyanosis, prolonged CPB time, lower weight, and low cardiac output syndrome postoperatively [9]. Special consideration should be on congenital heart defect patients, as drastic variations in kidney perfusion may occur, depending on the type of defect being corrected.

S. S. Waikar et al. (eds.), *Core Concepts in Acute Kidney Injury*,
https://doi.org/10.1007/978-1-4939-8628-6_12

Table 12.1 List of perioperative risk factors associated with AKI and cardiac surgery

Preoperative	Intraoperative	Postoperative
Diabetes	Use of furosemide and other diuretics on bypass	Sepsis
Hypertension	Cardiopulmonary bypass time (CPB)	Use of vasopressors
Hyperlipidemia	Use of inotropes	Use of inotropes
Anemia	Low hematocrit during CPB	Anemia
Advanced age	Aortic cross-clamp time	Blood transfusion
Peripheral vascular disease	Need to return to CPB	Diuretic administration
Previous stroke	Hypoperfusion	Hypovolemia
Smoking history	Reperfusion injury	
Liver disease	Hypovolemia	
Chronic kidney disease		

12.2 Pathophysiology

As previously mentioned, CPB provides a unique stress to the kidneys during surgery. Non-pulsatile blood flow alters organ perfusion, contributing to a state of hypoperfusion in the renal medulla. If exposed to CPB, VAD placement, ECMO, or another source of external hemodynamic support (i.e., intra-aortic balloon pump (IABP)), one must ensure that adequate mean arterial pressure (MAP) is preserved. Maintaining sufficient end-organ perfusion pressure throughout the body while on bypass can be quite difficult, and its assessment is both challenging and sometimes inaccurate, particularly in the presence of vasoplegia and/or dampened radial arterial line signals. This may increase the risk for end-organ ischemia and in turn lead to a prerenal component of AKI. Also, given the extent of the surgery, excessive sympathetic tone may increase the levels of circulating endogenous and exogenous catecholamines such as norepinephrine, which may cause vasoconstriction of the renal arteries with subsequent decreased renal blood flow (RBF) [10]. The increase in sympathetic activity also increases renin production which may further reduce RBF [11]. One must also consider the iatrogenic effects of vasopressors administered to support a target MAP (Table 12.2). Interestingly, therapies that increase RBF above basal levels do not routinely decrease AKI. An increase in RBF increases solute delivery to renal tubules and consequently tubule oxygen requirements for solute resorption. If an increase in RBF increases glomerular perfusion to a greater extent than tubule perfusion, increases in RBF may actually increase medullary ischemia and AKI [12]. Therefore, the focus should remain on maintaining renal perfusion by avoiding cardiac failure and hypotension, but not renal hyper-perfusion.

Table 12.2 Vasoactive agents and effect on renal blood flow

Vasoactive medication	Effect on renal blood flow
Dopamine	↑↑
Dobutamine	↑
Fenoldopam	↑↑↑
Epinephrine	↓↓
Norepinephrine	↔
Vasopressin	↓

With the significant amount of systemic inflammation induced by sternotomy and CPB, indirect damage to the kidneys is common. Although the mechanisms by which inflammation leads to AKI are not fully understood, several theories have been proposed [11, 13]. A hypothesis of relevance for cardiac surgery is that an initial insult to the vascular or tubular endothelial cells from ischemia due to hypoperfusion, reperfusion injury, and/or hemolysis leaves the kidney susceptible to inflammatory infiltration and injury. Leukocytes including neutrophils, macrophages, and lymphocytes are now readily able to infiltrate the kidneys leading to the recruitment of various cytokines and chemokines [13]. Thus, direct damage from these inflammatory mediators ensues and causes injury to the kidneys.

Plasma-free hemoglobin rises rapidly during CPB due to erythrocyte trauma from rotor heads, oxygenators, pump suckers, and filters.

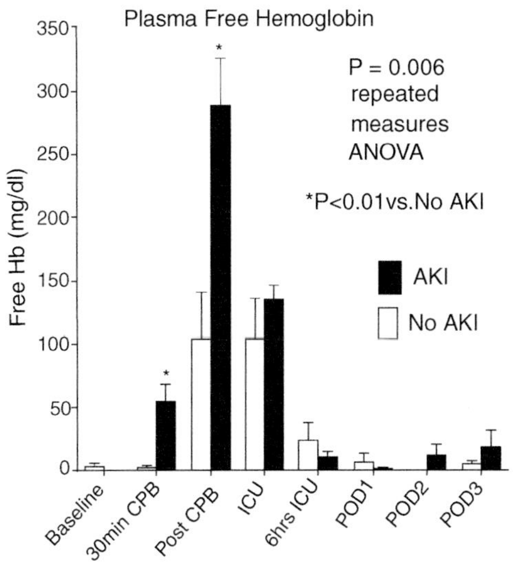

Fig. 12.1 Plasma-free hemoglobin (Hb) concentrations prior to surgery (baseline), 30 min into CPB, immediately following CPB, at ICU admission, 6 h after ICU admission, and on postoperative days 1, 2, and 3 in 10 patients that developed AKI and 10 risk-matched control patients that did not develop AKI. Free Hb concentrations were significantly higher during surgery in patients that developed postoperative AKI

Haptoglobin stores are rapidly exhausted, and free hemoglobin injures the kidneys via redox cycling and free iron-induced reactive oxygen species production, lipid peroxidation, heme protein with Tamm-Horsfall protein precipitating in the collecting system, and renal vasoconstriction [14–16]. In a clinical study, patients that developed AKI had more than twice the concentration of free hemoglobin in the plasma as non-AKI patients, despite similar risk factors and CPB durations (150 min) (Fig. 12.1) [17].

12.3 Prevention

Given the high incidence and negative outcomes associated with AKI, especially following cardiac surgery, preventive strategies are of the utmost importance given that up to 30% of cases of AKI may be preventable [18]. Fluid management during and after the operation, as well as maintaining adequate urine output, should be considered preoperatively with a plan set in place prior to the induction of the patient. Surgeons can assist with AKI prevention by limiting (or perhaps avoiding) CPB and reducing aortic cross-clamp times. Other strategies such as the use of bicarbonate and individualized hemodynamic management throughout the perioperative period may potentially play a role in preventing AKI, although large clinical trials have not demonstrated an overall benefit, particularly for bicarbonate therapy which should continue to be considered an experimental treatment.

The plan for fluid management should begin with assessing the patient's preoperative fluid balance. Determination as to whether the patient is hypovolemic, euvolemic, or hypervolemic can provide the clinician initial guidance. A strategy which aims for euvolemia is typically desired during the perioperative period with a few exceptions (i.e., relative hypervolemia in cases of cardiac tamponade, hypertrophic cardiomyopathy, etc.). Several monitors may assist the clinician in maintaining euvolemia including pulse pressure variation (PPV), stroke volume variation (SVV), central venous pressure (CVP), and echocardiography. Generally speaking, these monitors are more beneficial when used in a dynamic fashion (i.e., to assess the effect of a fluid bolus). The typical cardiac surgical patient will have an arterial line, central venous line, and transesophageal echocardiography probe in place intraoperatively enabling the real-time gathering and interpretation of these data elements. The use of goal-directed therapy (GDT) during cardiac surgery which aims to utilize one or more of these monitoring techniques to guide fluid and/or pressor/inotrope support has been investigated. Some studies have suggested benefits showing a reduction in overall complications when using GDT [19, 20]. One study specifically investigating GDT and AKI found that targeting stroke volume optimization with fluid challenges reduced the incidence of AKI [21]. The amount of literature on GDT and its effect on AKI are not extensive; however, whether or not GDT truly influences AKI after cardiac surgery has yet to be fully elucidated, and as with GDT in other settings, the type of fluid and/or vasoactive agent to use is not well established.

Prevention planning should include the consideration of whether to use colloid and/or crystalloid as integral components of the IV fluid prescription plan. As for the various types of colloid, albumin and hydroxyethyl starch have both been shown to be hazardous when considering AKI as an outcome [22, 23]. Although, the debate regarding whether or not there is benefit or harm with colloid use in surgical patients is still ongoing [24]. The type of crystalloid may be more important than previously appreciated [25]. The animal [26], human volunteer [27], and clinical observational evidence [24, 28] that IV fluid solutions containing high levels of chloride are harmful continues to accumulate. The interventional studies [29, 30] conducted to date have also suggested either an adverse effect or no benefit, although it is true that a definitive randomized controlled trial has not yet been conducted. Limiting fluids which remain in the circulation for a shorter time period may be a good strategy, although concerns for hypovolemia should be considered. With more liberal fluid administration, the dilution of clotting factors, platelets, and other blood products as well as extravascular accumulation such as pulmonary edema may arise. Hypovolemia for prolonged periods of time is known to cause AKI, while hemodilution with hypervolemia similarly has a net negative effect on the kidneys.

Regarding medications and the prevention of AKI, the discontinuation of angiotensin-converting enzyme inhibitors (ACE-Is), angiotensin receptor blockers (ARBs), nonsteroidal anti-inflammatory drugs (NSAIDs), metformin, and diuretics a couple of days before surgery is normally recommended. Several medications have been investigated for intraoperative use as part of a preventive strategy. Several studies suggested a benefit with the use of calcium channel blockers including nifedipine, nicardipine, and diltiazem [31–33], although the use of these medications has not gained popularity over the years. The use of fenoldopam in septic patients may reduce mortality and the need for dialysis in critically ill patients in the intensive care unit (ICU) [34]. This may be attributed to the increase in RBF observed with the use of this medication. Within cardiac surgery, some studies suggest benefit when using fenoldopam intraoperatively [35, 36]; however, others have found no advantage and also demonstrated a higher rate of hypotension [37]. One might expect comparable results from dopamine, but at low-dose infusions, perfusion to the kidneys may be blunted and therefore associated with worse outcomes [38]. Diuretics including furosemide and mannitol do not prevent AKI but may preserve urine output perioperatively [39, 40]. The use of sodium bicarbonate to prevent AKI in cardiac surgery patients is somewhat controversial. One study demonstrated that sodium bicarbonate may reduce the incidence of severe AKI and the need for renal replacement therapy (RRT) [41], while others showed harm in patients receiving sodium bicarbonate with reports of increased risk for AKI and higher in-hospital mortality rates [42]. Given these findings, alkalinization of urine with a bicarbonate infusion during cardiac surgery is not recommended or commonly practiced [43].

Reducing the amount of time on bypass and under general anesthesia is preferred, but unfortunately this is not always possible. A prolonged duration of CPB secondary to redo sternotomy or complex surgery may increase the duration of renal hypoperfusion and, depending on the type of procedure, may increase the time in which the patient's blood volume is exposed to processes that contribute to a systemic inflammatory response. When appropriate and feasible, the use of off-pump coronary artery bypass is preferred by some as this technique is thought to be associated with a lower incidence of AKI [44, 45]. This may also hold true for transcatheter aortic valve replacement (TAVR) in comparison with on-pump aortic valve replacement (AVR) and should be considered as an option in high-risk patients. Typically the surgical candidates for TAVR possess more comorbidities than the patient population undergoing surgical AVR making studies comparing the two techniques difficult to complete. As indications for TAVR extend into moderate and perhaps low-risk AVR patients, this may become more important in the future. There is evidence to suggest better hemodynamic control with TAVR [46], and a lower rate of systemic inflammatory response (SIRS) [47], but whether or not TAVR is associated with a lower incidence of AKI is currently unknown.

12.4 Treatment

When prevention strategies fail, knowing how to effectively treat AKI can help to minimize some of the devastating long-term complications associated with this insult. Before treating AKI, one must make the correct diagnosis. The diagnosis of AKI should be made as early as possible followed by the initiation of an appropriate treatment strategy. Multiple criteria for the diagnosis of AKI are available [48, 49]. Typically the incorporation of both serum creatinine (SCr) and UOP data assist with the diagnosis. Using SCr may be based on the change from the baseline or reaching a threshold value. Cutoffs in UOP can help to further categorize kidney impairment. The RIFLE (risk, injury, failure, loss of function, and end-stage renal disease) criteria make use of both SCr and UOP to characterize AKI. An issue when using SCr and/or UOP to diagnose AKI is that the timing may be late as damage to the kidneys reflected by an increase in SCr typically takes several days. This could result in prolonging the time to reach a diagnosis of AKI leading to potentially worse outcomes. The more recent KDIGO (Kidney Disease Improving Global Outcomes) criteria are an acceptable way to confirm the diagnosis of AKI.

Using KDIGO, AKI is defined as any of the following [48]:

- Increase in SCr by ≥0.3 mg/dL (≥26.5 mmol/L) within 48 h
- Increase in SCr to ≥1.5 times baseline, which is known or presumed to have occurred within the prior 7 days
- Urine volume ≤0.5 mL/kg/h for 6 h

Given the limitations with current lab studies to assist with the diagnosis of AKI, clinicians and researchers are actively seeking more efficient ways to diagnose AKI. The utilization of biomarkers may be a way to diagnose AKI before lab values such as SCr and UOP truly reflect damage to the kidneys. Many novel biomarkers have been studied in AKI, both for diagnosis and risk stratification. Some of these, including NGAL, KIM 1, IL 18, NAG, and GST, are only available as research tools. Several are available commercially however (cystatin C, TIMP2/IGFBP7), and their place in the diagnostic and risk stratification process for AKI is evolving.

After making the diagnosis of AKI, establishing the type of AKI is crucial. The treatment strategy will be reflective of the type of AKI in the patient. The details and differences between prerenal, intrarenal, and postrenal AKI have been discussed previously in great detail.

Strategies for treatment of prerenal AKI are focused on reestablishing a status of euvolemia in the patient. This should be done quickly, but overcompensating may actually worsen the patient's condition. Several considerations should be made before treatment as the type of fluid administered is dependent on the patient's condition. Is the patient anemic, coagulopathic, or thrombocytopenic? If so, blood products, with minimal crystalloid, should be administered. The decision between packed red blood cells, fresh frozen plasma, cryoprecipitate, and/or platelets will be guided by whether or not the patient is actively bleeding, and the presence of abnormal lab values and individualized appropriate target values should be established for each patient. Clues which may suggest the need for blood products include increased chest tube output and hemodynamic instability (hypotension and tachycardia). The mistake of administering crystalloid in the setting of ongoing bleeding may ultimately worsen the patient's condition and extend the time before AKI is effectively managed.

The use of diuretics to treat AKI is somewhat controversial. Loop diuretics have several mechanisms one would assume to be protective against AKI such as decreasing oxygen consumption at the loop of Henle and possibly providing higher thresholds for ischemia in the kidney. This unfortunately is not the case as studies specific to cardiac surgery patients have found furosemide to have no reduction in AKI and even showed that furosemide could be harmful to patients [40, 50].

While the routine intraoperative use of loop diuretics is generally not recommended, a circumstance where it should be considered is in the postoperative volume-overloaded patient. Cardiac surgery has high transfusion rates which can sometimes lead to volume overload in the perioperative period. As with loop diuretics, the use of mannitol is also not recommended for treatment of AKI following cardiac surgery.

Clinicians should not neglect nutrition when treating AKI. Patients undergoing cardiac surgery are often nutritionally depleted, and oral (or enteral) feeding should be started as early as possible postoperatively. This is supported by evidence suggesting increased mortality in malnourished patients with AKI [51]. In concert with the KDIGO guidelines, goals of 20–30 kcal/kg/day in patients with any stage of AKI should be maintained [48]. Tighter glycemic control in these patients may also be beneficial in patients developing AKI [52]. Aiming for glucose ≤150 mg/dL is an appropriate target while avoiding episodes of hypoglycemia (≤110 mg/dL).

Contingent on the extent of kidney injury, the use of dialysis may be necessary. In emergent situations of severe acidosis, electrolyte imbalance, volume overload, or uremia following cardiac surgery, RRT should be started immediately. Some clinicians may postpone the initiation of RRT in hopes that the patient will recover renal function without invasive measures. Others believe that an early return to normal blood chemistry and early initiation of dialysis prevents further deterioration. Clinical trials of early versus late initiation of RRT have been inconclusive. Many factors should be considered in this type of situation including clinical context, trends of laboratory values, and anticipated benefit from RRT. The decision to implement hemodialysis (HD) versus continuous veno-venous hemofiltration (CVVH) should be guided by the hemodynamic stability of the patient.

Conclusions

Acute kidney injury developing soon after cardiac surgery is typically mild, but common. Its appearance is a predictor of subsequent adverse outcomes, particularly impaired renal function, and if severe (which fortunately is rare) it can lead to increased mortality. Attempts to stratify the risk for AKI in cardiac surgery patients focus on pre-existing comorbidities such as diabetes, CKD, advanced age, and complexity of surgery. The diagnosis of AKI is likely to advance in the coming years as the role of newly approved diagnostic tests becomes clearer, and new advances in prevention and treatment are keenly awaited as the studies that will lead to their approval are ongoing. For now, efforts to minimize the impact of AKI on outcomes after cardiac surgery focus on the identification and mitigation of those risk factors which are modifiable.

References

1. Chawla LS, Amdur RL, Shaw AD, Faselis C, Palant CE, Kimmel PL. Association between AKI and long-term renal and cardiovascular outcomes in United States veterans. Clin J Am Soc Nephrol. 2014;9(3):448–56. https://doi.org/10.2215/CJN.02440213; Epub 2013 Dec 5.
2. Lagny MG, Jouret F, Koch JN, Blaffart F, Donneau AF, Albert A, Roediger L, Krzesinski JM, Defraigne JO. Incidence and outcomes of acute kidney injury after cardiac surgery using either criteria of the RIFLE classification. BMC Nephrol. 2015;16:76. https://doi.org/10.1186/s12882-015-0066-9.
3. Parolari A, Pesce LL, Pacini D, Mazzanti V, Salis S, Sciacovelli C, Rossi F, Alamanni F, MRGoCS Outcomes. Risk factors for perioperative acute kidney injury after adult cardiac surgery: role of perioperative management. Ann Thorac Surg. 2012;93(2):584–91. https://doi.org/10.1016/j.athoracsur.2011.09.073.
4. Lopez-Delgado JC, Esteve F, Torrado H, Rodríguez-Castro D, Carrio ML, Farrero E, Javierre C, Ventura JL, Manez R. Influence of acute kidney injury on short- and long-term outcomes in patients undergoing cardiac surgery: risk factors and prognostic value of a modified RIFLE classification. Crit Care. 2013;7(6):R293. https://doi.org/10.1186/cc13159.
5. Gomez H, Ince C, De Backer D, Pickkers P, Payen D, Hotchkiss J, Kellum JA. A unified theory of sepsis-induced acute kidney injury: inflammation, microcirculatory dysfunction, bioenergetics, and the tubular cell adaptation to injury. Shock. 2014;41(1):3–11. https://doi.org/10.1097/SHK.0000000000000052.
6. Pickering JW, James MT, Palmer SC. Acute kidney injury and prognosis after cardiopulmonary bypass: a meta-analysis of cohort studies. Am J Kidney Dis. 2015;65(2):283–93. https://doi.org/10.1053/j.ajkd.2014.09.008; Epub Nov 5.

7. Li S, Krawczeski CD, Zappitelli M, Devarajan P, Thiessen-Philbrook H, Coca SG, Kim RW, Parikh CR, TRIBE-AKI Consortium. Incidence, risk factors, and outcomes of acute kidney injury after pediatric cardiac surgery: a prospective multicenter study. Crit Care Med. 2011;39(6):1493–9. https://doi.org/10.1097/CCM.0b013e31821201d3.
8. Axelrod DM, Sutherland SM. Acute kidney injury in the pediatric cardiac patient. Paediatr Anaesth. 2014;24(9):899–901. https://doi.org/10.1111/pan.12448.
9. Li S, Krawczeski CD, Zappitelli M, Devarajan P, Thiessen-Philbrook H, Coca SG, et al. Incidence, risk factors, and outcomes of acute kidney injury after pediatric cardiac surgery: a prospective multicenter study. Crit Care Med. 2011;39(6):1493–9.
10. Fujii T, Kurata H, Takaoka M, Muraoka T, Fujisawa Y, Shokoji T, Nishiyama A, Abe Y, Matsumura Y. The role of renal sympathetic nervous system in the pathogenesis of ischemic acute renal failure. Eur J Pharmacol. 2003;481:241–8.
11. Sreedharan R, Devarajan P, Van Why S. Pathogenesis of acute renal failure. In: Avner E, Harmon W, Niaudet P, Yoshikawa N, editors. Pediatric nephrology. Heidleberg: Springer; 2009. p. 1579–602.
12. Ricksten SE, Bragadottir G, Redfors B. Renal oxygenation in clinical acute kidney injury. Crit Care. 2013;7(2):221. https://doi.org/10.1186/cc12530.
13. Schrier CLEaRW. Pathophysiology of ischemic acute renal injury. In: Schrier RW, editor. Diseases of the kidney and urinary tract. 8th ed. Philadelphia, PA: Lippincott Williams & Wilkins; 2007. p. 930–61.
14. Loebl EC, Baxter CR, Curreri PW. The mechanism of erythrocyte destruction in the early postburn period. Ann Surg. 1973;178(6):681–6.
15. Ronco C, Bellomo R, Kellum JA. Acute Kidney Injury. Contrib Nephrol. 2007;156:340–53.
16. Keene WR, Jandl JH. The sites of hemoglobin catabolism. Blood. 1965;26:705–19.
17. Billings FT 4th, Ball SK, Roberts LJ 2nd, Pretorius M. Postoperative acute kidney injury is associated with hemoglobinemia and an enhanced oxidative stress response. Free Radic Biol Med. 2011;50(11):1480–7. https://doi.org/10.1016/j.freeradbiomed.2011.02.011; Epub Feb 18.
18. Vijayan A, Miller SB. Acute renal failure: prevention and nondialytic therapy. Semin Nephrol. 1998;18:523–32.
19. Giglio M, Dalfino L, Puntillo F, et al. Haemodynamic goal-directed therapy in cardiac and vascular surgery. A systematic review and meta-analysis. Interact Cardiovasc Thorac Surg. 2012;15(5):878–87. https://doi.org/10.1093/icvts/ivs323; Epub 2012 Jul 24.
20. Aya HD, Cecconi M, Hamilton M, Rhodes A. Goal-directed therapy in cardiac surgery: a systematic review and meta-analysis. Br J Anaesth. 2013;110(4):510–7. https://doi.org/10.1093/bja/aet020; Epub 2013 Feb 27.
21. Thomson R, Meeran H, Valencia O, Al-Subaie N. Goal-directed therapy after cardiac surgery and the incidence of acute kidney injury. J Crit Care. 2014;29(6):997–1000. https://doi.org/10.1016/j.jcrc.2014.06.011; Epub Jun 23.
22. Frenette AJ, Bouchard J, Bernier P, Charbonneau A, Nguyen LT, Rioux JP, Troyanov S, Williamson DR. Albumin administration is associated with acute kidney injury in cardiac surgery: a propensity score analysis. Crit Care. 2014;8(6):602. https://doi.org/10.1186/s13054–014–0602–1.
23. Myburgh JA, Finfer S, Bellomo R, Billot L, Cass A, Gattas D, Glass P, Lipman J, Liu B, McArthur C, McGuinness S, Rajbhandari D, Taylor CB, Webb SA, Investigators C, AaNZICSCT Group. Hydroxyethyl starch or saline for fluid resuscitation in intensive care. N Engl J Med. 2012;367(20):1901–11. https://doi.org/10.1056/NEJMoa1209759; Epub 2012 Oct 17
24. Raghunathan K, Murray PT, Beattie WS, Lobo DN, Myburgh J, Sladen R, Kellum JA, Mythen MG, Shaw AD, ADQI XII Investigators Group. Choice of fluid in acute illness: what should be given? An international consensus. Br J Anaesth. 2014;113(5):772–83. https://doi.org/10.1093/bja/aeu301.
25. Kim JY, Joung KW, Kim KM, Kim MJ, Kim JB, Jung SH, Lee EH, Choi IC. Relationship between a perioperative intravenous fluid administration strategy and acute kidney injury following off-pump coronary artery bypass surgery: an observational study. Crit Care. 2015;19:350. https://doi.org/10.1186/s13054–015–1065–8.
26. Lai EY, Onozato ML, Solis G, Aslam S, Welch WJ, Wilcox CS. Myogenic responses of mouse isolated perfused renal afferent arterioles: effects of salt intake and reduced renal mass. Hypertension. 2010;55(4):983–9. https://doi.org/10.1161/HYPERTENSIONAHA.109.149120; Epub 2010 Mar 1.
27. Chowdhury AH, Cox EF, Francis ST, Lobo DN. A randomized, controlled, double-blind crossover study on the effects of 1-L infusions of 6% hydroxyethyl starch suspended in 0.9% saline (voluven) and a balanced solution (Plasma Volume Redibag) on blood volume, renal blood flow velocity, and renal corti. Ann Surg. 2014;259(5):881–7. https://doi.org/10.1097/SLA.0000000000000324.
28. Krajewski ML, Raghunathan K, Paluszkiewicz SM, Schermer CR, Shaw AD. Meta-analysis of high- versus low-chloride content in perioperative and critical care fluid resuscitation. Br J Surg. 2015;102(1):24–36. https://doi.org/10.1002/bjs.9651; Epub 2014 Oct 30.
29. Yunos NM, Bellomo R, Hegarty C, Story D, Ho L, Bailey M. Association between a chloride-liberal vs chloride-restrictive intravenous fluid administration strategy and kidney injury in critically ill adults. JAMA. 2012;308(15):1566–72. https://doi.org/10.1001/jama.2012.13356.
30. Young P, Bailey M, Beasley R, Henderson S, Mackle D, McArthur C, McGuinness S, Mehrtens J, Myburgh J, Psirides A, Reddy S, Bellomo R, SPLIT Investigators; ANZICS CTG. Effect of a buffered crystalloid solution vs saline on acute kidney injury

among patients in the intensive care unit: the SPLIT randomized clinical trial. JAMA. 2015;314(16):1701–10. https://doi.org/10.1001/jama.2015.12334.
31. Antonucci F, Calo L, Rizzolo M, Cantaro S, Bertolissi M, Travaglini M, Geatti O, Borsatti A, D'Angelo A. Nifedipine can preserve renal function in patients undergoing aortic surgery with infrarenal crossclamping. Nephron. 1996;74(4):668–73.
32. Bergman AS, Odar-Cederlöf I, Westman L. Renal and hemodynamic effects of diltiazem after elective major vascular surgery—a potential renoprotective agent? Ren Fail. 1995;17(2):155–63.
33. Colson P, Ribstein J, Séguin JR, Marty-Ane C, Roquefeuil B. Mechanisms of renal hemodynamic impairment during infrarenal aortic cross-clamping. Anesth Analg. 1992;75(1):18–23.
34. Tumlin JA, Finkel KW, Murray PT, Samuels J, Cotsonis G, Shaw AD. Fenoldopam mesylate in early acute tubular necrosis: a randomized, double-blind, placebo-controlled clinical trial. Am J Kidney Dis. 2005;46(1):26–34.
35. Zangrillo A, Biondi-Zoccai GG, Frati E, Covello RD, Cabrini L, Guarracino F, Ruggeri L, Bove T, Bignami E, Landoni G. Fenoldopam and acute renal failure in cardiac surgery: a meta-analysis of randomized placebo-controlled trials. J Cardiothorac Vasc Anesth. 2012;26(3):407–13. https://doi.org/10.1053/j.jvca.2012.01.038; Epub Mar 28.
36. Landoni G, Biondi-Zoccai GG, Marino G, Bove T, Fochi O, Maj G, Calabrò MG, Sheiban I, Tumlin JA, Ranucci M, Zangrillo A. Fenoldopam reduces the need for renal replacement therapy and in-hospital death in cardiovascular surgery: a meta-analysis. J Cardiothorac Vasc Anesth. 2008;22(1):7–33. https://doi.org/10.1053/j.jvca.2007.07.015; Epub Nov 7.
37. Bove T, Zangrillo A, Guarracino F, Alvaro G, Persi B, Maglioni E, Galdieri N, Comis M, Caramelli F, Pasero DC, Pala G, Renzini M, Conte M, Paternoster G, Martinez B, Pinelli F, Frontini M, Zucchetti MC, Pappalardo F, Amantea B. Effect of fenoldopam on use of renal replacement therapy among patients with acute kidney injury after cardiac surgery: a randomized clinical trial. JAMA. 2014;312(21):2244–53. https://doi.org/10.1001/jama.2014.13573.
38. Lauschke A, Teichgräber UK, Frei U, Eckardt KU. 'Low-dose' dopamine worsens renal perfusion in patients with acute renal failure. Kidney Int. 2006;69(9):1669–74.
39. Pass LJ, Eberhart RC, Brown JC, Rohn GN, Estrera AS. The effect of mannitol and dopamine on the renal response to thoracic aortic cross-clamping. J Thorac Cardiovasc Surg. 1988;95(4):608–12.
40. Lassnigg A, Donner E, Grubhofer G, Presterl E, Druml W, Hiesmayr M. Lack of renoprotective effects of dopamine and furosemide during cardiac surgery. J Am Soc Nephrol. 2000;11(1):v97–104.
41. Bailey M, McGuinness S, Haase M, Haase-Fielitz A, Parke R, Hodgson CL, Forbes A, Bagshaw SM, Bellomo R. Sodium bicarbonate and renal function after cardiac surgery: a prospectively planned individual patient meta-analysis. Anesthesiology. 2015;122(2):294–306. https://doi.org/10.1097/ALN.0000000000000547.
42. Schiffl H. Prevention of acute kidney injury by intravenous sodium bicarbonate: the end of a saga. Crit Care. 2014;18(6):672. https://doi.org/10.1186/s13054-014-0672-0.
43. McGuinness SP, Parke RL, Bellomo R, Van Haren FM, Bailey M. Sodium bicarbonate infusion to reduce cardiac surgery-associated acute kidney injury: a phase II multicenter double-blind randomized controlled trial. Crit Care Med. 2013;41(7):1599–607. https://doi.org/10.1097/CCM.0b013e31828a3f99.
44. Nigwekar SU, Kandula P, Hix JK, Thakar CV. Off-pump coronary artery bypass surgery and acute kidney injury: a meta-analysis of randomized and observational studies. Am J Kidney Dis. 2009;54(3):413–23. https://doi.org/10.1053/j.ajkd.2009.01.267; Epub May 5.
45. Seabra VF, Alobaidi S, Balk EM, Poon AH, Jaber BL. Off-pump coronary artery bypass surgery and acute kidney injury: a meta-analysis of randomized controlled trials. Clin J Am Soc Nephrol. 2010;5(10):1734–44. https://doi.org/10.2215/CJN.02800310; Epub 2010 Jul 29.
46. Kamperidis V, van Rosendael PJ, de Weger A, Katsanos S, Regeer M, van der Kley F, Mertens B, Sianos G, Ajmone Marsan N, Bax JJ, Delgado V. Surgical sutureless and transcatheter aortic valves: hemodynamic performance and clinical outcomes in propensity score-matched high-risk populations with severe aortic stenosis. JACC Cardiovasc Interv. 2015;8(5):670–7. https://doi.org/10.1016/j.jcin.2014.10.029.
47. Lindman BR, Goldstein JS, Nassif ME, Zajarias A, Novak E, Tibrewala A, Vatterott AM, Lawler C, Damiano RJ, Moon MR, Lawton JS, Lasala JM, Maniar HS. Systemic inflammatory response syndrome after transcatheter or surgical aortic valve replacement. Heart. 2015;101(7):537–45. https://doi.org/10.1136/heartjnl-2014-307057; Epub 2015 Jan 20.
48. Khwaja A. KDIGO clinical practice guidelines for acute kidney injury. Nephron Clin Pract. 2012;120:c79–84.
49. Bellomo R, Ronco C, Kellum JA, Mehta RL, Palevsky P, Acute Dialysis Quality Initiative workgroup. Acute renal failure—definition, outcome measures, animal models, fluid therapy and information technology needs: the Second International Consensus Conference of the Acute Dialysis Quality Initiative (ADQI) Group. Crit Care. 2004;8(4):R204–12; Epub 2004 May 24.
50. Lombardi R, Ferreiro A, Servetto C. Renal function after cardiac surgery: adverse effect of furosemide. Ren Fail. 2003;25:775–86.
51. Fiaccadori E, Lombardi M, Leonardi S, et al. Prevalence and clinical outcome associated with preexisting malnutrition in acute renal failure: a prospective cohort study. J Am Soc Nephrol. 1999;10:581–93.
52. Palevsky PM, Murray PT. Acute kidney injury and critical care nephrology. NephSAP. 2006;5(2):72–120.

Rare and Overlooked Causes of Acute Kidney Injury

13

José A. Morfín and Shruti Gupta

13.1 Introduction

While prerenal acute kidney injury (AKI) and acute tubular injury remain the most common causes of AKI in the community and hospital setting, respectively, there is increasing recognition of more subtle and rare causes of AKI. In this chapter, we describe some of the rarer etiologies of AKI. We discuss cholemic nephropathy, which is seen in the setting of cirrhosis or acute liver failure and may be difficult to distinguish from acute tubular injury and hepatorenal syndrome. We describe anticoagulation-related nephropathy, in which patients who are taking warfarin or other novel oral anticoagulants develop obstructing tubular red cell casts leading to AKI. Oxalate nephropathy is another rare cause of AKI that is increasingly being recognized in those with high dietary intake of oxalate, post-gastric bypass, or in the setting of short gut syndrome. There are several drugs that can trigger drug-related crystalluria, whereby precipitation of intratubular drug crystals leads to AKI and oliguria. Methotrexate and acyclovir are well-known causes of drug-related crystalluria, but antibiotics like ciprofloxacin and possibly even vancomycin may be offenders as well. Abdominal compartment syndrome occurs when intra-abdominal pressures rise, often in the setting of trauma, hemorrhage, or gut edema; this condition is often lethal if not diagnosed in a timely fashion. Patients with a significant burden of atherosclerotic disease are at high risk of cholesterol embolization, particularly in the setting of angiography. This condition is sometimes misdiagnosed as contrast-induced nephropathy, but its course and clinical presentation are markedly different. Finally, numerous street drugs, like cocaine, K2, and marijuana, are a growing cause of AKI in the younger population.

One common thread among all of the aforementioned causes of kidney injury is that they often go unrecognized until it is too late. This is the case because these conditions may lack supportive clinical or laboratory findings, and the urine sediment is often nondiagnostic. It is therefore critical to maintain a high index of suspicion for all of these rarer causes of AKI, so that they can be diagnosed and managed in a timely fashion.

J. A. Morfín (✉)
Division of Nephrology, Department of Internal Medicine, University of California Davis School of Medicine, Sacramento, CA, USA
e-mail: jmorfin@ucdavis.edu

S. Gupta
Division of Renal Medicine, Department of Medicine, Brigham and Women's Hospital, Boston, MA, USA
e-mail: sgupta21@bwh.harvard.edu

S. S. Waikar et al. (eds.), *Core Concepts in Acute Kidney Injury*,
https://doi.org/10.1007/978-1-4939-8628-6_13

13.2 Bile Acid Nephropathy

Bile acid nephropathy was first described in the 1920s as cholemic nephrosis by Haessler, given the association of severe jaundice with acute kidney injury; however, until recently, this entity has been largely under-recognized in the literature for many decades [1]. Furthermore, the underlying mechanisms are not totally clear, and there are no accepted diagnostic criteria for cholemic nephrosis. It is therefore important to review and understand the clinical features of bile acid nephropathy given the incidence of hyperbilirubinemia in many disease states, while also bearing in mind that there are often many other contributors to AKI in the setting of liver failure.

Bile acids are steroid acids with different molecular forms that are synthesized in the liver. They are conjugated with taurine or glycine in the liver, thereby forming toxic and carcinogenic bile salts. Hyperbilirubinemia can occur in the setting of a number of clinical conditions such as cirrhosis, cholestatic or obstructive jaundice, acute hepatic jaundice with severe acute liver damage, and hemolytic anemia. In both animal models and human subjects, biliary salts have been shown to induce tubular injury, particularly in the proximal tubule; the ensuing Fanconi-related tubular effects (glucosuria, phosphaturia, uricosuria, and tubular proteinuria) are reversible with normalization of bilirubin levels [2, 3]. Van Slambrouck et al. performed a clinicopathologic study of 44 patients with severe liver injury and identified the precipitation of biliary casts in the distal tubules, with the majority of the cases associated with higher total and direct bilirubin concentrations [4]. It has been hypothesized that in low albumin states, bile acids are preferentially unbound, thereby allowing them to be filtered by the glomerulus with subsequent increased tubular exposure. Furthermore, the increased and prolonged exposure of bilirubin in the tubules can lead to precipitation of biliary casts more distally in the nephron [4].

The clinical identification of bile acid nephropathy can be challenging, since hyperbilirubinemia is commonly associated with hepatorenal syndrome (HRS) and its associated hemodynamic permutations of a low effective circulatory volume state and kidney hypoperfusion. However, bile salts have been demonstrated to cause direct acute kidney injury in the absence of hypoperfusion and/or hemodynamic changes, further supporting a causal effect on kidney injury [5, 6]. Upon ligating bile ducts, mice develop acute tubular injury within 3 days, followed by progressive interstitial injury and tubulo interstitial fibrosis after a longer period (3–8 weeks) [7]. To this end, there have been several case reports of acute kidney injury in the setting of severe cholestatic jaundice in young men using anabolic steroids, in the absence of hemodynamic instability [8]. In each of these cases, the pathognomonic histologic findings of bile casts on kidney biopsy were observed, as well as a modest improvement in kidney function with restoration of normal bilirubin levels [4, 9].

The clinical features associated with bile acid nephropathy include oliguria, bilirubin levels greater than 20 mg/dL, hypoalbuminemia, and acidosis in the setting of acute kidney injury [4, 8]. Urinalysis often lacks significant proteinuria or hematuria, though direct urine microscopy may reveal coarse pigmented granular casts and heavily pigmented renal tubular epithelial cell casts (see Fig. 13.1a) [4]. A kidney biopsy may be indicated if the clinical suspicion remains high and other etiologies are being entertained. Kidney histology of bile acid nephropathy may reveal a tubular epithelium showing cytoplasmic vacuolization with pigmented protein reabsorption droplets [4] (see Fig. 13.1b). In addition, bile casts within the distal tubular show a luminal "myeloma-like" process that leads to tubular obstruction (see Fig. 13.1c). This obstructive tubular process may further delay recovery of kidney function, even after improvement in bilirubin levels. The clinical management is geared toward supportive measures. Therapies like steroids, cholestyramine, ursodeoxycholic acid, and lactulose have shown to have minimal effect [10]. Nevertheless, the recognition of bile acid nephropathy may be helpful in deciding on candidacy for dual liver-kidney transplantation versus liver transplantation alone.

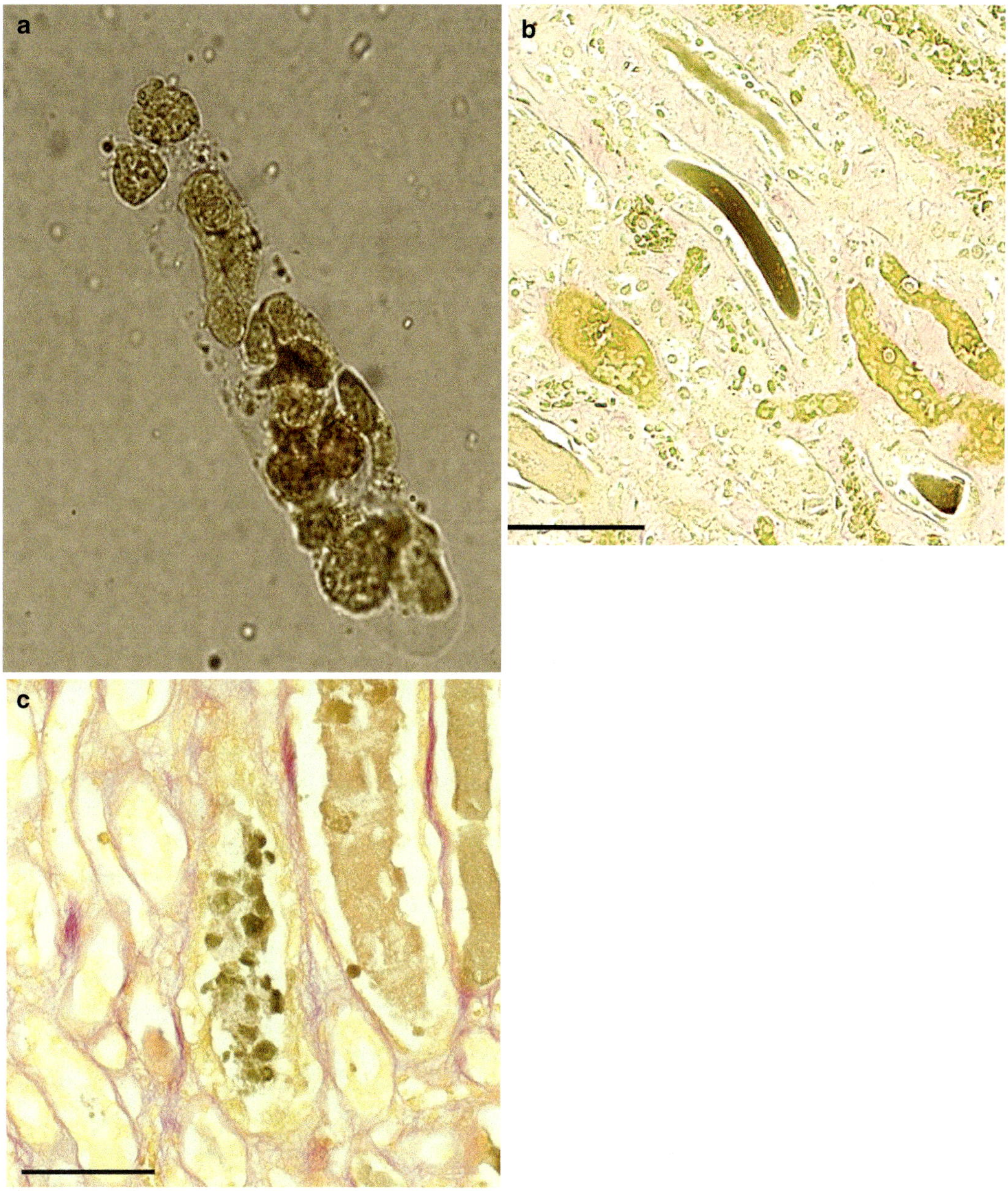

Fig. 13.1 Bile nephropathy. (**a**) Urine sediment (heavily pigmented renal tubular epithelial cell cast, original magnification, ×40). From: Luciano RL, Castano E, Moeckel G, Perazella MA. Bile acid nephropathy in a bodybuilder abusing an anabolic androgenic steroid. Am J Kidney Dis. 2014 Sep;64(3):473–6. doi: 10.1053/j.ajkd.2014.05.010. Epub 2014 Jun 18; used with permission. (**b**) Hall stain confirms the presence of bilirubin in several tubular casts. (**c**) Pigmented sloughed tubular epithelial cells can also be identified (Hall stain). From: van Slambrouck CM, Salem F, Meehan SM, Chang A. Bile cast nephropathy is a common pathologic finding for kidney injury associated with severe liver dysfunction. *Kidney Int*. 2013;84(1):192–197; used with permission

13.3 Anticoagulation-Related Nephropathy

Warfarin, a vitamin K antagonist, has been used as an anticoagulant for many clinical indications, ranging from atrial fibrillation to hypercoagulable states. Furthermore, warfarin has been increasingly substituted with novel non-vitamin K oral anticoagulants (NOAC) such as direct thrombin inhibitors and factor Xa inhibitors; as a result, the term anticoagulation-related nephropathy (ARN) has been used in the literature to include a broader range of anticoagulants and their associated effects on the kidney [11]. ARN can be overlooked since anticoagulation is often administered in patients with extensive comorbid conditions, many of whom have other reasons to have AKI.

Warfarin-induced nephropathy was first described by Brodsky as a type of acute kidney injury occurring within 1 week of a supratherapeutic international normalized ratio (INR), with or without the evidence of hemorrhage [12]. Typically, this process is observed within the first 8 weeks after initiating anticoagulation. On pathology, there may be histological evidence of disruption of the glomerular filtration barrier and an association with obstructing tubular red blood cell casts (see Fig. 13.2a, b) [12, 13]. The pathogenesis remains unclear, as molecular mechanisms have yet to be defined. However, given the histologic findings, it is hypothesized that disruption of the glomerular filtration barrier leads to hemorrhage into the Bowman's space and renal tubules. As a result, red blood cell casts form in the renal tubules, causing obstruction, ischemia, and eventual obliteration [12, 13].

At the molecular level, thrombin, which is a vitamin K-dependent coagulation factor, activates signaling proteinase-activated receptors (PARs) that are expressed in endothelial cells [14]. Thrombin has been postulated to be the common link between vitamin K antagonists and direct thrombin inhibitors in ARN, as decreased thrombin activity leads to breakdown of the endothelial barrier through the depletion of PARs, thereby leading to glomerular hemorrhage [14]. To further support this hypothesis as a "proof in concept," the administration of PAR antagonists to animal models with chronic kidney disease reproduces the ARN, while administration of vitamin K attenuates it [14, 15].

The risk of ARN appears to be heightened at an INR >3.0, and it is associated with comorbidities such as older age, diabetes mellitus, hypertension, and cardiovascular disease [13]. Patients may present with or without overt hemorrhage

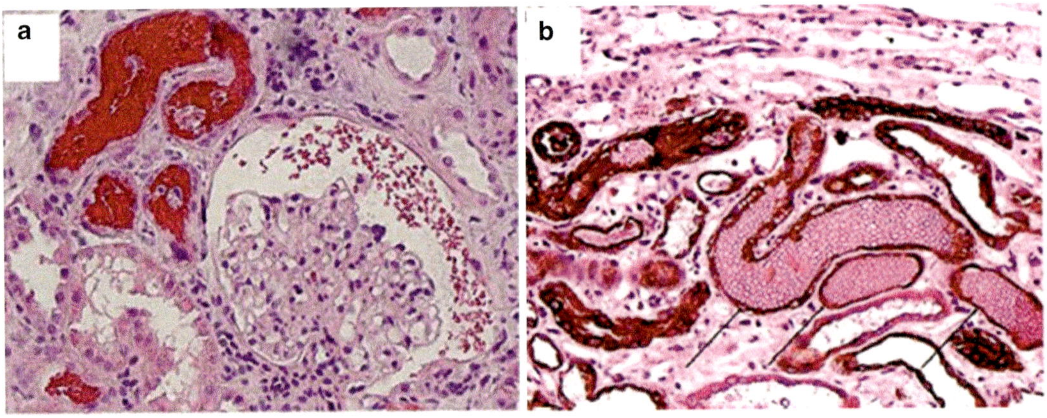

Fig. 13.2 Anticoagulation nephropathy. (**a**) Numerous RBCs and RBC occlusive casts were noticed in tubules and Bowman space (hematoxylin and eosin stain; original magnification ×200). (**b**) Immunohistochemical stain for cytokeratin AE1/AE3 (arrows, dark brown) highlights distal tubules with occlusive RBC casts (counterstain with hematoxylin/eosin; original magnification ×200). From: Brodsky SV, Satoskar A, Chen J, et al. Acute Kidney Injury During Warfarin Therapy Associated With Obstructive Tubular Red Blood Cell Casts: A Report of 9 Cases. *Am J Kidney Dis*. 2009;54(6):1121–1126; used with permission

but often manifest with a rise in serum creatinine even several weeks out from having supra-therapeutic levels of anticoagulation [13, 15]. In one data registry analysis, there appears to be a higher mortality risk with ARN, with approximately one third of patients with CKD and ARN dying within 1 month after the onset of this condition [13]. Clinical management is therefore geared toward timely adjustment of the anticoagulant dose to the proper target range, especially in patients with CKD, who are at highest risk for ARN. In the setting of hemorrhage, immediate reversal is necessary to limit toxicity and renal tubular obstruction. A high index of suspicion should be maintained in conditions of unexplained AKI in the setting of CKD with concomitant anticoagulation usage, especially if there is clinical evidence of persistent supra-therapeutic levels. A kidney biopsy may be necessary to make diagnosis; however, this is often deferred due to the bleeding risk, and a presumptive diagnosis is made on clinical grounds. Lastly, in cases of AKI thought to be secondary to novel non-vitamin K oral anticoagulants (NOAC) such as direct thrombin inhibitors (including, but not limited to dabigatran), hemodialysis has been shown to improve NOAC drug elimination [16, 17]. Prognosis is variable, with most patients experiencing stabilization or improvement of renal function; however, in Brodsky's study of nine patients, six did not recover from their AKI [13].

13.4 Acute Oxalate Nephropathy

Hyperoxalosis is defined by an excess of systemic oxalate and can lead to significant kidney injury. It can occur through both primary and secondary processes. Primary hyperoxaluria represents a group of genetic disorders characterized by inborn errors of glyoxylate metabolism, resulting in high oxalate levels [18]. Secondary oxalosis encompasses a broader range of etiologies which are usually classified into four major categories: increased dietary oxalate, increased oxalate absorption and metabolism, decreased oxalate elimination, and vitamin deficiencies [19]. Due to its heterogeneity and lack of obvious clinical and laboratory findings, acute oxalate nephropathy may be overlooked in the clinical evaluation of acute kidney injury.

Under normal physiologic conditions, oxalate is derived from glyoxylate, ascorbic acid and dietary intake. Anywhere from 2 to 20% of oxalate is absorbed in the gastrointestinal tract, with the colon believed to be the major site of absorption [8]. When present at high concentrations, oxalate can form a variety of salts, including calcium oxalate, which is insoluble in the urine and leads to direct tubular injury with crystallization in the tubules [20, 21]. Oxalate is found in large quantities in many plants, such as beets, spinach, black tea, and rhubarb. The average oxalate intake in an American diet, estimated to be 150–500 mg/day, is threefold higher than the recommended daily allowance by the Academy of Nutrition and Dietetics [21]. High intake can lead to systemic effects, accumulation of oxalate in the urine, and nephrolithiasis. There have been several case reports of acute kidney injury from starfruit [21] and black tea [22] as a result of up to a tenfold increase of daily oxalate intake.

Enteric hyperoxalosis occurs secondary to malabsorptive states and can be associated with a variety of conditions, including small intestinal resection, use of orlistat [23], short gut post gastric bypass surgery [24], and/or chronic pancreatitis [25]. The pathophysiology is related to the inability of the small intestine to absorb fatty acids, which results in increased calcium saponification and subsequent decreased availability of calcium in the intestine [24]. The decrease in free intestinal calcium leads to higher levels of unbound oxalate in the colon, which is readily absorbed and then filtered and excreted by the kidneys. In addition, the active metabolism of ethylene glycol and high doses of vitamin C can also increase systemic oxalate levels [21]. To this end, impairment of GFR due to pre-existing CKD or an acute decrement in GFR will further increase circulating oxalate accumulation.

The clinical evaluation should include a detailed dietary and medical history. The urinalysis may reveal hematuria or small amounts of proteinuria (<500 mg/day) in cases of nephrolithiasis; however, often the urine is unrevealing.

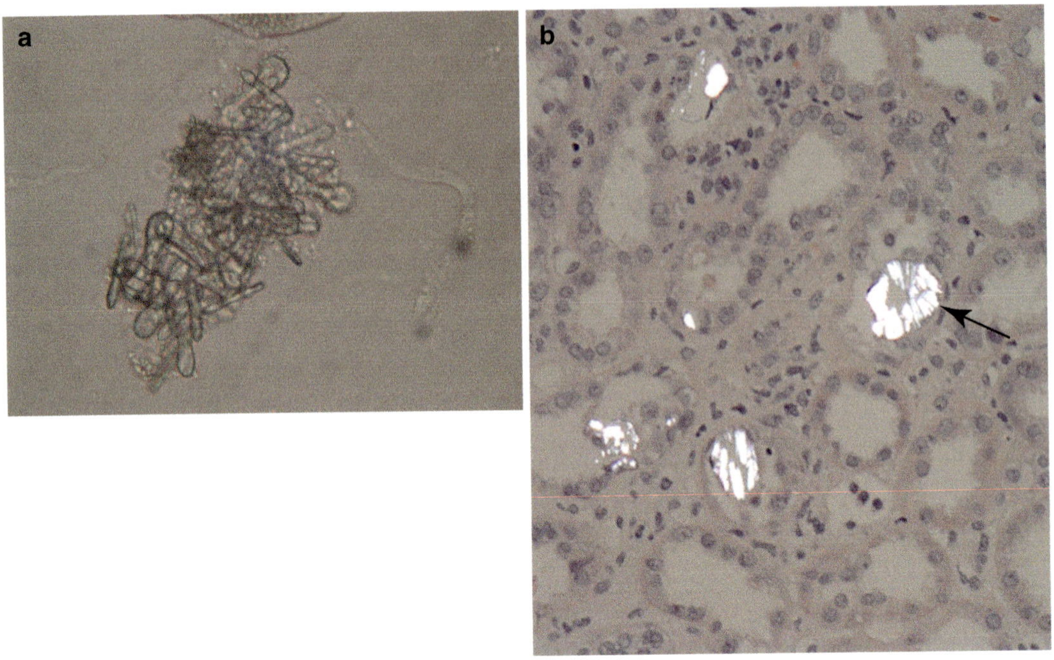

Fig. 13.3 Acute oxalosis. (**a**) Urine microscopy. Calcium oxalate monohydrate crystals (dumbbell, hairpin, hexagonal shapes) in clumps in a patient with ethylene glycol ingestion (original picture). (**b**) Kidney biopsy, light microscopy (H&E stain in a patient with chronic pancreatitis reveals acute tubular necrosis, along with intratubular calcium oxalate deposition, which shows positive birefringence under polarized light)

Direct urine microscopy in the setting of acute kidney injury may reveal calcium oxalate crystals, which come in two forms: envelope-shaped calcium oxalate dihydrate crystals and the more commonly visualized calcium oxalate monohydrate crystals. The latter tend to appear more heterogeneous and may take dumbbell, hairpin, and hexagonal shapes (see Fig. 13.3a). A 24-h urine collection in steady state for unexplained and asymptomatic kidney injury may be helpful to measure for excess excretion of calcium and oxalate. If this initial evaluation fails to reveal a diagnosis and there remains a high index of suspicion for acute oxalate nephropathy, a kidney biopsy may be appropriate to further clarify the diagnosis. The pathognomonic histologic finding is acute tubular necrosis with intratubular, birefringent calcium oxalate crystals (see Fig. 13.3b).

Management of hyperoxaluria is generally supportive once the underlying cause has been identified. In the case of idiopathic and enteric hyperoxaluria, patients should adhere to a low oxalate diet. In cases of persistent enteric hyperoxalosis, management includes the use of binding therapy to lower intestinal absorption of oxalate, high fluid intake (>1.5 L/m^2/day), and calcium citrate supplementation. Intestinal recolonization with oxalate-degrading bacteria such as *Oxalobacter formigenes* has been trialed with some success [25, 26].

13.5 Drug-Related Crystalluria

Drug-related crystalluria is a process triggered by the administration of a number of different drugs, many of which have been implicated in causing acute kidney injury (AKI) [27]. These medications are typically administered intravenously at high doses in order to achieve high plasma concentrations. In addition, the AKI risk is elevated in hypovolemic states, and in the setting of a depressed glomerular filtration rate, and poor metabolite solubility profile [28]. Characteristically, this condition leads to precipitation of intratubular drug crystals, leading to AKI and oliguria [27, 28]. Patients are generally asymptomatic, and kidney injury is detected typically on the basis of a chemistry panel. Occasionally, patients may present with renal colic symptoms within 1–7 days after initiation of the offending drug [28]. It is important to identify and understand the key features of those drugs which are most likely to cause crystal-induced acute kidney injury. Early recognition by clinical history and manual urine microscopy may facilitate timely treatment and important dose adjustments, thereby mitigating the risk of acute kidney injury. The following is a compilation of the "usual offenders," listed by drug class, describing their clinical indications and pharmacologic and crystallization profiles.

Acyclovir is an antiviral drug that is typically used to treat herpes, and renal excretion accounts for 60–90% of its elimination [27]. Urine microscopy will reveal classic needle-shaped crystals which are birefringent under polarized light [29] (see Fig. 13.4a). When administered intravenously, empiric isotonic fluids should be given to increase urine volume and reduce the risk of drug crystal precipitation. In addition, both dose adjustment for GFR and prolonging the infusion rate up to 2 hours have been shown to reduce the risk of AKI [30]. Hemodialysis has been used to in cases of acyclovir-induced neurotoxicity since the drug is dialyzable; however, there is no clear role for dialysis in the setting of AKI, since it has not been shown to reverse or limit duration of injury [31].

Sulfonamides are one of the oldest and most commonly used classes of antibiotics. They contain a sulfonamide group, such as sulfamethoxazole or sulfadiazine. Both sulfamethoxazole and sulfadiazine are relatively insoluble in acidic urine, especially when used in high doses to treat infections like *Pneumocystis jiroveci* and toxoplasmosis [32]. In addition, it has been reported that close to one third of patients treated with sulfadiazine are at risk of developing AKI [31, 33]. The risk of crystal precipitation is dose-related and is typically seen with sulfadiazine 4–6 g/day and sulfamethoxazole 50–100 mg/kg/day [33]. Urine microscopy may reveal crystals that resemble a "shock of wheat" (see Fig. 13.4b). Treatment is aimed at urinary alkalinization to a pH >7.15, which increases sulfadiazine solubility by more than 20-fold [33, 34]. Intravenous isotonic bicarbonate solution should be given prophylactically when using high doses of sulfonamides, with close monitoring for signs of fluid overload and/or systemic metabolic alkalosis. Hemodialysis has no utility in sulfonamide removal and hence is only indicated for fluid and solute management in AKI.

Ciprofloxacin is a fluoroquinolone antibiotic commonly used for the treatment of gram-negative bacterial infections. It has been implicated in cases of acute interstitial nephritis, but its role in causing crystalluria has not been readily recognized [35]. Case reports have described ciprofloxacin-induced crystalluria in the elderly, presumably because this represents a high risk group due to demographic features and lower GFR [35–37]. Concurrent use of ACE inhibitors and/or diuretics will increase the risk of AKI [38]. Urine microscopy may reveal needle-shaped birefringent crystals in round conglomerates [35], though they can assume many shapes. The crystals are composed of a ciprofloxacin salt with a lamellar structure (see Fig. 13.4c) [36, 39]. They typically precipitate in the setting of an alkaline pH; it is therefore critical that patients maintain euvolemia, and alkalinization of the urine is avoided.

Methotrexate is the most commonly drug used for the treatment of rheumatoid arthritis, and approximately 90% is excreted in the urine [40]. High doses of methotrexate can precipitate in the tubules and cause direct tubular injury [40, 41]. The resulting crystals often form clumps, and they appear as numerous brownish and gold crystals under direct urine microscopy (see Fig. 13.4d). Like sulfonamides, the risk of methotrexate-induced nephrotoxicity is increased in acidic urine due to the drug's insolubility, as well as in the setting of volume depletion, since this increases methotrexate levels in the tubular fluid [40]. The risk of methotrexate nephrotoxicity is also higher when there is sustained elevation in its plasma concentration; leucovorin, a reduced form of folic acid, can be effective as a "chemoprotectant" [41]. More recently, glucarpidase has been used when the plasma level exceeds

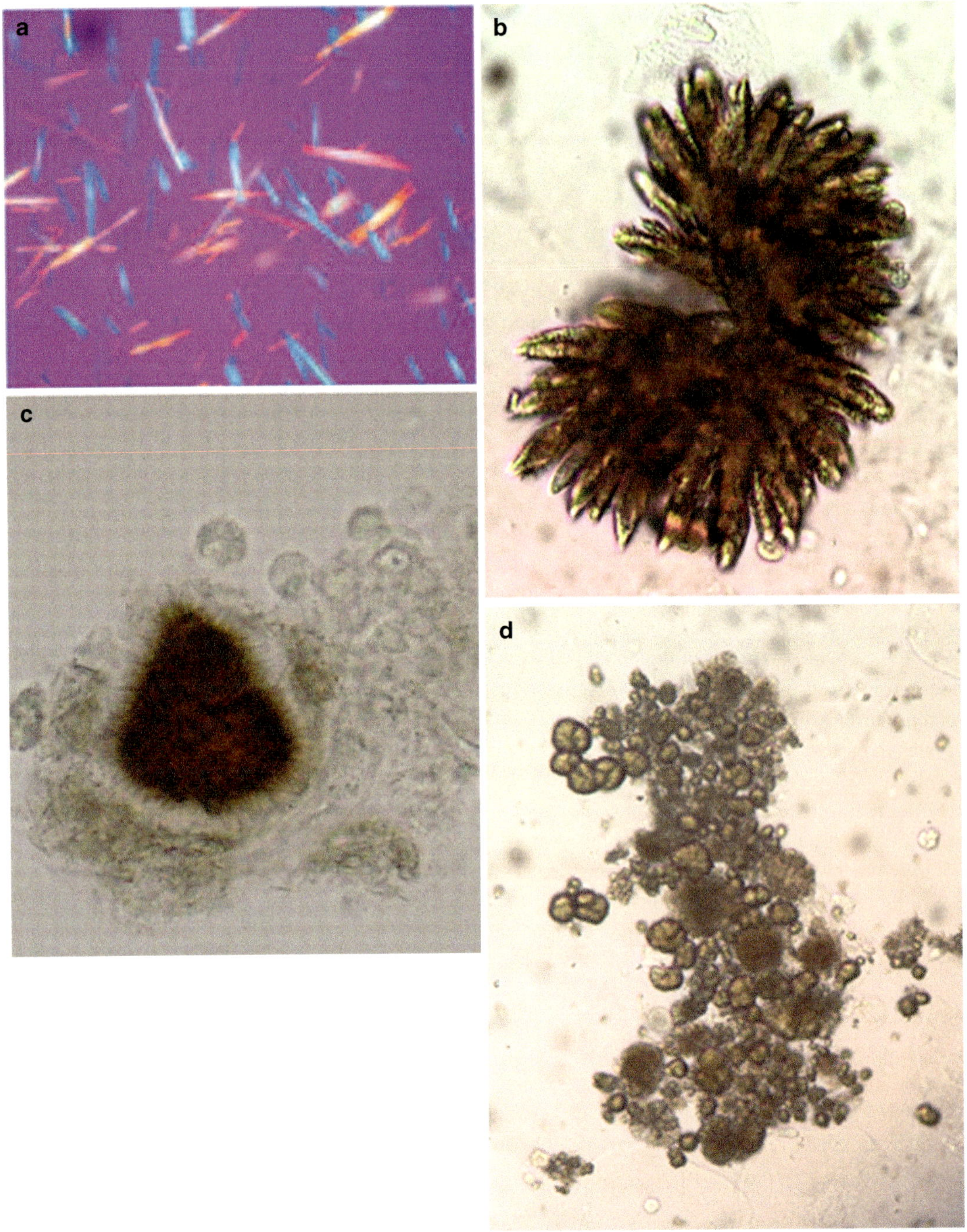

Fig. 13.4 Drug crystalluria. (**a**) Acyclovir, with multiple needles crystals which show positive birefringence under polarized light. From: Roberts D, Myles W, Smith B, et al. Acute kidney injury due to crystalluria following acute valacyclovir overdose. *Kidney Int*. 2011;79:574; used with permission. (**b**) Sulfamethazole crystals in a "shock of wheat" appearance. From: Gorlitsky BR, Perazella MA. Shocking urine. Kidney International (2015) 87, 865; doi:10.1038/ki.2014.317 used with permission. (**c**) Ciprofloxacin, needle-shaped birefringent crystals in round conglomerates in renal epithelial cells. From: Sedlacek M, Suriawinata A, Schoolwerth A, et al. Ciprofloxacin crystal nephropathy—a "new" cause of acute renal failure. *Nephrol Dial Transpl*. 2006;21:2339; used with permission. (**d**) Numerous clumps of brownish/gold methotrexate crystals. From: Pazhayattil GS. A case of crystalline nephropathy, Kidney International (2015) 87(6):1265–66; used with permission

1 mmol/L, as it rapidly metabolizes methotrexate to inactive metabolites. Lastly, hemodialysis does not play a major role in the management of methotrexate-induced AKI or crystalluria, since methotrexate is largely protein bound and has a large volume of distribution [42, 43].

With the widespread use of vancomycin for the treatment of resistant strains of *Staphylococcus aureus*, there are increasing reports of vancomycin-induced nephrotoxicity. There is controversy regarding the nature and extent of vancomycin's nephrotoxicity due to confounding factors, such as hypovolemia and coadministration of aminoglycosides. However, evidence suggest that vancomycin treatment is associated with a 2.45 relative risk of AKI, though the strength of evidence is moderate according to one meta-analysis [44]. Total vancomycin doses >4 g and high troughs have been associated with nephrotoxicity [45]. The mechanism of nephrotoxicity is due to free radical-mediated injury, though most biopsies performed in cases of vancomycin-associated AKI demonstrate acute interstitial nephritis rather than tubular injury [46, 47]. AKI due to crystal-induced injury has also been posited as one form of vancomycin nephrotoxicity; a recent study suggests that the mechanism may be related to obstructive tubular casts composed of nanospheric vancomycin and uromodulin aggregates [48]. Regardless of the mechanism of injury, management is usually supportive and involves drug discontinuation and the institution of renal replacement therapy if needed.

13.6 Abdominal Compartment Syndrome

Abdominal compartment syndrome is a serious yet often under-recognized condition that is associated with a wide array of clinical conditions. According to consensus definitions by the World Society of the Abdominal Compartment Syndrome, intra-abdominal pressure (IAP) is the steady-state pressure within the abdominal cavity, with an IAP of 5–7 mmHg considered normal in critically ill patients [49]. Intra-abdominal hypertension (IAH) is defined by a sustained elevation in IAP greater than or equal to 12 mmHg. Abdominal compartment syndrome (ACS) is usually characterized by a sustained IAP greater than 20 mmHg, though the defining feature is new-onset organ failure. IAH and ACS share the same underlying pathophysiology and represent two points along a continuum. It is critical to identify primary and secondary processes that may be contributing to IAH in order to prevent progression to ACS, as this condition can cause splanchnic ischemia, oliguric acute kidney injury, and even death.

ACS used to be seen predominantly in the setting of blunt trauma but has since been identified with many surgical and medical conditions, including intra-abdominal hemorrhage, intestinal obstruction, pancreatitis, and gut edema. Patients who requires large-volume fluid resuscitation can develop bowel distension and ascites, both of which can increase intra-abdominal pressure [50]. In a prospective study of 40 patients who developed septic shock and received more than 5 L of fluid resuscitation, 83% developed IAH and 25% developed ACS [51]. Burn patients may also be at particularly high risk of intra-abdominal hypertension and abdominal compartment syndrome compared to other groups of critically ill patients, with the percentage of total body surface area affected by burns correlating with mean IAP [52].

Regardless of the etiology, the underlying pathophysiology is the same. Increased IAP compromises venous return, cardiac output, and systemic oxygen delivery [53]. Furthermore, there is decreased diaphragmatic movement secondary to visceral edema, which leads to increased intrathoracic pressure and reduced venous return. Due to the absence of valves, the increased pressure is transmitted to the inferior vena cava, along with the hepatic and renal vein. Decreased venous return leads to arterial hypotension and tissue ischemia, with loss of capillary and membrane integrity. ACS ultimately leads to multi-organ dysfunction, and once this occurs, almost all patients have evidence of kidney injury [54].

The renal effects of increased IAP were first reported in 1876, when Wendt reported the association of oliguria with intra-abdominal pressure

[55]. Subsequently, Bradley and Bradley conducted a study in which they directly measured renal vein pressure and IVC pressure as a surrogate marker of IAP [56].As IAP was raised by external compression, renal plasma flow dropped, as did average glomerular filtration rate. All patients ultimately became oliguric. Studies have since shown that attempts to reverse decreased cardiac output with volume does not improve renal function [57]. Acute kidney injury secondary to ACS is likely driven in part by elevation in renal vein and intraparenchymal pressures [58]. However, there are likely other factors contributing to AKI, including renal artery vasoconstriction due to activation of the sympathetic nervous system and the renin-angiotensin axis, as well as the release of inflammatory cytokines.

In those at high risk of developing ACS, it is crucial to monitor serial bladder pressures using an indwelling Foley catheter, as physical examination is unreliable in making the diagnosis. In studies of blunt trauma victims, physical examination was only 56% sensitive, with a positive predictive value of 35% [59]. Bladder pressures remain the gold standard and should be monitored while the patient is supine, using an instillation of 25 mL of saline. While bladder pressures are accurate, it is important to bear in mind that patients with chronic ascites and those on peritoneal dialysis may have chronically elevated bladder pressures. Furthermore, those with neurogenic bladder and pelvic fractures and hematomas may not have accurate measurements because checking bladder pressures requires free movement of the bladder wall [60].

IAH leading to ACS can be lethal if it is not recognized quickly, with estimates of mortality ranging from 40 to 100% [61]. Definitive treatment for ACS is surgical decompression via laparotomy, though there is limited data on outcomes post-decompression. In one prospective cohort study of 33 patients who underwent decompressive laparotomy, 28-day mortality was 36% [62]. Non-survivors tended to be older and had greater dependence on mechanical ventilation. Among those with IAH who have not yet progressed to ACS, medical treatment may be an option. For instance, there may be benefit to relieving tense ascites through a therapeutic paracentesis or placing percutaneous drains for abscesses or hematomas [63, 64]. Diuretics may also be trialed to augment urine output and mobilize edema, though oliguria in ACS may be unresponsive to diuretics. The role of renal replacement therapy is not well-elucidated, but may be beneficial for fluid removal and relief of intra-abdominal pressure.

13.7 Atheroembolic Disease

Atheroembolic renal disease (AERD) is a systemic disease that can result in kidney injury due to occlusion of renal arteries, arterioles, and glomerular capillaries with cholesterol plaques. Large arteries like the aorta are the principle source of these atherosclerotic plaques, and because the renal arteries originate from the aorta, they are a prime target of cholesterol embolization. The release of cholesterol plaques can occur spontaneously, or secondary to instrumentation or use of thrombolytic agents. Because atherosclerotic disease can be diffuse and can manifest as carotid disease, peripheral arterial disease, coronary disease, or renovascular disease, identifying the source of atheroembolic plaques may be challenging. It is therefore important to maintain a high index of suspicion for AERD in those with predisposing factors.

The epidemiology of atheroembolic disease is not well-defined, in part because there are limited prospective data on this condition. Retrospective studies suggest that 1–2% of renal biopsies have features of AERD, though the low incidence in these studies may be due to selection bias [65, 66]. In those over 60 years old, the prevalence is closer to 4–6.5% [67]. AERD has been nicknamed the "great masquerader," because the diagnosis can only be confirmed with biopsy, which demonstrates cholesterol crystals in the renal vessels or glomeruli [68]. Because there is often reluctance to biopsy older patients with atherosclerotic disease, the incidence of AERD may be underreported because of the lack of confirmatory biopsies. Furthermore, renal failure is often mistakenly attributed to other conditions such as acute tubular necrosis or radiocontrast nephropathy.

Clinically, the disease can manifest as a sudden decrement in renal function, or it can have a more smoldering course; unlike contrast nephropathy, where recovery begins within 3–5 days, patients with AERD usually manifest with a slowly progressive decline in renal function or incomplete recovery. Predisposing factors for AERD include atherosclerotic disease, advanced age, male gender, Caucasian race, use of anticoagulants or thrombolytics, and recent invasive vascular procedures [69]. Up to 77% of cases of AERD may be iatrogenic, perhaps due to a rise in the number of vascular procedures and anticoagulation [70, 71]. Angiography is the most common iatrogenic cause, with AERD occurring in up to 80% of subjects; guidewires and catheters can scrape vessel walls and disrupt cholesterol plaques [72]. Anticoagulants and thrombolytics are rarely the sole precipitating factors for AERD but can contribute to embolization by dissolving superficial clots that stabilize atherosclerotic plaques.

Cholesterol emboli can affect multiple different organs, mimicking a systemic vasculitis. For instance, patients can present with digital ischemia (Fig. 13.5), cerebral infarction, mesenteric ischemia, and retinal emboli (referred to as Hollenhorst plaques). When Hollenhorst plaques are present, tissue biopsy sampling is not necessary, highlighting the importance of fundoscopy. Skin lesions are the most common extra- renal manifestation, occurring in up to 35% of cases [73]. The classic cutaneous manifestation is *livedo reticularis*, a purple net-like rash that develops principally in the lower extremities but can also occur on the buttocks or abdominal wall (see Fig. 13.5). Laboratory test findings are nondiagnostic and include elevated inflammatory markers, thrombocytopenia, anemia, and hypocomplementemia. Eosinophilia may be transiently seen in up to 80% of patients and is thought to occur due to immunologic activation by the exposed emboli [72, 74].

Urinalysis is often bland and unrevealing; renal biopsy is therefore considered the most definitive means of diagnosing AERD. Classically,

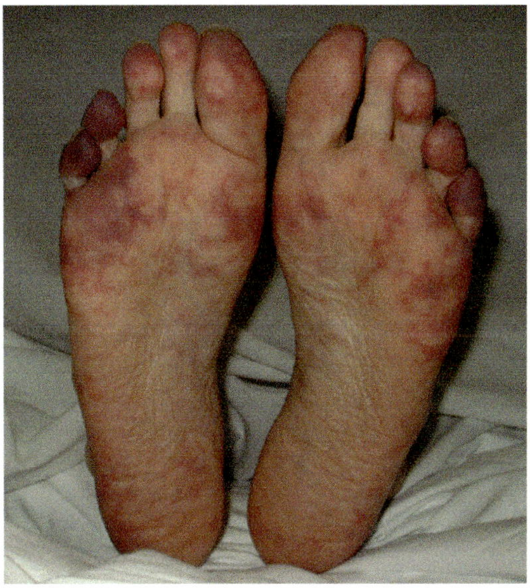

Fig. 13.5 Atheroembolic disease. Digital ischemia, "blue toes" with associated livedo reticular skin changes on the plantar aspect of the feet

histology reveals occlusion of the arcuate and interlobular arteries, as well as the glomerular capillaries with slit-like cholesterol clefts. Cholesterol crystals are dissolved by formalin fixation, leaving biconvex, needle-shaped clefts appearing as "ghosts" in their wake [75, 76]. In the acute phase, red blood cells, fibrin, and inflammatory cells infiltrate and surround the occluded vessels. Chronic lesions are surrounded by perivascular fibrosis and chronic inflammatory cells. Because of ongoing ischemic injury, glomerular sclerosis and interstitial fibrosis may be found in the late stages of the disease.

Because there is no specific therapy for AERD, management consists of mitigating cardiovascular risk factors, preventing recurrent embolization, and reducing the extent of ischemic damage. Hypertension and hyperlipidemia should be managed appropriately. Withdrawal of anticoagulant therapy should be considered after carefully weighing the risks and benefits. Because cholesterol crystal embolization is fundamentally a foreign body reaction to cholesterol crystals, anti-inflammatory agents have been trialed in small case series with variable success. Some studies have shown that steroids may be beneficial in the treatment of AERD [77–79], but a prospective study of 354 patients demonstrated no improvement in renal or patient outcomes with steroid administration [80]. Though there are few outcome studies in patients with AERD, renal prognosis is poor. One prospective study found that 37% of patients of 95 studied needed dialysis, with only 14 patients regaining enough renal function to come off of it [71]. Those patients who had pre-existing CKD and hypertension were more likely to remain dialysis-dependent, while those who were treated with statins were more likely to regain renal function. Further research is greatly needed in order accurately diagnose, prevent, and treat this complex condition.

13.8 Drugs of Abuse and AKI

Drugs of abuse, both illegal and legal, are becoming more of a presence in the United States. While cocaine has been implicated as a cause of kidney injury, there are a number of other drugs that are associated with a variety of nephrotoxic effects. These include synthetic cannabinoids, opioids, anabolic steroids, ecstasy, and bath salts. Some of the deleterious effects of these drugs include alterations in hemodynamics, acute tubular injury, rhabdomyolysis, and glomerular pathology. While the global burden of these drugs is increasing, there is still a dearth of literature on the nephrotoxicity of drugs of abuse, most likely because of underreporting.

Synthetic cannabinoids, marketed under a variety of names including "K2," are widely available, yet their harmful effects are not well-understood. These drugs were originally manufactured for research purposes but have become popular recreational drugs. Often marketed as herbal products, they are readily available, often mistakenly considered safe, and are not detected by routine drug screens. A number of disparate, chemically unrelated compounds fall under the larger umbrella of synthetic cannabinoids and all have one feature in common: they all bind to cannabis receptors. Recently, there have been a surge of case reports and case series of AKI among cannabis users [81–84]. Patients often present with a constellation of symptoms including abdominal or flank pain, along with nausea and vomiting. Those with AKI tend to be young males, which is likely due to the fact that most users tend to be men. Renal biopsies, when performed, show acute tubular injury with tubular cell apical blebbing and cytoplasmic vacuolization [82]. However, acute interstitial nephritis is also seen in some cases. The underlying etiology of the AKI is not quite clear; though ischemic acute tubular injury secondary to hypovolemia has been postulated to be one cause, many of the cases did not have physical signs of hypovolemia, like tachycardia or hypotension [81]. Cannabis receptors have been detected in renal tubular cells, podocytes and endothelial cells, which may implicate this as an alternate pathway of injury [85, 86]. In one case series, a cannabis product used by 5 of the 16 patients contained a metabolite known as XLR-11, raising the possibility that this could be the offending agent [83]. As with most other causes of acute tubular injury, treatment is largely supportive, though steroids can be considered in those who manifest AIN [87].

The United States has the highest prevalence of cocaine dependence, and this highly addictive drug has numerous nephrotoxic effects [88]. Cocaine is a well-known cause of rhabdomyolysis, which can lead to acute kidney injury due to direct tubular damage from myoglobin. However, it can also impair hemodynamics through multiple pathways. Cocaine triggers vasoconstriction of the glomerular circulation by activating the sympathetic nervous system and renin-angiotensin-aldosterone axis. The drug reduces renal blood flow through the vasoconstrictive effects of endothelin-1 [89]. Because of these hemodynamic effects, patients often present with hypertension and tachycardia. With regards to renal pathology, chronic administration of cocaine to rats can lead to nonspecific glomerular, interstitial, and tubular cell lesions [90]. Recently, there have been reports of ANCA-associated vasculitis among those who use cocaine that has been cut with levamisole, a nicotinic acetylcholine receptor antagonist [91, 92]. Almost all of these patients are seropositive for anti-myeloperoxidase ANCA, and at least half have anti-proteinase 3 positivity as well.

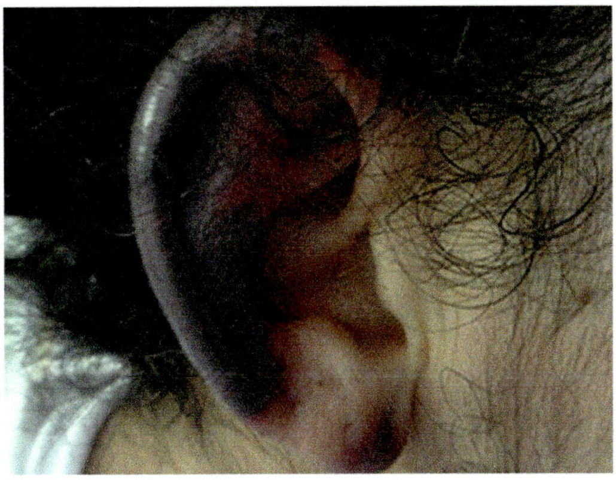

Fig. 13.6 Levamisole-laced cocaine with associated cutaneous necrotizing vasculitis involving the right ear helix. From: www.medscape.com; used with permission

Clinically, they may present with constitutional symptoms and a cutaneous necrotizing vasculitis that often involves the earlobes (see Fig. 13.6) [87]. Despite its wide spectrum of deleterious effects on the kidney, cocaine has not been found to be associated with chronic kidney disease [93]. However, there is a need for more prospective, epidemiologic data to fully address this question.

Ecstasy, also known as MDMA, is an amphetamine derivative that is typically used as a recreational drug among college-aged individuals because of its mood-enhancing effects. While it may induce feelings of euphoria, it has been associated with a spectrum of nephrotoxic effects, including AKI and hyponatremia. In severe cases of MDMA toxicity, cardiovascular collapse, rhabdomyolysis, and hyperthermia can ensue [94]. Non-traumatic rhabdomyolysis is the most likely scenario associated with the development of AKI, and it is thought to be due to seizure activity or direct toxic effects on skeletal myocytes [95]. While many of the mechanisms underlying MDMA's toxicities are not totally clear because ecstasy pills may be adulterated with other compounds, they are likely mediated by activation of the sympathetic system, serotonin syndrome, and arginine vasopressin (AVP) release [96]. Ecstasy is a potent stimulator of AVP release, which is why the most common renal toxicity associated with ecstasy use is hyponatremia. This complication is often seen in young women who are first-time users of the drug and take a single dose [97]. Hyponatremia is often exacerbated by excessive free water intake, as amphetamines also stimulate thirst. Even small doses can result in a rise in AVP levels and a fall in serum sodium. In severe cases of MDMA-induced symptomatic hyponatremia, cerebral edema, seizures, and coma can occur. These patients should be managed in the intensive care setting with appropriate monitoring of urine output, serum sodium, and serum and urine osmolality.

The misusc of opioids has become so rampant that it is has been dubbed the "opioid epidemic" or "opioid crisis." According to the Centers for Disease Control and Prevention, the total economic burden of prescription opioids alone is $78.5 billion in the United States [98]. Opioid overdose can result in AKI due to dehydration, rhabdomyolysis, and urinary retention [99]. The lack of well-designed, prospective studies as well as disparate findings on renal pathology among heroin users has called into question whether there is truly an entity known as heroin-associated nephropathy (HAN). Heroin has been associated with focal segmental sclerosis, particularly in black individuals; however, renal biopsies in 19 white heroin users showed a spectrum of findings, with 13 of the patients showing evidence of membranoproliferative glomerulonephritis (MPGN) [100]. All of the patients had positive serologies for hepatitis C infection (HCV), and therefore the authors concluded that white heroin addicts most likely have HCV-associated MPGN. It is therefore still unclear whether drug use is causal or it is related to demographics or genetic characteristics of individuals who use heroin [101].

References

1. Haessler H, Rous P, Broun G. The renal elimination of bilirubin. J Exp Med. 1922;35:533–52.
2. Topuzlu C, WM S. Effect of bile infusion on the dog kidney. N Engl J Med. 1966;274:760–3.
3. Wardle EN. Renal failure in obstructive jaundice—pathogenic factors. Postgrad Med J. 1975;51:512–4. https://doi.org/10.1136/pgmj.51.598.512.
4. van Slambrouck CM, Salem F, Meehan SM, Chang A. Bile cast nephropathy is a common pathologic finding for kidney injury associated with severe liver dysfunction. Kidney Int. 2013;84(1):192–7. https://doi.org/10.1038/ki.2013.78.

5. Bairaktari E, Liamis G, Tsolas O, Elisaf M. Partially reversible renal tubular damage in patients with obstructive jaundice. Hepatology. 2001;33(6):1365–9. https://doi.org/10.1053/jhep.2001.25089.
6. Sitprija V, Kashemsant U, Sriratanaban A, Arthachinta S, Poshyachinda V. Renal function in obstructive jaundice in man: cholangiocarcinoma model. Kidney Int. 1990;38(5):948–55. https://doi.org/10.1038/ki.1990.296.
7. Fickert P, Krones E, Pollheimer MJ, et al. Bile acids trigger cholemic nephropathy in common bile-duct-ligated mice. Hepatology. 2013;58(6):2056–69. https://doi.org/10.1002/hep.26599.
8. Alkhunaizi AM, ElTigani MA, Rabah RS, Nasr SH. Acute bile nephropathy secondary to anabolic steroids. Clin Nephrol. 2016;85(2):121–6. https://doi.org/10.5414/CN108696.
9. Tabatabaee SM, Elahi R, Savaj S. Bile cast nephropathy due to cholestatic jaundice after using stanozolol in 2 amateur bodybuilders. Iran J Kidney Dis. 2015;9(4):331–44.
10. Betjes MGH, Bajema I. The pathology of jaundice-related renal insufficiency: cholemic nephrosis revisited. J Nephrol. 2006;19(2):229–33.
11. Brodsky SV, Satoskar A, Chen J, et al. Acute kidney injury during warfarin therapy associated with obstructive tubular red blood cell casts: a report of 9 cases. Am J Kidney Dis. 2009;54(6):1121–6. https://doi.org/10.1053/j.ajkd.2009.04.024.
12. Ware K, Brodsky P, Satoskar AA, et al. Warfarin-related nephropathy modeled by nephron reduction and excessive anticoagulation. J Am Soc Nephrol. 2011;22(10):1856–62. https://doi.org/10.1681/asn.2010101110.
13. Brodsky SV, Nadasdy T, Rovin BH, et al. Warfarin-related nephropathy occurs in patients with and without chronic kidney disease and is associated with an increased mortality rate. Kidney Int. 2011;80(2):181–9. https://doi.org/10.1038/ki.2011.44.
14. Wheeler DS, Giugliano RP, Rangaswami J. Anticoagulation-related nephropathy. J Thromb Haemost. 2016;14(3):461–7. https://doi.org/10.1111/jth.13229.
15. Ryan M, Ware K, Qamri Z, et al. Warfarin-related nephropathy is the tip of the iceberg: direct thrombin inhibitor dabigatran induces glomerular hemorrhage with acute kidney injury in rats. Nephrol Dial Transplant. 2014;29(12):2228–34. https://doi.org/10.1093/ndt/gft380.
16. Shafi ST, Negrete H, Roy P, Julius CJ, Sarac E. A case of dabigatran-associated acute renal failure. WMJ. 2014;112:173–5; quiz 176.
17. Chang DN, Dager WE, Chin AI. Removal of dabigatran by hemodialysis. Am J Kidney Dis. 2013;61(3):487–9. https://doi.org/10.1053/j.ajkd.2012.08.047.
18. Diallo O, Janssens F, Hall M, Avni EF. Type 1 primary hyperoxaluria in pediatric patients: renal sonographic patterns. AJR Am J Roentgenol. 2004;183(6):1767–70. https://doi.org/10.2214/ajr.183.6.01831767.
19. Nasr SH, D'Agati VD, Said SM, et al. Oxalate nephropathy complicating Roux-en-Y Gastric bypass: an underrecognized cause of irreversible renal failure. Clin J Am Soc Nephrol. 2008;3(6):1676–83. https://doi.org/10.2215/CJN.02940608.
20. Chen CL, Fang HC, Chou KJ, Wang JS, Chung HM. Acute oxalate nephropathy after ingestion of star fruit. Am J Kidney Dis. 2001;37(2):418–22. https://doi.org/10.1053/ajkd.2001.21333.
21. Sunkara V, Pelkowski TD, Dreyfus D, Satoskar A. Acute kidney disease due to excessive Vitamin C ingestion and remote roux-en-y gastric bypass surgery superimposed on CKD. Am J Kidney Dis. 2015;66(4):721–4. https://doi.org/10.1053/j.ajkd.2015.06.021.
22. Seyd F, Mena-Gutierrez A, Ghaffar U. A case of iced-tea nephropathy. N Engl J Med. 2015;372(14):1377–8. https://doi.org/10.1056/NEJMc1500455.
23. MA W, MM B, Gomes T, et al. Orlistat and acute kidney injury: an analysis of 953 patients. Arch Intern Med. 2011;171(7):702–10. https://doi.org/10.1001/archinternmed.2011.103.
24. Whitson JM, Stackhouse GB, Stoller ML. Hyperoxaluria after modern bariatric surgery: case series and literature review. Int Urol Nephrol. 2010;42(2):369–74. https://doi.org/10.1007/s11255-009-9602-5.
25. Hoppe B, Leumann E, von Unruh G, Laube N, Hesse A. Diagnostic and therapeutic approaches in patients with secondary hyperoxaluria. Front Biosci. 2003;8:e437–43. http://www.ncbi.nlm.nih.gov/pubmed/12957811.
26. Escribano J, Balaguer A, Pagone F, Feliu A, Figuls MRI. Pharmacological interventions for preventing complications in idiopathic hypercalciuria. Cochrane Database Syst Rev. 2009;1:CD004754. https://doi.org/10.1002/14651858.CD004754.pub2.
27. Perazella MA. Crystal-induced acute renal failure. Am J Med. 1999;106(4):459–65. https://doi.org/10.1016/S0002-9343(99)00041-8.
28. Brigden D, Rosling AE, Woods NC. Renal function after acyclovir intravenous injection. Am J Med. 1982;73(1 PART 1):182–5. https://doi.org/10.1016/0002-9343(82)90087-0.
29. Roberts D, Myles W, Smith B, et al. Acute kidney injury due to crystalluria following acute valacyclovir overdose. Kidney Int. 2011;79:574.
30. Sawyer MH, Webb DE, Balow JE, Straus SE. Acyclovir-induced renal failure. Clinical course and histology. Am J Med. 1988;84(6):1067–71. http://www.ncbi.nlm.nih.gov/pubmed/3376977.
31. Krieble B, Rudy D, Glick M, et al. Case report: acyclovir neurotoxicity and nephrotoxicity-the role for hemodialysis. Am J Med Sci. 1993;305(1):36.
32. Berns JS, Cohen RM, Stumacher RJ, Rudnick MR. Renal aspects of therapy for human immunodeficiency virus and associated opportunistic infections. J Am Soc Nephrol. 1991;1(9):1061–80.
33. Carbone LG, Bendixen B, Appel GB. Sulfadiazine-associated obstructive nephropathy occurring in a patient with the acquired immunodeficiency

syndrome. Am J Kidney Dis. 1988;12(1):72–5. https://doi.org/10.1016/S0272-6386(88)80076-3.
34. Simon DI, Brosius FC 3rd, Rothstein DM. Sulfadiazine crystalluria revisited. The treatment of Toxoplasma encephalitis in patients with acquired immunodeficiency syndrome. Arch Intern Med. 1990;150(11):2379–84. http://www.ncbi.nlm.nih.gov/entrez/query.fcgi?cmd=Retrieve&db=PubMed&dopt=Citation&list_uids=2241449.
35. Chopra N, Fine P, Price B, et al. Bilateral hydronephrosis from ciprofloxacin induced crystalluria and stone formation. J Urol. 2000;164:438.
36. Sedlacek M, Suriawinata A, Schoolwerth A, et al. Ciprofloxacin crystal nephropathy—a "new" cause of acute renal failure. Nephrol Dial Transpl. 2006;21:2339.
37. Montagnac R, Briat C, Schillinger F, Sartelet H, Birembaut P, Daudon M. Fluoroquinolone induced acute renal failure. General review about a case report with crystalluria due to ciprofloxacin. Nephrol Ther. 2005;1(1):44–51. https://doi.org/10.1016/j.nephro.2005.02.005.
38. Fogazzi GB, Garigali G, Brambilla C, Daudon M. Ciprofloxacin crystalluria. Nephrol Dial Transplant. 2006;21(10):2982–3. https://doi.org/10.1093/ndt/gfl320.
39. Stratta P, Lazzarich E, Canavese C, Bozzola C, Monga G. Ciprofloxacin crystal nephropathy. Am J Kidney Dis. 2007;50(2):330–5. https://doi.org/10.1053/j.ajkd.2007.05.014.
40. Abelson HT, Fosburg MT, Beardsley GP, et al. Methotrexate-induced renal impairment: clinical studies and rescue from systemic toxicity with high-dose leucovorin and thymidine. J Clin Oncol. 1983;1(3):208–16.
41. Pitman SW, Frei E. Weekly methotrexate-calcium leucovorin rescue: effect of alkalinization on nephrotoxicity; pharmacokinetics in the CNS; and use in CNS non-Hodgkin's lymphoma. Cancer Treat Rep. 1977;61(4):695–701. https://doi.org/10.1017/CBO9781107415324.004.
42. Widemann BC, Adamson PC. Understanding and managing methotrexate nephrotoxicity. Oncologist. 2006;11(6):694–703. https://doi.org/10.1634/theoncologist.11-6-694.
43. Garella S. Extracorporeal techniques in the treatment of exogenous intoxications. Kidney Int. 1988;33(3):735.
44. Ray AS, Haikal A, Hammoud KA, Yu ASL. Vancomycin and the risk of AKI: a systematic review and meta-analysis. Clin J Am Soc Nephrol. 2016;11(12):2132–40. https://doi.org/10.2215/CJN.05920616.
45. Lodise TP, Lomaestro B, Graves J, Drusano GL. Larger vancomycin doses (at least four grams per day) are associated with an increased incidence of nephrotoxicity. Antimicrob Agents Chemother. 2008;52(4):1330–6. https://doi.org/10.1128/AAC.01602-07.
46. Eisenberg ES, Robbins N, Lenci M. Vancomycin and interstitial nephritis. Ann Intern Med. 1981;95(5):658.
47. Wai AO, Lo AMS, Abdo A, Marra F. Vancomycin-induced acute interstitial nephritis. Ann Pharmacother. 1998;32(11):1160–4. http://www.embase.com/search/results?subaction=viewrecord&from=export&id=L28543461.
48. Luque Y, Louis K, Jouanneau C, et al. Vancomycin-associated cast nephropathy. J Am Soc Nephrol. 2017;28(6):1723–8. https://doi.org/10.1681/ASN.2016080867.
49. Malbrain MLNG, Cheatham ML, Kirkpatrick A, et al. Results from the international conference of experts on intra-abdominal hypertension and abdominal compartment syndrome. I. Definitions. Intensive Care Med. 2006;32:1722–32. https://doi.org/10.1007/s00134-006-0349-5.
50. Regueira T, Hasbun P, Rebolledo R, et al. Intraabdominal hypertension in patients with septic shock. Am Surg. 2007;73(9):865–70.
51. Daugherty EL, Liang H, Taichman D, Hansen-Flaschen J, Fuchs BD. Abdominal compartment syndrome is common in medical intensive care unit patients receiving large-volume resuscitation. J Intensive Care Med. 2007;22(5):294–9. https://doi.org/10.1177/0885066607305247.
52. Wise R, Jacobs J, Pilate S, et al. Incidence and prognosis of intra-abdominal hypertension and abdominal compartment syndrome in severely burned patients: pilot study and review of the literature. Anestezjol Intens Ter. 2016;48(2):95–109. https://doi.org/10.5603/AIT.a2015.0083.
53. Maerz L, Kaplan LJ. Abdominal compartment syndrome. Crit Care Med. 2008;36(Suppl):S212–5. https://doi.org/10.1097/CCM.0b013e318168e333.
54. Malbrain MLNG, Chiumello D, Pelosi P, et al. Incidence and prognosis of intraabdominal hypertension in a mixed population of critically ill patients: a multiple-center epidemiological study*. Crit Care Med. 2005;33(2):315–22. https://doi.org/10.1097/01.CCM.0000153408.09806.1B.
55. Wendt E. Ueber den einfluss des intraabdominalenn druckes auf die absonderungsgeschwindigkeit des harnes. Arch Physiol Heilkd 1876;57(527).
56. Bradley SE, Bradley GP. The effect of increased intra-abdominal pressure on renal function in man. J Clin Invest. 1947;26(5):1010–22. https://doi.org/10.1172/JCI101867.
57. Harman PK, Kron IL, McLachlan HD, Freedlender AE, Nolan SP. Elevated intra-abdominal pressure and renal function. Ann Surg. 1982;196(5):594–7. https://doi.org/10.1097/00000658-198211000-00015.
58. Doty JM, Saggi BH, Sugerman HJ, et al. Effect of increased renal venous pressure on renal function. J Trauma. 1999;47(6):1000–3. http://www.ncbi.nlm.nih.gov/pubmed/10608524
59. Kirkpatrick AW, Brenneman FD, McLean RF, Rapanos T, Boulanger BR. Is clinical examination an accurate indicator of raised intra-abdominal pressure in critically injured patients? Can J Surg. 2000;43(3):207–11.
60. Malbrain MLNG. Different techniques to measure intra-abdominal pressure (IAP): time for a critical

re-appraisal. Intensive Care Med. 2004;30(3):357–71. https://doi.org/10.1007/s00134–003–2107–2.
61. Strang SG, Van Lieshout EM, Van Waes OJ, Verhofstad MH. Prevalence and mortality of abdominal compartment syndrome in severely injured patients: a systematic review. J Trauma Acute Care Surg. 2016;81(3):585–92. https://doi.org/10.1097/TA.0000000000001133.
62. De Waele JJ, Hoste EAJ, Malbrain MLNG. Decompressive laparotomy for abdominal compartment syndrome—a critical analysis. Crit Care. 2006;10(2):1–9. https://doi.org/10.1186/cc4870.
63. Parra M, Al-Khayat H, Smith H, et al. Paracentesis for resuscitation-induced abdominal compartment syndrome. J Trauma. 2006;60:1119–21.
64. Reckard JM, Chung MH, Varma MK, Zagorski SM. Management of intraabdominal hypertension by percutaneous catheter drainage. J Vasc Interv Radiol. 2005;16(7):1019–21. https://doi.org/10.1097/01.RVI.0000157781.67279.72.
65. Jones DB, Iannaccone PM. Atheromatous emboli in renal biopsies. An ultrastructural study. Am J Pathol. 1975;78(2):261–76. http://www.pubmedcentral.nih.gov/articlerender.fcgi?artid=1912470&tool=pmcentrez&rendertype=abstract.
66. Greenberg A, Bastacky SI, Iqbal A, Borochovitz D, Johnson JP. Focal segmental glomerulosclerosis associated with nephrotic syndrome in cholesterol atheroembolism: clinicopathological correlations. Am J Kidney Dis. 1997;29(3):334–44. https://doi.org/10.1016/s0272–6386(97)90193–1.
67. Preston RA, Stemmer CL, Materson BJ, Perez-Stable E, Pardo V. Renal biopsy in patients 65 years of age or older. An analysis of the results of 334 biopsies. J Am Geriatr Soc. 1990;38(6):669–74.
68. Darsee JR. Cholesterol embolism: the great masquerader. South Med J. 1979;72(2):174–80. http://www.ncbi.nlm.nih.gov/entrez/query.fcgi?cmd=Retrieve&db=PubMed&dopt=Citation&list_uids=371003.
69. Scolari F, Ravani P. Atheroembolic renal disease. Lancet. 2010;375(9726):1650–60. https://doi.org/10.1016/S0140–6736(09)62073–0.
70. Scolari F, Tardanico R, Zani R, et al. Cholesterol crystal embolism: a recognizable cause of renal disease. Am J Kidney Dis. 2000;36(6):1089–109. https://doi.org/10.1053/ajkd.2000.19809.
71. Scolari F, Ravani P, Pola A, et al. Predictors of renal and patient outcomes in atheroembolic renal disease: a prospective study. J Am Soc Nephrol. 2003;14(6):1584–90. https://doi.org/10.1097/01.ASN.0000069220.60954.F1.
72. Thadhani RI, Camargo CA Jr, Xavier RJ, Fang LS, Bazari H. Atheroembolic renal failure after invasive procedures. Natural history based on 52 histologically proven cases. Medicine (Baltimore). 1995;74(6):350–8. http://www.ncbi.nlm.nih.gov/pubmed/7500898
73. Falanga V, MJ F, WN K. THe cutaneous manifestations of cholesterol crystal embolization. Arch Dermatol. 1986;122(10):1194–8. https://doi.org/10.1001/archderm.1986.01660220112024.
74. Kasinath B, Corwin A, Bidwani S, et al. Eosinophilia in the diagnosis of atheroembolic disease. Am J Nephrol. 1987;7:173–7.
75. Lusco MA, Najafian B, Alpers CE, Fogo AB. AJKD atlas of renal pathology: cholesterol emboli. Am J Kidney Dis. 2016;67(4):e23–4. https://doi.org/10.1053/j.ajkd.2016.02.034.
76. Modi K, Rao V. Atheroembolic renal disease. JASN. 2001;12(8):1781–7.
77. Koga J-I. Cholesterol embolization treated with corticosteroids: two case reports. Angiology. 2005;56(4):497–501. https://doi.org/10.1177/000331970505600420.
78. Matsumura T, Matsumoto A, Ohno M, et al. A case of cholesterol embolism confirmed by skin biopsy and successfully treated with statins and steroids. Am J Med Sci. 2006;331(5):280–3. https://doi.org/10.1097/00000441-200605000-00010.
79. Mann SJ, Sos TA. Treatment of atheroembolization with corticosteroids. Am J Hypertens. 2001;14(8 I):831–4. https://doi.org/10.1016/S0895-7061(01)02183-5.
80. Scolari F, Ravani P, Gaggi R, et al. The challenge of diagnosing atheroembolic renal disease: clinical features and prognostic factors. Circulation. 2007;116(3):298–304. https://doi.org/10.1161/CIRCULATIONAHA.106.680991.
81. Kazory A, Aiyer R. Synthetic marijuana and acute kidney injury: an unforeseen association. Clin Kidney J. 2013;6(3):330–3. https://doi.org/10.1093/ckj/sft047.
82. Bhanushali GK, Jain G, Fatima H, Leisch LJ, Thornley-Brown D. AKI associated with synthetic cannabinoids: a case series. Clin J Am Soc Nephrol. 2013;8(4):523–6. https://doi.org/10.2215/CJN.05690612.
83. Report MW. Acute kidney injury associated with synthetic cannabinoid use—multiple states, 2012. MMWR Morb Mortal Wkly Rep. 2013;62(6):93–8. https://doi.org/10.3109/15563650.2013.770870.
84. Srisung W, Jamal F, Prabhakar S. Synthetic cannabinoids and acute kidney injury. Proc (Bayl Univ Med Cent). 2015;28(4):475–7.
85. Barutta F, Corbelli A, Mastrocola R, et al. Cannabinoid receptor 1 blockade ameliorates albuminuria in experimental diabetic nephropathy. Diabetes. 2010;59(4):1046–54. https://doi.org/10.2337/db09–1336.
86. Jenkin KA, McAinch AJ, Grinfeld E, Hryciw DH. Role for cannabinoid receptors in human proximal tubular hypertrophy. Cell Physiol Biochem. 2010;26:879–86. https://doi.org/10.1159/000323997.

87. Pendergraft WF, Herlitz LC, Thornley-Brown D, Rosner M, Niles JL. Nephrotoxic effects of common and emerging drugs of abuse. Clin J Am Soc Nephrol. 2014;9(11):1996–2005. https://doi.org/10.2215/CJN.00360114.
88. Pomara C, Cassano T, D'Errico S, et al. Data available on the extent of cocaine use and dependence: biochemistry, pharmacologic effects and global burden of disease of cocaine abusers. Curr Med Chem. 2012;19(33):5647–57. https://doi.org/10.2174/092986712803988811.
89. Sáez CG, Olivares P, Pallavicini J, et al. Increased number of circulating endothelial cells and plasma markers of endothelial damage in chronic cocaine users. Thromb Res. 2011;128(4):e18–23. https://doi.org/10.1016/j.thromres.2011.04.019.
90. Barroso-Moguel R, Mendez-Armenta M, Villeda-Hernandez J. Experimental nephropathy by chronic administration of cocaine in rats. Toxicology. 1995;98(1–3):41–6. https://doi.org/10.1016/0300-483X(94)02954-S.
91. McGrath MM, Isakova T, Rennke HG, Mottola AM, Laliberte KA, Niles JL. Contaminated cocaine and antineutrophil cytoplasmic antibody-associated disease. Clin J Am Soc Nephrol. 2011;6(12):2799–805. https://doi.org/10.2215/CJN.03440411.
92. Graf J, Lynch K, Yeh CL, et al. Purpura, cutaneous necrosis, and antineutrophil cytoplasmic antibodies associated with levamisole-adulterated cocaine. Arthritis Rheum. 2011;63(12):3998–4001. https://doi.org/10.1002/art.30590.
93. Akkina SK, Ricardo AC, Patel A, et al. Illicit drug use, hypertension, and chronic kidney disease in the US adult population. Transl Res. 2012;160(6):391–8. https://doi.org/10.1016/j.trsl.2012.05.008.
94. Hall AP, Henry JA. Acute toxic effects of "Ecstasy" (MDMA) and related compounds: overview of pathophysiology and clinical management. Br J Anaesth. 2006;96(6):678–85. https://doi.org/10.1093/bja/ael078.
95. Rusyniak DE, Tandy SL, Hekmatyar SK, et al. The role of mitochondrial uncoupling in 3,4-methylene dioxymethamphetamine-mediated skeletal muscle hyperthermia and rhabdomyolysis. J Pharmacol Exp Ther. 2005;313(2):629–39. https://doi.org/10.1124/jpet.104.079236.
96. Steinkellner T, Freissmuth M, Sitte HH, Montgomery T. The ugly side of amphetamines: short-and long-term toxicity of 3,4-methylenedioxymethampheta mine (MDMA, "Ecstasy"), methamphetamine and d-amphetamine. Biol Chem. 2011;392(1–2):103–15. https://doi.org/10.1515/BC.2011.016.
97. Campbell GA, Rosner MH. The agony of ecstasy: MDMA (3,4-methylenedioxymethamph etamine) and the kidney. Clin J Am Soc Nephrol. 2008;3(6):1852–60. https://doi.org/10.2215/CJN.02080508.
98. Florence CS, Zhou C, Luo F, Xu L. The economic burden of prescription opioid overdose, abuse, and dependence in the United States, 2013. Med Care. 2016;54(10):901–6. https://doi.org/10.1097/MLR.0000000000000625.
99. Mallappallil M, Sabu J, Friedman EA, Salifu M. What do we know about opioids and the kidney? Int J Mol Sci. 2017;18(1). https://doi.org/10.3390/ijms18010223.
100. do Sameiro Faria M, Sampaio S, Faria V, Carvalho E. Nephropathy associated with heroin abuse in Caucasian patients. Nephrol Dial Transplant. 2003;18(11):2308–13. https://doi.org/10.1093/ndt/gfg369.
101. Jaffe JA, Kimmel PL. Chronic nephropathies of cocaine and heroin abuse: a critical review. Clin J Am Soc Nephrol. 2006;1(4):655–67. https://doi.org/10.2215/CJN.00300106.

14 Acute Kidney Injury in the Tropics: Epidemiology, Presentation, Etiology, Specific Diseases, and Treatment

Sreejith Parameswaran and Vivekanand Jha

14.1 Introduction

The characteristics of acute kidney injury (AKI), including etiology and outcomes, are highly variable and are dictated to a great extent by the setting in which AKI develops. The etiology and outcomes of AKI developing in hospitalized patients (hospital-acquired AKI—HAAKI) are different from AKI developing in the community (community-acquired AKI—CAAKI), especially in the tropical climate [1]. Environmental and socioeconomic factors play a major role in human health and disease development in the tropics. A majority of AKI in the tropics is CAAKI, mostly as a consequence of the prevailing disease epidemiology and the variability in appropriateness of response by the local health system.

S. Parameswaran
Department of Nephrology, Jawaharlal Institute of Postgraduate Medical Education and Research, Pondicherry, India

V. Jha (✉)
George Institute for Global Health India, New Delhi, India

George Institute for Global Health, University of Oxford, UK
e-mail: vjha@pginephro.org

14.2 The Tropical Ecosystem as a Driver of Disease

Approximately 40% of world population lives in the tropics, defined geographically as area between approximately 23° on either side of the equator, where the sun is directly overhead at least once during the year. Tropical climate is characterized by high ambient temperature; some tropical regions receive heavy rains, while others get little precipitation. The rainy tropical ecosystem promotes the survival of pathogenic microorganisms outside the human host and is suitable for proliferation of parasites and vermin that cause disease or act as reservoirs, intermediate hosts, and vectors. On the other hand, water scarcity in the arid regions increases the susceptibility of kidneys to relatively minor insults. The tropics are home to a number of poisonous snakes and arthropods. Flooding of burrows in the rainy season forces snakes to come to the surface at a time when large numbers of workers are in the fields for planting or harvesting crops, leading to a spike in the incidence of bite victims. Seasonal variation in the incidence of AKI due to tropical infections and snake envenomation is a common feature throughout the tropics.

Quality of drinking water plays a major role in the pattern of kidney disease in the tropics. A number of conditions that are associated with of AKI in the tropics (see below) can be causally linked to contaminated water. The leaching of

S. S. Waikar et al. (eds.), *Core Concepts in Acute Kidney Injury*,
https://doi.org/10.1007/978-1-4939-8628-6_14

minerals and organic compounds into the fragile tropical soil during rains leads to waterlogging and contamination of fields [2] and also promote waterborne diseases. Transmission by direct contact and aerosols is also more likely because of overcrowding and poor living conditions in the tropics.

Tropical countries differ from those in temperate regions in socioeconomic terms as well. Despite occupying less than 10% of the land mass and only 20% of world population, countries in temperate regions account for 52% of the world's gross national product [3]. Almost all of the tropical countries are classified by the World Bank into low or low-middle income categories. The healthcare systems in the poor tropical countries exhibit several limitations in the form of limited and unevenly distributed medical resources, lack of specialized care, high costs, fear and suspicion of modern medicine, and continued reliance on traditional health systems. The harmful consequences are both secondary to denial or delay of appropriate treatment, and the use of potentially toxic ingredients of indigenous remedies is toxic that can lead to AKI.

The combined effect of a high disease burden and poor economic performance is reflected in the lower life expectancy and high infant and maternal mortality rates in tropical countries. Even after correction for the level of income, the infant mortality rate in the tropical zone is 52% higher and the life expectancy 8% lower than those in temperate zones [3]. Tropical regions also have high fertility rates, which result in a high proportion of children in the population but at the cost of fewer resources per child. Conversely, illness depletes household savings, reduces productivity, decreases learning ability, and leads to a diminished quality of life, thereby perpetuating or even increasing poverty [4].

Economic considerations prevent the implementation of technological solutions that might be feasible in affluent nontropical countries. For example, advanced and expensive treatments, such as continuous renal replacement therapy, are eschewed in favor of cheaper and less complex peritoneal dialysis, resulting in trade-off with efficiency, flexibility, and personalization.

14.3 Epidemiology of AKI in the Tropics

14.3.1 Incidence

Paucity of community-wide reports on AKI from tropical countries has hampered efforts to estimate its burden and compare the pattern, presentation, and outcome with that from other parts of the world. The available reports are single-center studies conducted at academic institutions, which may not be truly representative of the true characteristics of AKI, especially in rural settings. Patients are referred in advanced stages of illness, often with complications, and those developing AKI in rural communities may not reach hospitals at all. Most of the available studies have used different denominators to calculate the incidence of AKI or described single entities like "obstetric AKI" or "AKI due to leptospirosis." The absence of uniform definitions and use of inconsistent terminology has added another layer of complexity. All this makes estimation of disease burden and accurate comparisons difficult.

AKI is recognized as the most common renal emergency in tropical countries. However, the reported incidence has been variable and in general lower compared to other regions. In 2013, the International Society of Nephrology started the *0by25* (zero preventable deaths due to AKI by 2025) initiative, with focus on LMIC. A meta-analysis done as a part of this initiative included a large number of studies that have not been published in mainstream journals and provided the most comprehensive documentation yet of the incidence of AKI in different parts of the world (Table 14.1) [5].

An important finding from this meta-analysis was that with uniform definition and better

Table 14.1 Incidence of AKI from different regions of the world

Tropics		Other regions	
South Asia	7.5%	North America	22.3%
Middle Africa	23.5%	Europe	20.8–25.2%
East Africa	13.5%	Australia and NZ	16.9%
South America	31%		

reporting from the LMIC, the incidence of AKI in tropical countries no longer seems to be low, as had been reported earlier. In fact, in regions from where reports are gradually becoming available, the burden of AKI in hospitalized patients seems to be equivalent. Also, patients with more severe stages of AKI had high mortality, similar to other reports (42% and 46%, unadjusted odds ratio 12.5 and 19.7, respectively) [5]. The report confirmed the higher incidence of CAAKI in the developing countries, delayed presentation, and greater likelihood of not receiving RRT despite being indicated due to lack of resources and being discharged from the hospital to home, rather than to a step-down facility.

The International Society of Nephrology 0by25 Global Snapshot [6] provided a unique, though limited, picture of AKI around the globe. The snapshot provided significant insights into differences in epidemiology of AKI between countries in different socioeconomic categories and reaffirmed previous concepts about epidemiology of AKI in the low-income tropical countries. The distinguishing features of patients with AKI in LIC and LMIC were young age, low prevalence of preexisting CKD, presentation with more severe stages of AKI and relative prevalence of AKI associated with sepsis, obstetric complications, and animal envenomation. Lack of resources and inability to afford therapy meant that a significant proportion of patients could not receive dialysis despite being indicated. Although the overall mortality was higher, the survivors were more likely to show complete recovery from AKI in LLMIC.

14.3.2 Setting of AKI

In most nontropical countries, AKI is encountered largely among patients already admitted in hospital, either with multi-organ failure in the intensive care units or after major surgical procedures. Tropical countries of Africa, South and Southeast Asia, and Latin America, however, encounter a double burden of AKI—both CAAKI and HAAKI. The characteristics of HAAKI encountered in ICUs of large urban tropical centers are largely similar to the high-income countries, with relatively accessible sophisticated healthcare systems, even though these ICUs may also have patients with AKI secondary to tropical diseases. In rural areas, CAAKI secondary to diarrheal disease, envenomation from snakebite, leptospirosis, malaria, or obstetric complications predominate [6]. The rural healthcare infrastructure is usually inadequate with limited or no facilities for renal replacement therapy (RRT) and lack of specialized doctors. Hospitals that have infrastructure are overwhelmed with large number of patients, especially with seasonal surge of infectious diseases like leptospirosis.

14.3.3 Age and Sex

The mean age of patients with AKI in the tropics is 37–47 years, in contrast to mean of over 65 years in nontropical countries. Individuals with tropical CAAKI have few, if any, underlying diseases that might increase their AKI risk [7]. While there is no sex difference in the incidence of AKI from other regions, literature on tropical AKI consistently report lower incidence in females, with female/male ratio ranging from 1:1.5 to 1:5. This is unlikely to be a true difference and may be attributable to sociocultural factors with males accessing healthcare facilities more frequently than females. Of note is the consistently high prevalence of obstetric AKI.

14.4 Etiology of AKI in the Tropics and Comparison with Temperate Regions

Unlike AKI in high-income countries, AKI in the tropics is usually the predominant presenting feature following a specific condition (e.g., snakebite) or a specific infection (e.g., malaria), and not a part of a general multi-organ failure syndrome.

The causes of CAAKI in tropical countries can be broadly divided into those caused by infections; animal, plant, or chemical toxins; and obstetric complications (Table 14.2). Some of these causes have been well characterized and studied, whereas for others, the numbers of affected patients are small and only a temporal association suggests a cause and effect relationship. Reliable estimates of the importance of the different causes of AKI are difficult to make, as these vary from region to region. Diarrheal illness and malarial AKI are major public health threats in most tropical countries, whereas leptospirosis, typhus, and envenomation are the main

Table 14.2 Causes of acute kidney injury in the tropics

Vector-borne infections	Malaria (*Plasmodium falciparum*, *Plasmodium vivax*, or *Plasmodium knowlesi*, transmitted by *Anopheles* mosquito)
	Dengue fever (dengue virus, transmitted by *Aedes* mosquito)
	Scrub typhus (*Orientia tsutsugamushi*, transmitted by trombiculid mites)
	Hemorrhagic Rift Valley fever (RVF virus, transmitted by *Aedes* or *Culex* mosquitoes)
Direct infections	Leptospirosis (*Leptospira interrogans*)
	Hantaviruses, also known as hemorrhagic fever with renal syndrome (Puumala and Hantaan viruses)
	Zygomycosis
Diarrheal diseases	Viral diarrhea (rotavirus, Norwalk agent)
	Enterotoxigenic or enteroinvasive *Escherichia coli*
	Bacillary (*Shigella*) dysentery
	Cholera
Other infections	Melioidosis (*Burkholderia pseudomallei*)
	Typhoid (*Salmonella typhi*)
	Chlamydia (*Chlamydia trachomatis*)
	Legionellosis (*Legionella pneumophila*)
	Human immunodeficiency virus
Plant and fungal toxins	Herbal medicines
	Impila tuber
	Djenkol beans
	Marking nut
	Mushroom
	Star fruit and other oxalate-rich plants
	Plant-derived toxins used as insecticides and to kill fish
Animal poisons	Snakebites
	Wasp, hornet, and bee stings
	Spider bite
	Jellyfish sting
	Scorpion sting
	Carp gallbladder or bile
Chemical nephrotoxins	Ethylene glycol, propylene glycol
	Paraphenyldiamine
	Ethylene dibromide
	Copper sulfate
	Chromic acid
Environmental factors	Heat stroke
	Natural disasters
Obstetric complications	Postabortal sepsis
	Ante- and postpartum hemorrhage
	Preeclampsia
Other causes	Intravascular hemolysis resulting from glucose-6-phosphate 1-dehydrogenase deficiency

Adapted from Jha and Parameswaran, Nat Rev Nephrol 9: 278–290, 2013

causes of AKI in South Asia; malaria and indigenous herbal remedies are the most common causes of AKI in Africa; and leptospirosis, dengue fever, envenomation, and obstetric complications are the main causes of AKI in Latin American countries.

Knowledge of etiological factors is helpful in eliciting appropriate history and coming to a quick diagnosis. Certain facts like intake of toxic plants or indigenous medicines may be thought of as irrelevant and hence not volunteered, while others like a clandestine abortion may be even suppressed due to social or cultural reasons.

14.5 AKI Syndromes in the Tropics

CAAKI in the tropics can be part of a constellation of manifestations, presenting as specific patterns of AKI "syndromes" in the tropics, which help the clinician in deciding a diagnostic approach (Table 14.3).

- Fever—AKI syndrome due to tropical infections (fever + jaundice + AKI, fever + hemorrhagic manifestations + AKI)
- Envenomation and poisonings (including snakebite, illicit liquor, and industrial chemicals)
- Obstetric AKI
- AKI related to use of indigenous or herbal medicines

Table 14.3 Common differential diagnosis of tropical acute febrile illness with AKI

Pattern of organ involvement with tropical febrile illness	Differential diagnosis
Fever + jaundice	Leptospirosis, malaria, dengue, hantavirus, rickettsiosis
Biphasic fever + conjunctival suffusion + thrombocytopenia + transaminitis	Leptospirosis
Continuous fever + severe respiratory symptoms leading to ARDS	Hantavirus
Fever + severe myalgia + thrombocytopenia + acalculous cholecystitis	Dengue fever
Fever + maculopapular rash + "eschar"	Scrub typhus
Fever + splenomegaly + thrombocytopenia	Malaria
Fever + exposure to unpasteurized milk products	Brucellosis
Fever + diarrhea	Bacterial or viral gastroenteritis

14.5.1 Febrile Illness with Acute Kidney Injury

A large number of patients with tropical infections develop AKI in the setting of an undifferentiated febrile illness. In the absence of obvious evidence of common bacterial infections like respiratory tract infection or urinary tract infection, specific tropical infections need to be considered in the differential diagnosis of patients with AKI in the setting of acute febrile illness in the tropics or in travelers returning from the tropics. AKI is encountered in over 40% of these cases and increases the mortality and morbidity risk [8]. Upto 92% of patients hospitalized with AKI in a tertiary care hospital in India had fever from a tropical infection (Table 14.4).

AKI in the setting of tropical febrile illnesses can have additional manifestations related to other organ systems like the liver, nervous system, and heart, coagulopathy, and thrombocytopenia. Identification of these syndromes helps in narrowing the list of diagnostic possibilities. The

Table 14.4 Etiology of AKI in children in India [42]

Infections	92 (55%)
Pneumonia	24 (14%)
Diarrhea	13 (8%)
Sepsis	13 (8%)
Dengue	10 (6%)
Scrub typhus	3 (2%)
Leptospirosis malaria	1 (1%)
Malaria	1 (1%)
Acute glomerular diseases	28 (17%)
Underlying renal diseases	10 (6%)
Underlying cardiac diseases	8 (5%)
Envenomations	7 (4%)
Hemolytic uremic syndrome	6 (4%)
Drugs	2 (1%)
Others	13 (8%)

Table 14.5 Etiology of febrile illness with AKI [7]

Diagnosis	Number of cases (%)
Scrub typhus	188 (51.2)
Falciparum malaria	38 (10.4)
Enteric fever	32 (8.7)
Dengue	28 (7.6)
Mixed malaria	24 (6.5)
Leptospirosis	12 (3.3)
Spotted fever	7 (1.9)
Vivax malaria	6 (1.6)
Hantaan virus infection	1 (0.3)
Undifferentiated	31 (8.4)
Total	367

common differential diagnosis of tropical acute febrile illness based on organ involvement is summarized in Table 14.5.

14.6 Specific Diseases

14.6.1 Envenomation from Animal, Plant, or Chemical Toxins

Encounters with animals and insects are common in the tropics, due to their ubiquitous distribution; the nature of work of the inhabitants of the region, who are largely engaged in farming activities; and lack of sufficient protective gear. Envenomation following snakebite and insect stings accounts for a significant proportion of AKI in tropical countries. Usually the bite or sting is obvious, but it is important to consider this diagnosis even in the absence of overt history if the clinical manifestation are suggestive, because it is well known that snakebites can happen while the subject is asleep, or without the subject recognizing that she has been bitten by a snake, or made contact with a toxic plant. This is also important in the case of children with AKI (Table 14.6).

Table 14.6 Animal, plant, and chemical toxins that can cause AKI in the tropics

Animal poisons	Plant and fungal toxins	Chemical toxins
Snakebites	Herbal medicines	PPD
Wasp, hornet, and bee stings	Impila tubers	Ethylene or propylene glycol
Spider bite	Djenkol beans	Bromide
Jellyfish sting	Marking nut	Chromium
Scorpion sting	Mushroom	Copper sulfate
Carp gallbladder or bile	Plant-derived toxins used as insecticides and to kill fish	
	Oxalate-containing plants	

14.6.2 Snake Envenomation

There are more than 2000 species of snakes worldwide, of which approximately 450 are poisonous. It is estimated that out of the 2.4 million people bitten annually by poisonous snakes, approximately 100,000 die. About 45% of these deaths are reported from India [9]. AKI is an important contributor of these deaths. An additional 400,000 suffer nonfatal severe health consequences, such as AKI, amputation, infection, tetanus, scarring, contractures, and other sequelae attributable to envenomation [10]. Most instances of snake envenomation occur in tropical parts of Asia, Africa, and Latin America [11].

About 12% of all venomous snakebites are complicated by AKI, nearly all of whom following bites by colubrids, elapids, or hydrophids (Fig. 14.1). The species of the snake and the quantity of venom injected determine the clinical manifestations. Viper bites are characterized by florid local swelling, blistering, pain, tender regional lymphadenopathy, hemolysis, bleeding, and hypotension. Sea snake venom is myotoxic, and affected individuals develop myalgia and muscle weakness. Oliguria can develop within a few hours after the bite, or may be delayed for 3–4 days.

AKI is multifactorial in origin, with direct tubular toxicity, pigment-mediated tubular injury secondary to intravascular hemolysis or rhabdomyolysis, disseminated intravascular coagulation, or endothelial injury being the major causative factors. Fluid losses secondary to gastrointestinal symptoms or local infections can also contribute.

Grossly, the kidneys are swollen and appears "flea-bitten" secondary to petechial hemor-

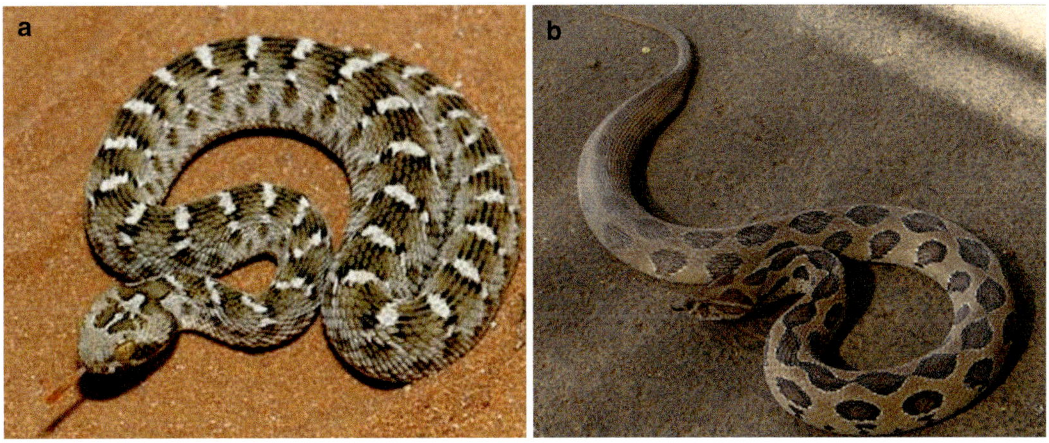

Fig. 14.1 Two common varieties of viper snakes that cause AKI in South Asia. (**a**) Saw-scaled viper (*Echis carinatus*) and (**b**) Russell's viper (*Daboia russelii*)

rhages. Histology shows acute tubular necrosis with intratubular pigment casts in 70–80% of patients, other lesions being thrombotic microangiopathy, mesangiolysis, interstitial inflammation, glomerulonephritis, vasculitis, and renal infarction. Acute cortical necrosis, the most severe form of AKI, is seen in approximately 20–25% of patients after a Russell's viper or Saw-scaled viper bite.

Management consists of wound care, administration of antivenom and supportive treatment. Early antivenom administration prevents or attenuates the development of hematological abnormalities or rhabdomyolysis and AKI. There is no consensus on the dose of antivenom or the duration of therapy. One approach in the case of hemotoxic bites has been to titrate the dose according to the whole-blood clotting time. Some recent studies, however, have shown that the outcomes are similar even with the use of a fixed lower dose of antivenom. Supportive measures include judicious volume replacement, inoculation with antitetanus immunoglobulin, and appropriate management of bleeding risk by the use of fresh frozen plasma as needed. Patients bitten by myotoxic snakes need aggressive fluid therapy and urinary alkalinization to prevent intratubular precipitation of myoglobin. Mortality from snakebite envenomation is estimated to be up to 35%. A substantial proportion, especially those with patchy or diffuse cortical necrosis and thrombotic microangiopathy, is left with varying degrees of renal insufficiency.

14.6.3 Insect Stings

Insects like honeybees, wasps, yellow jackets, and hornets are common in the tropics, and hence stings from these insects are also encountered not infrequently. AKI typically results in individuals who sustain multiple stings from a swarm of insects like honey bees or wasps, resulting in injection of a large dose of toxins. Kidney injury is usually secondary to hemolysis or rhabdomyolysis, though direct toxicity has also been proposed. Less commonly, AKI has been described following isolated stings secondary to anaphylactic reactions or thrombotic microangiopathy [12]. Apart from AKI, proteinuria and nephritic and nephrotic syndromes have also been reported after insect stings [13–15]. The diagnosis is usually obvious. Management is largely supportive and symptomatic, including short course of steroids, antihistamines, fluid replacement, and RRT if necessary.

14.6.4 Obstetric AKI

AKI related to complications of pregnancy (obstetric AKI) has been all but eliminated from developed nontropical economies due to system-wide improvements in healthcare delivery. In contrast, obstetric AKI continues to be encountered in many tropical countries due to suboptimal antenatal care, frequent out-of-hospital childbirth, and unsafe abortion practices.

Obstetric AKI shows a bimodal temporal distribution: the first peak, attributable to hyperemesis gravidarum and septic abortion, is seen in the first trimester. Preeclampsia, eclampsia, placental abruption, postpartum hemorrhage, and puerperal sepsis develop close to term or following delivery and account for the second peak of AKI in third trimester or in the immediate postpartum period. There is a significant variation, however, in the frequency and outcome of obstetric AKI in different parts of tropics. In India, the contribution of obstetric AKI declined from 22% of all cases of AKI in the 1970s to approximately 8% in the 1990s. This decline was attributed to legalization of abortion and improvements in antenatal care [16]. In other parts of the tropics, however, obstetric AKI continues to be prevalent and has a poor prognosis even today. Septic abortion is the cause of AKI in 52% of patients in Ethiopia [17], and in Argentina and Nigeria, gynecological and obstetric complications still account for about one third of patients with AKI [18–20]. In one hospital in Pakistan, of 100 patients with obstetric AKI seen over a 3year period, over 90% needed dialysis, 7% died in hospital, and only 44% were off dialysis at discharge [21]. About 20% of all patients develop acute cortical necrosis, the most catastrophic variety of AKI. In recent years, atypical hemolytic uremic syndrome, secondary to genetic abnormalities in complement regulatory proteins, has been recognized in several cases of third trimester and postpartum AKI (Ramachandran R, unpublished). It is important to identify these cases because they respond well to eculizumab.

14.6.5 Indigenous Medicine and Herb Use and AKI

The use of indigenous remedies of herbal or animal origin is an integral part of traditional cultures in many parts of sub-Saharan Africa and Asia. AKI resulting from ingestion of plant, fungal, and animal nephrotoxins is common in countries in these regions. A variety of renal lesions including acute tubular necrosis, acute cortical necrosis, and interstitial nephritis have been reported [22]. Even some of the commonly ingested tropical plant foods can have toxic effects if consumed without proper preparation (Fig. 14.2). An example is the consumption of beans from the djenkol plant, a delicacy in several Southeast Asian countries [23]. Ingestion of a large amount of uncooked beans, especially in individuals with a low fluid intake, can cause oliguric AKI secondary to the intratubular precipitation of djenkolic acid crystals. The breath and urine of these patients have a characteristic, sulfurous odor, and the needlelike crystals can be seen in urine under light microscopy. Increased fluid intake and urinary alkalinization with sodium bicarbonate help to dissolve the crystals.

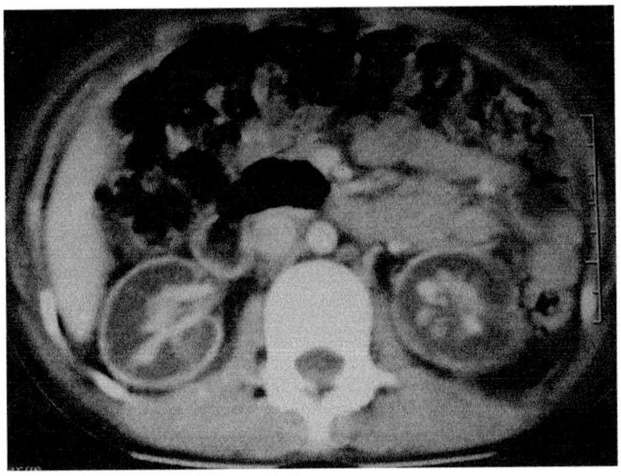

Fig. 14.2 Contrast-enhanced CT scan of a patient with acute cortical necrosis shows non-enhancing renal cortex bound on the outside by a rim of enhancing subcapsular region and on the inside by enhancing medulla

About 25–60% of all cases of AKI from medical causes in hospitals in sub-Saharan Africa are associated with the use of traditional herbal medicines. Such medicines are usually prepared under nonstandard conditions and are not tested for efficacy and safety, the ingredients are variable, and dosage and route of administration are often not standardized.

A large number of cases of AKI in Africa have been associated with use of extracts of impila tubers, which are taken either orally or as an enema for their purgative and vermifugal effects [24]. Atractyloside, an alkaloid that inhibits ATP synthesis, is thought to be the active component. Symptoms appear 1–4 days after consumption and include abdominal pain, vomiting, seizures, oliguria, and jaundice. The mortality rate for impilarelated AKI is over 50%.

Potentially toxic substances like paint thinners, turpentine, chloroxylenol, ginger, pepper, soap, vinegar, copper sulfate, and potassium permanganate are often added to plant extracts in an effort to potentiate their effect [23].

The raw gallbladder or bile of sheep, freshwater carp, and grass carp are used for medicinal purposes in rural areas of the Middle East and South and Southeast Asia [25, 26] and can cause a syndrome of acute hepatic failure and renal failure. Oliguric AKI develops within 48 h and lasts 2–3 weeks. Susceptibility to AKI varies according to the species of fish, the amount of bile ingested, and patient-specific factors. An association has been found between the size of the fish and the severity of the toxic effect. The prognosis is usually good, and mortality has been described only in those who present late and already have multi-organ failure.

14.6.6 Paraphenyldiamine Nephrotoxicity

Paraphenyldiamine (PPD) is used in Africa, Middle East, and Indian subcontinent as a coloring agent, especially as hair dye. Clinical manifestations include cervicofacial edema, high colored urine, oliguria, edema, shock, and oliguric AKI. Direct toxicity, rhabdomyolysis, and hypovolemia contribute to AKI. PPD poisoning is the chief cause of AKI in some tropical African countries.

14.6.7 Infections

14.6.7.1 Malaria

Malaria continues to be a public health challenge throughout the tropical belt. The African region accounted for most global cases of malaria (88%), followed by the Southeast Asia (10%) and the Eastern Mediterranean (2%). In 2015, there were an estimated 438,000 malaria deaths worldwide, with 90% in Africa [27]. Although *P. falciparum* infection accounts for most case of malaria-related AKI, *P. vivax* and *P. knowlesi* infections have also been reported to lead to AKI in recent years [28, 29].

AKI is seen in approximately 1–4% of all patients with *P. falciparum* malaria. The incidence increases to 60% in those with severe disease [27, 30]. Patients with severe parasitemia and children under the age of 5 years, pregnant women, and individuals with HIV or AIDS are at an increased risk [31, 32]. Mortality may be as high as 45%. About 70% of all deaths occur in children below the age of 5. The pathogenesis of malarial AKI is related to clogging of the microvasculature as a result of reduced deformability and increased stickiness of the parasitized erythrocytes that causes them to adhere to each other, other circulating cells, and the vascular endothelium.

The standard method of making a diagnosis is by demonstration of the asexual forms of the parasite in a thick finger-prick blood smear. Simple card tests that use antibodies to detect specific parasitic antigens allow quick diagnosis in the field where microscopy facilities or trained personnel are not available. The sensitivity and specificity of these tests are variable.

Artemisinin-based combination therapies are the recommended treatment for severe malaria with AKI [33]. Early effective antimicrobial treatment and timely renal replacement therapy are associated with improved survival and recovery of renal function in patients with malaria-induced AKI. A comparative study showed continuous renal replacement therapy to be better than peritoneal dialysis in malarial AKI.

14.6.7.2 Leptospirosis

Caused by the spirochete *Leptospira interrogans*, leptospirosis is the most widespread zoonosis in the world and an occupational hazard in fishermen, coal miners, sewage, abattoir, and farm workers throughout the tropics. Human infection occurs when organisms in contaminated water, soil, or vegetation enter abraded skin and exposed mucosa.

The disease presents with a biphasic febrile illness. Renal involvement is seen in the second phase and often presents with cholestatic jaundice and hemorrhagic manifestations (Weil's syndrome). AKI develops in 20–85% of cases and is oliguric in about half. Diagnosis is based on demonstration of anti-leptospira antibodies, either a single titer of >1:400 or a fourfold increase. Nucleic acid based testing has allowed identification of greater number of cases.

Renal injury is caused by direct invasion of the renal tissue by the organism and liberation of bacterial enzymes, metabolites, and endotoxins. Grossly, the kidneys are swollen and bile stained. The main light-microscopic lesion is a tubulointerstitial nephritis, with mononuclear cells and eosinophilic infiltration.

Leptospirosis is self-limiting, and mild cases recover with supportive treatment. Antibiotic therapy can shorten the duration of illness. The elderly and those with multi-organ involvement are at risk of adverse outcome.

Recent data suggests that leptospirosis may have long-term consequences for kidney health. In a community-based study, subjects with high leptospira antibody titers (indicating past infection) were more likely to show a decline in eGFR over a 2-year follow-up.

14.6.7.3 Scrub Typhus

Scrub typhus, caused by a gram-negative bacterium *Orientia tsutsugamushi*, is endemic in Asia and a grossly under-recognized cause of tropical febrile illness. The infection is transmitted to humans by trombiculid mites. A recent study [34] from India, employing a novel PCR-based diagnostic technique, showed that 24% of all patients presenting with unexplained febrile illness and/or multi-system involvement had scrub typhus. AKI was present in over 50% and was an important predictor of mortality. Vascular endothelial cell injury is thought to be the predominant mechanism of injury. Histology shows mesangial hyperplasia, acute tubular necrosis, or tubulointerstitial nephritis. Management entails a short course of doxycycline and supportive care. It has a fatality rate of 30% if untreated.

14.6.7.4 Diarrheal Diseases

AKI related to infective diarrheal diseases continues to be a major problem in tropical countries with poor sanitation, especially among the pediatric population and the elderly [35]. AKI related to diarrheal diseases is more frequent in rural areas and urban slums with inadequate provision of safe drinking water. The incidence increases during summer and rainy seasons. During the 1980s, 35–50% of all children who required dialysis for AKI in India had diarrhea-related AKI [36, 37]. The current incidence of diarrhea-related AKI requiring dialysis has declined to 8% as a result of the improved sanitation and widespread use of oral rehydration solutions [8].

Infective diarrhea may result from a variety of viral, bacterial, and protozoal infections. The clinical presentation provides clues to the identity of the causative pathogen. Early vomiting is a feature of rotavirus infection. Loose, watery stools indicate infection with enterotoxigenic *E. coli* or *Vibrio cholerae*. Fever, cramps, and tenesmus accompanied by bloody diarrhea suggest infection with *Shigella*, *Salmonella*, or enteroinvasive *E. coli*. Diagnosis requires stool microscopy, as with cholera or certain parasites and culture for other organisms.

Early and adequate fluid replacement using WHO-recommended oral rehydration solution (ORS) is the cornerstone of management. The ORS can be easily prepared at home by adding six (6) level teaspoons of sugar and half (1/2) level teaspoon of salt to 1 L of clean drinking or boiled water and then cooled (five cup full, with each cup about 200 mL). This will yield a solution with 75 mmol/L sodium, 65 mmol/L chloride, 20 mmol/L potassium, 10 mmol/L citrate, and 75 mmol/L of anhydrous glucose, with a resultant osmolarity of 245 mosm/L [38]. Intravenous rehydration might be required in patients with severe dehydration, persistent vomiting, or paralytic ileus. Hypokalemia may worsen during rehydration. The mortality rate associated with diarrhea-related AKI remains high in some tropical regions. In a study from Malaysia, the mortality rate was 2.1 per 1000 admissions [39].

In contrast, other tropical countries have practically eliminated diarrhea-associated AKI. An example is the nurse-led program developed by the International Centre for Diarrhoeal Disease Research, Dhaka, Bangladesh, that has achieved a mortality rate of <1%.

14.6.7.5 HIV and AKI

HIV continues to be a major global public health issue and a leading global cause of infectious disease-related mortality, having claimed more than 34 million lives so far. In 2014, about 1.2 million people died from HIV-related causes [40]. The number of new HIV cases and AIDS-related deaths is declining, however. Between 2000 and 2015, new HIV infections and AIDS-related deaths fell by 35% and 24%, respectively. Approximately 36.9 million people were living with HIV globally at the end of 2014, 70% in sub-Saharan Africa [41].

AKI is encountered in over 50% of patients hospitalized with HIV infection [41]. Patients with HIV-AIDS are at high risk of AKI from various factors. Opportunistic infections, especially tuberculosis, volume depletion from chronic diarrhea due to intestinal parasites, the use of nephrotoxic antiretroviral drugs, and contrast agents for medical imaging increase the risk of AKI. HIV infection can give rise to AKI secondary to thrombotic microangiopathy.

AKI in patients with HIV has consequences beyond the acute episode, including an increased risk of cardiovascular events, end-stage renal disease (ESRD), and increased mortality [42]. Antiretroviral drugs used in highly active antiretroviral therapy (HAART), such as tenofovir and indinavir, can cause AKI. AKI in HIV-infected patients (in the HAART era) is associated with a sixfold increase in mortality [41]. Prevention of AKI requires attention to common risk factors like volume depletion and avoidance of nephrotoxic drugs, especially in individuals with preexisting CKD. Management entails maintaining a high index of suspicion, prompt correction of volume deficits, and attention to the list of medications.

14.6.7.6 Dengue Fever

Dengue fever is a mosquito-borne tropical viral infection caused by the dengue virus, often causing flu-like illness and occasionally causing severe disease with complications including AKI. The incidence of dengue has increased exponentially and more than half of the world population is at risk [43]. Dengue is found in tropical and subtropical climates worldwide, mostly in urban and semi-urban areas. The reported incidence of AKI in patients with dengue fever varies from 0.9% among Thai children [44] to 10.8% in reports from India [45]. Dengue was the cause of AKI in 4% of patients in an ICU in Brazil [46]. AKI usually develops in patients with severe disease (dengue hemorrhagic fever) and is frequently associated with hypotension, rhabdomyolysis, hemolysis, or sepsis. There is no specific treatment, and management is essentially supportive in nature. Prevention depends on effective vector control.

14.6.7.7 Post-Infectious Glomerulonephritis

Post-infectious glomerulonephritis (PIGN) is the result of an immunological process triggered by an infection afflicting the kidney, resulting in immune-complex-mediated glomerulonephritis. Though classically associated with streptococcal infection, PIGN can follow any bacterial, viral, fungal, or parasitic infection. Manifestation can be with asymptomatic urinary abnormalities, acute nephritic illness, hypertension, or rapidly progressive glomerulonephritis (more common in adults). While the incidence of PIGN has declined in the high-income countries, it continues to be a common condition in the tropical LMIC, where the burden of infection due to nephritogenic bacteria continues to be high. The burden of group A streptococcal infections was estimated to be 24.3 cases per 100,000 person-years in adults and 2 cases per 100,000 person-years in children in the developing countries [47], compared to 6 and 0.3 cases per 100,000 person-years, respectively, in developed regions. PIGN is primarily seen among children and young adults in developing countries with a male preponderance of 2–3:1, while the patients in the developed world tend to be adults [48]. In a study from India, PIGN was identified as the cause in 86.7% of children who presented with nephritic illness [49] and PIGN accounted for 16.9% of AKI [50].

14.7 Prevention and Treatment

Community-acquired tropical AKI is largely preventable but requires public health policy initiatives and resources directed toward improvement of basic health needs, such as the provision of safe drinking water, improved sanitation, infection control through eradication of parasites and disease-carrying vectors, improvements in the conditions of farm workers, and the provision of good antenatal and obstetric care.

Vector control using an integrated vector management strategy is the most effective way to prevent transmission of vector-borne diseases. This is based on employing a range of interventions, such as rational use of pesticides and mosquito nets on the basis of local knowledge about vectors, disease determinants, and engagement with local communities and other stakeholders within a public health regulatory and legislative framework. Improving public awareness of the need for use of safe water, safe handling and use of pesticides and other nephrotoxins should be attempted by sustained campaigns in mass media.

Since most cases of tropical AKI are encountered in the community where trained healthcare personnel are scarce, nonphysician healthcare workers (NPHW) must be trained to look for early warning signs of AKI, identify those at highest risk for appropriate triage, and prompt referral of patients who need specialist care at secondary or tertiary hospitals. Availability of point-of-care tests will be helpful in this process. The few tests in development include those that measure salivary urea nitrogen or work on an algorithm based on urine color. Early institution of rehydration therapy may limit the severity of AKI. The ISN *0by25* initiative is implementing a clinical trial that will test the hypothesis that NPHW-driven algorithmic triaging will lead to improved outcomes. Figure 14.3 shows a suggested algorithm for risk stratification and referral using locally appropriate point-of-care tests.

In addition to the severity of the disease, poor healthcare systems and the lack of infrastructure are believed to contribute to mortality and morbidity from AKI in the tropics. Even though HD is available in most tropical countries (with the possible exception of a few sub-Saharan African nations), facilities are concentrated in large cities that are often unable to cope with the huge demand for their services. Peritoneal dialysis is often resorted to, especially in remote areas [51] and for small children [52]. In view of the simplicity of technique and minimal technical requirements, the ISN, in association with the International Pediatric Nephrology Association, International Society for Peritoneal Dialysis, and the Sustainable Kidney Care Foundation, is implementing the Saving Young Lives project in tropical countries of Africa and Southeast Asia. Under this project, children with AKI are treated with PD [53].

14.8 Future Challenges

Tropical societies are likely to face major challenges to kidney health as a result of climate change and water scarcity. According to the UK-based risk analysis firm Maplecroft, the top 10 countries at "extreme risk" from climate change are all tropical countries.

Kidneys are likely to be particularly vulnerable to heat stress and the predicted reemergence of water- and vector-borne infectious diseases. Another area of concern is the evolution in the virulence of disease-causing organisms, as noted by emergence of kidney injury in vivax malaria and scrub typhus. This is compounded by emergence of antimicrobial resistance. Degradation of ecosystem and air and water pollution will increase the risk of exposure to environmental toxins that can cause AKI.

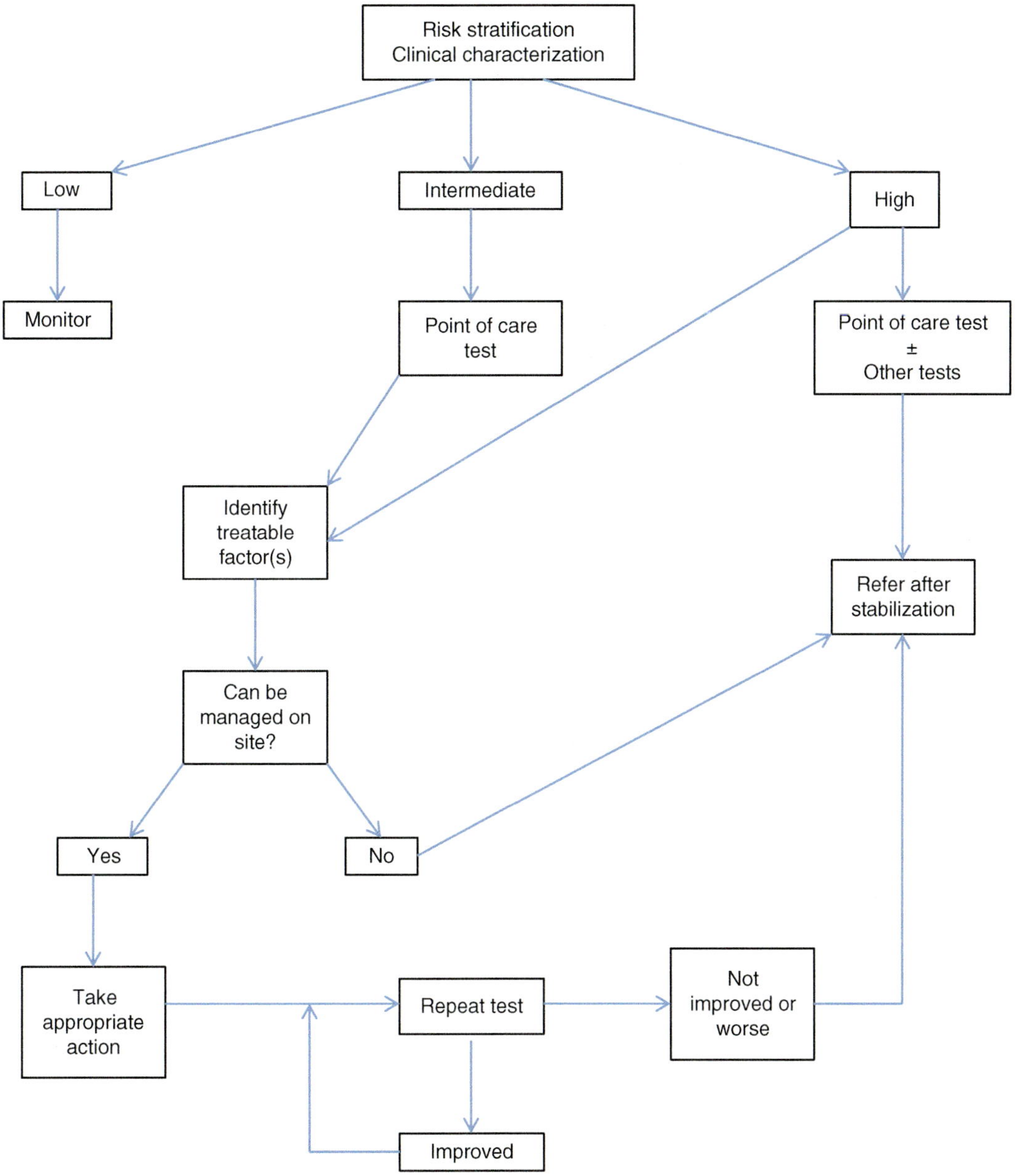

Fig. 14.3 A suggested algorithm for risk stratification, triaging, and referral of community-acquired tropical acute kidney injury

References

1. Cerda J, Bagga A, Kher V, Chakravarthi RM. The contrasting characteristics of acute kidney injury in developed and developing countries. Nat Clin Pract Nephrol. 2008;4:138–53.
2. Tiessen H, Cuevas E, Salcedo IH. Organic matter stability and nutrient availability under temperate and tropical conditions. Adv Geoecol. 1997;31:415–22.
3. Sachs JM. Why tropical countries are underdeveloped. The National Bureau of Economic Research Working Paper Series [online]. 2001. http://www.nber.org/w8119.html.
4. WHO. Health Topics [online]. 2011. http://www.who.int/topics/poverty/en/.
5. Mehta RL, Cerdá J, Burdmann EA, et al. International Society of Nephrology's 0by25 initiative for acute kidney injury (zero preventable deaths by 2025): a human rights case for nephrology. Lancet. 2015;385(9987):2616–43.
6. Mehta RL, Burdmann EA, Cerdá J, et al. Recognition and management of acute kidney injury in the International Society of Nephrology 0by25 global snapshot: a multinational cross-sectional study. Lancet. 2016;387(10032):2017–25.
7. Jha V, Parameswaran S. Community-acquired acute kidney injury in tropical countries. Nat Rev Nephrol. 2013;9:278–90.
8. Basu G, Chrispal A, Boorugu H, et al. Acute kidney injury in tropical acute febrile illness in a tertiary care Centre—RIFLE criteria validation. Nephrol Dial Transplant. 2011;26(2):524–31.
9. Mohapatra B, Warrell DA, Suraweera W, et al. Snakebite mortality in India: a nationally representative mortality survey. PLoS Negl Trop Dis. 2011;5:e1018.
10. http://www.who.int/mediacentre/factsheets/fs373/en/
11. Kasturiratne A, Wickremasinghe AR, de Silva N, et al. The global burden of snakebite: a literature analysis and modelling based on regional estimates of envenoming and deaths. PLoS Med. 2008;5:e218.
12. Kumar V, Nada R, Kumar S, et al. Acute kidney injury due to acute cortical necrosis following a single wasp sting. Ren Fail. 2013;35:170–2.
13. Abdulkader RC, Barbaro KC, Barros EJ, Burdmann EA. Nephrotoxicity of insect and spider venoms in Latin America. Semin Nephrol. 2008;28:373–82.
14. Cuoghi D, Venturi P, Cheli E. Bee sting and relapse of nephrotic syndrome. Child Nephrol Urol. 1988;9:82–3.
15. Vikrant S, Patial RK. Acute renal failure following multiple honeybee stings. Indian J Med Sci. 2006;60:202–4.
16. Chugh KS, Sakhuja V, Malhotra HS, et al. Changing trends in acute renal failure in third-world countries—Chandigarh study. Q J Med. 1989;73:1117–23.
17. Zewdu W. Acute renal failure in Addis Abeba, Ethiopia: a prospective study of 136 patients. Ethiop Med J. 1994;32:79–87.
18. Chijioke A, Makusidi AM, Rafiu MO. Factors influencing hemodialysis and outcome in severe acute renal failure from Ilorin, Nigeria. Saudi J Kidney Dis Transpl. 2012;23:391–6.
19. Okunola OO, Ayodele OE, Adekanle AD. Acute kidney injury requiring hemodialysis in the tropics. Saudi J Kidney Dis Transpl. 2012;23:1315–9.
20. Firmat J, Zucchini A, Martin R, et al. A study of 500 cases of acute renal failure (1978–1991). Ren Fail. 1994;16:91–9.
21. Ali A, Ali MA, Ali MU, et al. Hospital outcomes of obstetrical-related acute renal failure in a tertiary care teaching hospital. Ren Fail. 2011;33:285–90.
22. Luyckx VA, Steenkamp V, Stewart MJ. Acute renal failure associated with the use of traditional folk remedies in South Africa. Ren Fail. 2005;27:35–43.
23. Segasothy M, Swaminathan M, Kong NC, et al. Djenkol bean poisoning (djenkolism): an unusual cause of acute renal failure. Am J Kidney Dis. 1995;25:63–6.
24. Hutchings A, Terblanche SE. Observations on the use of some known and suspected toxic Liliiflorae in Zulu and Xhosa medicine. S Afr Med J. 1989;75:62–9.
25. Centers for Disease Control and Prevention. Hepatic and renal toxicity among patients ingesting sheep bile as an unconventional remedy for diabetes mellitus-Saudi Arabia-1995. MMWR Morb Mortal Wkly Rep. 1996;45:941–3.
26. Park SK, Kim DG, Kang SK, et al. Toxic acute renal failure and hepatitis after ingestion of raw carp bile. Nephron. 1990;56:188–93.
27. http://www.who.int/malaria/media/world-malaria-report-2015/en/
28. Naqvi R, Ahmad E, Akhtar F, et al. Outcome in severe acute renal failure associated with malaria. Nephrol Dial Transplant. 2003:1820–3.
29. Prakash J, Singh AK, Kumar NS, et al. Acute renal failure in Plasmodium vivax malaria. J Assoc Physicians India. 2003;51:265–7.
30. Mehta KS, Halankar AR, Makwana PD, et al. Severe acute renal failure in malaria. J Postgrad Med. 2001;47:24–6.
31. Mishra SK, Das BS. Malaria and acute kidney injury. Semin Nephrol. 2008;28:395–408.
32. Jha V, Chugh KS. In: Ronco C, Bellomo R, Kellum J, editors. Critical care nephrology. Philadelphia: Saunders Elsevier; 2009. p. 850–6.
33. WHO. Guidelines for the treatment of malaria. 2015. http://www.who.int/malaria/publications/atoz/9789241549127/en/.
34. Kumar V, Kumar V, Yadav AK, et al. Scrub typhus is an under-recognized cause of acute febrile illness with acute kidney injury in India. PLoS Negl Trop Dis. 2014;8(1):e2605.
35. Hayat A, Kamili MA, Samia R, et al. Peritoneal dialysis for adults with acute renal failure: an underutilized modality. Saudi J Kidney Dis Transpl. 2007;18:195–9.
36. Choudhry VP, Srivastava RN, Vellodi A, et al. A study of acute renal failure. Indian Pediatr. 1980;17:405–10.

37. Chugh KS, Narang A, Kumar L, et al. Acute renal failure amongst children in a tropical environment. Int J Artif Organs. 1987;10:97–101.
38. WHO Drug information. Vol. 16, No. 2, 2002. http://apps.who.int/medicinedocs/en/d/Js4950e/2.4.html
39. Lee WS, Ooi TL. Deaths following acute diarrhoeal diseases among hospitalised infants in Kuala Lumpur. Med J Malaysia. 1999;54:303–9.
40. http://www.who.int/mediacentre/factsheets/fs360/en/
41. Wyatt CM, Arons RR, Klotman PE, et al. Acute renal failure in hospitalized patients with HIV: risk factors and impact on in-hospital mortality. AIDS. 2006;20:561–5.
42. Choi AI, Li Y, Parikh C, et al. Long-term clinical consequences of acute kidney injury in the HIV-infected. Kidney Int. 2010;78:478–85.
43. WHO Dengue and severe dengue Fact sheet. 2017. http://www.who.int/mediacentre/factsheets/fs117/en/
44. Laoprasopwattana K, Pruekprasert P, Dissaneewate P, et al. Outcome of dengue hemorrhagic fever-caused acute kidney injury in Thai children. J Pediatr. 2010;157:303–9.
45. Mehra N, Patel A, Abraham G, et al. Acute kidney injury in dengue fever using acute kidney injury network criteria: incidence and risk factors. Trop Dr. 2012;42:160–2.
46. Daher EDF, Silva Junior GB, Vieira APF, et al. Acute kidney injury in a tropical country: a cohort study of 253 patients in an infectious diseases intensive care unit. Rev Soc Bras Med Trop. 2014;47:86–9.
47. Carapetis JR, Steer AC, Mulholland EK, et al. The global burden of group a streptococcal diseases. Lancet Infect Dis. 2005;5(11):685–94.
48. Kanjanabuch T, Kittikowit W, Eiam-Ong S. An update on acute postinfectious glomerulo-nephritis worldwide. Nat Rev Nephrol. 2009;5:259–69.
49. Gunasekaran K, Krishnamurthy S, Mahadevan S, et al. Clinical characteristics and outcome of post-infectious glomerulonephritis in children in southern India: a prospective study. Indian J Pediatr. 2015;82(10):896–903.
50. Krishnamurthy S, Mondal N, Narayanan P, et al. Incidence and etiology of acute kidney injury in southern India. Indian J Pediatr. 2013;80(3):183–9.
51. Mohandas N, Chellapandian D. Value of intermittent peritoneal dialysis in rural setup. Indian J Perit Dial. 2004;6:19–20.
52. Kohli HS, Arora P, Kher V, et al. Daily peritoneal dialysis using a surgically placed Tenckhoff catheter for acute renal failure in children. Ren Fail. 1995;17:51–6.
53. Smoyer WE, Finkelstein FO, McCulloch MI, et al. "Saving young lives" with acute kidney injury: the challenge of acute dialysis in low-resource settings. Kidney Int. 2016;89(2):254–6.

Pediatric Acute Kidney Injury: Diagnosis, Epidemiology, and Treatment

15

Elizabeth A. K. Hunt and Michael A. Ferguson

15.1 Introduction

Acute kidney injury (AKI) is classically defined as an abrupt decrease in glomerular filtration rate (GFR), often associated with derangements in metabolic and volume balance.

Recent efforts to standardize AKI definitions have led to a more a robust understanding of populations at risk for AKI as well as the impact on those affected with respect to clinical outcomes. It is now well established that AKI is a common occurrence in hospitalized children, both in the intensive care unit and general inpatient setting. In addition, there is emerging evidence that AKI of any severity confers a higher risk of morbidity and mortality in the short-term as well as an increased likelihood of developing chronic kidney disease (CKD) over the long-term. This chapter provides an overview of the current understanding of pediatric AKI with respect to diagnosis, epidemiology, treatment, and outcomes.

E. A. K. Hunt
Department of Pediatrics, Division of Pediatric Nephrology, University of Vermont Medical Center, Larner College of Medicine at UVM, Burlington, VT, USA
e-mail: liz.hunt@uvmhealth.org

M. A. Ferguson (✉)
Division of Nephrology, Department of Medicine, Boston Children's Hospital, Harvard Medical School, Boston, MA, USA
e-mail: michael.ferguson@childrens.harvard.edu

15.2 Diagnosis of AKI: Definitions and Limitations

Multiple definitions and classification schema for AKI have been developed for use in adults (see Chap. 2), all of which have been studied for use in pediatrics. The RIFLE (risk, injury, failure, loss, end-stage kidney disease) criterion was developed by the Acute Dialysis Quality Initiative group in 2004 [1] in an attempt to standardize the definition of AKI by stratifying patients based on changes in serum creatinine and/or urine output. The pediatric RIFLE (pRIFLE) criteria were adapted from the RIFLE criteria in 2007 [2] and used changes in estimated glomerular filtration as calculated with the Schwartz formula rather than changes in serum creatinine to stratify severity. Subsequently, pRIFLE has been studied and validated primarily in critically ill children [2–4] and children who have undergone cardiac surgery [5, 6]. In general, pRIFLE has been shown to be a useful classification system for not only diagnosing AKI but also for providing prognostic information with respect to morbidity and mortality in those affected.

More recently, the Acute Kidney Injury Network (AKIN) modified the RIFLE criteria to include an absolute increase in serum creatinine concentration of $\geq$0.3 mg/dL from baseline. The AKIN criteria have not been modified specifically for use in children, though have been used in multiple pediatric studies, primarily in the ICU

S. S. Waikar et al. (eds.), *Core Concepts in Acute Kidney Injury*,
https://doi.org/10.1007/978-1-4939-8628-6_15

Table 15.1 Comparison of AKI diagnostic criteria

Definition	AKI stages		
pRIFLE	R: eGFR[a] decreased by 25%	I: eGFR[a] decreased by 50%	F: eGFR[a] decreased by 75% or eGFR* <35 mL/mn/1.73m^2
AKIN	1: Increase in sCr of ≥50% or Absolute increase in sCr of ≥0.3 mg/dL	2: Increase in sCr of ≥100%	3: Increase in sCr ≥200%
KDIGO	1: Increase in sCr ≥50% or Absolute increase in sCr of ≥0.3 mg/dL	2: Increase in sCr of ≥100%	3: Increase in sCr of ≥200% or eGFR ≤35 mL/min/1.73m^2 (if age <18 year)

pRIFLE pediatric RIFLE, *AKIN* Acute Kidney Injury Network, *KDIGO* kidney disease improving global outcomes, *eGFR* estimated glomerular filtration rate, *sCr* serum creatinine
[a]eGFR calculated using the bedside Schwartz formula

setting [7–9]. More recently, the KDIGO definition was published in 2012 and defines and stages AKI according to changes in serum creatinine and urine output [10]. There were no specific adjustments made for children. As it is the newest definition, there are fewer studies using it in children; however, there is a general movement toward adopting this definition, and the most recent, larger-scale studies have used the KDIGO definition. Currently, there is not one universally accepted AKI definition, making comparison of findings across studies challenging. It should be noted that all of the above AKI definitions include urine output criteria. However, due to the difficulty in obtaining accurate measurements of urine output, particularly in retrospective studies, these data are often not available. Thus, there is limited data regarding the etiology, outcomes, and impact of pediatric AKI as defined by urine output. Table 15.1 compares the definitions described.

Clinically, AKI is generally diagnosed following an increase in serum creatinine or a decrease in urine output. Unfortunately, these metrics have significant limitations and result in delayed recognition of AKI, especially in children. Changes in serum creatinine are not timely markers of kidney injury because a sudden drop in GFR to a constant low level is typically reflected by a gradual increase in serum creatinine until the patient reaches a new steady state [11]. In general, patients with more severe AKI take longer to reach a new steady state, which delays determination of the severity of injury [12]. The rate of rise is further altered by factors unrelated to renal function, such as volume of distribution, tubular secretion of creatinine, as well as creatinine generation. Thus, at the time a patient is noted to have AKI, the GFR may be much lower than that estimated using the serum creatinine. The inverse is true as AKI resolves and GFR recovers. The improvement in serum creatinine lags behind and as a result renal function may be underestimated during the phase of renal recovery.

In addition, there is day-to-day and site-to-site variability between serum creatinine levels which complicate interpretation of serum creatinine changes. This is especially problematic in children as there is more variation in patients with lower serum creatinine [13, 14].

15.3 Novel Biomarkers for the Diagnosis of AKI

Over the last decade, there has been considerable effort dedicated to the discovery and characterization of novel biomarkers that may allow for increased sensitivity and specificity for the detection of AKI (see Chap. 3). A number of these biomarkers, including neutrophil gelatinase-associated lipocalin (NGAL), kidney injury molecule-1 (KIM-1), interleukin-18 (IL-18), and liver-type fatty acid binding protein (L-FABP), have been studied in the pediatric population. Some of the most important early studies characterizing these biomarkers in humans included pediatric patients at risk for AKI in the setting of cardiac corrective or palliative surgery. In many respects, this cohort represents an ideal population to study given the ability to recruit subjects prospectively and closely approximate the timing of AKI onset. Early studies suggested that some of these biomarkers had superior performance characteristics for the early detection of AKI. For example, Mishra et al. [15] reported that urinary NGAL levels in excess of 50 mc/L 2 h after cardiopulmonary bypass (CBP) were predictive of development of AKI, diagnosed by increased serum creatinine 24–72 h after CPB with a nearly perfect under the receiver-operating characteristic curve of 0.998 (sensitivity 1.00, specificity 0.98). Secondary analyses of a subset of samples from Mishra's original study demonstrated that urinary IL-18 [16], KIM-1 [17], and L-FABP [18] were also early predictive biomarkers of AKI after CPB, though with less robust performance characteristics than NGAL. Numerous additional studies have further characterized candidate AKI biomarkers in a variety of pediatric populations including premature infants, newborns, critically ill older children, and those exposed to nephrotoxins.

Despite the work described above, serum creatinine remains the metric most widely used clinically to diagnose AKI. There remains optimism that further efforts toward biomarker discovery and validation will eventually enable earlier diagnosis of AKI, ultimately leading to improved outcomes. The inclusion of diverse pediatric populations in future research in this area will be critically important. It is quite likely that biomarker profiles in children with or at risk for AKI will vary depending on age and stage of development and will prove quite distinct from those in adults, particularly those with significant comorbidities (diabetes, hypertension, etc.).

15.4 Pediatric AKI Etiology and Risk Factors

A comparison of historical and more recent studies of AKI in children indicates a clear shift in AKI etiology over the last two to three decades. Data from the 1980s–1990s suggest that AKI was most commonly caused by primary renal disease, including hemolytic uremic syndrome (HUS) and glomerulonephritis, with secondary causes of renal disease, including sepsis and burns, which is less common [19, 20]. Over time, secondary causes of AKI have become increasingly more common. In a single-center study, Williams et al. [21] noted a sharp increase of oncologic diagnoses as a cause of AKI from 1978–1988 when compared to 1988–1998 (8% vs. 17%) with HUS simultaneously becoming less common (38% vs. 22%). Studies performed more recently clearly demonstrate that this trend has continued and that AKI in childhood is now most commonly caused by some other systemic illness (sepsis, cardiac disease, oncologic disease) and medically related therapies (ECMO, surgery, nephrotoxic medications) as opposed to primary kidney disease [2, 22–24]. It is likely that with improvements in critical care more children are surviving to develop AKI, explaining the evolution in terms of underlying etiology.

Today, it is clear that sicker children are at increased risk for AKI. Multiple studies have shown that illness severity (often as measured by the pediatric risk of mortality [PRISM] score) is associated with AKI [2, 25–27]. In burn patients, higher body surface area (BSA) was associated with increased AKI risk [25]. Other risk factors include sepsis [2, 25, 28], hematologic/malignant diagnoses [29], and cardiac surgery (with more complex cardiac surgeries being associated with increased risk) [30]. Not surprisingly, children receiving longer courses of aminoglycosides [29] and those receiving increasing number of nephrotoxic medications concomitantly [31] have an increased risk of AKI.

In adults, there are clear data that preexisting CKD increases risk for developing AKI; however, there are limited prospective studies in children, and retrospective studies have yielded conflicting results. That being said, given the reduced renal reserve present in those with CKD, it seems logical that those with CKD would be at a higher risk for AKI in the setting of intercurrent illness, nephrotoxic medication exposure, and/or surgical intervention.

15.5 Epidemiology of Pediatric AKI and Short-Term Outcomes

Determining the epidemiology of AKI in children is complicated by the different criteria used to define AKI as well as lack of available baseline serum creatinine values in many of the populations studied. The reported incidence of AKI varies by population and definition. The most studied pediatric patient population is those who are critically ill. There is increasing recognition that infants should be considered as a distinct population. Epidemiology of this population will be reviewed separately.

Wide ranges in the incidence of AKI (10–82%) have been reported in critically ill children using pRIFLE criteria [2, 4, 27]. Multiple studies have demonstrated that AKI as defined by pRIFLE criteria is associated with increased mortality (which generally increases with stage of AKI) and increased length of stay, even after adjusting for illness severity and other known risk factors [2–4, 25, 32]. These studies also generally report that there is increased need for renal replacement therapy (RRT) with increasing stages of AKI.

Using AKIN criteria, incidences are typically slightly lower than with pRIFLE, ranging from 33 to 65% in critically ill patients [32–34]. There is less data regarding the incidence of AKI in critically ill children using KDIGO criteria, but there are several large, good-quality studies. Selewski et al. found an incidence of 24.5% in a combined pediatric intensive care unit (PICU)/cardiac intensive care unit (CICU) cohort [26], and Sutherland et al. found an incidence of 42% in a PICU population [33]. For both KDIGO and AKIN definitions, AKI in PICU patients was associated with increased mortality and length of stay even in multivariate analysis. Increases in mortality are particularly impressive when using KDIGO criteria. Selewski [26] and Sutherland [33] reported an increased mortality in those with AKI when compared with those without AKI from 1.1% to 11.1% and 2.3% to 15.3%, respectively. There is only one large-scale prospective study of AKI in the pediatric ICU (PICU) population, which is the AWARE study that included 32 PICUs worldwide. Kaddourah et al. defined AKI using KDIGO criteria and found an overall incidence of 26.9% (15.3% stage 1, 6.3% stage 2, and 5.3% stage 3). Severe AKI (stage 2 or 3) was associated with increased risk of death (OR 2.41–5.14) after adjustment for illness severity score (PRISM-III, PIM-2, or PELOD depending on the center). Stage 1 was not associated with increased mortality, but any AKI was (OR ranging from 1.87 to 3.91 depending on illness severity score.) Patients with stage 1 AKI had longer ICU stays and longer mechanical ventilation than those with no AKI [35].

There is less data regarding the incidence and outcomes of AKI in the noncritically ill or general pediatric population. Logically, one would expect a lower incidence than in critically ill children; however, the incidence still appears to be significant. Patients receiving ≥72 h of aminoglycosides had an AKI incidence of 56% using pRIFLE and 45.2% using AKIN criteria [34]. A similar study of patients administered aminoglycosides reported incidences of 33% using pRIFLE and 20% using AKIN [29]. In a retrospective review of hospitalized children at higher risk for AKI (defined as having a baseline creatinine within 3 months before hospital admission), Sutherland and colleagues [33] reported an overall incidence of 51.1% using pRIFLE, 37.3% using AKIN, and 40.3% using KDIGO. Surprisingly, the incidence of AKI in the ICU and non-ICU population was similar across all definitions (pRIFLE, 51.3% vs. 51.0%; AKIN, 39.9% vs. 37.6%; KDIGO, 42% vs. 40.5%). There was no significant association between AKI and mortality in the non-ICU population; however, AKI was associated with longer lengths of stay across all definitions, and lengths of stay increased with AKI stage, except that patients with pRIFLE stage 3 was shorter than those with stage 2. An additional study which used ICD-9 diagnosis codes in a nationally representative sample of noncritically ill hospitalized children reported a much lower incidence of 0.39% [24]. This dramatic difference in reported incidence is likely related to the fact that many patients who meet criteria for AKI don't receive an appropriate diagnosis. In one study of noncritically ill children receiving nephrotoxins, 58% more patients were classified as having AKI using pRIFLE criteria when compared to ICD-9 codes [36], suggesting that strict reliance on administrative data to identify cases of AKI in retrospective studies is unreliable.

15.6 Special Population: Neonates

There is emerging consensus that neonates should be considered separately from other children due to differences in renal physiology after birth and during the first few months of life as well as the potential for interruption of nephrogenesis in premature infants. Nephrogenesis begins at week 5 of gestation with a full complement of nephrons typically achieved reached by 34–36 weeks [37]. There are limited studies of kidneys of premature infants, but those that exist suggest that prematurity, IUGR, and AKI all result in decreased nephrogenesis and that former premature infants are at increased risk for CKD, proteinuria, and hypertension as they age. The normal GFR in term neonates at birth is 10–20 mL/min/1.73 m^2 and increases to 30–40 mL/min/1.73 m^2 by 2 weeks of life. The initial GFR is lower and improves more slowly in preterm infants [38]. In addition, immediately after birth, the infant's serum creatinine reflects maternal creatinine. Thus, interpreting changes in creatinine can be challenging in the neonatal period, and this population may require different standards to diagnose AKI.

AKI appears to be quite common in neonatal intensive care unit (NICU) patients. Studies of very low and extremely low birth weight infants (defined as birth weight of <1500 g and < 1000 g, respectively) reported incidences between 12.5 (using an alternative definition of urine output <1 mL/kg/h for at least 24 h or serum creatinine >1.5 mg/dL) and 39.8% (using KIDGO definition) [39, 40]. Two studies of newborns undergoing therapeutic cooling for treatment of significant perinatal asphyxia reported incidences of 38% using KDIGO and 41.7% using AKIN [41, 42]. Extracorporeal membranous oxygenation (ECMO) is also associated with AKI as defined by RIFLE criteria with one study suggesting an incidence of 64% [43]. The incidence of AKI defined by AKIN is also high in newborns and infants requiring cardiac corrective or palliative surgery, with rates reported as high as 62% in those <28 days [44] and 52% in those <90 days [45]. Other reported risk factors include low birth weight, low gestational age, maternal and infant NSAID use, and sepsis as well as the presence of signs of perinatal stress including low APGARs, low cord pH, asystole, and intubation at birth [46–50]. As in older children, outcomes for infants with AKI appear to be worse after adjustment for confounders with studies showing increased mortality, hospital length of stay, and increased likelihood of abnormal brain MRI at 7–10 days of life [39, 42, 46, 49, 51, 52].

In 2012, Askenazi and Jetton [53] proposed a standardized classification system for neonatal AKI based on the KDIGO definition. The neonatal modified KDIGO criteria are described in Table 15.2. In 2013, a group of neonatologists and pediatric nephrologists reached consensus that this definition represented a reasonable starting point to provide standardization for future studies. Utilization of this definition moving forward will help facilitate comparison of findings across studies.

Table 15.2 Neonatal modified KDIGO AKI criteria

Stage	Creatinine	Urine output
0	No change in sCr or increase <0.3 mg/dL	≥0.5 mL/kg/h
1	sCr increase of ≥0.3 mg/dL within 48 h or sCr increase ≥1.5–1.9 × baseline sCr within 7 days	<0.5 mL/kg/h for 6–12 h
2	sCr rise ≥2–2.9 × baseline sCr	<0.5 mL/kg/h for ≥12 h
3	sCr rise ≥3 × baseline sCr or sCr ≥2.5 mg/dL or RRT initiated	<0.3 mL/kg/h for ≥24 h or anuria for ≥12 h

sCr serum creatinine, *RRT* renal replacement therapy

15.7 Management of Pediatric AKI

To date, there is no clear evidence that any intervention decreases the likelihood of children developing AKI or hastens recovery from it. As a result, treatment is generally supportive and involves removing or treating any known triggers of AKI and attempting to avoid added renal injury. Avoiding further nephrotoxin exposure and ensuring adequate renal perfusion are important to avoid further damage and to promote renal recovery. In addition, meticulous attention to fluid status with strict monitoring of intake and output and daily weights is helpful to prevent volume excess. Prompt reduction of fluid rates in children with oliguria/anuria is critical as even modest degrees of volume overload may contribute to respiratory or cardiac compromise due to smaller body size.

There is a growing body of evidence that volume excess contributes to poor outcomes in critically ill children who require renal replacement therapy (RRT). Multiple small, single-center studies of PICU patients undergoing continuous renal replacement therapy (CRRT) have shown that patients who do not survive AKI tend to have a higher percent fluid overload, but multivariate analysis including illness severity scores has generally showed borderline association [54–56]. Two larger studies reported more compelling results. A prospective study of 297 children undergoing CRRT at 13 centers showed an adjusted odds ratio (OR) mortality of 1.03 (1.01–1.05) for fluid overload, suggesting a 3% increase in mortality for each 1% fluid overload. When fluid overload was dichotomized into <20% and ≥20%, the adjusted OR was 8.5 [57]. This was corroborated by a retrospective single-center study of 190 children undergoing CRRT in which a multivariate analysis showed that percent fluid overload was associated with mortality. Hazard ratio for death was also increased, even when adjusted for timing of CRRT initiation and illness severity score [58]. Some of these studies also suggest that earlier initiation of CRRT may be associated with improved survival. Further research is needed to better understand optimal timing of CRRT initiation and what degree of fluid overload requires RRT initiation.

Once a patient is determined to have severe AKI, they may require RRT for solute clearance as well as fluid removal. Indications for initiation include fluid overload, electrolyte or acid-base derangements refractory to medical therapy, and symptomatic uremia. Patients may also require RRT for removal of nephrotoxins such as CT contrast, which can further exacerbate AKI. The treatment modality of choice depends on patient characteristics as well as center expertise. In patients who are more stable and are likely to tolerate more rapid fluid shifts, intermittent hemodialysis (IHD) is an option. This modality provides the most efficient clearance and is most amenable to running without anticoagulation. Traditionally, it is initiated in a stepwise fashion with progressively increased urea reduction on successive days to avoid dialysis disequilibrium syndrome. The length of treatment time depends on patient size, access, and clearance desired. When patients are acutely ill, HD treatments are generally provided daily.

If patients are less stable or are unlikely to tolerate more rapid fluid shifts, CRRT is often a better choice for RRT. Short-term clearance is lower with CRRT due to lower blood and dialysate flows, but over time, CRRT can be adjusted to provide comparable clearance to HD, and fluid removal can be continuously adjusted, which permits optimizing provision of nutrition and transfusions. CRRT can provide clearance through diffusion and/or convection, and modalities and protocols are institution dependent. Close attention to electrolyte balance is critical as pateints can develop hypokalemia and hypophosphatemia depending on dialysate solutions and replacement fluids. Also, medications need to be dosed appropriately for all forms of RRT, especially antibiotics and sedation.

Pediatric-specific considerations for both IHD and CRRT include catheter selection, blood flow rate, and treatment time, all of which are determined by patient size and clinical stability. In addition attention must be paid to the priming solution. Options include saline, albumin, or blood. In small patients, if the extracorporeal circuit volume is more than 10% of the patient's estimated blood volume, the circuit should be primed with blood to prevent hemodilution leading to instability. In unstable patients who do not require priming with blood, priming with albumin may be of utility. In most other patients, saline can be used for priming. Generally, anticoagulation for RRT is provided with citrate or heparin. Other agents are available for those with complicating factors precluding the use of heparin. Occasionally, in patients with coagulopathies, CRRT can be provided without anticoagulation though circuit survival may be compromised in this setting.

Peritoneal dialysis (PD) is another option for RRT in AKI. It is often the modality of choice in infants due to the challenges of placing a large catheter for hemodialysis and challenges maintaining blood flows necessary for dialysis machines. In addition, infants typically require a blood prime for both HD and CRRT, which can result in sensitization, complicating future transplantation. PD eliminates this blood exposure, allows gradual fluid removal, and does not require anticoagulation. The challenges of PD include catheter leakage (which is more common when initiated in the acute setting) and lack of precise control over fluid removal and clearance. When PD is initiated acutely, lower dwell volumes are employed to avoid leaking around the catheter prior to healing. In this setting, solute clearance through PD is not as efficient as that achieved with HD or CRRT. PD is contraindicated in patients with recent abdominal surgery or infection and is relatively contraindicated in patients with VP shunts.

Given the described advantages and limitations of each modality, the modality of dialysis for those with AKI should be determined based on the above-noted factors, the local expertise and resources available, and the expected length of therapy required whenever possible.

15.8 Long-Term Outcomes

There is limited information about long-term outcomes of children after AKI, though emerging reports suggest significant chronic sequelae. Mammen et al. [59] showed an incidence of chronic kidney disease (CKD), defined as estimated GFR <60 mL/min/1.73 m^2 and/or albuminuria, of 10.3% at 1–3-year follow-up. Another 46.8% were deemed at risk for CKD due to findings of more mild reductions in GFR (60–90 mL/min/1.72 m^2), hypertension, and/or hyperfiltration. The study was small (n = 126), but there were no differences between those with CKD and those without in terms of underlying diagnoses, severity of illness scores, or nephrotoxin exposure. Patients with more severe AKI (AKIN stage 3) demonstrated an increased trend toward CKD development, though this did not reach statistical significance. There were significantly more patients who required dialysis that developed CKD. Askenazi [60] and colleagues reported 3–5-year outcomes of a cohort of children who developed AKI at a single center between 1998 and 2001. Of 174 patients who survived to hospital discharge, 32 subsequently died, and 16 developed end-stage renal disease. Of the 126 remaining survivors, 29 (23%) were recruited to participate in a study to assess renal injury. Of these children, 59% had at least one sign of chronic renal injury, including microalbuminuria (31%), hyperfiltration (31%), decreased GFR (14%), and hypertension (21%). Of concern, a pediatric nephrologist was involved in the care of only 35% of patients with evidence of chronic renal injury. These small, relatively short-term follow-up studies not only indicate that children with a history of AKI are at significantly increased risk for developing CKD over time but also suggest they are likely under-recognized and not being followed appropriately for such complications. Larger prospective studies are necessary to confirm these findings.

Conclusion

AKI is common in hospitalized children and associated with poorer outcomes, including increased mortality in ICU patients and increased length of stay in ICU and non-ICU patients. In addition, childhood survivors of childhood AKI are at high risk for complications including CKD, hypertension, and proteinuria. Future investigations should include established standardized definitions of pediatric AKI to further clarify at-risk populations and long-term outcomes. It will be important to study children from a variety of populations, as AKI susceptibility and recovery is very likely to be unique depending on age, developmental stage, as well as the presence of preexisting comorbidities.

References

1. Bellomo R, Ronco C, Kellum JA, Mehta RL, Palevsky P. Acute Dialysis Quality Initiative w. Acute renal failure—definition, outcome measures, animal models, fluid therapy and information technology needs: the Second International Consensus Conference of the Acute Dialysis Quality Initiative (ADQI) Group. Crit Care. 2004;8(4):R204–12. https://doi.org/10.1186/cc2872.
2. Akcan-Arikan A, Zappitelli M, Loftis LL, Washburn KK, Jefferson LS, Goldstein SL. Modified RIFLE criteria in critically ill children with acute kidney injury. Kidney Int. 2007;71(10):1028–35. https://doi.org/10.1038/sj.ki.5002231.
3. Bresolin N, Bianchini AP, Haas CA. Pediatric acute kidney injury assessed by pRIFLE as a prognostic factor in the intensive care unit. Pediatr Nephrol. 2013;28(3):485–92. https://doi.org/10.1007/s00467-012-2357-8.
4. Schneider J, Khemani R, Grushkin C, Bart R. Serum creatinine as stratified in the RIFLE score for acute kidney injury is associated with mortality and length of stay for children in the pediatric intensive care unit. Crit Care Med. 2010;38(3):933–9. https://doi.org/10.1097/CCM.0b013e3181cd12e1.
5. dos Santos El Halal MG, Carvalho PR. Acute kidney injury according to pediatric RIFLE criteria is associated with negative outcomes after heart surgery in children. Pediatr Nephrol. 2013;28(8):1307–14. https://doi.org/10.1007/s00467-013-2495-7.
6. Ricci Z, Di Nardo M, Iacoella C, Netto R, Picca S, Cogo P. Pediatric RIFLE for acute kidney injury diagnosis and prognosis for children undergoing cardiac surgery: a single-center prospective observational study. Pediatr Cardiol. 2013;34(6):1404–8. https://doi.org/10.1007/s00246-013-0662-z.
7. Bagga A, Bakkaloglu A, Devarajan P, Mehta RL, Kellum JA, Shah SV, et al. Improving outcomes from acute kidney injury: report of an initiative. Pediatr Nephrol. 2007;22(10):1655–8. https://doi.org/10.1007/s00467-007-0565-4.
8. Mehta RL, Kellum JA, Shah SV, Molitoris BA, Ronco C, Warnock DG, et al. Acute Kidney Injury Network: report of an initiative to improve outcomes in acute kidney injury. Crit Care. 2007;11(2):R31. https://doi.org/10.1186/cc5713.
9. Ozcakar ZB, Yalcinkaya F, Altas B, Ergun H, Kendirli T, Ates C, et al. Application of the new classification criteria of the Acute Kidney Injury Network: a pilot study in a pediatric population. Pediatr Nephrol. 2009;24(7):1379–84. https://doi.org/10.1007/s00467-009-1158-1.
10. Khwaja A. KDIGO clinical practice guidelines for acute kidney injury. Nephron Clin Pract. 2012;120(4):c179–84. https://doi.org/10.1159/000339789.
11. Moran SM, Myers BD. Course of acute renal failure studied by a model of creatinine kinetics. Kidney Int. 1985;27(6):928–37.
12. Waikar SS, Bonventre JV. Creatinine kinetics and the definition of acute kidney injury. J Am Soc Nephrol. 2009;20(3):672–9. https://doi.org/10.1681/ASN.2008070669.
13. Carobene A, Ceriotti F, Infusino I, Frusciante E, Panteghini M. Evaluation of the impact of standardization process on the quality of serum creatinine determination in Italian laboratories. Clin Chim Acta. 2014;427:100–6. https://doi.org/10.1016/j.cca.2013.10.001.
14. Komenda P, Beaulieu M, Seccombe D, Levin A. Regional implementation of creatinine measurement standardization. J Am Soc Nephrol. 2008;19(1):164–9. https://doi.org/10.1681/ASN.2007020156.
15. Mishra J, Dent C, Tarabishi R, Mitsnefes MM, Ma Q, Kelly C, et al. Neutrophil gelatinase-associated lipocalin (NGAL) as a biomarker for acute renal injury after cardiac surgery. Lancet. 2005;365(9466):1231–8. https://doi.org/10.1016/S0140-6736(05)74811-X.
16. Parikh CR, Mishra J, Thiessen-Philbrook H, Dursun B, Ma Q, Kelly C, et al. Urinary IL-18 is an early predictive biomarker of acute kidney injury after cardiac surgery. Kidney Int. 2006;70(1):199–203. https://doi.org/10.1038/sj.ki.5001527.
17. Han WK, Waikar SS, Johnson A, Betensky RA, Dent CL, Devarajan P, et al. Urinary biomarkers in the early diagnosis of acute kidney injury. Kidney Int. 2008;73(7):863–9. https://doi.org/10.1038/sj.ki.5002715.
18. Portilla D, Dent C, Sugaya T, Nagothu KK, Kundi I, Moore P, et al. Liver fatty acid-binding protein as a biomarker of acute kidney injury after cardiac surgery. Kidney Int. 2008;73(4):465–72. https://doi.org/10.1038/sj.ki.5002721.
19. Andreoli SP. Acute renal failure. Curr Opin Pediatr. 2002;14(2):183–8.
20. Flynn JT. Choice of dialysis modality for management of pediatric acute renal failure. Pediatr Nephrol. 2002;17(1):61–9. https://doi.org/10.1007/s004670200011.
21. Williams DM, Sreedhar SS, Mickell JJ, Chan JC. Acute kidney failure: a pediatric experience over 20 years. Arch Pediatr Adolesc Med. 2002;156(9):893–900.
22. Ball EF, Kara T. Epidemiology and outcome of acute kidney injury in New Zealand children. J Paediatr Child Health. 2008;44(11):642–6. https://doi.org/10.1111/j.1440-1754.2008.01373.x.

23. Hui-Stickle S, Brewer ED, Goldstein SL. Pediatric ARF epidemiology at a tertiary care center from 1999 to 2001. Am J Kidney Dis. 2005;45(1):96–101.
24. Sutherland SM, Ji J, Sheikhi FH, Widen E, Tian L, Alexander SR, et al. AKI in hospitalized children: epidemiology and clinical associations in a national cohort. Clin J Am Soc Nephrol. 2013;8(10):1661–9. https://doi.org/10.2215/CJN.00270113.
25. Palmieri T, Lavrentieva A, Greenhalgh D. An assessment of acute kidney injury with modified RIFLE criteria in pediatric patients with severe burns. Intensive Care Med. 2009;35(12):2125–9. https://doi.org/10.1007/s00134-009-1638-6.
26. Selewski DT, Cornell TT, Heung M, Troost JP, Ehrmann BJ, Lombel RM, et al. Validation of the KDIGO acute kidney injury criteria in a pediatric critical care population. Intensive Care Med. 2014;40(10):1481–8. https://doi.org/10.1007/s00134-014-3391-8.
27. Slater MB, Anand V, Uleryk EM, Parshuram CS. A systematic review of RIFLE criteria in children, and its application and association with measures of mortality and morbidity. Kidney Int. 2012;81(8):791–8. https://doi.org/10.1038/ki.2011.466.
28. Plotz FB, Bouma AB, van Wijk JA, Kneyber MC, Bokenkamp A. Pediatric acute kidney injury in the ICU: an independent evaluation of pRIFLE criteria. Intensive Care Med. 2008;34(9):1713–7. https://doi.org/10.1007/s00134-008-1176-7.
29. Zappitelli M, Moffett BS, Hyder A, Goldstein SL. Acute kidney injury in non-critically ill children treated with aminoglycoside antibiotics in a tertiary healthcare centre: a retrospective cohort study. Nephrol Dial Transplant. 2011;26(1):144–50. https://doi.org/10.1093/ndt/gfq375.
30. Lex DJ, Toth R, Cserep Z, Alexander SI, Breuer T, Sapi E, et al. A comparison of the systems for the identification of postoperative acute kidney injury in pediatric cardiac patients. Ann Thorac Surg. 2014;97(1):202–10. https://doi.org/10.1016/j.athoracsur.2013.09.014.
31. Moffett BS, Goldstein SL. Acute kidney injury and increasing nephrotoxic-medication exposure in noncritically-ill children. Clin J Am Soc Nephrol. 2011;6(4):856–63. https://doi.org/10.2215/CJN.08110910.
32. Kavaz A, Ozcakar ZB, Kendirli T, Ozturk BB, Ekim M, Yalcinkaya F. Acute kidney injury in a paediatric intensive care unit: comparison of the pRIFLE and AKIN criteria. Acta Paediatr. 2012;101(3):e126–9. https://doi.org/10.1111/j.1651-2227.2011.02526.x.
33. Sutherland SM, Byrnes JJ, Kothari M, Longhurst CA, Dutta S, Garcia P, et al. AKI in hospitalized children: comparing the pRIFLE, AKIN, and KDIGO definitions. Clin J Am Soc Nephrol. 2015;10(4):554–61. https://doi.org/10.2215/CJN.01900214.
34. Zappitelli M, Parikh CR, Akcan-Arikan A, Washburn KK, Moffett BS, Goldstein SL. Ascertainment and epidemiology of acute kidney injury varies with definition interpretation. Clin J Am Soc Nephrol. 2008;3(4):948–54. https://doi.org/10.2215/CJN.05431207.
35. Kaddourah A, Basu RK, Bagshaw SM, Goldstein SL, AWARE Investigators. Epidemiology of acute kidney injury in critically ill children and young adults. N Engl J Med. 2017;376(1):11–20. https://doi.org/10.1056/NEJMoa1611391.
36. Schaffzin JK, Dodd CN, Nguyen H, Schondelmeyer A, Campanella S, Goldstein SL. Administrative data misclassifies and fails to identify nephrotoxin-associated acute kidney injury in hospitalized children. Hosp Pediatr. 2014;4(3):159–66. https://doi.org/10.1542/hpeds.2013-0116.
37. Hinchliffe SA, Sargent PH, Howard CV, Chan YF, van Velzen D. Human intrauterine renal growth expressed in absolute number of glomeruli assessed by the disector method and Cavalieri principle. Lab Investig. 1991;64(6):777–84.
38. Vieux R, Hascoet JM, Merdariu D, Fresson J, Guillemin F. Glomerular filtration rate reference values in very preterm infants. Pediatrics. 2010;125(5):e1186–92. https://doi.org/10.1542/peds.2009-1426.
39. Carmody JB, Swanson JR, Rhone ET, Charlton JR. Recognition and reporting of AKI in very low birth weight infants. Clin J Am Soc Nephrol. 2014;9(12):2036–43. https://doi.org/10.2215/CJN.05190514.
40. Viswanathan S, Manyam B, Azhibekov T, Mhanna MJ. Risk factors associated with acute kidney injury in extremely low birth weight (ELBW) infants. Pediatr Nephrol. 2012;27(2):303–11. https://doi.org/10.1007/s00467-011-1977-8.
41. Kaur S, Jain S, Saha A, Chawla D, Parmar VR, Basu S, et al. Evaluation of glomerular and tubular renal function in neonates with birth asphyxia. Ann Trop Paediatr. 2011;31(2):129–34. https://doi.org/10.1179/146532811X12925735813922.
42. Selewski DT, Jordan BK, Askenazi DJ, Dechert RE, Sarkar S. Acute kidney injury in asphyxiated newborns treated with therapeutic hypothermia. J Pediatr. 2013;162(4):725–9 e1. https://doi.org/10.1016/j.jpeds.2012.10.002.
43. Zwiers AJ, de Wildt SN, Hop WC, Dorresteijn EM, Gischler SJ, Tibboel D, et al. Acute kidney injury is a frequent complication in critically ill neonates receiving extracorporeal membrane oxygenation: a 14-year cohort study. Crit Care. 2013;17(4):R151. https://doi.org/10.1186/cc12830.
44. Alabbas A, Campbell A, Skippen P, Human D, Matsell D, Mammen C. Epidemiology of cardiac surgery-associated acute kidney injury in neonates: a retrospective study. Pediatr Nephrol. 2013;28(7):1127–34. https://doi.org/10.1007/s00467-013-2454-3.
45. Blinder JJ, Goldstein SL, Lee VV, Baycroft A, Fraser CD, Nelson D, et al. Congenital heart surgery in infants: effects of acute kidney injury on outcomes. J Thorac Cardiovasc Surg. 2012;143(2):368–74. https://doi.org/10.1016/j.jtcvs.2011.06.021.

46. Askenazi DJ, Koralkar R, Hundley HE, Montesanti A, Patil N, Ambalavanan N. Fluid overload and mortality are associated with acute kidney injury in sick near-term/term neonate. Pediatr Nephrol. 2013;28(4):661–6. https://doi.org/10.1007/s00467–012–2369–4.
47. Cataldi L, Leone R, Moretti U, De Mitri B, Fanos V, Ruggeri L, et al. Potential risk factors for the development of acute renal failure in preterm newborn infants: a case-control study. Arch Dis Child Fetal Neonatal Ed. 2005;90(6):F514–9. https://doi.org/10.1136/adc.2004.060434.
48. Cuzzolin L, Fanos V, Pinna B, di Marzio M, Perin M, Tramontozzi P, et al. Postnatal renal function in preterm newborns: a role of diseases, drugs and therapeutic interventions. Pediatr Nephrol. 2006;21(7):931–8. https://doi.org/10.1007/s00467–006–0118–2.
49. Koralkar R, Ambalavanan N, Levitan EB, McGwin G, Goldstein S, Askenazi D. Acute kidney injury reduces survival in very low birth weight infants. Pediatr Res. 2011;69(4):354–8. https://doi.org/10.1203/PDR.0b013e31820b95ca.
50. Mathur NB, Agarwal HS, Maria A. Acute renal failure in neonatal sepsis. Indian J Pediatr. 2006;73(6):499–502.
51. Askenazi DJ, Griffin R, McGwin G, Carlo W, Ambalavanan N. Acute kidney injury is independently associated with mortality in very low birthweight infants: a matched case-control analysis. Pediatr Nephrol. 2009;24(5):991–7. https://doi.org/10.1007/s00467–009–1133-x.
52. Sarkar S, Askenazi DJ, Jordan BK, Bhagat I, Bapuraj JR, Dechert RE, et al. Relationship between acute kidney injury and brain MRI findings in asphyxiated newborns after therapeutic hypothermia. Pediatr Res. 2014;75(3):431–5. https://doi.org/10.1038/pr.2013.230.
53. Jetton JG, Askenazi DJ. Update on acute kidney injury in the neonate. Curr Opin Pediatr. 2012;24(2):191–6. https://doi.org/10.1097/MOP.0b013e32834f62d5.
54. Foland JA, Fortenberry JD, Warshaw BL, Pettignano R, Merritt RK, Heard ML, et al. Fluid overload before continuous hemofiltration and survival in critically ill children: a retrospective analysis. Crit Care Med. 2004;32(8):1771–6.
55. Selewski DT, Cornell TT, Blatt NB, Han YY, Mottes T, Kommareddi M, et al. Fluid overload and fluid removal in pediatric patients on extracorporeal membrane oxygenation requiring continuous renal replacement therapy. Crit Care Med. 2012;40(9):2694–9. https://doi.org/10.1097/CCM.0b013e318258ff01.
56. Selewski DT, Cornell TT, Lombel RM, Blatt NB, Han YY, Mottes T, et al. Weight-based determination of fluid overload status and mortality in pediatric intensive care unit patients requiring continuous renal replacement therapy. Intensive Care Med. 2011;37(7):1166–73. https://doi.org/10.1007/s00134–011–2231–3.
57. Sutherland SM, Zappitelli M, Alexander SR, Chua AN, Brophy PD, Bunchman TE, et al. Fluid overload and mortality in children receiving continuous renal replacement therapy: the prospective pediatric continuous renal replacement therapy registry. Am J Kidney Dis. 2010;55(2):316–25. https://doi.org/10.1053/j.ajkd.2009.10.048.
58. Modem V, Thompson M, Gollhofer D, Dhar AV, Quigley R. Timing of continuous renal replacement therapy and mortality in critically ill children*. Crit Care Med. 2014;42(4):943–53. https://doi.org/10.1097/CCM.0000000000000039.
59. Mammen C, Al Abbas A, Skippen P, Nadel H, Levine D, Collet JP, et al. Long-term risk of CKD in children surviving episodes of acute kidney injury in the intensive care unit: a prospective cohort study. Am J Kidney Dis. 2012;59(4):523–30. https://doi.org/10.1053/j.ajkd.2011.10.048.
60. Askenazi DJ, Feig DI, Graham NM, Hui-Stickle S, Goldstein SL. 3–5 year longitudinal follow-up of pediatric patients after acute renal failure. Kidney Int. 2006;69(1):184–9. https://doi.org/10.1038/sj.ki.5000032.

16 Post-renal Acute Kidney Injury: Epidemiology, Presentation, Pathophysiology, Diagnosis, and Management

Valary T. Raup, Steven L. Chang, and Jairam R. Eswara

16.1 Introduction

Postobstructive renal damage has many etiologies but can be simply defined as a mechanical inability for urine to pass through the urinary system resulting in kidney damage. This obstruction can occur at any point along the urinary tract, from the tip of the urethra to within the kidney itself. Etiologies can be intrinsic and extrinsic and partial and complete and can occur at any time. Here, we present the epidemiology, pathophysiology, presentation, and treatment of postobstructive renal damage.

16.2 Epidemiology

Most cases of obstructive uropathy are diagnosed in an outpatient setting with the discovery of an elevated creatinine on routine labs [1]. Thus, the prevalence of obstructive renal injury is difficult to assess, as many individuals may have silent obstruction that is asymptomatic. In 1950, an autopsy study was performed in 59,064 individuals of all ages, and hydronephrosis was found in 3.1% of the population [2]. When stratified by age, hydronephrosis at time of autopsy has been reported in 2–2.5% of children, largely attributed to congenital etiologies, and there were no differences in gender in this population. In individuals aged 20–60 years, females were more likely to have hydronephrosis, which was thought to be due to transient obstruction during pregnancy or the increased likelihood of developing gynecologic malignancies at a younger age. In contrast, among individuals older than 60 years, males were more likely to have hydronephrosis due to prostatic hyperplasia and urologic malignancies [3, 4].

16.3 Pathophysiology

Obstructive uropathy causes numerous functional changes within the kidney. These changes are mediated by both humoral and physical factors

V. T. Raup · S. L. Chang · J. R. Eswara (✉)
Division of Urology, Department of Surgery, Brigham and Women's Hospital, Harvard Medical School, Boston, MA, USA
e-mail: vraup@partners.org; slchang@bwh.harvard.edu; jeswara@partners.org

S. S. Waikar et al. (eds.), *Core Concepts in Acute Kidney Injury*,
https://doi.org/10.1007/978-1-4939-8628-6_16

secondary to the obstruction and are dependent upon duration and severity of obstruction. It is, therefore, worth considering obstructive uropathy as comprising several pathophysiological entities including unilateral and bilateral disease and short-term and long-term obstruction. A brief review of glomerular filtration is warranted.

Glomerular filtration rate (GFR) can be thought of as the product of the permeability factor K_f and the difference between the transglomerular hydrostatic pressure Δ[DELTA] P = (P_{GC} − P_T) and the transglomerular oncotic pressure Δ[DELTA] π[pi] = (π[pi]$_{GC}$ − π[pi]$_T$) where GC and T represent the glomerular capillary and tubule, respectively:

$$\mathrm{GFR} = K_f\left(\Delta[\mathrm{DELTA}]P - \Delta[\mathrm{DELTA}]\right)$$

Since the oncotic pressure in Bowman's space is negligible, π[pi]$_T$ = 0 and Δ[DELTA] π[pi] = π[pi]$_{GC}$.

Renal blood flow (RBF) is also an important determinant in glomerular filtration, and this is dependent upon a number of vasoactive substances as well as physical parameters.

16.3.1 Unilateral Ureteral Obstruction

Experiments by Vaughn and others showed a triphasic response in renal blood flow within the first 18 h after unilateral ureteral obstruction (UUO). In the first phase, the increase in tubular pressure caused by the obstruction is mitigated by the increase in renal blood flow leading to only a slight decrease in GFR. The increase in RBF lasts approximately 2 h and is secondary to tubuloglomerular feedback (TGF), which may be mediated by several factors including prostaglandins (PGE_2), nitric oxide (NO), and the renin-angiotensin-aldosterone pathway [5–10].

After an initial increase in RBF and GFR, both decline secondary to a rise in afferent arteriolar resistance [11]. This vasoconstriction is mediated, at least in part, by angiotensin II since angiotensin-converting enzyme (ACE) inhibitors blunt the effect [12]. Thromboxane (TXA_2) is also an important mediator of postobstructive vasoconstriction, and TXA_2 may be generated from within the kidney or by macrophages that have migrated to the kidney during obstruction [13–17]. Endothelin may also play a role: it has been shown in a swine model that during unilateral obstruction, endothelin production is increased in the affected kidney and that endothelin antagonists blunt the reduction in RBF and GFR in rats [18, 19].

Renal recovery from unilateral obstruction depends upon the duration and extent. After 24 h of complete UUO, GFR is reduced 50% in dogs and 25% in rats with a concomitant decrease in RBF. Regional differences in blood flow are also seen. A significant decrease in perfusion of the superficial cortex with increased juxtamedullary glomerular perfusion has been noted in rats [20]. The mechanism is unknown but likely involves tubuloglomerular feedback [21].

16.3.2 Bilateral Ureteral Obstruction

There are significant differences in the pathophysiology of unilateral and bilateral ureteral obstruction (BUO). While there is a significant increase in RBF initially with unilateral obstruction, the increase in RBF associated with bilateral obstruction is more modest [22]. This typically lasts 90 min and is followed by a marked reduction in RBF and GFR that is longer and more pronounced than with UUO. The factors involved in mediating this response are the same as for UUO, with NO involved in initial vasodilation and angiotensin II and TXA_2 involved in vasoconstriction [23]. Another distinction between UUO and BUO is the distribution of regional blood flow after obstruction. While in UUO there is a preferential distribution of blood from the outer to the inner cortex, in BUO there is an increase in cortical blood flow at the expense of medullary flow [24, 25].

Ureteral pressure is higher and persists longer in BUO than UUO, lasting at least 24 h in BUO compared 4–5 in UUO [26]. Ureteral pressure remains high in BUO due to prolonged vasodilation of the afferent arteriole and vasoconstriction of the efferent arteriole. This appears to be secondary to the accumulation of vasoactive substances such as atrial natriuretic peptide (ANP) [15]. This is not seen in UUO since the nonobstructed kidney can excrete the excess ANP keeping levels low. Elimination of excretory function leads to expansion of intravascular volume and subsequent increase in ANP secretion from the right atrium primarily. Once the bilateral obstruction is relieved, there is a significantly greater diuresis compared to UUO because of the volume expansion and accumulation of urea and other solutes. Pathologic postobstructive diuresis only occurs after release of BUO and is also due to the lack of a functional kidney and persistent secretion of ANP leading to natriuresis [27].

16.3.3 Alteration of Renal Function

In addition to alterations in RBF and GFR, there are a number of other metabolic alterations that take place after ureteral obstruction. Among these are a derangement of concentrating ability, sodium transport, potassium transport, and acidification, but these are all predicated upon a shift from aerobic to anaerobic metabolism.

Renal obstruction alters cellular metabolism by shifting blood to the nutrient-rich outer cortex from the relatively hypoxic and nutrient-poor medulla. Given the high metabolic needs of the thick ascending limb within the medulla, it is acutely sensitive to changes in blood flow, and, consequently, ureteral obstruction can lead to a shift from aerobic metabolism to anaerobic metabolism with reduced ATP levels and increased ADP and AMP [28–31].

The changes in RBF and oxidative metabolism affect the ability of the kidney to concentrate urine. Normally controlled by vasopressin, the aquaporin-2 (AQP2)-mediated water permeability of the collecting duct is altered in ureteral obstruction, and the mechanism may involve cyclooxygenase 2 or the inflammasome [32]. It has been hypothesized that vasopressin resistance is the cause, although there is conflicting evidence to support this [25, 33]. Regardless of the mechanism, the concentrating defect has an early onset (it can be seen as early as 6 min after obstruction) and can persist for many hours [34].

As described previously, the secretion of ANP can lead to altered sodium transport and natriuresis after BUO. Other factors may also play a role in altered sodium reabsorption in UUO including decreased expression of sodium transporters on the cell surface [35]. In addition, expression of sodium transporters may be altered during ureteral obstruction as well [36, 37].

Potassium transport is altered during ureteral obstruction and is dependent upon the nature of the obstruction [20]. After release of UUO, there is a decrease in K^+ excretion likely due to decreased distal delivery of Na^+. This is in distinction to the increase in K^+ secretion seen after relief of BUO, which is due to the increased delivery of Na^+ and water to the collecting duct as well as elevation in ANP [38].

16.3.4 Urinary Acidification

Ureteral obstruction leads to a disorder in urinary acidification that has been demonstrated in both humans and animal models. Relief of ureteral obstruction does not increase bicarbonate secretion, suggesting that proximal reabsorption is still intact. Nevertheless, urinary pH does not decrease after acid loading suggestive of a defect in distal nephron H^+ transport. The exact mechanism is unknown and may be secondary to a defect in the H^+-ATPase, H^+/K^+-antiporter, or the Cl^-/HCO_3^- antiporter. Ureteral obstruction leads to a decrease in apical expression of the H^+-ATPase among intercalated cells of the cortical collecting duct [39–41].

16.4 Etiology

The causes of post-renal acute kidney injury may be divided anatomically based on location. Upper tract causes of renal obstruction include renal etiologies and ureteral etiologies. Lower tract causes of post-renal obstruction include bladder, prostatic, and urethral etiologies. Table 16.1 provides a non-exhaustive list of the more common causes of urinary obstruction.

Table 16.1 Etiology of urinary obstruction

Location of obstruction	Examples
Renal	
Malignant	Wilms' tumors, renal cell carcinoma, transitional cell carcinomas, multiple myeloma, metastatic disease
Nonmalignant	Polycystic kidney disease, renal cysts, peripelvic cysts
Others	Infections, trauma, vascular anomalies
Ureteral	Renal stones, transitional cell carcinoma of the ureters, extrinsic compression, retroperitoneal fibrosis, amyloidosis, infections
Bladder	Bladder cancer, prostate cancer extension, posterior urethral valves
Prostate	Prostate cancer, benign prostatic hypertrophy, prostatitis
Urethra	Strictures, foreign objects, phimosis

16.4.1 Renal

Renal etiologies include malignant causes such as Wilms' tumors, renal cell carcinomas, or transitional cell carcinomas affecting the collecting system. Other neoplastic causes include metastatic disease that has spread to the kidneys or other malignancies such as multiple myeloma. Nonneoplastic renal causes include polycystic kidney disease, renal cysts, and peripelvic cysts. Inflammatory conditions such as tuberculosis and *Echinococcus* infections can also cause post-renal obstruction. Other rare causes include sloughed papillae, trauma, and renal artery aneurysms.

16.4.2 Ureteral

The most common cause of post-renal obstruction worldwide is pregnancy; however, this is usually asymptomatic, self-limiting, and generally not a cause of renal failure. Another common cause of post-renal obstruction worldwide is the presence of a renal stone obstructing one or both ureters. Malignant causes include intrinsic cancers such as transitional cell carcinomas of the ureters, while extrinsic compression is commonly seen secondary to pelvic or intra-abdominal malignancies. Inflammatory processes such as tuberculosis, amyloidosis, schistosomiasis, retroperitoneal fibrosis, and abscesses can also compress the ureter.

16.4.3 Bladder, Prostate, and Urethra

Malignancies involving the bladder can lead to compression of either the ureters or the urethra which can lead to post-renal acute kidney injury. This is also true of malignancies of the prostate, urethra, and penis. While prostate cancer is prevalent, it generally affects the peripheral zones of the prostate and only rarely leads to compression of the urinary tract. Congenital anomalies such as posterior urethral valves, commonly seen in the perinatal period, can lead to a post-renal obstructive picture, as can phimosis and hydrocolpos. It is important to note that posterior urethral valves identified in a neonate is a medical emergency and needs to be decompressed immediately. Finally, benign processes such as benign prostatic hyperplasia and urethral strictures are also common causes of post-renal acute kidney injury.

16.5 Presentation/Diagnosis

Obstructive uropathy often presents as some combination of flank or abdominal pain, hematuria, uremic symptoms, occasionally signs of infection when this is present, or rarely decreased urine output. Identification of elevated creatinine and/or hydronephrosis on routine surveillance or workup of other issues can also lead to the diagnosis.

The preferred screening test for hydronephrosis is renal ultrasound, but up to 24% of patients can have hydronephrosis in the absence of obstruction [42, 43]. Figure 16.1 provides an example of a renal ultrasound showing hydronephrosis. Bilateral hydronephrosis, especially with a fairly acute development, suggests an obstruction at the level of the bladder neck or bilateral ureteral orifices. Differentiation often requires the provider obtain a good medical his-

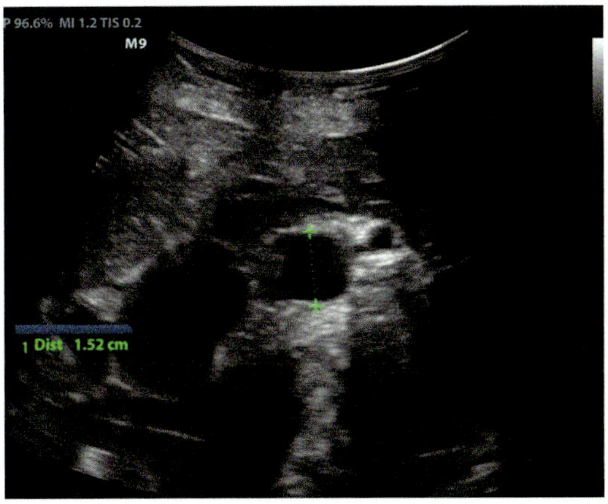

Fig. 16.1 Renal ultrasound showing hydronephrosis

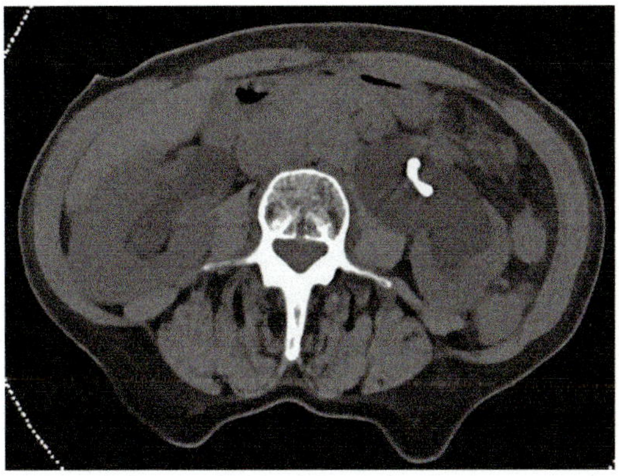

Fig. 16.2 Axial CT scan showing bilateral hydronephrosis with ureteral stent curl present on the left

tory but also typically requires further imaging studies. Plain radiography is useful if renal calculi are a possible cause of obstruction or to assess stent position if one has been placed. CT urogram allows for better visualization of the anatomy and possible cause, but contrast administration is often contraindicated due to elevated serum creatinine. A noncontrast CT can also be obtained and will give the diagnosis of hydronephrosis but may not elucidate its etiology. MRI may also be useful if a soft tissue etiology of obstruction is suspected or if creatinine prohibits a CT urogram, and a CT or MRI may be necessary for surgical planning. Figure 16.2 provides an example of an axial CT scan showing bilateral hydronephrosis with ureteral stent curl present on the left. Figures 16.3 and 16.4 show coronal CT scans in patients with bilateral ureteral obstruction due to pelvic malignancies. Figure 16.4 again has a ureteral stent in place on the left.

In cases in which contrast is contraindicated or the remaining function of the kidney is in question, renal radionuclide studies may be indicated, such as Tc99-MAG3 or Tc99-DTPA scans. Figures 16.5 and 16.6 provide an example of a MAG3 scan with renal obstruction on the right. If intrinsic urologic pathology is suspected, stent placement is deemed necessary, or if the patient is having surgery for another reason, retrograde pyelograms should be considered. Although rarely used nowadays, the Whitaker perfusion pressure-flow (PPF) study can be used to assess possible upper urinary tract obstruction in patients with equivocal results from other testing, suspected intermittent obstruction, suspected obstruction with poor kidney function, pain with negative renal radionuclide studies, and gross dilation with positive renal radionuclide studies [44]. The Whitaker test is performed by inserting a nephrostomy tube, obtaining intrarenal and

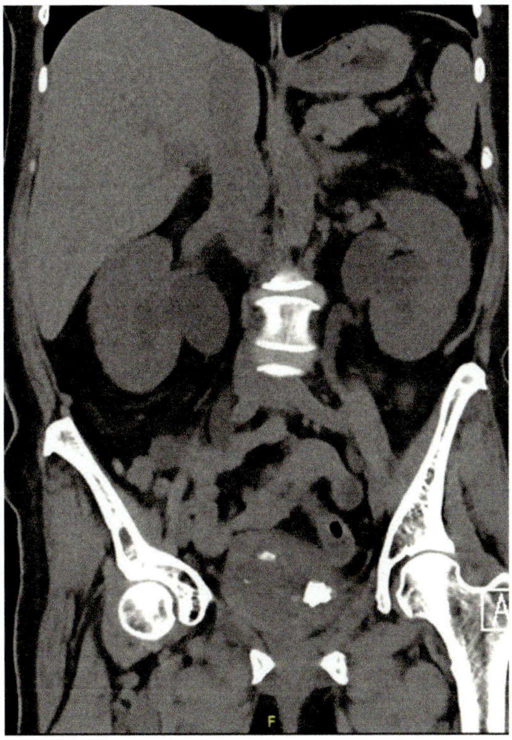

Fig. 16.3 Coronal CT scan showing bilateral ureteral obstruction due to pelvic malignancy

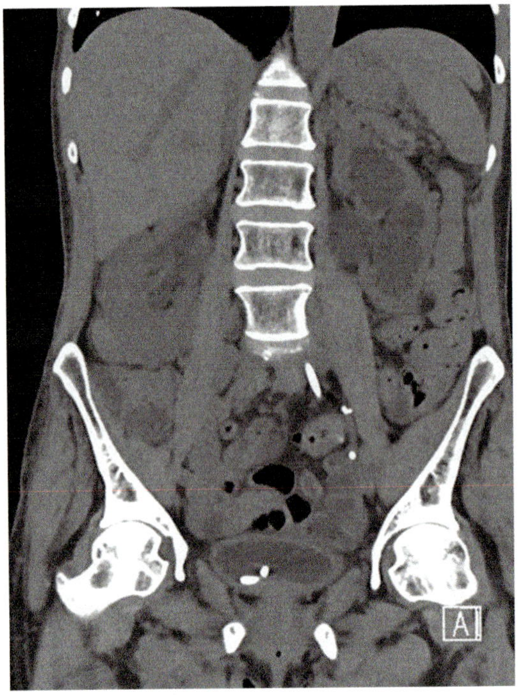

Fig. 16.4 Coronal CT scan showing bilateral ureteral obstruction due to pelvic malignancy with ureteral stent in place on the left

intravesical pressure measurements, and then perfusing the kidney percutaneously with contrast while measuring pressures [45]. This test is classically used in children but can serve a purpose in adult patients as well. It is important to remember, however, that hydronephrosis can lessen over time as renal filtration decreases from the affected kidney.

While imaging such as CT and ultrasound provide anatomical detail of the abdomen and pelvis thereby assessing the entire urinary tract, urodynamics can provide a functional assessment of the lower urinary tract. Assessing for bladder outlet obstruction, typically from prostatic obstruction or urethral stricture disease, is essential as these are reversible causes of urinary tract obstruction. Urodynamics pressure assessments of the bladder allow determination of bladder contractility as well as inference of bladder outlet obstruction.

Urodynamics testing involves the placement of pressure-sensing catheters in the bladder and the rectum or vagina. The pressure detected by the bladder catheter represents the sum of the detrusor pressure (from bladder contraction) and

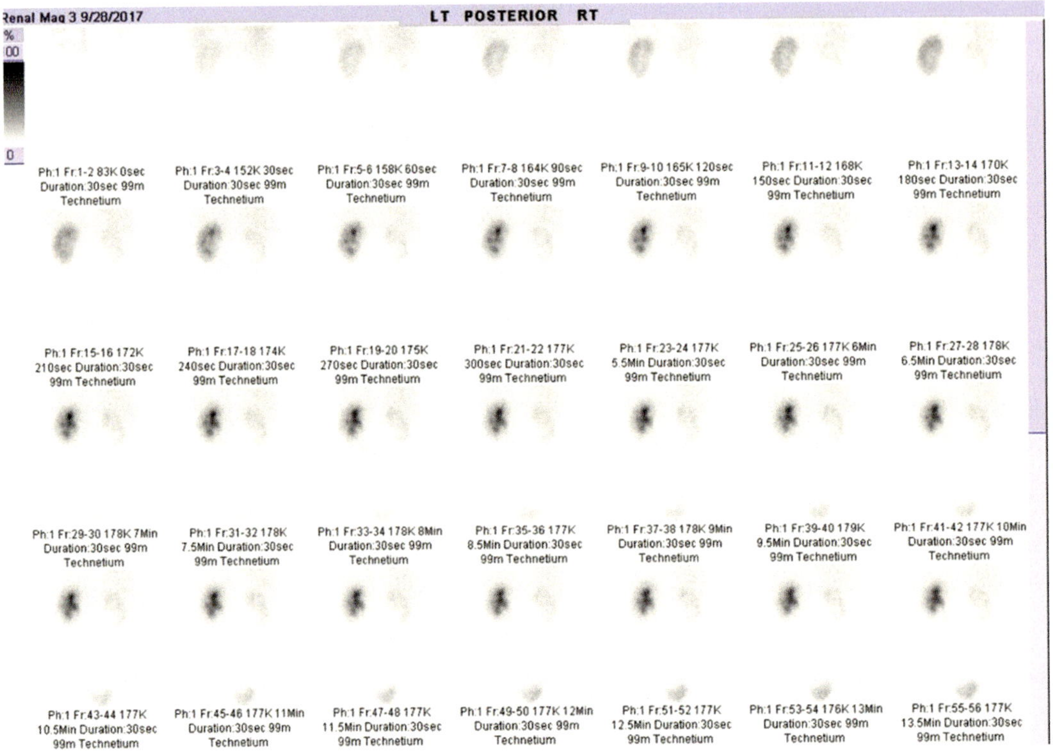

Fig. 16.5 MAG-3 renal scan showing renal obstruction on the right

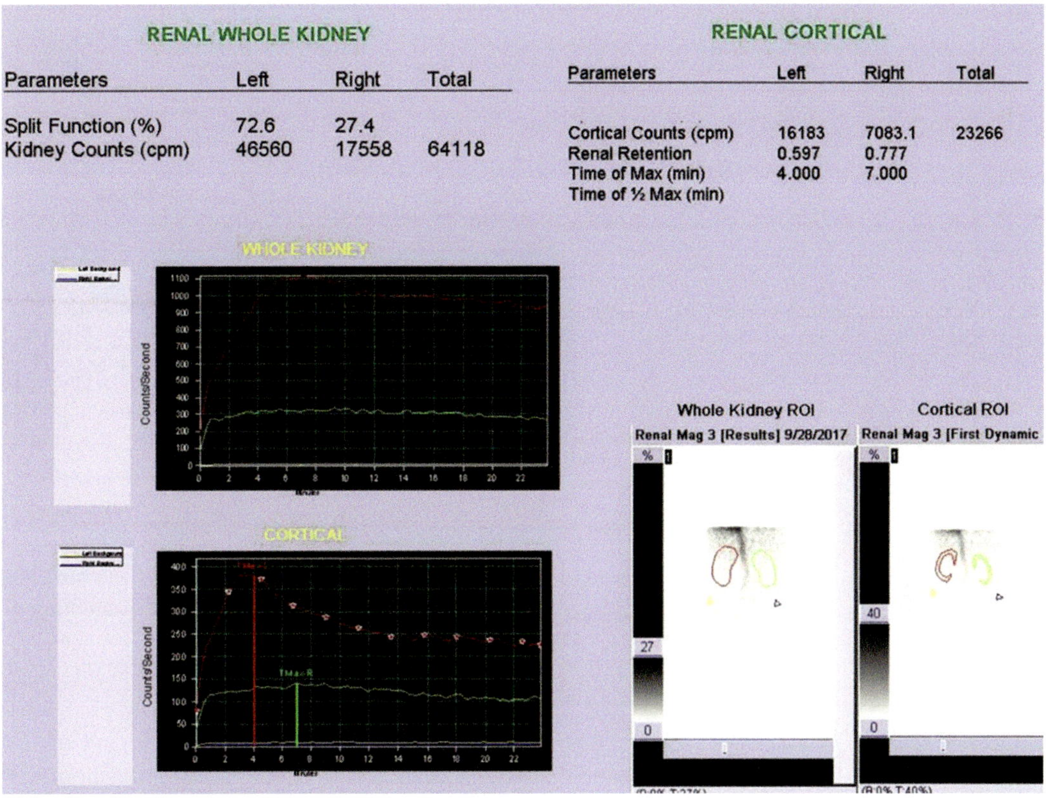

Fig. 16.6 MAG-3 renal scan showing renal obstruction on the right

the abdominal pressure. Subtracting the abdominal pressure as measured by the rectal/vaginal catheter allows calculation of bladder pressure. Simultaneous fluoroscopic imaging to determine the shape of the bladder and urethra, called videourodynamics, can enhance standard urodynamics. This can be useful in patients with neurogenic bladder or who have surgically augmented bladders. The anatomic detail of videourodynamics can support these diagnoses.

Urodynamics includes a series of clinical tests, such as uroflowmetry, filling cystometry, pressure-flow studies, assessment of urethral closure, and electromyographic measurement of the urethral sphincter muscle. Urodynamics is useful when considering the following clinical situations: [1] conservative treatment has failed; [2] when considering invasive treatment; [3] assessing the pressure of the bladder or urinary reservoir; and [4] determining the efficacy of intervention.

Figure 16.7 represents a sample urodynamic tracing from a patient with bladder outlet obstruction. The third tracing from the top represents the calculated bladder pressure. The increase in bladder pressure toward the right of the graph represents the bladder contracting during voiding. Note the relatively high rise in bladder pressure compared to the low flow rate (long blue arrow, below), which indicates bladder outlet obstruction. Also note the presence of a second void (short blue arrow) since the first was incomplete, another indication of bladder outlet obstruction.

16.6 Management

Management of post-renal acute kidney injury involves first relieving the obstruction, and this depends upon the anatomic location and etiology. Treatments are grouped based on anatomic location.

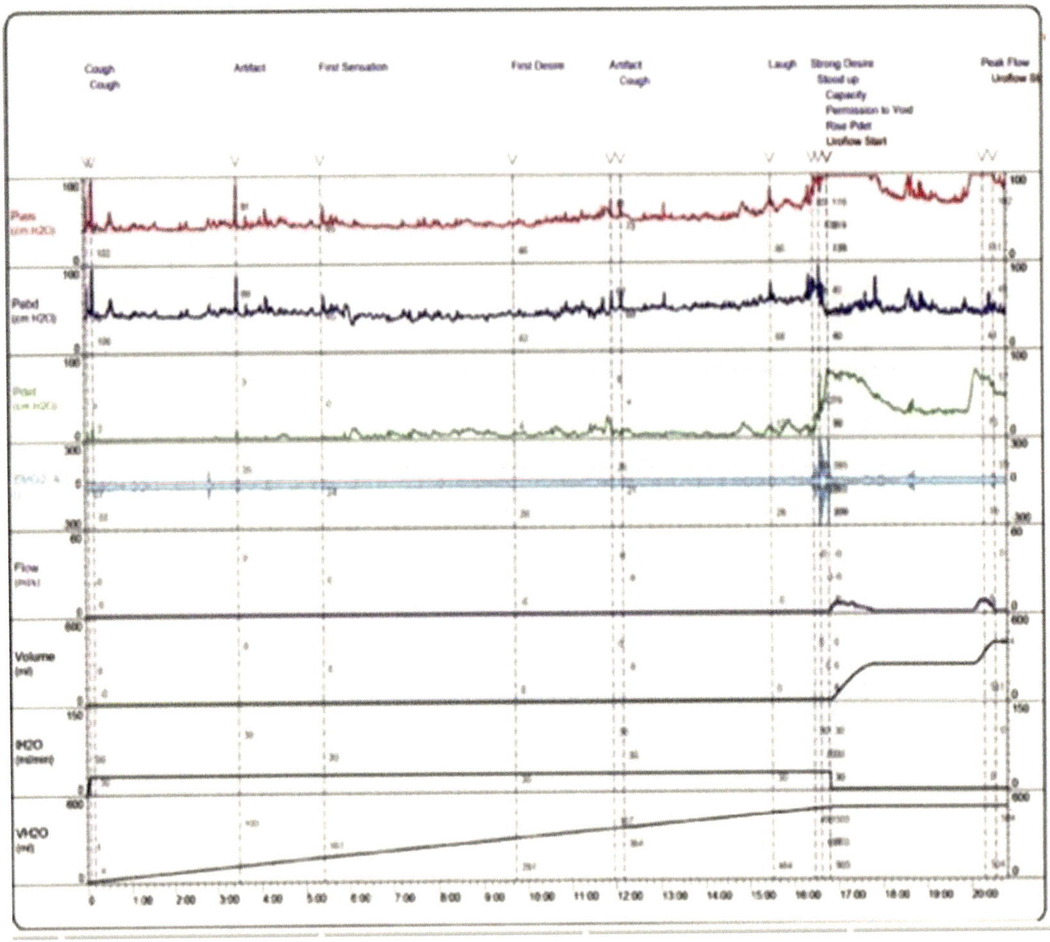

Fig. 16.7 Urodynamic tracing showing bladder outlet obstruction. The third tracing from the top represents the calculated bladder pressure. The increase in bladder pressure toward the right of the graph represents the bladder contracting during voiding. Note the relatively high rise in bladder pressure compared to the low flow rate (long blue arrow, below), which indicates bladder outlet obstruction. Also note the presence of a second void (short blue arrow) since the first was incomplete, another indication of bladder outlet obstruction

16.6.1 Kidney and Ureter

For most upper urinary tract obstruction, the treatment options in the acute setting are similar. Whether the origin is the kidney or the ureter, relief of the obstruction can be achieved by placing either a ureteral stent or percutaneous nephrostomy tube. Intervention is warranted if there is evidence of renal failure or infection, if the obstruction appears bilateral, or if the patient has pain that is intractable to pain medications. Both ureteral stents and percutaneous nephrostomy tubes can achieve decompression of the urinary tract; however, extrinsic compression of the ureter from either malignant or nonmalignant causes can sometimes lead stents to fail. Should a ureteral stent fail due to extrinsic compression, a percutaneous nephrostomy tube would be necessary to decompress the urinary tract. If the etiology of compression is such that it is likely to progress significantly without good treatment options, such as refractory peritoneal carcinomatosis or unresectable pelvic mass, percutaneous nephrostomy tubes should be considered as initial intervention.

16.6.2 Bladder, Prostate, and Urethra

Obstruction of the urinary tract due to a bladder etiology can be relieved in one of several ways. If the obstruction is due to mass compression of the ureteral orifice or bladder outlet, it is best treated by endoscopic transurethral resection of the mass and placement of either a ureteral stent or Foley catheter. The same is true of prostatic obstruction. This is best relieved in the acute phase by placement of a urethral catheter or suprapubic tube. Subsequent treatment often includes medical or surgical therapy to increase the diameter of the bladder outlet and thereby improve urinary flow. Urethral strictures are also best treated endoscopically in the acute setting by either urethral dilation or endoscopic urethrotomy with placement of Foley catheter in order to allow urinary drainage. In particularly challenging cases, a suprapubic tube may be necessary.

References

1. Gottlieb RH, Weinberg EP, Rubens DJ, Monk RD, Grossman EB. Renal sonography: can it be used more selectively in the setting of an elevated serum creatinine level? Am J Kidney Dis. 1997;29(3):362–7.
2. Bell ET. Renal diseases. Philadelphia: Lea & Febiger; 1950.
3. Campbell MF. Urinary obstruction. In: Campbell MF, Harrison JH, editors. Urology. Philadelphia: Saunders; 1970. p. 1772–93.
4. Tan PH, Chiang GS, Tay AH. Pathology of urinary tract malformations in a paediatric autopsy series. Ann Acad Med Singap. 1994;23:838–43.
5. Allen JT, Vaughan ED, Gillenwater JY. The effect of indomethacin on renal blood flow and urethral pressure in unilateral ureteral obstruction in a awake dogs. Investig Urol. 1978;15:324–7.
6. Gaudio KM, Siegel NJ, Hayslett JP, Kashgarian M. Renal perfusion and intratubular pressure during ureteral occlusion in the rat. Am J Phys. 1980;238(3):F205–9.
7. Salvemini D, Seibert K, Masferrer JL, Misko TP, Currie MG, Needleman P. Endogenous nitric oxide enhances prostaglandin production in a model of renal inflammation. J Clin Invest. 1994;93(5):1940–7.
8. Miyajima A, Chen J, Poppas DP, Vaughan ED Jr, Felsen D. Role of nitric oxide in renal tubular apoptosis of unilateral ureteral obstruction. Kidney Int. 2001;59(4):1290–303.
9. Lanzone JA, Gulmi FA, Chou SY, et al. Renal hemodynamics in acute unilateral ureteral obstruction: contribution of endothelium-derived relaxing factor. J Urol. 1995;153:2055–9.
10. Wang W, Luo R, Lin Y, Wang F, Zheng P, Levi M, Yang T, Li C. Aliskiren restores renal AQP2 expression during unilateral ureteral obstruction by inhibiting the inflammasome. Am J Physiol Renal Physiol. 2015;308(8):F910–22. https://doi.org/10.1152/ajprenal.00649.2014; Epub 2015 Feb 18.
11. Siegel NJ, Feldman RA, Lytton B, Hayslett JP, Kashgarian M. Renal cortical blood flow distribution in obstructive nephropathy in rats. Circ Res. 1977;40(4):379–84.
12. Ichikawa I, Purkerson ML, Yates J, Klahr S. Dietary protein intake conditions the degree of renal vasoconstriction in acute renal failure caused by ureteral obstruction. Am J Phys. 1985;249(1 Pt 2):F54–61.
13. Klotman PE, Smith SR, Volpp BD, Coffman TM, Yarger WE. Thromboxane synthetase inhibition improves function of hydronephrotic rat kidneys. Am J Phys. 1986;250(2 Pt 2):F282–7.
14. Loo MH, Egan D, Vaughan ED Jr, Marion D, Felsen D, Weisman S. The effect of the thromboxane A2 synthesis inhibitor OKY-046 on renal function in rabbits following release of unilateral ureteral obstruction. J Urol. 1987;137(3):571–6.
15. Purkerson ML, Blaine EH, Stokes TJ, et al. Role of atrial peptide in the natriuresis and diuresis that follows relief of obstruction in rat. Am J Phys. 1989;256:F583–9.
16. Schreiner GF, Harris KP, Purkerson ML, et al. Immunological aspects of acute ureteral obstruction: immune cell infiltrate in the kidney. Kidney Int. 1988;34:487–93.
17. Harris KP, Schreiner GF, Klahr S. Effect of leukocyte depletion on the function of the postobstructed kidney in the rat. Kidney Int. 1989;36(2):210–5.
18. Kelleher JP, Shah V, Godley ML, Wakefield AJ, Gordon I, Ransley PG, Snell ME, Risdon RA. Urinary endothelin (ET1) in complete ureteric obstruction in the miniature pig. Urol Res. 1992;20(1):63–5.
19. Syed N, Gulmi FA, Chou SY, Mooppan UM, Kim H. Renal actions of endothelin-1 under endothelin receptor blockade by BE-18257B. J Urol. 1998;159(2):563–6.
20. Harris RH, Yarger WE. The pathogenesis of post-obstructive diuresis: the role of circulating natriuretic and diuretic factors, including urea. J Clin Invest. 1975;56:880–7.
21. Tanner GA. Tubuloglomerular feedback after nephron or ureteral obstruction. Am J Phys. 1985;248(5 Pt 2):F688–97.
22. Gulmi FA, Matthews GJ, Marion D, et al. Volume expansion enhances the recovery of renal function and prolongs the diuresis and natriuresis after release of bilateral ureteral obstruction: a possible role for atrial natriuretic peptide. J Urol. 1995;153:1276–83.
23. Reyes AA, Klahr S. Renal function after release of ureteral obstruction: role of endothelin and the renal artery endothelium. Kidney Int. 1992;42:632–8.

24. Jaenike JR. The renal functional defect of postobstructive nephyropathy: the effects of bilateral ureteral obstruction in the rat. J Clin Invest. 1972;51:2999–3006.
25. Solez K, Ponchak S, Buono RA, et al. Inner medullary plasma flow in the kidney with ureteral obstruction. Am J Phys. 1976;231:1315–21.
26. Yarger WE, Aynedjian HS, Bank N. A micropuncture study of postobstructive diuresis in the rat. J Clin Invest. 1972;51(3):625–37.
27. Li P, Oparil S, Novak L, Cao X, Shi W, Lucas J, Chen YF. ANP signaling inhibits TGF-beta-induced Smad2 and Smad3 nuclear translocation and extracellular matrix expression in rat pulmonary arterial smooth muscle cells. J Appl Physiol (1985). 2007;102(1):390–8; Epub 2006 Oct 12.
28. Stecker JF, Gillenwater JY. Experimental partial ureteral obstruction. I. Alteration in renal function. Investig Urol. 1971;8:377–85.
29. Middleton GW, Beamon CR, Panko WB, Gillenwater JY. Effects of ureteral obstruction on the renal metabolism of alpha-ketoglutarate and other substrates in vivo. Investig Urol. 1977;14(4):255–62.
30. Nito H, Descoeudres C, Kurokawa K, Massry SG. Effect of unilateral obstruction on renal cell metabolism and function. J Lab Clin Med. 1978;91(1):60–71. No abstract available.
31. Klahr S, Schwab SJ, Stokes TJ. Metabolic adaptations of the nephron in renal disease. Kidney Int. 1986;29(1):80–9. Review. No abstract available.
32. Nilsson L, Madsen K, Topcu SO, Jensen BL, Frøkiær J, Nørregaard R. Disruption of cyclooxygenase-2 prevents downregulation of cortical AQP2 and AQP3 in response to bilateral ureteral obstruction in the mouse. Am J Physiol Renal Physiol. 2012;302(11):F1430–9. https://doi.org/10.1152/ajprenal.00682.2011; Epub 2012 Mar 7.
33. Li C, Wang W, Kwon TH, et al. Downregulation of AQP1, -2, and -3 after ureteral obstruction is associated with a long-term urine-concentrating defect. Am J Physiol Renal Physiol. 2001;281:F163–71.
34. Jaenike JR, Bray GA. Effects of acute transitory urinary obstruction in the dog. Am J Phys. 1960;199:1219–22.
35. Zeidel ML. Hormonal regulation of inner medullary collecting duct sodium transport. Am J Phys. 1993;265(2 Pt 2):F159–73. Review.
36. Rokaw MD, Sarac E, Lechman E, West M, Angeski J, Johnson JP, Zeidel ML. Chronic regulation of transepithelial Na+ transport by the rate of apical Na+ entry. Am J Phys. 1996;270(2 Pt 1):C600–7.
37. Kwon TH, Laursen UH, Marples D, Maunsbach AB, Knepper MA, Frokiaer J, Nielsen S. Altered expression of renal AQPs and Na(+) transporters in rats with lithium-induced NDI. Am J Physiol Renal Physiol. 2000;279(3):F552–64.
38. Sonnenberg H, Wilson DR. The role of the medullary collecting ducts in postobstructive diuresis. J Clin Invest. 1976;57:1564–74.
39. Purcell H, Bastani B, Harris KP, Hemken P, Klahr S, Gluck S. Cellular distribution of H(+)-ATPase following acute unilateral ureteral obstruction in rats. Am J Phys. 1991;261(3 Pt 2):F365–76.
40. Valles PG, Manucha WA. Kidney Int. 2000;58:1641–51.
41. Wang CJ, Huang SW, Chang CH. Efficacy of an alpha1 blocker in expulsive therapy of lower ureteral stones. J Enourol. 2008;22:41–6.
42. Ellenbogen PH, Scheible FW, Talner LB, Leopold GR. Sensitivity of gray scale ultrasound in detecting urinary tract obstruction. AJR Am J Roentgenol. 1978;130(4):731.
43. Kamholtz RG, Cronan JJ, Dorfman GS. Obstruction and the minimally dilated renal collecting system: US evaluation. Radiology. 1989;170(1 Pt 1):51.
44. Lupton EW, George NJ. The Whitaker test: 35 years on. BJU Int. 2010;105(1):94–100.
45. Oates J, O'Flynn K. The Whitaker test. In: Payne S, Eardley I, O'Flynn K, editors. Imaging and technology in urology. London: Springer; 2012. p. 157–60.

Cardiorenal Acute Kidney Injury: Epidemiology, Presentation, Causes, Pathophysiology, and Treatment

17

Claudio Ronco and Luca Di Lullo

17.1 Introduction

Cardiovascular disease and major cardiovascular events represent the main cause of death in both acute and chronic kidney disease patients.

Kidney and heart failure are common and frequently coexist; this organ-organ interaction, also called organ cross talk, leads to a well-known definition of cardiorenal syndrome (CRS). A novel consensus definition and classification about CRS was proposed in 2008 by the Acute Dialysis Quality Initiative workgroup [1] (Table 17.1) and identified five CRS subtypes according to disease onset.

Here we'll describe cardiovascular involvement in patients with acute kidney injury (AKI). Also known as type-3 CRS or acute reno-cardiac CRS, it occurs when AKI contributes to and/or precipitates the development of acute cardiac injury.

AKI may directly or indirectly produce an acute cardiac event, and it can be associated to volume overload, metabolic acidosis, and electrolyte disorders such as hyperkalemia and hypocalcemia; coronary artery disease, left ventricular dysfunction, and fibrosis have been also described in patients with AKI with consequent direct negative effects on cardiac performance [2, 3].

C. Ronco
International Renal Research Institute, S.Bortolo Hospital, Vicenza, Italy

L. Di Lullo (✉)
Department of Nephrology and Dialysis, L. Parodi-Delfino Hospital, Colleferro, Italy

17.2 Definition of Type-3 Cardiorenal Syndrome

17.2.1 Acute Kidney Disease

As previously described, type-3 cardiorenal syndrome is characterized by acute worsening of kidney function leading to heart disease. The spectrum of cardiac dysfunction includes acute decompensated heart failure (ADHF), acute coronary syndrome (ACS), and arrhythmias as defined by RIFLE (risk, injury, failure, loss, and end-stage kidney disease) and AKIN (Acute Kidney Injury Network) criteria [4, 5].

AKIN criteria contributed to previous RIFLE ones adding serum creatinine increase of 0.3 mg/dL, or more, in a time-lapse of 48 h [6]; at present time RIFLE and AKIN criteria are validated in over half-million patients worldwide [7].

AKI actually represents an independent cardiovascular risk factor for mortality in hospitalized patients especially in those on renal replacement therapy (RRT).

AKI is particularly preeminent in over 65 aged patients with infections at admission, underlying cardiovascular disease, hepatic cirrhosis, respiratory distress, chronic heart failure, and hematologic neoplasia.

S. S. Waikar et al. (eds.), *Core Concepts in Acute Kidney Injury*,
https://doi.org/10.1007/978-1-4939-8628-6_17

Table 17.1 Classification of cardiorenal syndrome

Type	Denomination	Description	Example
1	Acute cardiorenal	Heart failure leading to AKD	Acute coronary syndrome leading to acute heart and kidney failure
2	Chronic cardiorenal	Chronic heart failure leading to kidney failure	Chronic heart failure
3	Acute nephrocardiac	AKD leading to acute heart failure	Uremic cardiomyopathy AKD related
4	Chronic nephrocardiac	Chronic kidney disease leading to heart failure	Left ventricular hypertrophy and diastolic heart failure due to kidney failure
5	Secondary	Systemic disease leading to heart and kidney failure	Sepsis, vasculitis, diabetes mellitus

AKI is prevalent and incident in intensive care units (ICU), mainly due to sepsis, major surgery proceedings, hypovolemic status with low cardiac output heart failure, and drugs' management [8].

Based on recent findings, AKI seems to involve almost 70% patients in ICUs (among these, 5–25% can develop severe AKI) with mortality rates ranging from 50 to 80% [8].

17.2.2 Acute Cardiac Dysfunction

Acute cardiac dysfunction includes a broad spectrum of cardiac diseases from ADHF to ACS, arrhythmias, and cardiogenic shock; to better define what we mean with "acute cardiac dysfunction," we have to relate to the European Society of Cardiology and American College of Cardiology Foundation guidelines [9, 10].

ADHF still represents the most common acute cardiac dysfunction syndrome all over the world, and it can be defined as new-onset, gradual or rapid, worsening of preexistent heart failure with signs and symptoms requiring immediate therapy [11]. The main pathophysiologic pathway is represented by increased ventricular filling pressures in the presence or absence of cardiac output's decrease. Increased filling pressures lead to pulmonary and systemic congestion irrespective of both underlying (chronic ischemic heart disease) and incoming (severe hypertensive disease) clinical events [11].

Cardiac valvular disease, atrial fibrillation, arterial hypertension, as well as noncardiac comorbidities (renal dysfunction, diabetes, anemia) and medications (especially nonsteroidal anti-inflammatory drugs and glitazones) can contribute to ADHF development [11].

Renal dysfunction affects mortality rates in ADHF patients from 1.9 (mild renal disease) to 7.6% (severe renal dysfunction) according to the Acute Decompensated Heart Failure National Registry database [12].

Adverse prognostic factors are mainly represented by low ejection fraction, low systolic blood pressure, hyponatremia, and older age.

Independent predictive 1-year mortality risk factors are provided by older age, male sex, low systolic blood pressure at hospital admission, renal dysfunction, and inflammatory status as underlined by elevated serum levels of C-reactive protein (CRP) [13].

Probably AKI and ADHF could be identified as two sides of the same coin, and a vicious cycle is established: AKI leads to heart dysfunction and heart disease affects progressive kidney failure (Fig. 17.1).

17.3 Epidemiology of Type-3 CRS

Defining incidence and prevalence of type-3 CRS is quite difficult due to lack of epidemiologic data at present time.

At the same time, it's possible to collect data derived from single-population studies; among them a 2147 per million population AKI incidence was reported in northern Scotland population-based study [14].

Another prospective, multicenter, community-based study in 748 AKI patients reported common death's causes: infections (48%), hypovolemic shock (45.9%), respiratory distress (22.2%), heart disease (15%), disseminated intravascular coagulation (6.3%), gastrointestinal bleeding (4.5%), and stroke (2.7%).

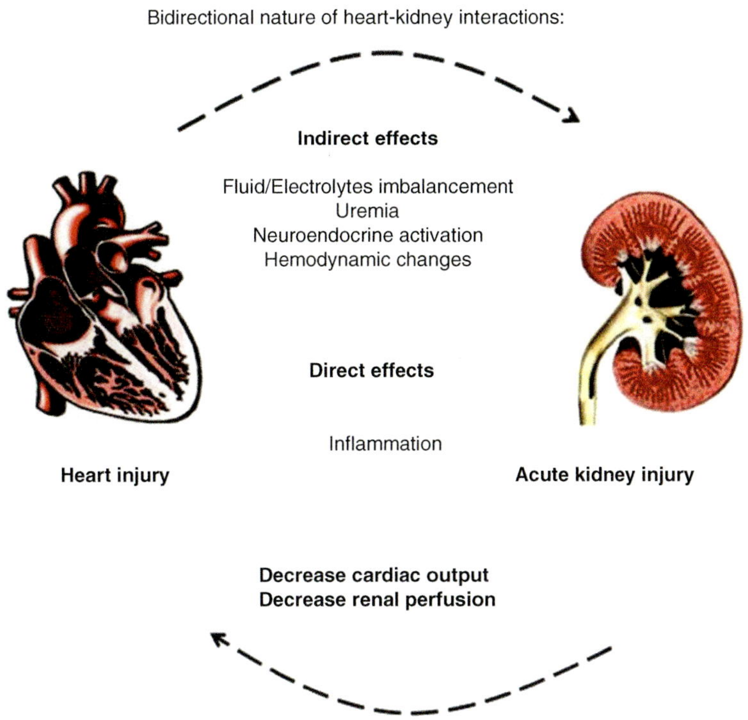

Fig. 17.1 Pathophysiology of type-3 CRS and the potential vicious cycle

In more recent retrospective AKI study following traumatic disease, cardiac arrest was reported as the cause of death in 20% of patients. Other causes of death were cerebrovascular accidents (46%), sepsis (17%), multiple organ dysfunction syndrome (7.3%), and respiratory insufficiency (3.2%) [15].

Cardiac failure is certainly the most common cause of death in end-stage renal disease patients [16] with higher incidence than hepatic failure, massive transfusion, older age (>60 years), and respiratory and neurologic failure [17].

17.4 Pathophysiology of Type-3 CRS

It's clearly established that kidneys play a crucial role in regulating body water and blood volume; at the same time, kidneys are involved in electrolyte balance (such as sodium and potassium levels), help in regulating blood pH, and provide for excretion of nitrogen and other toxic molecules.

Kidney holds neuroendocrine functions as underlined by the production of erythropoietin and renin to regulate both erythropoiesis and systemic blood pressure.

Kidney is also mainly involved in the excretion of the majority of drugs, and tubular cells may be provided to regulate leukocyte activation and cytokine production in inflammatory processes [18].

As kidney's function is impaired, acid-base and electrolyte imbalance, fluid overload (i.e., pulmonary edema, pleural effusion), atrial distension (leading to arrhythmias, since to atrial fibrillation), gut mucosal edema, hematologic dysfunction (anemia, platelet and white blood cell dysfunction), and altered drug excretion occur [19].

As well, platelet and leukocyte dysfunction, together with delayed wound healing, may encourage infectious processes 'till to sepsis also due to widespread inflammation [19].

Pathophysiologic cross-link between kidney injury and heart dysfunction has to be clearly understood.

Table 17.2 Summary of potential contributing causes for AKI contributing to type-3 CRS

Prototypical condition	
Contrast-induced AKI	Post-inflammatory GN
Drug-induced AKI	Rhabdomyolysis
Major surgery	Acute pyelonephritis
Cardiac surgery	Post-obstructive uropathy

Table 17.3 Summary of susceptibilities for type-3 CRS

Risk-modifying factors	
Age	Congestive heart failure
Sex	Pulmonary disease
Coronary artery disease	Chronic kidney disease
Hypertension	Systemic vascular disease
Hypercholesterolemia	Systemic immune disease
Diabetes mellitus	Infection/sepsis

As it's clear that heart failure leads to decrease in tissue perfusion also involving renal physiology, on the other hand, AKI itself can affect heart by direct and indirect pathophysiologic mechanisms (Tables 17.2 and 17.3).

17.4.1 Direct AKI Effects on Heart Function

Pathophysiological interactions between the kidney and heart during AKI have been referred to "cardiorenal connectors" [20], like activation of immune (i.e., pro- and anti-inflammatory cytokine and chemokine release) and sympathetic nervous systems, hyperactivity of RAAS, and coagulation cascade.

Most of experimental available data are focused on immune cardiorenal connectors, especially on renal ischemia and reperfusion injury; animal models show that AKI encourages an immune response characterized by secretion of pro- and anti-inflammatory mediators such as structural and functional changes in immune cell responsiveness; leukocyte function is also affected with alterations in adhesion. It is well-known that leukocytes play an important role in cardiac dysfunction following acute coronary disease; blocking leukocyte activity can protect against myocardial damage [21].

Circulating levels of tumor necrosis factor-alpha (TNF-α), interleukin-1 (IL-1), and interleukin-6 (IL-6) seem to increase immediately after renal experimental ischemia, and, together with other cytokines as well as interferon-alpha (IFN-α), they have direct cardio-depressant effects underlined by the reduction in left ventricular ejection fraction and elevation of left ventricular end-diastolic and end-systolic volumes and areas [22].

Cytokine release can affect myocardial cells directly on their contractility or by close interactions with extracellular matrix leading to negative inotropic effects; complete cellular mechanisms are still unclear, but they probably involve secondary mediators such as sphingolipids, arachidonic acid, and intracellular Ca^{2+} alterations [2].

In animal models, infusion of TNF-α results in decrease of left ventricular diastolic pressure with secondary coronary vasoconstriction; more infusions cause time-dependent dysfunction (regional contractility alterations) of the left ventricle and its dilation lasting up to 10 days [23]. Together with left ventricular systolic dysfunction, several diastolic abnormalities are observed, including slow relaxation of left ventricle and raised left atrium filling pressure to indicate an increase in left ventricle diastolic stiffness. TNF-α acute infusion directly increases oxygen consumption by myocardial cells affecting contractility and excitation-contraction coupling [23].

In the presence of renal ischemia, rat hearts show increased expression of adhesion molecules such as ICAM-1 together with myocardial apoptosis (this is not true in case of bilateral nephrectomy) to prove that systemic inflammation, and not AKI, plays an immediate role in myocardial damage and dysfunction.

Also patients with chronic heart failure show increased levels of pro-inflammatory cytokines associated with higher rates of impaired left ventricle remodeling, chronic cachexia, and mortality [24].

In animal experiments, it has been shown that left ventricular dilation, increased left ventricular end-diastolic and end-systolic diameters, increased relaxation time, and decreased fractional shortening can occur 48 h after renal injury [25].

During AKI, a hyperactivity of SNS is also described with abnormal secretion of norepinephrine impairing myocardial activity by several ways: direct norepinephrine effect, impairment in Ca^{2+} metabolism, increase in myocardial oxygen demand with potential evolution to myocardial ischemia, myocardial cell β[beta]1-adrenergic-mediated apoptosis, stimulation of α1 receptors, and, finally, activation of RAAS. β[beta]1-adrenergic stimulus on juxtaglomerular cells simplifies renal blood flow reduction and stimulates further renin secretion by RAAS.

Abnormal and uncontrolled RAAS activation leads to angiotensin II release with consequent systemic vasoconstriction and elevation of vascular resistance; on the other hand, angiotensin II itself directly modifies myocardial structure promoting cellular hypertrophy and apoptosis [26].

In experimental model of renal ischemia, authors postulated how increased RAAS activity could be accountable for diminished coronary response to adenosine, bradykinin, and L-arginine [3].

These data probably underline that AKI could directly account for impaired coronary vasoreactivity and increased susceptibility to ischemia and other major cardiovascular events.

Other animal models allowed to discover how AKI can contribute to altered permeability of lung vessels, with resultant interstitial edema and bleeding, mediated by inflammatory mediators, altered expression of epithelial sodium channel, and aquaporin-5 expression [27].

As mentioned above, myocardial cell apoptosis and neutrophil activation greatly contribute to pathophysiologic pathways of coronary artery following AKI leading to lethal major cardiac events as can be seen in rat transgenic models [28].

Cardiac myocyte apoptosis and neutrophil infiltration represent two of the most important contributors to the pathophysiology of myocardial infarction during AKI [29].

Best evidence for a cardiorenal link between AKI and cardiac fibrosis is beta-galactoside-binding lectin galectin-3 whose mRNA expression is upregulated after renal ischemia; it is also implicated in the development of myocardial fibrosis and heart failure in AKI, and its inhibition can delay progression of myocardial fibrosis [30].

17.4.2 Indirect Effects of AKI on Heart Function

As renal function goes down, it can result in significant pathophysiological derangement, leading to cardiac injury.

First of all, oliguria can lead to sodium and water retention with consequent fluid overload and development of edema, cardiac overload, hypertension, pulmonary edema, and myocardial injury.

Furthermore, electrolyte imbalances (hyperkalemia primarily) can contribute to raised risk of fatal arrhythmias (see dedicated section) and sudden death.

Acidemia also can affect myocytes' metabolism, and it can be accountable for pulmonary vasoconstriction, increased right ventricular afterload, and negative inotropic effect.

Finally, sudden accumulation of uremic toxins (i.e., nitric oxide synthase-modulating guanidinesuccinic acid and methylguanidine) can lead to myocardial infarction and other organ and tissue dysfunction [31]. Uremia itself can directly affect myocardial cell contractility through myocardial depressant factors and promoting pericardial effusions and pericarditis [32].

Type-3 CRS is also characterized by lung, brain, and liver involvement. Lung injury is mediated by neutrophil's infiltration and cytokine release, while uremic encephalopathy represents AKI effects on the brain due to inflammation and volume overload.

Hepatic involvement is usually represented by development of hepatorenal syndrome.

As mentioned in previous paragraph concerning direct effects of AKI on cardiac function, neuroendocrine system is involved in type-3 CRS pathophysiology since both the kidney and heart can activate sympathetic nervous system (SNS) and renin-angiotensin-aldosterone system (RAAS) [33, 34].

In response to systemic and renal hemodynamic changes, baroreceptor and intrarenal chemoreceptors lead to SNS and RAAS activation; SNS activation directly affects intrarenal hemodynamics and stimulates renin incretion. SNS activation can lead to cardiomyocyte apoptosis and increases the release of neuropeptide Y, a vascular growth factor accountable for neointimal formation and following vasoconstriction [33, 34].

On the other hand, RAAS activation stimulates sodium reabsorption at proximal tubule and determines efferent arteriole constriction, leading to an increase of intraglomerular pressure and filtration fraction to maintain a valid glomerular filtration rate (GFR) despite decreased renal blood flow.

Overactivation of RAAS can also contribute to vasoconstriction due to angiotensin II production; angiotensin II provides direct negative effects on cardiovascular system, increasing preload and afterload, inducing apoptosis, and activating NADPH oxidase in endothelial cells, vascular smooth muscle cells, renal tubular cells, and cardiomyocytes. NDPH oxidase activation results in abnormal formation of reactive oxygen species [35–39].

17.4.3 Electrophysiological Effects

Electrolytes' alterations directly affect cellular membrane potentials with development of potential fatal arrhythmias. Classical ECG aspect of hyperkalemic patients is represented by tenting of T wave due to rapid and consistent changes in extracellular potassium levels leading to increased activity of potassium channel (and inactivation of sodium channel) with faster repolarization and inclination to arrhythmias.

Thus, hyperkalemia reduces resting membrane potentials (both atrial and ventricular) and induces ST-T segment abnormalities (i.e., elevations in V1 and V2) simulating an ischemic pattern. In some patients, hyperkalemia can simulate a Brugada-like pattern, characterized by right bundle branch block and persistent ST-T segment elevation in at least two precordial leads.

Hypercalcemia is accountable to short ventricular action potential duration during phase 2, and ECG shows shortening of QT interval; it can also produce ST-T segment abnormalities simulating ischemic pattern because Ca^{2+} plays a central role in regulation of cardiac cycle (contraction and relaxation) [40].

17.5 Diagnosis of Type-3 CRS

17.5.1 Ultrasound Diagnosis

Ultrasound evaluation of type-3 CRS patients shows several patterns both on kidney and heart examination.

Kidney size and echogenicity provide primary features to discern between acute and chronic nephropathies always remembering how kidney volume and longitudinal diameters correlate with patient height and body surface [41, 42] and that chronic renal failure does not exclude normal or enlarged kidneys (e.g., early stages of diabetic nephropathy, HIV-related glomerulonephritis, or cast nephropathy).

A hyperechogenic renal cortex with low cortico-medullary ratio is predictive of chronic nephropathy [41, 42] (Fig. 17.2). At the same time cortical hyperechogenicity can also present in acute tubular necrosis or systemic lupus erythematosus nephritis [41, 42]. In these cases,

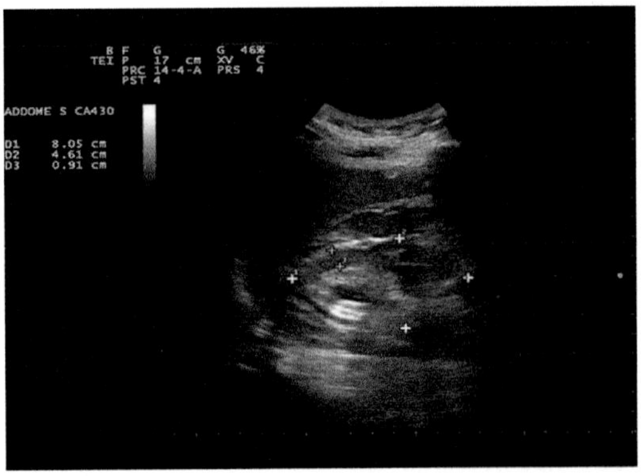

Fig. 17.2 A hyperechogenic renal cortex with low cortico-medullary ratio in AKI patients with acute renal failure

enlarged renal parenchyma may suggest a condition of edema in the acute setting.

Doppler and color Doppler evaluation can be crucial in the diagnosis and prognosis in the acute setting, mainly in relation to diastolic flow evaluation in interlobular arteries [43]. Renal ultrasound is also crucial in differential diagnosis of obstructive nephropathies.

Echocardiographic pattern is not diagnostic showing an increase in atrial volumes or areas as indices of volume overload or pleural or pericardial effusion, and it's often associated to lung comet evidence on thoracic ultrasound [44] (Figs. 17.3 and 17.4).

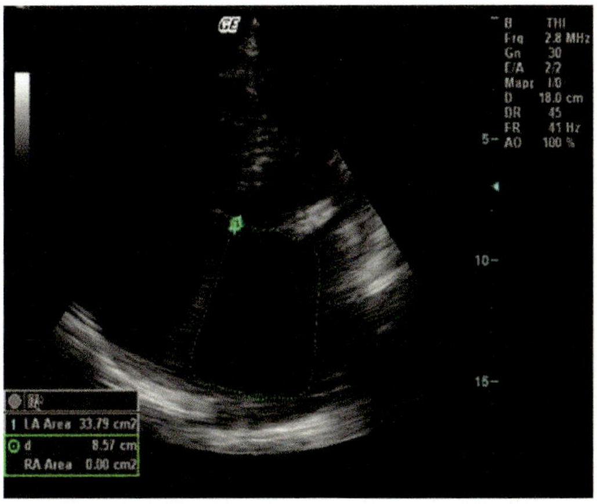

Fig. 17.3 Left atrium enlargement in AKI patient with acute renal failure

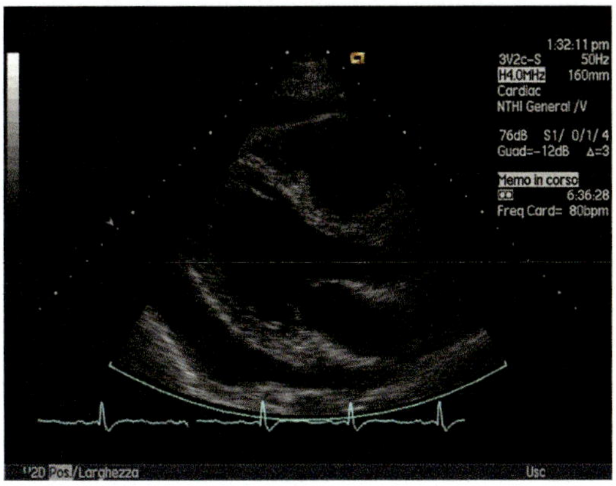

Fig. 17.4 Severe pericardial effusion in AKI patient with acute renal failure

17.5.2 Biochemical Diagnosis

17.5.2.1 Biomarkers of Type-3 CRS

During the last decades, and especially during the last 5–10 years, a large amount of potential biomarkers have been proposed for the diagnosis of type-3 CRS (Table 17.4). Among AKI novel biomarkers (each with pros and cons), some of them seem to be particularly interesting, such as neutrophil gelatinase-associated lipocalin (NGAL), kidney injury molecule-1 (KIM-1), interleukin-18 (IL-18), interleukin-6 (IL-6), cystatin C (Cys-C), N-acetyl-β[beta]-d-glucosaminidase, liver-type fatty acid-binding protein (L-FABP), netrin-1, klotho, and midkine.

On the other side, several cardiac biomarkers are routinely employed in clinical practice: biomarkers of myocardial necrosis, such as

Table 17.4 Potential biomarkers in acute kidney injury

Biomarkers of AKI, acute cardiac dysfunction, and type-3 CRS	
Potential biomarkers for early detection of AKI	NGAL KIM-1 Cystatin C IL-18 N-acetyl-β-D-glucosaminidase (NAG) L-FABP Netrin-1 Klotho Midkine
Potential biomarkers for differential diagnosis of AKI	KIM-1 IL-18 Potential for prognosis of AKI NGAL Cystatin C N-acetyl-β-D-glucosaminidase (NAG)
Potential biomarkers for inflammation and immune response	Urinary IL-18 Tumor necrosis factor receptor-1 (TNFR-1) Urinary vascular cell adhesion molecule-1 (VCAM-1) Monocyte chemoattractant protein-1 (MCP-1)
Early detection of acute cardiac dysfunction	BNP/NT-proBNP cTnT, cTnI Myoglobin Myeloperoxidase (MPO) C-reactive protein (CRP) H-FABP

troponins T (cTnT) and I (cTnI), and markers of heart failure such as B-type natriuretic peptide (BNP) and its inactive N-terminal fragment (NT-proBNP) [25].

17.5.2.2 AKI Biomarkers

NGAL is a protein of the lipocalin superfamily, and it is normally expressed (at low levels) by neutrophils and several epithelial cells (kidney, lung, stomach, and gut). NGAL seems to play an important role in limiting oxidative damage in acute and chronic kidney diseases, and it represents the earliest kidney biomarker of ischemic damage.

Cys-C is a cysteine protease inhibitor produced and secreted by all nucleated cells, and its blood levels are not affected by age, sex, race, or muscle mass. It's freely filtrated at glomerulus and completely reabsorbed by tubular cells and not secreted (it's not normally found in urine).

KIM-1 is a transmembrane glycoprotein, normally undetected in the urinary samples, which can be found in the urine after ischemic or nephrotoxic insult to proximal tubular cells; KIM-1 urinary levels seem to be highly specific for ischemic AKI (such as acute tubular necrosis, ATN) [25].

L-FABP is a protein mainly produced in the liver and expressed on hepatocytes and renal proximal tubular cells; it can be filtered by renal glomeruli and reabsorbed in the proximal tubular cells; if renal proximal tubular cells are injured, L-FABP urinary levels rapidly increase [45] but later in respect of NGAL.

IL-18 is a pro-inflammatory cytokine detected in the urine after ischemic tubular damage, associated with AKI mortality and sepsis.

Klotho is another proximal tubule transmembrane protein that inhibits renal phosphate excretion; AKI is characterized by an acute, but reversible, deficiency of klotho levels, and a reduction in klotho levels could be associated to AKI [46].

Netrin-1 is a laminin-like protein whose blood levels can increase in AKI patients; it can be detected in urine after 1–3 h after ischemia-reperfusion following renal injury [47].

Finally, midkine is a heparin-binding protein shown to increase its expression in ischemic renal injury; its urinary levels represent a sensitive biomarker for early AKI detection [48].

17.5.2.3 Cardiac Biomarkers

Cardiac biomarkers are commonly employed in daily clinical practice. BNP is a vasopeptide hormone released by the left ventricle in response to wall stress and modified by a prohormone (proBNP).

ProBNP and BNP are found in the kidney, and glomerular filtration process has a role in the clearance of NT-proBNP.

BNP/NT-proBNP ratio is the best diagnosis and prognostic markers in patients with acute renal failure [49].

The PRIDE study has highlighted how NT-proBNP levels in patients with eGFR <60 mL/min/1.73 m^2 are the best predictors of clinical outcomes [50].

BNP and NT-proBNP provide fundamental information in patients with renal dysfunction although it has been to remember that NT-proBNP seems to be reduced in patients undergoing hemodialysis by high-flux membranes.

Troponins are highly sensitive and specific for ischemic myocardial injury, and they correlate with outcomes in kidney disease patients [51, 52].

Heart-FABP (H-FABP) is a nonenzymatic protein increasing during cardiac ischemia, and it holds more than 80% sensitivity for diagnosis of acute myocardial infarction in the period of 30–210 min after symptoms' onset [53], faster than CK-MB activity and cardiac troponins, but it shows limited diagnostic value in kidney disease patients.

17.5.2.4 Biomarkers of Both the Heart and Kidney

Many biomarkers can be associated both to kidney and heart acute disease; higher levels of Cys-C seem to be associated with increased left ventricular mass and concentric left ventricular hypertrophy, and they could be and independent predictor of major cardiovascular events in a 12-month follow-up period of non-ST elevation acute coronary syndrome (ACS) patients [54].

IL-18, another AKI biomarker, has been indicated as associated with atherogenesis, coronary artery disease, lipidic plaque instability, and myocardial infarction; high IL-18 levels have also been described in acute decompensated heart failure (ADHF) patients with clear impact on long-term cardiovascular outcomes [55].

Combination of H- and L-FABP seems to play a role in defining both kidney and heart injury, since H-FABP levels have been correlated with BNP levels in patients with ADHF. Both serum H-FABP and urinary L-FABP may be able to detect ongoing myocardial damage involved in the progression of ACS [56].

Finally, serum H-FABP appears as an independent predictor of cardiac events on 1-year follow-up evaluation in patients with ACS, also showing a greater predictive capacity for cardiac events rather than cTnT [56].

17.6 Management Approach to Type-3 CRS Patients

To better provide complete management of type-3 CRS, the best treatment strategy is probably to identify various stages of the disease (according to RIFLE/AKIN criteria), from patients at high risk of developing AKI to stage 3 AKI patients, those who present kidney failure requiring renal replacement therapy.

17.6.1 Patients at High Risk of Developing AKI

Risk factors for developing AKI are age older than 75 years, CKD (estimated GFR 60 mL/min/1.73 m^2), cardiac failure, atherosclerotic peripheral vascular disease, liver disease, diabetes mellitus, nephrotoxic medications, hypovolemic status, and sepsis [7].

Avoiding or minimizing nephrotoxic medications and procedures is an important strategy to prevent AKI. Antibiotics (aminoglycosides) and contrast medium represent the main nephrotoxic agents employed in intensive care units, and their employment should be reduced. Combination therapy with vancomycin and aminoglycoside or angiotensin-converting enzyme inhibitors, non-steroidal anti-inflammatory drugs, and diuretics can lead to renal tubular injury and volume depletion.

Preventing hypoperfusion is a cornerstone to avoid an acute kidney injury, and volume depletion should be corrected. A vasopressor may be added after adequate volume resuscitation in hypotensive patients to maintain mean arterial pressure. Strict monitoring of fluid balance is fundamental to avoid volume overload, especially in patients with higher filling pressures and signs of right heart dysfunction due to increased preload [7].

17.6.2 Stage 1 (Risk)

Patients at risk are confident with AKI criteria, and they can develop severe AKI until acute renal failure. These patients should be treated as previous group (patients at high risk). In addition, they need urine analysis, routine blood tests, biomarkers, and ultrasound to investigate etiology, make diagnosis, and plan the treatment. Underlying and correctable diseases should be treated. Close monitoring and supportive care should be provided [25].

17.6.3 Stage 2 (Injury)

Stage 2 patients are characterized by high risk of morbidity/mortality due to renal injury. Patients need conservative therapy, and functional hemodynamic monitoring to guide resuscitation, especially pulse pressure variation in ventilated patients, should be considered. Clinicians have to provide optimal intravascular volume status, mean arterial pressure, cardiac output, and oxygen carrying capacity (e.g., hemoglobin). Maintenance of electrolytes and acid-base homeostasis should be ensured. Drug dosing and their blood levels have to be in the therapeutic range to avoid incorrect storage [25].

17.6.4 Stage 3 (Failure)

At this stage, the patient is at the highest risk of death and has a high probability of extrarenal complications including CRS. RRT or extracorporeal kidney support should be considered if pharmacological therapy doesn't work, kidney injury is severe, or there is risk of developing life-threatening complications. The final chapter will be dedicated to renal replacement therapy [25].

Cardiac dysfunction may occur in any stage of AKI but mainly in stage 3 when patients also present higher cardiovascular risk. The European Society of Cardiology (ESC) and American College of Cardiology Foundation (ACCF)/American Heart Association (AHA) guidelines for ADHF [10, 11] have to be followed. Intravascular and extravascular volume control should be reached with diuretics and extracorporeal therapies. Prevention of left ventricular volume overload is critical to maintain adequate cardiac output and systemic perfusion.

Diuretics, especially loop diuretics, are the gold standard in ADHF and type-3 CRS therapy since they provide for the reduction of fluid overload and improve symptoms (beneficial effects on patients' dyspnea and edema); on the other side, inappropriate diuretic therapy can worsen the kidney's injury during AKI.

Therefore, diuretic therapy has been associated with increased risk of death in AKI patients showing no benefits in the kidneys' function recovery [57]. Despite of this clinical evidence, diuretics remain the first choice therapy in ADHF patients. Continuous infusion of furosemide has been recommended for improved efficacy as far as combination therapy thiazide diuretics.

17.7 Renal Replacement Therapy

Once pharmacological treatment fails in AKI patients and oligo-anuric renal failure is established, renal replacement therapy has to be started, and it represents a cornerstone in the management of severe kidney injury although several aspects of RRT remain still controversial.

The timing of RRT initiation is strongly dependent by clear impairment of renal function with electrolytes and acid-base imbalances, hypercreatininemia, and severe fluid overload not responsive to pharmacological treatment [58].

Clinicians are not always confident in estimating potential recovery from kidney injury, and this fact can complicate any decision in starting RRT.

As previously discussed, AKI biomarkers may be helpful to target which patients will recover renal function [59, 60].

Timing of RRT initiation can impact on clinical outcomes; for example, early application of RRT in patients with severe sepsis might be beneficial [18], but, at the same time, early "classic dose" of continuous veno-venous hemofiltration (CVVH) does not provide complete or partial renal recovery [61].

It's also demonstrated that avoiding or delaying RRT is strictly associated with higher mortality and increased hospitalization rates [62, 63].

Fluid overload represents a major outcome parameter in AKI patients on CRRT (continuous renal replacement therapy) [64]; starting RRT with low rates of fluid retention may improve renal and cardiovascular outcomes [64].

RRT can be stopped when improvement in renal function is clearly evident as pointed up by increased urine output and decrease in serum creatinine levels in patients with constant CRRT dose. A urine output of more than 400 mL/day can represent a cutoff value, while a 15–20 mL/min creatinine clearance could allow CRRT withdrawal [65].

CRRT and intermittent hemodialysis (IHD) both present pros and cons; when correctly applied, both CRRT and IHD can achieve good metabolic control in many randomized controlled trials and meta-analyses [66], although CRRT seems to be associated with best outcomes and more frequent renal recovery in critically ill patients in comparison with IHD [66].

Together with CRRT and IHD therapies, some "hybrid therapies" have been proposed, such as sustained low-efficiency (daily) dialysis (SLED) and extended daily dialysis in which IHD techniques are adapted to provide longer dialysis sessions [67–69].

Some clinical trials have not found any difference between SLED and CVVH in terms of cardiovascular stability and mortality rates, but SLED seems to be associated with short duration of mechanical ventilation [70].

Concerning RRT dose, it was largely underdosed in critically ill patients in the past decades; the Vicenza group trial proposed the milestone RRT dose of 35 mL/kg to be increased in septic patients [71].

Large multicenter randomized controlled trials demonstrated that increased RRT dose was not associated to better clinical and renal outcomes, and a dose of 20–30 mL/kg/h is the recommended "normal dose" for CRRT treatments [72].

In conclusion, despite multiple RRT device availability, clinicians have to tailor RRT therapy on single critically ill patients to provide the ideal blood purification treatment.

References

1. Ronco C, McCullough P, Anker SD, et al. Cardiorenal syndromes: report from the consensus conference of the acute dialysis quality initiative. Eur Heart J. 2010;31:703–11.
2. Prabhu SD. Cytokine-induced modulation of cardiac function. Circ Res. 2004;95(12):1140–53.
3. Kingma JG Jr, Vincent C, Rouleau JR, Kingma I. Influence of acute renal failure on coronary vasoregulation in dogs. J Am Soc Nephrol. 2006;17(5):1316–24.
4. Bagshaw SM, Cruz DN. Aspromonte N, et al, and for the Acute Dialysis Quality Initiative (ADQI) Consensus Group. Epidemiology of cardio-renal syndrome: workgroup statements from the 7th ADQI Consensus Conference. Nephrol Dial Transplant. 2010;25:1406–16.
5. Bellomo R, Ronco C, Kellum JA, Mehta RL, Palevsky PM, the ADQI Workgroup. Acute renal failure-definition, outcome measures, animal models, fluid therapy and information technology needs. The Second International Consensus Conference of the Acute Dialysis Quality Initiative (ADQI) Group. Crit Care. 2004;8:R204–12.
6. Mehta RL, Kellum JA, Shah SV, et al. Acute kidney injury network (AKIN): report of an initiative to improve outcomes in acute kidney injury. Crit Care. 2007;11:R31.
7. Lewington A, Kanagasundaram S. Kidney diseases: Improving Global Outcomes (KDIGO) acute kidney injury clinical practice guideline. Kidney Int. 2012;2(1):1–138.
8. Uchino S, Kellum JA, Bellomo R, et al. Beginning and Ending Supportive Therapy for the Kidney (BEST Kidney) investigators. Acute renal failure in critically ill patients: a multinational, multicenter study. JAMA. 2005;294:813–8.
9. Dickstein K, Cohen-Solal A, Filipatos G, et al. ESC guidelines for the diagnosis and treatment of acute and chronic heart failure 2008 of the European Society of Cardiology. Developed in collaboration with the Heart Failure Association of the ESC (HFA) and endorsed by the European Society of Intensive Care Medicine (ESICM). Eur J Heart Fail. 2008;10:933–89.
10. Jessup M, Abraham WT, Casey DE, et al. ACCF/AHA guidelines for the diagnosis and management of heart failure in adults: a report of the American College of Cardiology Foundation/American Heart Association Task Force on Practice Guidelines: developed in collaboration with the International Society for Heart and Lung Transplantation. Circulation. 2009;119:1977–2016.
11. Gheorghiade M, Zannad F, Sopko G, et al. Failure syndromes: current state and framework for future research. Circulation. 2005;112:3958–68.
12. Heywood JT, Fonarow GC, Costanzo MR, et al. High prevalence of renal dysfunction and its impact on outcome in 118465 patients hospitalized with acute decompensated heart failure: a report from the ADHERE database. J Card Fail. 2007;13:422–30.
13. Siirila-Waris K, Lassus J, Melin J, et al. Characteristics, otucomes, and predictors of 1 year mortality in patients hospitalized for acute heart failure. Eur Heart J. 2006;27:3011–7.
14. Ali T, Khan I, Simpson W, et al. Incidence and outcomes in acute kidney injury: a comprehensive population-based study. J Am Soc Nephrol. 2007;18:1292–8.
15. De Abreu KLS, Silva Junior GB, Carreto AGC, et al. Acute kidney injury after trauma: prevalence, clinical characteristics and RIFLE classification. Indian J Crit Care Med. 2010;14:121–8.
16. Raine A, Margreiter R, Brunner F, et al. Report on management of renal failure in Europe. XXII. Nephrol Dial Transplant. 1992;7(Suppl 2):7–35.
17. Schwilk B, Wiedeck H, Stein B, et al. Epidemiology of acute renal failure and outcome of haemodiafiltration in intensive care. Intensive Care Med. 1997;23:1204–11.
18. Song JH, Humes HD. Renal cell therapy and beyond. Semin Dial. 2009;22:603–9.
19. Wen X, Murugan R, Peng Z, Kellum JA. Pathophysiology of acute kidney injury: a new perspective. Contrib Nephrol. 2010;165:39–45.
20. Bongartz LG, Cramer MJ, Doevendans PA, Joles JA, Braam B. The severe cardiorenal syndrome: 'Guyton revisited'. Eur Heart J. 2005;26(1):11–7.
21. Ma XL, Lefer DJ, Lefer AM, Rothlein R. Coronary endothelial and cardiac protective effects of a monoclonal antibody to intercellular adhesion molecule-1 in myocardial ischemia and reperfusion. Circulation. 1992;86(3):937–46.

22. Blake P, Hasegawa Y, Khosla MC, Fouad-Tarazi F, Sakura N, Paganini EP. Isolation of "myocardial depressant factor(s)" from the ultrafiltrate of heart failure patients with acute renal failure. ASAIO J. 1996;42(5):M911–5.
23. Edmunds NJ, Lal H, Woodward B. Effects of tumour necrosis factor-alpha on left ventricular function in the rat isolated perfused heart: possible mechanisms for a decline in cardiac function. Br J Pharmacol. 1999;126(1):189–96.
24. Rauchhaus M, Doehner W, Francis DP, et al. Plasma cytokine parameters and mortality in patients with chronic heart failure. Circulation. 2000;102(25):3060–7.
25. Chuasuwan A, Kellum JA. Cardio-renal syndrome type 3: epidemiology, pathophysiology, and treatment. Semin Nephrol. 2012;32(1):31–9.
26. Kajstura J, Cigola E, Malhotra A, et al. Angiotensin II induces apoptosis of adult ventricular myocytes in vitro. J Mol Cell Cardiol. 1997;29(3):859–70.
27. Nath KA, Grande JP, Croatt AJ, et al. Transgenic sickle mice are markedly sensitive to renal ischemia-reperfusion injury. Am J Pathol. 2005;166(4):963–72.
28. Kelly KJ. Distant effects of experimental renal ischemia/reperfusion injury. J Am Soc Nephrol. 2003;14(6):1549–58.
29. Bryant D, Becker L, Richardson J, et al. Cardiac failure in transgenic mice with myocardial expression of tumor necrosis factor-alpha. Circulation. 1998;97:1375–81.
30. Liu YH, D'Ambrosio M, Liao TD, et al. N-acetyl-seryl-aspartyl-lysyl-proline prevents cardiac remodeling and dysfunction induced by galectin-3, a mammalian adhesion/growth-regulatory lectin. Am J Physiol Heart Circ Physiol. 2009;296(2):H404–12.
31. De Deyn PP, vanholder R, D'Hooge R. Nitric oxide in uremia: effects of several potentially toxic guanidino compounds. Kidney Int. 2003;63(84 Suppl):S25–8.
32. Scheuer J, Stezoski W. The effects of uremic compounds on cardiac function and metabolism. J Mol Cell Cardiol. 1973;5:287–300.
33. Jackson G, Gibbs CR, Davies MK, Lip GY. ABC of heart failure. Pathophysiology. Br Med J. 2000;320:167–70.
34. Li L, Lee EW, Ji H, Zukowska Z. Neuropeptide Y-induced acceleration of postangioplasty occlusion of rat carotid artery. Arterioscler Thromb Vasc Biol. 2003;23:1204–10.
35. Shah BN, Greaves K. The cardio-renal syndrome: a review. Int J Nephrol. 2011;2011:920195. https://doi.org/10.4061/2011/920195.
36. Qin F, Patel R, Yan C, Liu W. NADPH oxidase is involved in angiotensin II-induced apoptosis in H9C2 cardiac muscle cells: effects of apocynin. Free Radic Biol Med. 2005;40:236–46.
37. Chabrashvili T, Kitiyakara C, Blau J, et al. Effects of ANF II type 1 and 2 receptors on oxidative stress, renal NADPH oxidase, and SOD expression. Am J Physiol Regul Integr Comp Physiol. 2003;285:R117–24.
38. Nakagami H, Takemoto M, Liao JK. NADPH oxidase-derived superoxide anion mediates angiotensin II-induced cardiac hypertrophy. J Mol Cell Cardiol. 2003;35:851–9.
39. Griendling KK, Minieri CA, Ollerenshaw JD, Alexander RW. Angiotensin II stimulates NADH and NADPH oxidase activity in cultured vascular smooth muscle cells. Circ Res. 1994;74:1141–8.
40. Shannon TR, Pogwizd SM, Bers DM. Elevated sarcoplasmic reticulum Ca2+ leak in intact ventricular myocytes from rabbits in heart failure. Circ Res. 2003;93(7):592–4.
41. Licurse A, Kim MC, Dziura J, Forman HP, Formica RN, Makarov DV, Parikh CR, Gross CP. Renal ultrasonography in the evaluation of acute kidney injury: developing a risk stratification framework. Arch Intern Med. 2010;170:1900–7.
42. Ozmen CA, Akin D, Bilek SU, Bayrak AH, Senturk S, Nazaroglu H. Ultrasound as a diagnostic tool to differentiate acute from chronic renal failure. Clin Nephrol. 2010;74:46–52.
43. Darmon M, Schortgen F, Vargas F, Liazydi A, Schlemmer B, Brun-Buisson C, Brochard L. Diagnostic accuracy of Doppler renal resistive index for reversibility of acute kidney injury in critically ill patients. Intensive Care Med. 2011;37(1):68–76.
44. Di Lullo L, Floccari F, Granata A, D'Amelio A, Rivera R, Fiorini F, Malaguti M, Timio M. Ultrasonography: Ariadne's thread in the diagnosis of cardiorenal syndrome. Cardiorenal Med. 2012;2(1):11–7; Epub 2011 Nov 30.
45. Negishi K, Noiri E, Doi K, et al. Monitoring of urinary L-type fatty acid-binding protein predicts histological severity of acute kidney injury. Am J Pathol. 2009;174:1154–9.
46. Hu M-C, Shi M, Zhang J, et al. Klotho deficiency is an early biomarker of renal ischemia-reperfusion injury and its replacement is protective. Kidney Int. 2010;78:1240–51.
47. Reeves WB, Kwon O, Ramesh G. Netrin-1 and kidney injury. II. Netrin-1 is an early biomarker of acute kidney injury. Am J Physiol Renal Physiol. 2007;294:F731–F8.
48. Hayashi H, Sato W, Maruyama S, et al. Urinary Midkine as a biomarker of acute kidney injury: comparison with three major biomarkers; NAG, IL-18 and NGAL [abstract]. NDT Plus. 2009;2:ii, 1634, Suppl 2.
49. McCullough PA, Nowak RM, McCord J, et al. B-type natriuretic peptide and clinical judgment in emergency diagnosis of heart failure: analysis from Breathing Not Properly (BNP) Multinational Study. Circulation. 2002;106:416–22.
50. Wu AH, Jaffe AS, Apple FS, et al. National Academy of Clinical Biochemistry Laboratory Medicine practice guidelines: use of cardiac troponin and B-type natriuretic peptide or N-terminal proB-type natriuretic peptide for etiologies other than acute coronary syndromes and heart failure. Clin Chem. 2007;53:2086–96.

51. Januzzi JL Jr, Camargo CA, Anwaruddin S, et al. The N-terminal Pro-BNP investigation of dyspnea in the emergency department (PRIDE) study. Am J Cardiol. 2005;95:948–54.
52. Di Lullo L, Barbera V, Santoboni A, Bellasi A, Cozzolino M, De Pascalis A, Rivera R, Balducci A, Russo D, Ronco C. Troponins and chronic kidney disease. G Ital Nefrol. 2015;32(4).
53. Glatz JF, Vander Vusse FJ, Maessen JG, et al. Fatty acid-binding protein as marker of muscle injury: experimental fi and clinical application. Acta Anaesthesiol Scand Suppl. 1997;111:292–4.
54. Taglieri N, Fernandez-Berges DJ, Koenig W, et al. Plasma cystatin C for prediction of 1-year cardiac events in Mediterranean patients with non-ST elevation acute coronary syndromes. Atherosclerosis. 2010;209:300–5.
55. Furtado MV, Rossini AP, Campani RB, et al. Interleukin-18: an independent predictor of cardiovascular events in patients with acute coronary syndrome after 6 months of follow-up. Coron Artery Dis. 2009;20:327–31.
56. Liyan C, Jie Z, Xiaozhou H. Prognostic value of combination of heart-type fatty acid-binding protein and ischemia-modified albumin in patients with acute coronary syndromes and normal troponin T value. J Clin Lab Anal. 2009;23:14–8.
57. Mehta RL, Pascual MT, Soroko SH, et al. Diuretics, mortality, and nonrecovery of renal function in acute renal failure. JAMA. 2002;288:2547–53.
58. Bellomo R, Kellum JA, Ronco C. Acute kidney injury. Lancet. 2012;380:756–66.
59. Srisawat N, Murugan R, Lee M, Kong L, Carter M, Angus DC, et al. Plasma neutrophil gelatinase-associated lipocalin predicts recovery from acute kidney injury following community-acquired pneumonia. Kidney Int. 2011;80:545–52.
60. Srisawat N, Wen X, Lee M, Kong L, Elder M, Carter M, et al. Urinary biomarkers and renal recovery in critically ill patients with renal support. Clin J Am Soc Nephrol. 2011;6:1815–23.
61. Payen D, Mateo J, Cavaillon JM, Fraisse F, Floriot C, Vicaut E. Impact of continuous venovenous hemofiltration on organ failure during the early phase of severe sepsis: a randomized controlled trial. Crit Care Med. 2009;37:803–10.
62. Karvellas CJ, Farhat MR, Sajjad I, Mogensen SS, Leung AA, Wald R, et al. A comparison of early versus late initiation of renal replacement therapy in critically ill patients with acute kidney injury: a systematic review and meta-analysis. Crit Care. 2011;15:R72.
63. Clec'h C, Darmon M, Lautrette A, Chemouni F, Azoulay E, Schwebel C, et al. Efficacy of renal replacement therapy in critically ill patients: a propensity analysis. Crit Care. 2012;16:R236.
64. Bellomo R, Cass A, Cole L, Finfer S, Gallagher M, Lee J, et al. An observational study fluid balance and patient outcomes in the Randomized Evaluation of Normal vs Augmented Level of Replacement Therapy trial. Crit Care Med. 2012;40:1753–60.
65. Uchino S, Bellomo R, Morimatsu H, Morgera S, Schetz M, Tan I, et al. Discontinuation of continuous renal replacement therapy: a post hoc analysis of a prospective multicenter observational study. Crit Care Med. 2009;37:2576–82.
66. Schneider AG, Bellomo R, Bagshaw SM, Glassford NJ, Lo S, Jun M, et al. Choice of renal replacement therapy modality and dialysis dependence after acute kidney injury: a systematic review and meta-analysis. Intensive Care Med. 2013;39:987–97.
67. Berbece AN, Richardson RM. Sustained low-efficiency dialysis in the ICU: cost, anticoagulation, and solute removal. Kidney Int. 2006;70:963–8.
68. Kumar VA, Craig M, Depner TA, Yeun JY. Extended daily dialysis: a new approach to renal replacement for acute renal failure in the intensive care unit. Am J Kidney Dis. 2000;36:294–300.
69. Wu VC, Wang CH, Wang WJ, Lin YF, Hu FC, Chen YW, et al. Sustained low-efficiency dialysis versus continuous veno-venous hemofiltration for postsurgical acute renal failure. Am J Surg. 2010;199:466–76.
70. Schwenger V, Weigand MA, Hoffmann O, Dikow R, Kihm LP, Seckinger J, et al. Sustained low efficiency dialysis using a single-pass batch system in acute kidney injury-a randomized interventional trial: the REnal Replacement Therapy Study in Intensive Care Unit PatiEnts. Crit Care. 2012;16:R140.
71. Legrand M, Darmon M, Joannidis M, Payen D. Management of renal replacement therapy in ICU patients: an international survey. Intensive Care Med. 2013;39:101–8.
72. Bellomo R, Cass A, Cole L, Finfer S, Gallagher M, Lo S, et al. Intensity of continuous renal-replacement therapy in critically ill patients. N Engl J Med. 2009;361:1627–38.

Perioperative (Non-cardiac) Acute Kidney Injury: Epidemiology, Pathophysiology, Prevention, and Treatment

18

Paras Dedhia and Charuhas V. Thakar

18.1 Incidence and Trends

The incidence of acute kidney injury (AKI) is generally 5–7.5%, in all acute care hospitalizations and accounts for up to 20% of admissions to intensive care units (ICU). Of all the cases of AKI during hospitalization, approximately 30–40% are observed in operative settings. AKI during hospitalization is associated with increased risk of mortality, prolonged length of day, and significant hospitalization costs [1]. More recently, it has also been noted that AKI can have long-term consequences on the risk of chronic kidney disease as well as poor survival [2].

With limited treatment options, prevention of AKI or amelioration of its severity remains important cornerstones of improving outcomes. The purpose of the present review is to discuss the current knowledge regarding the epidemiology and risk factors, outcomes, diagnosis, and prevention and treatment of AKI during the perioperative period. Much of our knowledge about incidence and natural history of AKI in the perioperative setting is derived from the literature that focuses on cardiac and vascular surgery settings. Literature regarding non-cardiovascular surgery is more heterogeneous and represents other diverse surgical settings. We will be examining the topic of non-cardiac surgery by further classifying it based on specific type of clinical setting.

The recent KDIGO (Kidney Disease Improving Global Outcomes; www.kdigo.org) clinical practice guidelines for AKI have adopted the Acute Kidney Injury Network (AKIN) criteria to define AKI and classify it based on the severity of injury [3, 4]. According to these criteria, AKI is present when an abrupt (over 48 h) reduction in kidney function results in an absolute increase in serum creatinine of more than or equal to 0.3 mg/dL, a percentage increase in serum creatinine of more than or equal to 50% (1.5-fold increase from baseline), or a reduction in urine output (oliguria of less than 0.5 mL/kg/h for more than 6 h). AKI is further classified into three stages (arbitrarily) based on the severity of kidney injury, as indicated by either the degree of rise of serum creatinine or loss of urine output.

18.2 Pathophysiology

Traditionally serum creatinine is used as a surrogate marker for changes in glomerular filtration rate (GFR) to evaluate the renal function, and elevation of serum creatinine remains the present standard of care in determining rapid decline in eGFR occurring in patients with AKI.

P. Dedhia · C. V. Thakar (✉)
Division of Nephrology, Department of Internal Medicine, Kidney CARE Program, University of Cincinnati, Cincinnati, OH, USA
e-mail: paras.dedhia@uc.edu; Charuhas.thakar@uc.edu; Charuhas.thakar@va.gov

S. S. Waikar et al. (eds.), *Core Concepts in Acute Kidney Injury*,
https://doi.org/10.1007/978-1-4939-8628-6_18

The putative major mechanisms of perioperative AKI include (1) hypoperfusion, (2) nephrotoxic injury, and (3) sepsis/inflammation. All of these mechanisms have overlapping pathways that eventually lead to renal tubular epithelial injury, along with disruption of adjacent microcirculation and activation of inflammatory mediators, adhesion molecules, platelets, and thromboxane [5, 6].

The common causes of AKI include ischemia/hypoxia or nephrotoxicity. An underlying feature is a rapid decline in GFR usually associated with decreases in renal blood flow. Inflammation represents an important additional component of AKI leading to the extension phase of injury, which may be associated with insensitivity to vasodilator therapy. It is suggested that targeting the extension phase represents an area potential of treatment with the greatest possible impact. The underlying basis of renal injury appears to be impaired energetics of the highly metabolically active nephron segments (i.e., proximal tubules and thick ascending limb) in the renal outer medulla, which can trigger conversion from transient hypoxia to intrinsic renal failure. Injury to kidney cells can be lethal or sublethal. Sublethal injury represents an important component in AKI, as it may profoundly influence GFR and renal blood flow (Fig. 18.1).

AKI in perioperative settings also occurs in the context of multi-organ failure and sepsis, which involves hemodynamic alterations, inflammation, and direct injury to the tubular epithelium. Inflammation is an important component of this paradigm of injury, playing a considerable role in its pathophysiology. Significant progress has been made in defining major components of this process, yet the complex molecular and cellular interactions among endothelial cells, inflammatory cells, and the injured epithelium remain poorly understood.

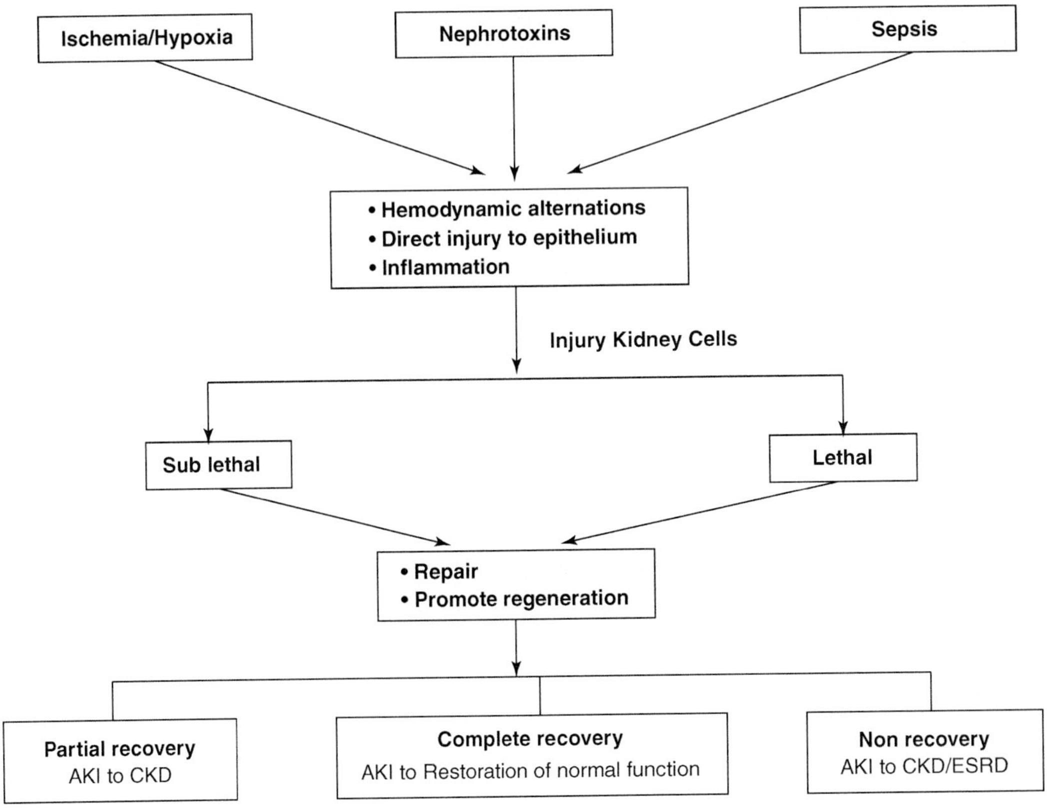

Fig. 18.1 Schematic of pathophysiology of acute kidney injury in perioperative settings

Recently researchers have come to realize the intrinsic capacity of the damaged proximal epithelium to repair itself by dedifferentiation and proliferation of surviving epithelial cells without a source of distinct progenitor cells. The nature of the recovery response is mediated by the degree to which sublethal cells can restore normal function and promote regeneration. The successful recovery from AKI depends on the degree to which these repair processes ensue and these may be compromised in variety of concomitant comorbid conditions along with age and preexisting CKD being more prevalent in the population under consideration.

Investigators have also identified potential pathophysiological links among injury, abnormal repair, and the pro-fibrotic sequelae of severe injury that may help to explain why in humans AKI is such a great risk factor for progression of CKD [6]. Recent data suggests that AKI represents a potential link to CKD in surviving patients [7].

18.3 Clinical Settings and Specific Syndromes

In this section, we will discuss different clinical settings of non-cardiac surgery and associated incidence, risk factors, and outcomes of AKI.

18.3.1 Major Abdominal Surgery

The epidemiology of AKI in this setting is heterogeneous and perhaps a reflection of smaller sample sizes and single-center analyses. In one recent review of all types of abdominal surgeries, it was reported that the overall incidence of AKI among intra-abdominal surgery patients was 1.1%, which varied from 0.2% in appendectomy and 0.3% in gastric bypass patients to 2.6% in small bowel resection and 3.5% in exploratory laparotomy patients. Of the patients who developed AKI, 31.3% died within 30 days, compared with 1.9% of those who did not develop AKI. After adjusting for comorbidities and operative factors, AKI was associated with a 3.5-fold increase in the risk of 30-day mortality (adjusted risk ratio, 3.51; 95% confidence interval [CI], 3.29–3.74). Among individual procedures, the estimated adjusted risk ratio of 30-day mortality associated with AKI ranged from 1.87 (95% CI, 1.62–2.17) in exploratory laparotomy to 31.6 (95% CI, 17.9–55.9) in gastric bypass [8].

When studied in patients undergoing non-cardiac surgery with normal preoperative renal function, the incidence of postoperative AKI was less than 1%; with AKI defined as an absolute level of estimated GFR less than 50 mL/min during the postoperative period (representing a 40% reduction from preoperative levels). In this study, Kheterpal et al. developed a preoperative renal-risk index in non-cardiovascular surgeries. The following were identified as independent risk factors for postoperative AKI: older age, emergency surgery, liver disease, high BMI, high-risk surgery, peripheral vascular disease, and COPD [9]. Higher risk scores were associated with a greater frequency of AKI, which ranged between 0.3 and 4.5% depending on the risk category (Table 18.1).

Another setting that has been studied in abdominal surgery includes those patients undergoing gastric bypass. This cohort of patients can present with a unique comorbidity profile including high body mass index (BMI), high prevalence of diabetes, hypertension, hyperlipidemia, and osteoarthritis. Additionally, due to the comorbid conditions, these patients are commonly exposed

Table 18.1 Incidence and risk factors of AKI after non-cardiovascular surgery [40]

Risk factors	Risk categories	Frequency of AKI
Age >59 years	0 risk factors (Class I)	0.3%
BMI >32	1 risk factor (Class II)	0.5%
Emergency surgery	2 risk factors (Class III)	1.3%
High-risk surgery	≥3 risk factors (Class IV)	4.3%
Peripheral vascular disease		
COPD		
Liver disease		

AKI acute kidney injury, *BMI* body mass index, *COPD* chronic obstructive pulmonary disease

to drugs such as angiotensin-converting enzyme inhibitors (ACE-I) or angiotensin receptor blockers (ARBs), diuretics, and nonsteroidal anti-inflammatory agents. In a single-center study, which examined over 300 gastric bypass surgeries, risk factors associated with postoperative AKI included higher BMI, hyperlipidemia, and preoperative use of ACE-I/ARB agents. At least in this analysis, the study did not find any interaction between combination of therapy between NSAID, diuretics, and ACE-I/ARB agents [10].

Abdominal Compartment Syndrome The incidence of intra-abdominal hypertension and abdominal compartment syndrome varies depending on population and surgical setting studied. The incidence of ACS is reported to be as high as 40.7% in surgical intensive care unit setting. Abdominal compartment syndrome can be classified as either primary or secondary, depending on occurrence of compartment syndrome in the setting of abdominal pathology and the setting of systemic disease, respectively. The most recent consensus guidelines, updated in 2013, defined IAH as sustained intra-abdominal pressure (IAP) of ≥12 mmHg. In the more severe form, ACS was defined as IAPs that rose to levels ≥20 mmHg and were associated with new organ dysfunction/failure [11]. Physical examination is not a very sensitive method to diagnose ACS. The World Society of Abdominal Compartment Syndrome (WSACS) recommends using bladder pressure for measurement of intra-abdominal pressure. In patients with ACS, maintaining abdominal perfusion pressure (mean arterial pressure—intra-abdominal pressure) at more than 50 mmHg has shown to be associated with better survival. Abdominal perfusion pressure has been demonstrated to be a better marker than MAP, IAP, arterial pH, base deficit, arterial lactate, and urine output in predicting survival from IAH and ACS [12].

In the updated 2013 guidelines, the WSACS suggested using a resuscitation protocol that attempted to avoid a positive cumulative fluid balance in critically ill or injured patients at risk for IAH/ACS once initial resuscitation had been achieved and the inciting issues addressed (grade 2c recommendation). Sedation and neuromuscular blockade provide additional tools for the medical management of IAH by increasing abdominal wall compliance. Removal of excessive fluids by drainage, diuresis, hemofiltration, and ultrafiltration are alternative potentially effective medical treatments for IAH. In patients with significant gaseous bowel distension, the use of prokinetics, nasogastric decompression, rectal drainage, and enemas may sustain minor reductions in IAP. Avoiding reverse Trendelenburg positioning or proning may prevent further increases in IAP.

IAH that has progressed to the point of ACS, i.e., organ failure, must be treated surgically. This typically presents clinically with IAP ≥20–25 mmHg in association with hypotension, raised airway pressures, impaired ventilation, or oliguria. Decompressive laparotomy (DL) is almost always effective and is associated with a rapid improvement in airway pressures, PaO2/FIO2 ratio, and urine output. When necessary, it can be performed at bedside for those too unstable to travel.

18.3.2 Orthopedic Surgery

Over the past decade, there has been a marked increase in the total number of total hip and knee arthroplasties performed in the United States. It is estimated that in the next decade, the demand for primary total hip arthroplasties will grow by 174% to 572,000, and the total knee arthroplasties are projected to grow by 673% to 3.48 million procedures [13].

Much of the literature regarding AKI in orthopedic surgery focused on traumatic hip fractures and has been represented as either case series or single-center studies. More recently, Kimmel et al. describe the incidence and outcomes of AKI in patients undergoing orthopedic surgery [14]. AKI occurred in 15% following elective total joint arthroplasty (TJA) in a population that was older and more obese and included patients with pre-existing renal dysfunction in comparison to the relatively younger, healthier patients studied by Weingarten et al. that exhibited an incidence of <2% in elective TJAs [15].

An observational cohort from the United Kingdom reported the incidence of AKI and its impact on short-term and long-term outcome following orthopedic surgery. The following were identified as independent risk factors for postoperative AKI: older age, male sex, diabetes, number of prescribed drugs, lower estimated glomerular filtration rate, use of ACE-I/ARB, and American Society of Anesthesiologists severity grade. Short-term survival was poor in AKI as compared to those without AKI. Even patients with mild (stage 1) AKI had impact on survival [16].

In a recent report based on national inpatient survey, Nadkarni and colleagues examined 7,235,251 discharges across the United States of patients undergoing elective hip or knee replacement for osteoarthritis from 2002 to 2012. The study found that 94,367 (1.3%) had developed AKI. Over a 10-year period, the incidence of AKI has risen fourfold (from 0.5% in 2002 to 1.8–1.9% in 2010–2012; $p < 0.0001$). Preoperative chronic kidney disease, which is prevalent in such patient population, was among the most important risk factor for AKI. Additionally, postoperative events including myocardial infarction, need for cardiac catheterization, sepsis, and need for transfusions were most commonly associated with AKI. Most importantly, patients with perioperative AKI were at a significantly high risk of hospital mortality (odds ratio, 11.32; $p < 0.0001$); and those who survived had two times greater risk of an adverse discharge (defined as nursing home or long-term acute care). It is expected that we will see more than doubling of hip and knee surgeries, and even a modest increase in the frequency of postoperative AKI can have significant impact on both the patient outcomes as well as resource utilization [17].

18.3.3 Burns Surgery

Patients experiencing trauma and burns are subject to many potential risk factors for AKI, including hypoperfusion, sepsis, nephrotoxins, intra-abdominal hypertension, transfusions, and exposure to iodinated contrast material. Studies of patients with burn injuries using the RIFLE classification have revealed an AKI incidence of approximately 25% [18–20]. These studies demonstrated high mortality rates in patients with AKI, especially in the failure category.

Palmieri et al. [21] examined the incidence of AKI, as defined by RIFLE criteria, in ICU burn patients and also identified risk factors of AKI, progression of AKI across RIFLE stages, and its impact on outcome. In this single-center eight-bed ICU, they assessed adults with a burn injury of 20% or more of a total body surface area percent (TBSA%). AKI occurred in 32 (53.3%) of the 60 patients with severe burns with the maximum RIFLE category: risk in 9 (28.1%), injury in 6 (18.8%), and failure in 17 (53.1%). Thirteen patients progressed to higher RIFLE I class of AKI. The progression to higher RIFLE class was associated with the higher extrarenal SOFA scores, the use of nephrotoxic drugs, the number of operations, the cumulative fluid balance prior the maximum RIFLE, and the presence of sepsis. Overall mortality in AKI was 34%. Patients who progressed to severe RIFLE category experienced a higher mortality rate (46%) compared to those who remained at the same (risk or injury) RIFLE class (7.7%).

In a more recent study, Stewart et al. [22] examined military burn causalities from Iraq and Afghanistan combat operations. AKI was classified by both AKIN and RIFLE classes. Age, sex, TBSA%, percentage of full-thickness burn, inhalation injury, and injury severity score were recorded. In over 700 patients, AKI prevalence rates by the RIFLE and AKIN criteria were 23.8% and 29.9%, respectively. After logistic regression, AKIN-2 (OR, 23.70; 95% CI, 2.32–242; $P = 0.008$) and AKIN-3 (OR, 130; 95% CI, 13.38–999; $P < 0.001$) were significantly associated with death. AKIN-3 and RIFLE injury and failure remained significant in the subset of patients with ≥20% TBSA. There was also a strong interaction between TBSA and the stage of AKI with respect to ventilator and ICU days.

These contemporary studies and historical literature point out that AKI is prevalent in casualties with burn injury and is independently associated with morbidity and mortality after adjustment for factors associated with injury severity. The key goals of care include timely resuscitation with appropriate fluids and avoiding nephrotoxic exposure in patients with higher severity of illness. Additionally, a proactive approach to anticipating complications such as rhabdomyolysis or abdominal compartment syndrome can prevent AKI.

Rhabdomyolysis Rhabdomyolysis is more commonly described in traumatic surgical settings. Direct crush injuries, lower extremity fractures, muscular vessel occlusion and impaired venous drainage, and vascular injuries with limb ischemia and reperfusion injury especially after revascularization are notable for the development of rhabdomyolysis. Burns and high-voltage injuries, pressure necrosis of the muscle after fall, prolonged immobilization, and surgical settings with prolonged and improper positioning may lead to muscle necrosis as well.

Muscle injury leading to rhabdomyolysis causes the release of a number of substances, including calcium, potassium, myoglobin, and uric acid. Myoglobin is filtered by the renal glomeruli and concentrated in the renal tubules, resulting in the characteristic red-brown or "tea-colored" urine. Several mechanisms of renal injury have been proposed, including renal tubule obstruction from myoglobin precipitation, oxidative injury from the release of iron and free radicals, and vasoconstriction leading to hypoperfusion [23]. The utility of monitoring creatine phosphokinase levels and serum or urine myoglobin levels remains controversial. Supportive therapy with aggressive volume resuscitation to maintain urine output of 150–200 mL/h is the mainstay of therapy. There are some reports to suggest that alkalization of urine by using sodium bicarbonate infusion could be cyto-protective. Diuretic use can be harmful if instituted prior to adequate volume resuscitation. In patients with established oligo-anuric AKI or refractory hyperkalemia and metabolic acidosis, renal replacement therapy is indicated. There is no clear role of instituting renal replacement therapy to remove potential nephrotoxins as a preventive or prophylactic measure.

18.3.4 Nonrenal Solid Organ Transplant Surgery

AKI is not uncommon in nonrenal solid organ transplant recipients. A national analysis [24] had revealed that the occurrence of AKI in the immediate postoperative period increases the long-term risk of CKD in these subjects. More importantly, AKI in the immediate postoperative period increases the risk of mortality, leading to the loss of patient as well as the newly transplanted organ. Transplant recipients are a particularly vulnerable group of patients to develop postoperative renal dysfunction for multiple reasons, including pre-existing renal impairment, infections, and the use of calcineurin inhibitors.

In liver transplant, almost a third of recipients develop AKI with up to 17% of patients requiring dialysis [25–27]. Multiple factors contribute to this high incidence of AKI. In the immediate postoperative period, prerenal azotemia and ATN are the main causes of AKI, whereas infection/sepsis and calcineurin inhibitor toxicity are more likely culprits in AKI cases after second week of transplant. Risk factors associated with AKI in liver transplant recipients include serum albumin <3.2 g/dL, baseline impaired renal function, dopamine use, and graft dysfunction; bacterial infection/sepsis is associated with late-onset AKI (2–4 weeks postoperatively).

AKI occurs in approximately 5–30% of recipients of thoracic organ transplantations. Many risk factors for AKI in cardiac transplant settings are similar to other cardiac surgery patients and include atherosclerosis, valvular disease, cigarette smoking, diabetes, and abnormal baseline renal function. Certain factors such as low baseline albumin and prolonged cold ischemia time are relatively unique to transplant settings only. The intraoperative use of cardiopulmonary bypass also contributes to the development of AKI. These include factors specifically related to the bypass procedure itself, such as cross-clamp time and duration of bypass. Cardiopulmonary bypass is also associated with the generation of free hemoglobin and iron through hemolysis that typically occurs during the procedure. Hemolysis can be caused by cardiotomy suction, occlusive

Table 18.2 Common risk factors for AKI after nonrenal solid organ transplant surgery

Liver transplant [28–30]	Cardiac transplant [31–33]
Preoperative factors	
Preoperative ARF (Cr >1.5 mg/dL) *Lower preoperative serum albumin (<3.2 mg/dL)* Urgent re-transplant Child-Pugh score Hematuria and/or proteinuria Advanced age Diabetes mellitus Need for high doses of diuretics High body mass index (BMI)	Low cardiac output Serum albumin Prior cardiac surgery Medication toxicity Diabetes Hepatitis C
Intraoperative factors	
Increasing use of fresh frozen plasma and cryoprecipitate (surrogate for coagulopathy) Higher number of platelet transfusions Intraoperative complications Increased use of pressors	Cardiopulmonary bypass time Organ ischemia time Transfusion requirements Hypotension/hypoperfusion Nephrotoxic agent exposure (antibiotics, radiographic contrast) Atheroembolism Hemolysis/pigment nephropathy
Postoperative factors	
Longer duration of pressors postoperatively *Longer duration of ventilator support* *Liver allograft dysfunction* Lower blood pressures through all aspects of the operation and postoperatively Higher pulmonary capillary wedge pressure pre-anhepatic and lower cardiac indices post-anhepatic CNI toxicity	Mechanical ventilation *Bacterial infection/*sepsis *Surgical reoperation* CNI toxicity Aggressive diuresis Graft dysfunction

roller pumps, turbulent flow in the oxygenator, and blood return through cell saver devices; this in turn may contribute to increased oxidative stress and renal tubular injury.

The risk of postoperative dialysis is slightly higher in cardiac transplant recipients than in those undergoing non-transplant surgery. However, length of stay and crude hospital mortality are similar regardless of the setting of cardiac surgery. This observation emphasizes the need for additional efforts to prevent kidney injury in heart transplant recipients given its impact on both the patient and the valuable organ. Detailed account of risk factors associated with AKI is shown in Table 18.2 [28–33].

Recently, Grimm et al. [34] found an incidence of postoperative renal failure necessitating dialysis in lung transplant patients to be 5.5%, which is consistent with previous studies. They described a Risk Stratification Score (RSS) that includes race, diagnosis, BMI, pre-existing renal function, diabetes, etc. and predicts a rate of renal failure of 3.1% in the lowest risk group, increasing up to 15.6% in the highest risk category.

18.3.5 Surgery for Kidney Cancer

Kidney cancer is a common malignancy in older adults. Radical nephrectomy (RN) or partial nephrectomy (PN) is now available as the gold standard of care depending on the size of the renal tumor. Patients undergoing surgical treatment for kidney cancer are likely to be older adults (>65 years of age) and suffer from diabetes, hypertension, or chronic kidney disease. Moreover, the surgical options include removal of functioning renal mass, placing patients at risk of both near-term and long-term renal complications. Epidemiological data indicates that, in patients without preoperative chronic kidney disease (CKD), the probability of incident CKD during a 3-year follow-up can reach up to 65% after radical nephrectomy and over 30% in those undergoing PN [35]. A plausible explanation is that given the age and comorbidity profile of an average patient with RCC, the compensatory ability of the remaining kidney could be limited (in RN), or the ischemic damage sustained by the remnant kidney in PN could lead to progressive decline in renal function. Much of the literature that has outlined these complications or risk factors have used the Clavien approach to grade postoperative complications—graded from levels I to V based on the degree of severity, where grade IV represents life-threatening organ failure and grade V represents death [36].

Approximately one in four patients undergoing nephrectomy will experience some postoperative complication during hospitalization. In a single-center study [37] of 150 patients undergoing PN, the frequency of postop complications (any grade) was 22% in laparoscopic approach versus 26% in open approach. Common renal complications during the postoperative period include fluid and electrolyte disturbances and AKI. The frequency of severe AKI requiring dialysis is relatively low, and in most reports, it is <5%. In patients undergoing radical or partial nephrectomy, several potential risk factors are known to be associated with AKI. These are shown in Table 18.3.

In patients undergoing PN, certain surgical approaches and techniques lead to subjecting of the kidney to warm or cold ischemia during surgery; cold ischemia is usually achieved by packing ice around the kidney undergoing PN. The optimal duration of ischemia that can be safely tolerated by the kidney remains unclear. It is extrapolated from animal models that approximately 30–45 min of ischemia followed by reperfusion is considered to be generally safe and provides optimal time required in achieving surgical efficacy for the treatment of these tumors. A recent study evaluating serial biopsies suggested that subjecting the human kidney to ischemia, lasting for 30 min or less, leads to mitochondrial swelling and cytological changes, which are potentially reversible [38, 39].

Table 18.3 Common causes of AKI associated with nephrectomy for RCC

Risk factors	Cause of AKI
Surgical technique – Renal pedicle clamp – Intra-abdominal hypertension – Warm and cold ischemia – Ureteral injury	– Hypoperfusion, ischemic injury – Obstructive uropathy
Perioperative factors – Renin-angiotensin blockers, diuretics, NSAID – Rhabdomyolysis	– Ischemic and toxic injury
Complications – Infection/sepsis – Bleeding	– Ischemic/inflammatory injury

Laparoscopic approaches to PN or RN, in some cases, can be associated with intra-abdominal hypertension (IAH). Typically, these procedures require induction of pneumoperitoneum to achieve pressures ranging from 20 to 25 mm of Hg. Experimental models that have studied the safety of this process indicate that IAH can impact the production of nitric oxide in renal microcirculation [40, 41]. Taken together, it can be hypothesized that a certain subgroup of patients may be vulnerable to sustain significant kidney injury/damage when exposed to prolonged IAH and other coexisting risk factors (e.g., preoperative CKD, intraoperative hypotension, preoperative use of drugs that may impair intrarenal hemodynamics and autoregulation).

18.3.6 Obstetrics and Gynecological Surgery

This clinical setting has not been well studied. There have been case reports of AKI, typically described as a result of surgical trauma to ureters, or due to endogenous and exogenous toxins.

In a recent study representing over 2000 patients undergoing major inpatient gynecological surgery (2000–2010), Vaught AJ et al. [42] described the incidence and outcomes of AKI. In this single-center analysis, AKI was defined by RIFLE criteria as an increase in serum creatinine greater than or equal to 50% from the reference creatinine. The authors used multivariable regression analyses to determine the association between perioperative factors, AKI, mortality, and cost. Main outcome measures were AKI, combined major adverse events (hospital mortality, sepsis, or mechanical ventilation), 90-day mortality, and hospital cost.

Overall frequency of AKI was 13%. Of women with benign tumor surgeries, 5% (43/801) experienced AKI compared with 18% (211/1159) of women with malignant disease ($P < 0.001$). Only 1.3% of the whole cohort had evidence of urologic mechanical injury. In a multivariable analysis, AKI patients had nine times greater odds of a major adverse event compared to patients without AKI (adjusted odds ratio 8.95, 95% confidence interval 5.27–15.22).

Contrary to common belief, AKI is rarely due to urological injury but likely similar to other surgeries is a multifactorial disease resulting from susceptibilities like age and cancer and exposures including intraoperative hypotension, bleeding, transfusions, and nephrotoxic medications. Remarkably, even small decline in kidney function after surgery is associated with risks for dying as well as increased costs of care.

18.4 Prevention and Treatment

Maintaining adequate renal perfusion and avoidance of the nephrotoxin are the mainstays of therapy for prevention of AKI in the perioperative setting. Traditionally, central venous pressure, mean arterial pressure, pulmonary artery occlusive pressure (wedge pressure), and cardiac output by pulmonary artery catheter were used to monitor hemodynamic status. Recent data from critical care literature demonstrated that these parameters are of limited utility and do not take into account functional and local hemodynamic status. Currently, the focus is on functional hemodynamic parameter to maintain adequate perfusion and avoid fluid overload which is shown to be associated with excess mortality. This hemodynamic parameter includes stroke volume variation, lactate clearance, abdominal perfusion pressure, esophageal Doppler or continuous transesophageal echocardiography, and ratio between the venoarterial carbon dioxide tension gradient and arteriovenous O_2 content gradient.

Multiple studies demonstrated the association between fluid overload and increase in mortality in both medical and surgical ICU settings [43]. The presence of fluid overload defined as 10% weight gain from admission weight is associated with increased mortality and higher morbidity in sepsis, acute respiratory distress syndrome (ARDS), general surgical patients, trauma, and cardiac surgery. The presence of hypervolemia at the time of renal replacement therapy (RRT) initiation in AKI is strongly associated with mortality in both pediatric and adult patient populations. Current data do not support the use of hydroxyethyl starch for volume expansion in critically ill patient which has been shown to be associated with increased incidence of mortality, after kidney injury, and increased need of renal replacement therapy.

Animal studies and small observational studies [44–46] have supported the use of balance crystalloid over normal saline to avoid hyperchloremic metabolic acidosis and increased incidence of AKI including the need for renal replacement therapy. From this translated pathophysiological data emanated the SPLIT clinical trial [47] further examining this question. This trial randomized 2278 patients admitted to the ICU to receive normal saline or Plasma-Lyte. Nearly all ICU patients requiring crystalloid were included. Overall, 57% of subjects were admitted to the ICU following elective surgery, whereas 14% of subjects were admitted from the emergency department. Patients in both groups received nearly the same volumes of crystalloid. The day before enrollment, patients received a median of 1 L of fluid (mostly balanced crystalloids) prior to being subjected to the stated ICU protocol. Subsequently patients in both groups received a median of 2000 mL of study fluid over their entire ICU stay. The primary outcome was proportion of patients with AKI (defined as a rise in serum creatinine level of at least twofold or a serum creatinine level of ≥ 3.96 mg/dL with an increase of ≥ 0.5 mg/dL); main secondary outcomes were incidence of RRT use and in-hospital mortality. In the buffered crystalloid group, 102 of 1067 patients (9.6%) developed AKI within 90 days after enrollment compared with 94 of 1025 patients (9.2%) in the saline group [absolute difference, 0.4% (95% CI, −2.1 to 2.9%); relative risk, 1.04 [95% CI, 0.80–1.36]; $P = 0.77$). The incidence of renal replacement therapy was also similar. This trial concluded that among patients receiving crystalloid fluid therapy in the ICU, use of a buffered crystalloid compared with saline did not reduce the risk of AKI.

A recent meta-analysis by Brienza et al. [48] concluded that protocolized therapies (regardless of the protocol) with specific physiological goals can significantly reduce postoperative AKI. A major problem in interpreting these studies is the lack of standardized hemodynamic and tissue oxygenation targets and management strategies used to verify the efficacy of these measures over standard perioperative care. A heterogeneous collection of study populations, types of surgical procedures, monitoring methods, and treatment strategies comprise this recent meta-analysis. The basic strategy of goal-directed therapy to prevent AKI in the perioperative period is based on protocols that avoid hypotension, optimize oxygen delivery, and include careful fluid management, vasopressors when indicated, and inotropic agents and blood products if needed [49].

Clinical trials and meta-analyses of patients with sepsis have shown that the use of synthetic colloids like gelatin, dextran, and HES is associated with higher incidence of increased AKI requiring RRT [50, 51]. In a retrospective study [52] of 1129 patients undergoing lung resection surgery, HES was associated with a higher risk of postoperative AKI (OR 1.5, 95% CI 1.1–2.1). A recent Cochrane review [53] determined that all HES products increase the risk in AKI and RRT in all patient populations, thus providing clear evidence to avoid these agents.

Multiple vasoactive agents such as dopamine, fenoldopam, or theophylline have been studied in the treatment of postoperative AKI but have failed to demonstrate any conclusive benefits in ameliorating kidney injury. But these results are largely extrapolated from cardiac surgery settings [54].

As for drug treatment in perioperative period, there have been several studies examining the role of antihypertensive agents and aspirin. The following are the results of some of the key studies in non-cardiac surgical settings.

Previous perioperative observational cohort studies have shown that aspirin reduces the risk for AKI, and in two randomized controlled trials of patients undergoing cardiac surgery, clonidine was also shown to prevent AKI. Recently, the Perioperative Ischemic Evaluation (POISE) trial found that neither aspirin nor clonidine reduced the risk for death or nonfatal myocardial infarction when administered perioperatively for non-cardiac surgery. In a sub-study of POISE-2 [55], Dr. Garg and his team evaluated the effect of both aspirin and clonidine on the risk for AKI. The risk for AKI was not significantly different between the aspirin and placebo groups (13.4% vs. 12.3%; adjusted relative risk [aRR], 1.10; 95% confidence interval [CI], 0.96–1.25). Similarly, there was no significant difference in the incidence of AKI between clonidine and placebo (13.0% vs. 12.7; aRR 1.03; 95% CI, 0.90–1.18]). However, both drugs were associated with other adverse events.

In terms of use of angiotensin-converting enzyme (ACE) inhibitors and angiotensin II receptor blockers (ARB), the preoperative use of ACE-I and ARB drugs is a risk factor for postoperative AKI in non-cardiac surgery when studied in specific surgical settings such as gastric bypass [10].

When examined in broader surgical settings, the message seems to be different. For example, a large population-based retrospective cohort study [56] was conducted on patients aged 66 years or older and who received major elective surgery in 118 hospitals in Ontario, Canada (1995–2010; $n = 237{,}208$). After adjusting for potential confounders, preoperative ACE-I/ARB use versus nonuse was associated with 17% lower risk of postoperative AKI-D (adjusted relative risk (RR), 0.83; 95% confidence interval (CI), 0.71–0.98) and 9% lower risk of all-cause mortality (adjusted RR, 0.91; 95% CI, 0.87–0.95).

The role of statins has also been of recent interest in terms of their effect on renal function in perioperative settings. Single-center analysis of electronic data of elective non-cardiac surgery [57] did not support the hypothesis that preoperative statin therapy in doses routinely used to treat hypercholesterolemia is associated with a change in the incidence of AKI, postoperative dialysis, or hospital mortality. Of the total group of 28,508 patients analyzed, the overall incidence of AKI was 6.1%, and not statistically different based on exposure to statin use. However this study did not account for the selection bias associated with the retrospective design.

A recent international, prospective, cohort study [58] of patients who were ≥45 years having inpatient non-cardiac surgery assessed the probability of receiving statins preoperatively using a multivariable logistic model and conducted a propensity score analysis to correct for confounding. Among patients undergoing non-cardiac surgery, preoperative statin therapy was independently associated with a lower risk of cardiovascular outcomes at 30 days. The preoperative use of statins was associated with lower risk of the primary outcome, a composite of all-cause mortality, myocardial injury after non-cardiac surgery (MINS), or stroke at 30 days [relative risk (RR), 0.83; 95% confidence interval (CI), 0.73–0.95; $P = 0.007$]. Statins were also associated with a significant lower risk of all-cause mortality (RR, 0.58; 95% CI, 0.40–0.83; $P = 0.003$), cardiovascular mortality (RR, 0.42; 95% CI, 0.23–0.76; $P = 0.004$), and MINS (RR, 0.86; 95% CI, 0.73–0.98; $P = 0.02$).

Brunelli et al. [59] examined a retrospective cohort of 98,939 patients who underwent a major open abdominal, cardiac, thoracic, or vascular procedure between 2000 and 2010. Statin users were pair-matched to nonusers on the basis of surgery type, baseline kidney function, days from admission until surgery, and propensity score based on demographics, comorbid conditions, and concomitant medications. Across various AKI definitions, statin use was consistently associated with a decreased risk: adjusted odds ratios (95% confidence intervals) varied from 0.74 (0.58–0.95) to 0.80 (0.71–0.90). Associations were similar among diabetics and nondiabetics and across strata of baseline kidney function.

Molnar et al. [60] conducted a population-based retrospective cohort study that included 213,347 older patients who underwent major elective surgery in the province of Ontario, Canada, from 1995 to 2008. During the first 14 postoperative days, 1.9% developed AKI and 0.5% required acute dialysis. The 30-day mortality rate was 2.8%. Prior to surgery, 32% of patients were taking a statin. After statistical adjustment for patient and surgical characteristics, statin use is associated with 16% lower odds of AKI (OR, 0.84; 95% CI, 0.79–0.90), 17% lower odds of acute dialysis (OR, 0.83; 95% CI, 0.72–0.95), and 21% lower odds of mortality (OR, 0.79; 95% CI, 0.74–0.85). Propensity score matching produced similar results.

Susan Lee et al. [61] collected data on 307,151 patients who had been *taking statins* before non-cardiac surgery between 2000 and 2014. The researchers found that 98,014 patients had not resumed taking statins in 2 days after their operation. However, the percentage of patients who did not resume taking statins within 2 days of surgery dropped over the study period. From 2000 to 2002, 46% of patients had not resumed their statins in 2 days after surgery. From 2012 to 2014, only 24% hadn't resumed taking statins by the second day. Lee and her colleagues then looked at mortality rates in 30 days after surgery. They found that the mortality rate was 2.6% among those who did not resume taking their statins in 2 days after surgery which was 40% higher than those who quickly resumed or never stopped taking their statins.

In summary, large observational studies provide insight into some commonly used prescribed drugs for their effect on renal function and mortality. Caution needs to be exercised in interpreting these studies as few are randomized and thus provide associative information rather than causal links. Table 18.4 summarizes some of the key medications/classes for their effects on renal function.

Table 18.4 Renal adverse effects of commonly used drugs in perioperative settings

Pharmacological agent/class	Potential nephrotoxic effects
Propofol infusions	Rhabdomyolysis, hyperkalemia, metabolic acidosis, and AKI
Lorazepam infusions	Propylene glycol toxicity Hyperosmolar anion gap metabolic acidosis, lactic acidosis, and renal dysfunction
Warfarin	Warfarin-related nephropathy (glomerular hemorrhage and formation of obstructing RBC casts and tubular injury)
Sodium phosphate-containing enema	Acute phosphate nephropathy
Hydroxyethyl starch	Increased risk of acute kidney injury, increase need of renal replacement therapy, and increased mortality in critically ill patients with sepsis
Contrast media	Acute tubular necrosis (ATN)
Antimicrobials	Acute tubular necrosis (ATN), acute interstitial nephritis (AIN), electrolyte disturbances
ACE-I/ARB	Increased risk of AKI in gastric bypass
Chloride-rich fluid resuscitation	Suggestion of increased AKI risk
Trimethoprim/sulfamethoxazole	Acute tubular necrosis (ATN), acute interstitial nephritis (AIN), hyperkalemia
Heparin derivatives	Hyperkalemia

18.5 Dialytic Therapies for AKI

There is no consensus regarding optimal timing to initiate renal replacement therapy for acute kidney injury in perioperative settings. Observational studies tend to favor early initiation of renal replacement therapy and shown to be associated with improved patient survival. Indications to initiate a replacement therapy in perioperative setting are similar to AKI in other settings and include hyperkalemia, refractory metabolic acidosis, volume overload, and signs and symptoms suggestive of uremia. Details of dialytic therapies are described elsewhere.

In hemodynamic unstable patients, we favor to start continuous renal replacement therapy (CRRT). Observational studies and limited data tend to favor early initiation of renal replacement therapy, and this strategy is shown to be associated with improved patient survival; however this needs to be validated in randomized controlled trial. KDIGO guidelines suggested CRRT rather than intermittent renal replacement therapy for hemodynamically unstable patients (grade 2B). We suggest CRRT rather than intermittent RRT for AKI patients with acute brain injury or other causes of increased intracranial pressure or generalized brain edema (grade 2B). In terms of type of solute removal, it is not clear whether hemofiltration is favorable over hemodialysis with a clear survival benefit. However, it is well demonstrated that hemofiltration-based therapies offer a higher success in removing middle to large-molecular-weight toxins compared to diffusive techniques which are excellent in removing small-molecular-weight substances. Thus, in non-cardiac surgery settings, the opinion would favor use of hemofiltration in settings such as burns, trauma, or sepsis.

The KDIGO clinical practice guidelines recommend using anticoagulation during RRT in AKI if a patient does not have an increased bleeding risk or impaired coagulation and is not already receiving systemic anticoagulation (1B). The risk of bleeding is considered high in patients with recent (within 7 days) or active bleeding, recent trauma or surgery (especially in head trauma and neurosurgery), recent stroke, intracranial arteriovenous malformation or aneurysm, retinal hemorrhage, uncontrolled hypertension, or presence of an epidural catheter.

As for the dose of dialysis, it has been well established that the minimum standard for delivering CRRT should entail a dose of 20 mL/kg/h and at least three times a week of intermittent dialysis [62, 63]. One of the caveats is that non-cardiac surgery is not as well represented in these trials. Additionally, the average BMI of the patients included in these trials was relatively lower than what is encountered in common practice, and hence careful attention needs to be paid to weight-based calculations for dose of CRRT.

With regard to anticoagulation in intermittent RRT, it is recommended using either unfractionated or low-molecular-weight heparin, rather than other anticoagulants (1C). For anticoagulation in CRRT, it is suggested to use regional citrate anticoagulation rather than heparin in patients who do not have contraindications for citrate. For anticoagulation during CRRT in patients who have contraindications for citrate, either unfractionated or low-molecular-weight heparin can be used, rather than other anticoagulants.

A major contraindication for the use of citrate anticoagulation is severely impaired liver function or shock with muscle hypoperfusion, both representing a risk of citrate accumulation. Markedly reduced citrate clearances and lower ionized calcium levels have been found in patients with acute liver failure or with severe liver cirrhosis.

References

1. Chertow GM, Burdick E, Honour M, Bonventre JV, Bates DW. Acute kidney injury, mortality, length of stay, and costs in hospitalized patients. J Am Soc Nephrol. 2005;16(11):3365–70.
2. Coca SG, Yusuf B, Shlipak MG, Garg AX, Parikh CR. Long-term risk of mortality and other adverse outcomes after acute kidney injury: a systematic review and meta-analysis. Am J Kidney Dis. 2009;53(6):961–73.
3. Mehta RL, Kellum JA, Shah SV, Molitoris BA, Ronco C, Warnock DG, et al. Acute kidney injury network: report of an initiative to improve outcomes in acute kidney injury. Crit Care. 2007;11(2):R31.
4. Molitoris BA, Levin A, Warnock DG, Joannidis M, Mehta RL, Kellum JA, et al. Improving outcomes from acute kidney injury. J Am Soc Nephrol. 2007;18(7):1992–4.
5. Garg AX, Kurz A, Sessler DI, Cuerden M, Robinson A, Mrkobrada M, et al. Perioperative aspirin and clonidine and risk of acute kidney injury: a randomized clinical trial. JAMA. 2014;312(21):2254.
6. Bonventre JV, Yang L. Cellular pathophysiology of ischemic acute kidney injury. J Clin Invest. 2011;121(11):4210–21.
7. Basile DP, Anderson MD, Sutton TA. Pathophysiology of acute kidney injury. Compr Physiol. 2012;2(2):1303–53.
8. Kim M, Brady JE, Li G. Variations in the risk of acute kidney injury across intraabdominal surgery procedures. Anesth Analg. 2014;119(5):1121–32.
9. Kheterpal S, Tremper KK, Englesbe MJ, O'Reilly M, Shanks AM, Fetterman DM, et al. Predictors of postoperative acute renal failure after noncardiac surgery in patients with previously normal renal function. Anesthesiology. 2007;107(6):892–902.
10. Thakar CV, Kharat V, Blanck S, Leonard AC. Acute kidney injury after gastric bypass surgery. Clin J Am Soc Nephrol. 2007;2(3):426–30.
11. Kirkpatrick AW, Roberts DJ, Waele JD, Jaeschke R, Malbrain MLNG, Keulenaer BD, et al. Intra-abdominal hypertension and the abdominal compartment syndrome: updated consensus definitions and clinical practice guidelines from the World Society of the Abdominal Compartment Syndrome. Intensive Care Med. 2013;39(7):1190–206.
12. Malbrain M. Abdominal perfusion pressure as a prognostic marker in intra-abdominal hypertension. In: Vincent PJ-L, editor. Yearbook of intensive care and emergency medicine 2002 [Internet]. Berlin, Heidelberg: Springer; 2002. p. 792–814. https://doi.org/10.1007/978-3-642-56011-8_71.
13. Kurtz S, Ong K, Lau E, Mowat F, Halpern M. Projections of primary and revision hip and knee arthroplasty in the United States from 2005 to 2030. J Bone Joint Surg Am. 2007;89(4):780–5.
14. Matlock D, Earnest M, Epstein A. Utilization of elective hip and knee arthroplasty by age and payer. Clin Orthop. 2008;466(4):914–9.
15. Parvizi J, Holiday AD, Ereth MH, Lewallen DG. The Frank Stinchfield Award. Sudden death during primary hip arthroplasty. Clin Orthop. 1999;369:39–48.
16. Bell S, Dekker FW, Vadiveloo T, Marwick C, Deshmukh H, Donnan PT, et al. Risk of postoperative acute kidney injury in patients undergoing orthopaedic surgery—development and validation of a risk score and effect of acute kidney injury on survival: observational cohort study. BMJ. 2015;351:h5639.
17. Nadkarni G, Patel A, Annapureddy N, Agarwal S, Simoes P, Konstantinidis I, et al. Incidence, risk factors, and outcome trends of acute kidney injury in elective total hip and knee replacement. Am J Orthop (Belle Mead NJ). 2016;45(1):E12–9.
18. Burris D, Rhee P, Kaufmann C, Pikoulis E, Austin B, Eror A, et al. Controlled resuscitation for uncontrolled hemorrhagic shock. J Trauma. 1999;46(2):216–23.
19. Lin G-S, Chou T-H, Wu C-Y, Wu M-C, Fang C-C, Yen Z-S, et al. Target blood pressure for hypotensive resuscitation. Injury. 2013;44(12):1811–5.
20. Plurad D, Brown C, Chan L, Demetriades D, Rhee P. Emergency department hypotension is not an independent risk factor for post-traumatic acute renal dysfunction. J Trauma. 2006;61(5):1120–7; discussion 1127–8.

21. Palmieri T, Lavrentieva A, Greenhalgh DG. Acute kidney injury in critically ill burn patients. Risk factors, progression and impact on mortality. Burns. 2010;36(2):205–11.
22. Stewart IJ, Tilley MA, Cotant CL, Aden JK, Gisler C, Kwan HK, et al. Association of AKI with adverse outcomes in burned military casualties. Clin J Am Soc Nephrol. 2011;7(2):199–206.
23. Thakar CV, Parikh CR. Perioperative kidney injury [Internet]. New York, NY: Springer; 2015. https://doi.org/10.1007/978-1-4939-1273-5.
24. Ojo AO, Held PJ, Port FK, Wolfe RA, Leichtman AB, Young EW, et al. Chronic renal failure after transplantation of a nonrenal organ. N Engl J Med. 2003;349(10):931–40.
25. Francoz C, Nadim MK, Baron A, Prié D, Antoine C, Belghiti J, et al. Glomerular filtration rate equations for liver-kidney transplantation in patients with cirrhosis: validation of current recommendations. Hepatology. 2014;59(4):1514–21.
26. Gonwa TA, Wadei HM. The challenges of providing renal replacement therapy in decompensated liver cirrhosis. Blood Purif. 2012;33(1–3):144–8.
27. Mindikoglu AL, Weir MR. Current concepts in the diagnosis and classification of renal dysfunction in cirrhosis. Am J Nephrol. 2013;38(4):345–54.
28. Cabezuelo JB, Ramírez P, Ríos A, Acosta F, Torres D, Sansano T, et al. Risk factors of acute renal failure after liver transplantation. Kidney Int. 2006;69(6):1073–80.
29. McCauley J, Van Thiel DH, Starzl TE, Puschett JB. Acute and chronic renal failure in liver transplantation. Nephron. 1990;55(2):121–8.
30. Yalavarthy R, Edelstein CL, Teitelbaum I. Acute renal failure and chronic kidney disease following liver transplantation. Hemodial Int. 2007;11:S7–12.
31. Greenberg A. Renal failure in cardiac transplantation. Cardiovasc Clin. 1990;20(2):189–98.
32. Boyle JM, Moualla S, Arrigain S, Worley S, Bakri MH, Starling RC, et al. Risks and outcomes of acute kidney injury requiring dialysis after cardiac transplantation. Am J Kidney Dis. 2006;48(5):787–96.
33. Ishani A, Erturk S, Hertz MI, Matas AJ, Savik K, Rosenberg ME. Predictors of renal function following lung or heart-lung transplantation. Kidney Int. 2002;61(6):2228–34.
34. Grimm JC, Lui C, Kilic A, Valero III V, Sciortino CM, Whitman GJR, et al. A risk score to predict acute renal failure in adult patients after lung transplantation. Ann Thorac Surg. 2015;99(1):251–7.
35. Huang WC, Levey AS, Serio AM, Snyder M, Vickers AJ, Raj GV, et al. Chronic kidney disease after nephrectomy in patients with renal cortical tumours: a retrospective cohort study. Lancet Oncol. 2006;7(9):735–40.
36. Dindo D, Demartines N, Clavien P-A. Classification of surgical complications. Ann Surg. 2004;240(2):205–13.
37. Hakimi AA, Rajpathak S, Chery L, Shapiro E, Ghavamian R. Renal insufficiency is an independent risk factor for complications after partial nephrectomy. J Urol. 2010;183(1):43–7.
38. Porpiglia F, Fiori C, Bertolo R, Angusti T, Piccoli GB, Podio V, et al. The effects of warm ischaemia time on renal function after laparoscopic partial nephrectomy in patients with normal contralateral kidney. World J Urol. 2011;30(2):257–63.
39. Parekh DJ, Weinberg JM, Ercole B, Torkko KC, Hilton W, Bennett M, et al. Tolerance of the human kidney to isolated controlled ischemia. J Am Soc Nephrol. 2013;24(3):506–17.
40. Wiesenthal JD, Fazio LM, Perks AE, Blew BDM, Mazer D, Hare G, et al. Effect of pneumoperitoneum on renal tissue oxygenation and blood flow in a rat model. Urology. 2011;77(6):1508.e9–1508.e15.
41. Dunn MD, McDougall EM. Renal physiology. Laparoscopic considerations. Urol Clin North Am. 2000;27(4):609–14.
42. Vaught A, Ozrazgat-Baslanti T, Javed A, Morgan L, Hobson C, Bihorac A. Acute kidney injury in major gynaecological surgery: an observational study. BJOG Int J Obstet Gynaecol. 2015;122(10):1340–8.
43. Bouchard J, Soroko SB, Chertow GM, Himmelfarb J, Ikizler TA, Paganini EP, et al. Fluid accumulation, survival and recovery of kidney function in critically ill patients with acute kidney injury. Kidney Int. 2009;76(4):422–7.
44. Shaw AD, Bagshaw SM, Goldstein SL, Scherer LA, Duan M, Schermer CR, et al. Major complications, mortality, and resource utilization after open abdominal surgery: 0.9% saline compared to Plasma-Lyte. Ann Surg. 2012;255(5):821–9.
45. Raghunathan K, Shaw A, Nathanson B, Stürmer T, Brookhart A, Stefan MS, et al. Association between the choice of IV crystalloid and in-hospital mortality among critically ill adults with sepsis*. Crit Care Med. 2014;42(7):1585–91.
46. Shaw AD, Raghunathan K, Peyerl FW, Munson SH, Paluszkiewicz SM, Schermer CR. Association between intravenous chloride load during resuscitation and in-hospital mortality among patients with SIRS. Intensive Care Med. 2014;40(12):1897–905.
47. Young P, Bailey M, Beasley R, Henderson S, Mackle D, McArthur C, et al. Effect of a buffered crystalloid solution vs. saline on acute kidney injury among patients in the intensive care unit: the SPLIT randomized clinical trial. JAMA. 2015;314(16):1701–10.
48. Brienza N, Giglio MT, Marucci M, Fiore T. Does perioperative hemodynamic optimization protect renal function in surgical patients? A meta-analytic study. Crit Care Med. 2009;37(6):2079–90.
49. Kidney Disease. Improving Global Outcomes (KDIGO) Acute Kidney Injury Work Group. KDIGO Clinical Practice guideline for acute kidney injury. Kidney Int. 2012;2:1–138.
50. Haase N, Perner A, Hennings LI, Siegemund M, Lauridsen B, Wetterslev M, et al. Hydroxyethyl starch 130/0.38–0.45 versus crystalloid or albumin in patients with sepsis: systematic review with

meta-analysis and trial sequential analysis. BMJ. 2013;f839:346.
51. Bayer O, Reinhart K, Sakr Y, Kabisch B, Kohl M, Riedemann NC, et al. Renal effects of synthetic colloids and crystalloids in patients with severe sepsis: a prospective sequential comparison. Crit Care Med. 2011;39(6):1335–42.
52. Ishikawa S, Griesdale DEG, Lohser J. Acute kidney injury after lung resection surgery: incidence and perioperative risk factors. Anesth Analg. 2012;114(6):1256–62.
53. Mutter TC, Ruth CA, Dart AB. Hydroxyethyl starch (HES) versus other fluid therapies: effects on kidney function. Cochrane Database Syst Rev. 2013;7:CD007594.
54. Thakar CV. Perioperative acute kidney injury. Adv Chronic Kidney Dis. 2013;20(1):67–75.
55. Garg AX, Kurz A, Sessler DI, et al. Perioperative aspirin and clonidine and risk of acute kidney injury: a randomized clinical trial. JAMA. 2014;312(21):2254–64.
56. Shah M, Jain AK, Brunelli SM, Coca SG, Devereaux PJ, James MT, et al. Association between angiotensin converting enzyme inhibitor or angiotensin receptor blocker use prior to major elective surgery and the risk of acute dialysis. BMC Nephrol. 2014;15(1):53.
57. Argalious MY, Dalton JE, Sreenivasalu T, O'Hara J, Sessler DI. The association of preoperative statin use and acute kidney injury after noncardiac surgery. Anesth Analg. 2013;117(4):916–23.
58. Berwanger O, Le Manach Y, Suzumura EA, Biccard B, Srinathan SK, Szczeklik W, et al. Association between pre-operative statin use and major cardiovascular complications among patients undergoing non-cardiac surgery: the VISION study. Eur Heart J. 2015;37(2):177–85.
59. Brunelli SM, Waikar SS, Bateman BT, Chang TI, Lii J, Garg AX, et al. Preoperative statin use and postoperative acute kidney injury. Am J Med. 2012;125(12):1195–204.e3.
60. Molnar AO, Coca SG, Devereaux PJ, Jain AK, Kitchlu A, Luo J, et al. Statin use associates with a lower incidence of acute kidney injury after major elective surgery. J Am Soc Nephrol. 2011;22(5):939–46.
61. 10.27.15. American Society of Anesthesiologists—Surgical patients should stay on cholesterol medications to reduce risk of death, study shows [Internet]. [cited 2015 Nov 29]. http://www.asahq.org/about-asa/newsroom/news-releases/2015/10/surgical-patients-should-stay-on-cholesterol-medications.
62. Intensity of renal support in critically ill patients with acute kidney injury. N Engl J Med. 2008;359(1):7–20.
63. Intensity of continuous renal-replacement therapy in critically ill patients. N Engl J Med. 2009;361(17):1627–38.

Part IV

Management

Non-dialytic Management of Acute Kidney Injury

19

John R. Prowle

19.1 Introduction

Acute kidney injury (AKI) is now estimated to complicate 13–18% of hospital admissions and has been associated with both short- and long-term risk of death and the development and progression of chronic kidney disease. In the UK it has been estimated that the hospital costs of acute kidney injury are estimated to be as much as £1.02 billion per year [1]. These figures reflect our better understanding of the adverse clinical associations of AKI of all severities and increased recognition of the significance of milder cases of AKI since the development and widespread adoption of consensus definitions of AKI over the last 12 years [2–4]. This revolution in our approach to AKI has also resulted in major changes in management. Historically management of *acute kidney failure* focused on the care of a much smaller group of individuals with severe kidney dysfunction and the treatment of severe metabolic abnormalities and the provision of renal replacement therapy (RRT). However, in contemporary practice we have identified a large group of patients with milder AKI, of which the vast majority will never require acute RRT, but who are still at significant risk of adverse short- and long-term outcomes. As a consequence, modern management of AKI without RRT has broadened from a focus on the medical management of the metabolic effects of advanced kidney failure to cover the recognition and management of deteriorating patients with early organ dysfunction and the identification and follow-up of a population defined by the acquisition of AKI during acute illness who may be at risk of long-term chronic kidney disease and cardiovascular morbidity.

J. R. Prowle
Critical Care and Perioperative Medicine Research Group, William Harvey Research Institute,
Barts and the London School of Medicine and Dentistry, Queen Mary University of London, London, UK
e-mail: j.prowle@qmul.ac.uk

19.2 Historical Perspective of Acute Kidney Injury

The first modern descriptions of acute kidney dysfunction date to World War II when patients with major crush injuries were recovered alive but, without effective RRT technology, later died with oliguric kidney injury and hyperkalaemia [5]. During the 1940s–1950s, the concept of acute kidney failure was thus developed with small case series of patients with advanced kidney dysfunction and life-threatening metabolic abnormalities in the context of predominantly single-organ dysfunction caused by rhabdomyolysis, haemolysis, or poisoning or as an outcome after an episode of sustained circulatory shock [6]. In the absence of RRT, management of these patients focused on prevention of uraemia, fluid overload and

S. S. Waikar et al. (eds.), *Core Concepts in Acute Kidney Injury*,
https://doi.org/10.1007/978-1-4939-8628-6_19

electrolyte abnormalities by highly restricted diets, excluding protein, almost all water and potassium together with bicarbonate supplementation [7, 8]. Such approaches did lead to survival of some patients with prolonged oliguric kidney failure to recover kidney function; however the adoption of effective haemodialysis technology in the 1950s, incorporating reliable vascular access and controlled ultrafiltration, rendered such techniques obsolete. The triumph of RRT technologies has, over time, led to the treatment of increasing sicker and comorbid patients with AKI complicating multi-organ failure in intensive care units now usually with continuous modalities of RRT. Conversely, the management of patients with AKI who are not on RRT has remained unsophisticated despite the fact that the vast majority of AKI diagnoses fall into this category.

19.3 Contemporary Concepts in Acute Kidney Injury

Until recently AKI management has been dominated by concepts applied to the causes and clinical presentation of acute kidney failure in the 1950s. However contemporary AKI cases are much more commonly of mixed aetiology with patients presenting with a wider spectrum of AKI severity. The commonest associations of AKI complicating critical illness are sepsis, major surgery, cardiogenic shock, hypovolaemia and nephrotoxin exposure [9]; however these conditions often co-exist and occur on the background of predisposing risk factors, the most potent of which are old age and pre-existing chronic kidney disease (CKD) [10]. Thus, current management of patients with AKI requires consideration of the severity of AKI, of co-existent acute and chronic conditions and of multiple causative factors for AKI. While any one causative acute condition or nephrotoxin could precipitate AKI in any patient if sufficiently severe or potent, the majority of cases of AKI now occur in a setting of multiple milder insults and/or nephrotoxic exposures on the background of baseline risk factors. As a consequence, management of most current AKI patients is more nuanced and requires broader consideration AKI in the context of overall clinical condition (Table 19.1). This individualized clinical approach can be summarized as recognition of patients most at risk of AKI at baseline, appropriate treatment directed at underlying conditions and the minimization of exposure to exogenous nephrotoxins (Table 19.2).

Table 19.1 Comparison of a "traditional" single-organ acute kidney failure patient with a typical acute kidney injury patient commonly encountered

	Traditional single-organ kidney failure	Typical contemporary AKI patient
Examples	Ethylene glycol poisoning Massive post-partum haemorrhage	Urosepsis in an elderly man with CKD, diabetes treated with gentamicin and undergoing a contrast CT scan for diagnostic workup
Causes of AKI	Single high-intensity exposure—potent nephrotoxic or prolonged shock	Multiple
Baseline risk factors	Often absent	Common
Co-existent organ failure	Absent or resolved	Common
Severity of AKI	Severe	Variable
Stage of AKI at presentation	Late	Often early
Histology	Classical acute tubular necrosis	Most often undetermined—when examined often apparently normal
Management	Treatment of metabolic abnormalities Institution of RRT for life-threatening consequences of advanced kidney failure	Care of deteriorating patient, avoidance of secondary organ injury and monitoring of organ function RRT as a part of multi-organ support in ICU

Table 19.2 Multifactorial aetiology of AKI

Baseline risks	Acute conditions	Exogenous nephrotoxins
Advanced age	Sepsis	Radiological contrast
Chronic kidney disease	Major surgery	Antibiotics
Diabetes mellitus	Cardiogenic shock	Chemotherapy
Heart failure	Volume depletion	Non-steroidal anti-inflammatories
Liver failure	Abdominal compartment syndrome	Calcineurin inhibitors
Vascular disease	Rhabdomyolysis	Hydroxyethyl starch
Genetic predisposition	Haemolysis	
Male Sex		
Management		
Recognize risk	Treat/mitigate conditions	Avoid/minimize exposure

Most contemporary AKI occurs in the setting of baseline risks and multiple medical, surgical or toxic acute kidney insults. An approach to the management of AKI in these patients thus requires (1) recognition of baseline risk, (2) treatment of underlying conditions and (3) minimization of nephrotoxin exposures

19.4 Diagnostic Considerations in Management of AKI

Timely and accurate diagnosis of AKI is an essential prerequisite to its appropriate management. Diagnosis of AKI is considered in more detail elsewhere in this volume, but, in brief, modern AKI diagnostic algorithms depend in the assessment of fold increases in serum creatinine (reflecting fold decreases in underlying GFR) from baseline (Table 19.3) and have demonstrated good correlation between severity of peak AKI stage and risk of death during acute illness [11, 12]. Even very mild changes in kidney function have been correlated with increased risk of death [13]—emphasizing the clinical importance of AKI but leaving open the question of whether mild AKI is a sensitive measure of illness severity and physiological reserve or directly participating in the ongoing disease process. Furthermore, in terms of driving clinical management, clinicians don't have access to the eventual peak creatinine measurement but receive results at a single time point during when the trajectory or serum creatinine and underlying kidney function may be unclear. Importantly, it takes time for creatinine to rise after an abrupt change in GFR, and the rate of these changes is dependent not only on the severity of kidney dysfunction but on acute and chronic determinants of muscle mass and creatinine generation which will be reduced with older age and chronic illness and may be further decreased in acute illness [14, 15]. Thus older, more comorbid and more acutely unwell patients may manifest slower rises in serum creatinine causing underestimation of the severity of AKI (Fig. 19.1). As a consequence, apparently mild AKI can represent significant underlying kidney dysfunction, particularly in the acutely unwell, and thus the importance of recognition of AKI risk factors, treatment of underlying conditions and avoidance of secondary kidney injury should be emphasized in all patients with an AKI diagnosis.

Table 19.3 Kidney Disease: Improving Global Outcomes (KDIGO) 2012 criteria for diagnosis and staging of AKI in adults [2]

Stage	Serum creatinine	Urine output
1	Increase ≥26 μmol/L within 48 h or increase ≥1.5 to 1.9 × reference SCr	<0.5 mL/kg/h for >6 consecutive hours
2	Increase ≥2 to 2.9 × reference SCr	<0.5 mL/kg/h for >12 h
3	Increase ≥3 × reference SCr or increase of ≥26 μmol/L to ≥354 μmol/L or commenced on renal replacement therapy (RRT) irrespective of stage	<0.3 mL/kg/h for >24 h or anuria for 12 h

Recognition of the importance of AKI diagnosis in enabling effective management has led many healthcare institutions to implement AKI electronic alerts (e-alerts) into laboratory

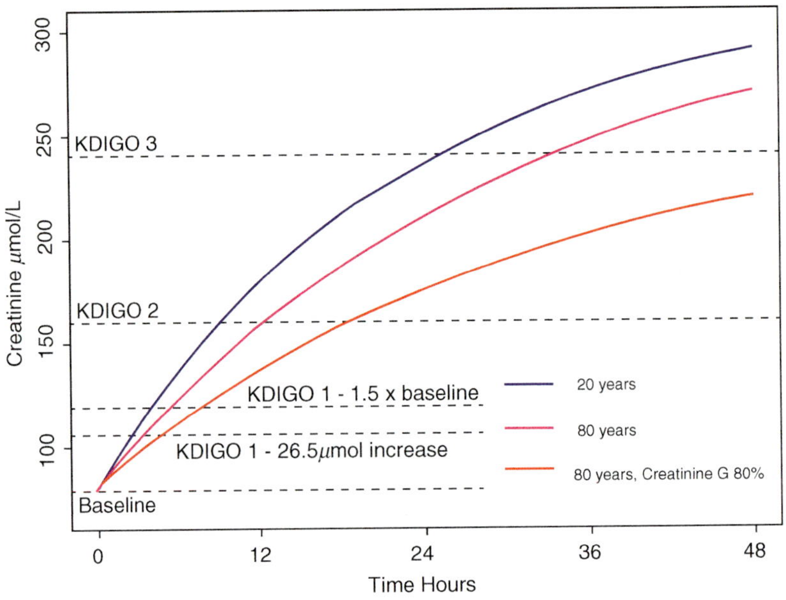

Fig. 19.1 Predicted creatinine profiles in male patients aged 80 and 20 with a baseline creatinine of 80 μmol/L and abrupt decline in GFR to 25% of baseline. AKI staging depends on time elapsed from change in GFR and occurs faster in younger patients with greater predicted muscle mass; a small acute fall in creatinine generation (G) with acute illness reduces that rate of rise and plateau creatinine confounding timely and accurate diagnosis of AKI. Despite apparently less severe rise in creatinine from an identical baseline, GFR is lower for the 80-year-old (80 falling to 20 mL/min/1.73 m^2) compared to the 20-year-old (120 falling to 30 mL/min/1.73 m^2). Prediction of AKI severity at early time points in illness is consequently difficult

information management systems to flag AKI diagnoses based on consensus creatinine criteria [2–4] to clinicians. Indeed, the adoption of such systems has now been mandated within the UK National Health Service. Systematic electronic AKI screening has resulted in the increased recognition of AKI as a widespread clinical problem strongly associated with adverse outcomes [16, 17] but also emphasizes that effective identification has to be coupled to effective management. A recent randomized trial of AKI e-alerting in a large teaching hospital population in the USA [18] failed to demonstrate decreased mortality, need for RRT or AKI progression in patients where clinicians were provided with an e-alert; however in this study the alerting was not linked to any specific management recommendations or training. Importantly the majority of alerts in the trial were associated with AKI defined by a 0.3 mg/dL (26.5 μmol/L) increase in creatinine within 48 h, and the authors have subsequently demonstrated that these small changes could arise from inter-assay variation in serum creatinine measurements particularly in patients with baseline CKD [19]. This finding has important implications for the response to stage 1 AKI suggested by small changes in serum creatinine, which may require confirmation AKI diagnosis by repeated creatinine measurement prior to immediate changes in patient management.

In recognition of the limitations of serum creatinine in the dynamic setting of early acute illness, the consensus AKI definitions have incorporated varying definition of oliguria into the diagnostic criteria for AKI. The role of urine output monitoring [20] is discussed at greater length elsewhere in this volume, but overall urine output may be most useful in conjunction with the serum creatinine criteria. Short duration of oliguria may represent physiological neurohormonal response to stress and/or transient haemodynamic changes in GFR, which may not signify parenchymal kidney injury per se, but certainly do indicate risk of both kidney and other organ injuries. Conversely sustained oliguria or anuria may represent a fall in GFR to a very low level prior to peak creatinine, conferring a worse prognosis and potentially implying that early RRT might be preferred over non-dialytic management. Finally, a large group of patients with established AKI and impaired renal concentrating capacity, but without complete loss of GFR, may sustain urine output out of the oliguric range. Thus in driving management, urine output plays a complementary role in suggesting risk of deterioration early on or greater severity in advanced AKI; again the emphasis in directing management should be placed on monitoring duration and changes in urine output after AKI is recognized in order to inform management decisions and response to therapy.

Because of the diagnostic limitations of creatinine changes and urine output, which is often not reliably measured outside of ICU, a number of putative biomarkers of AKI [21] have been identified over the last 10–15 years. These markers are promising because they may detect tubular injury before changes in GFR have even occurred and well before rises in serum creatinine, potentially enabling early risk stratification and preventative interventions that might lack benefit when employed after AKI have become overt. However, while of great potential to guide AKI management, as yet no biomarker-driven intervention has been demonstrated to alter clinical outcomes in patients with biomarker-defined AKI. Thus, at present biomarkers have no clear role in AKI management. This situation is likely to change over time, and evidence-based early non-dialytic treatment for AKI may be enabled by biomarker identification in the near future [22].

Lastly, diagnostic evaluation is of key importance in both identifying the specific cause of AKI and in guiding management. While less common than the multifactorial aetiology of secondary AKI complicating major illness, identification of processes such as urinary outflow obstruction or acute parenchymal injury is crucial. As well, specific management and/or speciality referral is indicated for these conditions. The diagnosis of AKI requires a detailed history and physical evaluation and the interpretation of a combination of tests to distinguish "multifactorial" AKI from a specific aetiology for AKI. For example, complete anuria or kidney dysfunction appears to antedate or is disproportionate in severity to systemic illness, as well as eliciting any clinical features suggestive of specific diagnoses such as systemic vasculitis or thrombotic microangiopathy. At a minimum, urinalysis and kidney imaging, with other tests aimed at specific diagnoses prompted by these findings and the clinical history, are recommended. Specific management of cases of urinary obstruction, autoimmune disease and other parenchymal kidney disease is beyond the scope of this chapter. This consideration of specific pathophysiology for AKI also extends to specific causes of AKI related to multi-organ failure, major injury and critical illness, specifically AKI in the setting of advanced cardiac or liver disease and AKI occurring in the setting of rhabdomyolysis or abdominal compartment syndrome.

19.5 Approaches to the Non-dialytic Management of AKI

In the 2012 Kidney Disease: Improving Global Outcomes (KDIGO) guidelines, an evidence-based approach to AKI management was proposed with recommendations for patients at risk of AKI during major illness and at increasing severity of AKI (Fig. 19.2). While important in conceptualizing an approach to AKI at all levels of severity that merges into AKI prevention in those at risk, the actual recommendations prior to institution of RRT are relatively sparse in content and really provide only blanket recommendations to provide good supportive care, monitor kidney function and intervene with RRT when clinically indicated. The general nature of these recommendations reflects the paucity of evidence for any specific clinical interventions in the management or prevention of AKI and the delay and imprecision in AKI diagnosis in determining actual underlying disease severity in the acute setting. Unfortunately, this leads clinicians with little effective guide when faced with responding to an early AKI diagnosis. In the author's opinion, the appropriate approach to any

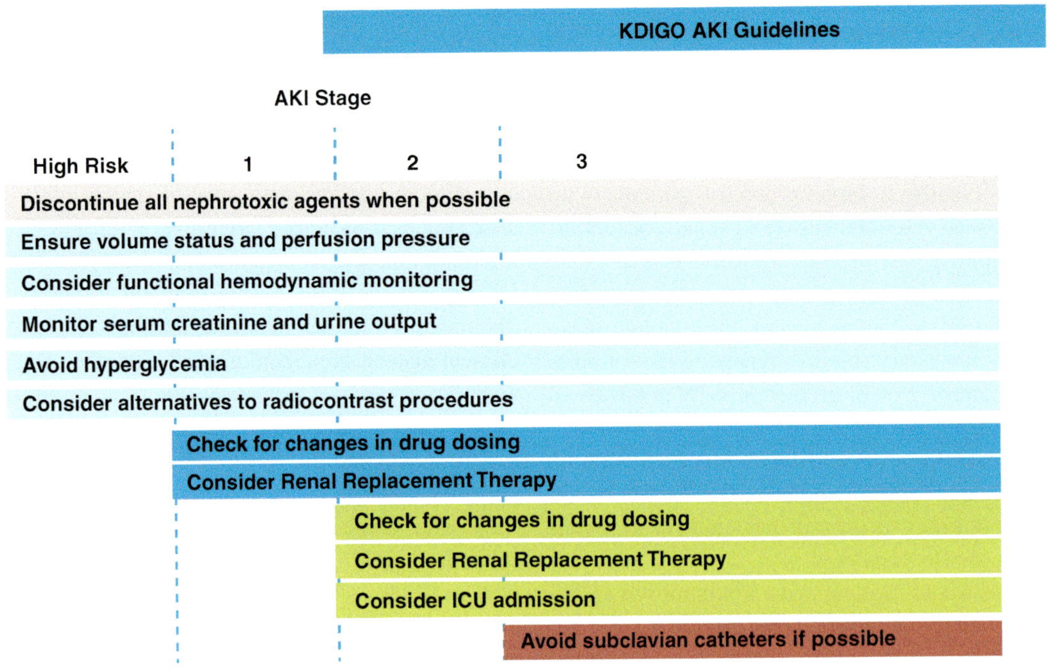

Fig. 19.2 Summary of Kidney Disease: Improving Global Outcomes (KDIGO) 2012 recommendations for the management of patients with or at risk of acute kidney injury [118]. Few interventions have a strong evidence base, and recommendations are predominantly based on expert recommendation for close monitoring, supportive haemodynamic management and avoidance of secondary organ injury

AKI diagnosis is one of establishing diagnosis, monitoring, providing appropriate supportive treatment and avoiding secondary organ injury (Table 19.4). Importantly, most of these processes are not kidney specific but form part of the general care of a deteriorating patient. It should be emphasized that a patient with a stage 1 AKI diagnosis has early organ dysfunction and is at risk of deterioration into multi-organ impairment; an AKI alert can therefore be considered a powerful indicator of a patient at increased risk of death requiring monitoring, treatment of any underlying condition and supportive care—more than one requiring treatment directed at the kidney in isolation. Seen in this light, the direct contribution of kidney dysfunction to outcome, as opposed to merely an association with disease severity, becomes less relevant as an objection to a targeted approach to the identification and management of early AKI patients in hospital as these patients are a well-defined population at increased risk of death, requiring a global assessment of their clinical condition. In an attempt to address the real-world needs of the clinician in approaching patients with AKI, the London Acute Kidney Injury Network has published pragmatic management guidelines (Fig. 19.3) [23]. This guideline emphasizes the role of AKI as an indicator of a deteriorating patient with early organ failure (a medical emergency) while also addressing the need not to miss treatable specific aetiologies. Several important points can be taken from this approach, most importantly, that all AKI patients are at increased risk of adverse outcomes and that, as severity and cause of AKI cannot be established from serum creatinine measurements single time point, a combined diagnostic and management approach is required in all patients. In the guideline the potential need to recheck a creatinine to confirm a diagnosis based on a 26.5 μmol/L increase is highlighted at the outset. An acronym STOP (sepsis/hypoperfusion, toxicity, obstruction, parenchymal kidney disease) is used to guide management providing, in order, for sepsis/hypoperfusion, early resuscitation and recognition and treatment of sepsis; for toxicity, the minimization

Table 19.4 Goals in the management of AKI encompass establishing diagnosis and severity, monitoring, best supportive care and avoidance of secondary injury; these can be divided into diagnostic goals and therapeutic changes

• *Diagnostic goals*
– Monitor kidney function in patients at risk of AKI from baseline risk factors and acute conditions
– Recognize AKI as a sign of an at risk/deteriorating patient
– Recognize features suggestive of specific AKI aetiologies requiring specific management or referral
– Recognize AKI baseline risks and AKI causes that may determine AKI prognosis
– Assess severity of AKI and confirm diagnosis in cases with small changes in serum creatinine
– Monitor AKI progression/recovery with creatinine and urine output
– Recognize life-threatening complication of AKI
– Assess recovery from AKI and impact on long-term health
• *Therapeutic goals*
– Manage patients in an appropriate setting for their level of illness and likely need to organ support with regular review
– Treat underlying conditions such as sepsis, hypovolaemia and shock
– Maintain tissue perfusion with judicious use of fluids and vasoactive medication if necessary
– Minimize/avoid exposure to nephrotoxins unless essential to the diagnosis or treatment of a causative underlying condition such as sepsis
– Avoid secondary injury to the kidneys or other organs in particular from fluid overload and accumulation of kidney-excreted medication
– Provide organ support with renal replacement therapy in a timely fashion when indicated

Many of these approaches are not specific to AKI but form part of the general care of the deteriorating patient

of ongoing nephrotoxic injury; and for obstruction or parenchymal kidney disease, the consideration and exclusion of causes of AKI with important specific treatments. Importantly this approach to initial management is followed by monitoring or response to treatment, attention to the avoidance of secondary organ injury and appropriate long-term follow-up.

19.6 Non-dialytic Interventions for AKI

An approach to the contemporary patient with AKI thus emphasizes the appropriate resuscitation of tissue perfusion in the face of potential underlying causes of organ dysfunction such as septic shock or hypovolaemia. Historical concepts such as distinguishing "prerenal failure" should be discarded in favour of an approach to the resuscitation of any AKI patients as individuals with early multi-organ impairment. As with any critically ill patient, this requires a balanced approach of fluid and vasoactive drugs titrated to physiological endpoints such as blood pressure and cardiac output while attempting to minimize inappropriate interventions which may be associated with adverse effects.

19.6.1 Fluid Management in AKI

Fluid therapy is often considered essential to the maintenance of renal perfusion and GFR and thus a first-line treatment in the prevention and management of AKI complicating major illness. However, importance of inflammation in the development of AKI is now well recognized [24, 25]. Conversely, the role of global renal ischemia in the pathogenesis AKI is less clear [26]. Consequently the clinical course of many or most cases of AKI may not be so readily affected by haemodynamic intervention aimed at increasing renal oxygen delivery.

In AKI, the rationale of fluid therapy is to restore systemic blood pressure and cardiac output; however, routine haemodynamic measurements (blood pressure, heart rate, central venous pressure) are poorly predictive of cardiac output and much less indicative of adequate renal perfusion. Furthermore, fluid therapy will only effectively treat systemic hypotension arising as a consequence of hypovolaemic shock [27–29]. Similarly, the response of the cardiovascular system to fluid therapy is highly variable depending on factors including cardiac function [30–32], regional blood flow distribution [33, 34] and capillary permeability [35]. This makes clinical

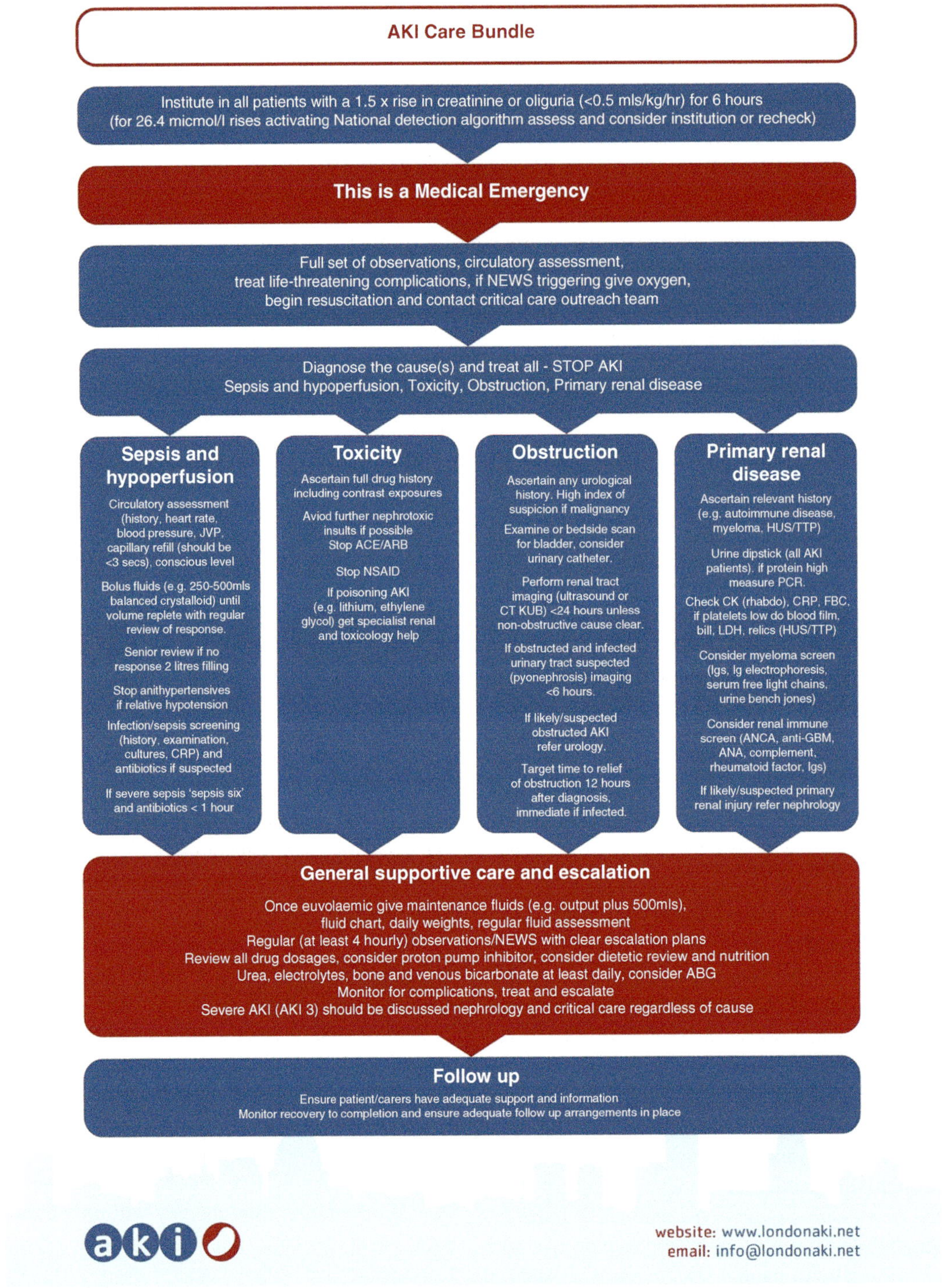

Fig. 19.3 AKI Care Bundle provided by the *London Acute Kidney Injury Network* (www.londonaki.net) [23]

management of volume replacement very challenging. Traditionally used measurements such as central venous pressure [36] and arterial lactate [37] lack evidence to support their ability to predict response particularly in key clinical situations such as septic shock. Actual measurements of cardiac output do provide some information on global perfusion allowing fluid and other haemodynamic interventions titrated against response. However, indiscriminate use of intravenous fluid to maximize cardiac output might not be beneficial. In animal models, administration of intravenous fluid may acutely improve systemic haemodynamics without improvement in renal oxygen delivery [38, 39]. However, while the physiological effects of fluid resuscitation are uncertain, one consequence is predictable: repeated volume challenges will inevitably lead to positive fluid balance [38, 40]. Invasive monitoring may, therefore, be required more to prevent excessive fluid administration, than to ensure adequate resuscitation.

Some evidence for the effects of fluid resuscitation on kidney function is available from studies examining perioperative goal-directed therapy (GDT) for haemodynamic resuscitation in major surgery. In a meta-analysis [41] of studies, use of perioperative GDT was associated with a significantly lower incidence of AKI; however, benefit was only apparent in those trials where goal-directed therapy did not result in greater quantity fluid administration. Furthermore, only studies incorporating inotropic drugs in GDT protocols were associated with a significantly less postoperative AKI. These data suggest that while maintenance of cardiac output may be important in reducing incidence of AKI at a time of physiological demand, if these strategies overall result in excessive fluid administration, this benefit is not present. In short, if some patients benefit from receiving extra fluids when indicated, others may also benefit by avoiding excess fluid which they do not require. Importantly, outside the setting of surgery, three recent multicentre randomized studies [42–44] did not demonstrate a survival benefit from goal-directed resuscitation in patients presenting with septic shock, and in these studies there was also no apparent benefit from GDT in the occurrence of severe AKI. These results suggest that in a setting where kidney injury may have already occurred at presentation, the clinical course of AKI may not be readily modified and, consequently, that resuscitation strategies may need to focus most on avoidance of further harm.

Considerable evidence exists to associate fluid overload with adverse outcome in patients with AKI. Physiologically, fluid overload manifests as interstitial volume expansion and increased venous pressure. The kidney, as an encapsulated organ, is particularly vulnerable to raised interstitial and venous pressures which will decrease renal blood flow and GFR [45]. At its most extreme, these effects mediate the well-described association between fluid overload, the development of the abdominal compartment syndrome and the occurrence of AKI [46–48]. However, there is evidence that in less extreme situations both renal venous congestion and renal interstitial oedema can play an important role in the initiation and maintenance of AKI, and fluid overload is likely to exacerbate these effects by increasing venous pressure and renal volume [49].

A number of studies have consistently demonstrated an association between positive fluid balances and adverse outcomes in AKI [50–52]. While it is difficult to separate the indirect association of fluid overload as a marker of physiological instability from any direct causative role with adverse renal and patient outcomes, fluid overload has remained independently associated with adverse outcomes in studies attempting to account for the confounding effects of illness severity and haemodynamic instability [53–57]. Fluid accumulation appears to be important both in determining both risk of AKI early after surgery [58, 59] and risk of death in adults [57] and children [56, 60] requiring RRT, suggesting an important role at all stages of AKI. Conversely there is a lack of evidence associating greater fluid administration with better outcomes in AKI despite the well-established belief that fluid therapy benefits kidney function [61].

When considering the role of fluid therapy in the management of AKI, it is important to address the composition as well as the quantity of fluid administered. Colloid solutions have long been advocated for resuscitation with the intention of providing greater magnitude and duration of plasma volume expansion, potentially limiting eventual fluid overload. However, modern commercially available solutions are lost from the circulation within hours [62]. Thus, most fluids administered as iso-oncotic colloid in the ICU lead to clinically insignificant decreases in the total quantity of fluid administered [63–67]. Furthermore evidence now exists that hydroxyethyl starch (HES) solutions have significant nephrotoxicity; meta-analyses examining 6%, 130 kDa HES solutions for resuscitation of patients with sepsis [68], HES solutions in critically ill patients requiring volume resuscitation [69] and colloids versus crystalloids for fluid resuscitation in critically ill patients [70] have all concluded that HES solutions are associated with increased risk of AKI. Thus, HES solutions should be avoided in all patients with or at risk of AKI as potential nephrotoxins with no clear clinical benefit over crystalloids.

A further debate exists over the use of balanced versus unbuffered crystalloid solutions and the risk of AKI. Multiple studies have shown that saline fluid resuscitation is associated with hyperchloraemia and metabolic acidosis [71]. In observational and interventional studies, the use of balanced solutions in surgery and in the ICU has been associated with decreased need for RRT or incidence of AKI [72, 73]. A reduction in renal blood flow associated with hyperchloraemia provides a physiological rationale for these associations [74–76]. However a recent cluster randomized study [77] failed to demonstrate reduction in need for RRT in critically ill patients treated with balanced solutions compared with saline, although overall volumes infused were small. Thus initial resuscitation in patients with or at risk of AKI could be with crystalloid of any composition, but if there is a rational need for ongoing fluid therapy, then use of a balanced solution to avoid the potential adverse effects of hyperchloraemic acidosis can be justified.

Overall fluid management in AKI involves a complex balance between treatment of true hypovolaemia and avoidance of the adverse effects of fluid overload. However, all too often clinical management emphasizes the avoidance of any chance of hypovolaemia without consideration of the very major adverse effect of fluid loading and the physiological rationale of the therapy. To combat these thought processes, a strategy for fluid management after the initial first few hours of treatment has been suggested [49] (Fig. 19.4). This approach emphasizes that only patients with ongoing evidence of hypoperfusion might require ongoing resuscitation and that demonstration of an inadequate cardiac output that is reversible by fluid therapy is then also required to justify ongoing volume expansion. Furthermore, given the propensity of critically ill and AKI patients to develop fluid overload when an active requirement for fluid therapy is not present, attention should then shift to the recognition and management of fluid accumulation as a vital part of the prevention of the adverse effects of fluid overload on organ systems including the kidney.

19.6.2 Vasopressor Therapy in AKI

While vasoconstrictors were regarded as potentially harmful when AKI was considered a predominantly ischemia phenomena, most available evidence now favours moderate vasopressor use in vasodilatory shock. Use of norepinephrine has been shown to improve kidney function in experimental septic AKI [78, 79] and to restore urine output in clinical septic shock [80]. Increasing mean arterial pressure up to 75 mmHg has been shown to increase renal oxygen delivery and GFR during AKI in adults [81], and a persistently lower blood pressure has been associated with persistence or worsening of AKI in the context of sepsis [82]. Consideration should be given to a patient's baseline blood pressure when selecting blood pressure targets as relative hypotension has been associated with development of AKI in hospital [83]. Similarly, in a small study of patients with septic shock admitted to the ICU, it was not the achieved blood pressure that predicted the

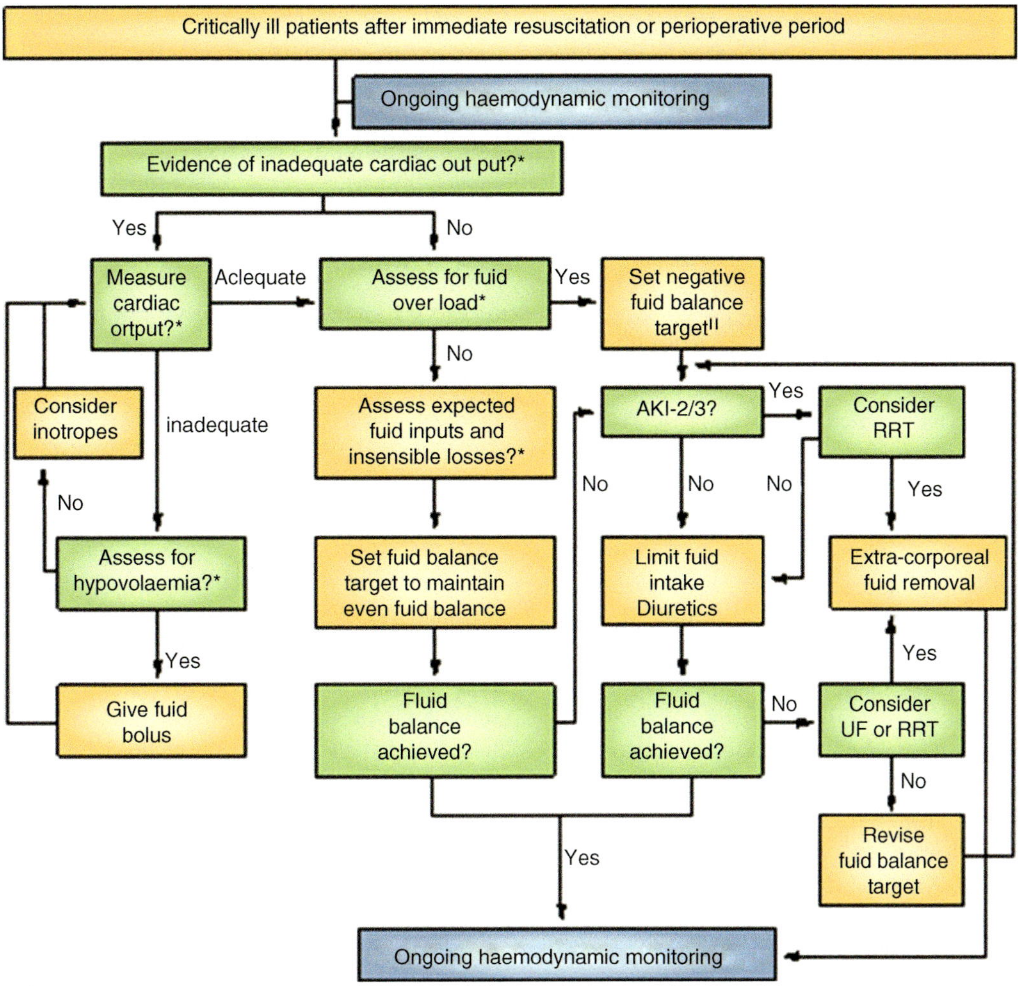

Fig. 19.4 Fluid and haemodynamic management after the initial phase of critical illness. Throughout this pathway a clinically appropriate arterial blood pressure is targeted using vasopressors, if required. In addition to fluid overload, in AKI, RRT may be required for other indications including hyperkalaemia, acidaemia or severe uraemia. Reproduced with permission from: Prowle JR, Kirwan CJ, Bellomo R. Fluid management for the prevention and attenuation of acute kidney injury. *Nat Rev Nephrol.* 2014 [49]. *Increased vasopressor requirement, new or worsening organ dysfunction, tachycardia, lactic acidosis or clinical examination. ‡Measure cardiac index, stroke volume, ejection volume, oxygen delivery or venous saturation of oxygen. Ensure oxygen delivery is adequate to clinical need. §Clinical examination, serial weights, cumulative fluid balance, chest X-ray or ventilation parameters. Lung ultrasound, echocardiography, abdominal pressure measurements and bioimpedance analysis may provide added information. ‖Based on relative fluid overload, haemodynamic stability and expected speed of vascular refilling. ¶Maintenance intravenous fluid is rarely needed where no large ongoing fluid losses are present and feeding established. Replacement should be titrated to volume and expected composition of fluid losses. #Interpretation of stroke volume, pulse pressure, corrected aortic systolic flow time, intrathoracic blood volume index, low central venous or pulmonary artery pressure, echocardiography or fluid responsiveness to passive leg raises or fluid challenges. Abbreviations: *AKI* acute kidney injury, *RRT* renal replacement therapy, *UF* ultrafiltration

development or worsening of AKI, but the magnitude of the difference between baseline and achieved blood pressure and time spent with an achieved blood pressure more than >20% below baseline [84]. These findings have been borne out in a large multicentre study examining vasopressor targets in septic shock where a higher blood pressure target of 75–80 mmHg did not increase survival compared to a lower target of 65–70 mmHg, but was associated with a lower need for RRT in a predefined group with chronic hypertension [85]. Thus, early consideration should be given to use of vasopressors in AKI patients with persistent hypotension unresponsive to initial fluid resuscitation as such an approach may both protect kidney function and prevent unnecessary fluid administration. However, blood pressure targets may need to be tailored to the clinical context. In patients with chronic hypertension and early AKI, higher targets may be justified. However, in sicker patients requiring high-dose vasopressors, haemodynamic management should be aimed at maintaining adequate vital organ perfusion with the least harm to the patient as we know higher targets aren't associated with better overall survival and RRT likely to be inevitably required if oliguria arises.

19.6.3 Specific Vasoactive Drugs for AKI

A wide variety of specific pharmacological interventions for the treatment of AKI have been proposed and shown benefit in animal models or uncontrolled case series; however none has established benefit in large prospective clinical studies and entered established clinical practice [86]. Particular focus has been placed on vasoactive medication that might preferentially benefit renal perfusion. Historically low-dose dopamine was commonly administered to critically ill patients in the belief that it reduces the risk of kidney failure by increasing kidney blood flow via dopamine-1 receptor agonism; however in a landmark placebo-controlled study published in 2000, Bellomo et al. demonstrated no improvement in serum creatinine or need for RRT in critically ill patients randomized to so-called *renal-dose dopamine*—effectively removing this treatment from the management of AKI [87]. Given our current understanding that global ischaemia is unlikely to be a major factor in the pathogenesis of most cases of AKI, the failure of this strategy is unsurprising. Nevertheless, considerable interest has persisted in the use of fenoldopam, a selective D1 agonist that may also have anti-inflammatory properties, in the prevention or treatment of AKI in high-risk settings—with suggestion of preventative benefit in small studies [88]. However, a recent multicentre randomized controlled study demonstrated no benefit from fenoldopam in prevention of AKI progression or need for RRT in patients with early AKI after cardiac surgery [89]. In contrast to the failure of vasodilators, it has been suggested that the vasopressor, vasopressin, might have some beneficial effect over noradrenaline in early septic AKI perhaps by better preserving intra-glomerular pressure in septic shock [90]; however results of a multicentre randomized controlled study [91] examining the early use of vasopressin in septic shock targeting a kidney endpoint have now been presented with a negative result at the primary endpoint. Finally preliminary studies with levosimendan, a calcium-sensitizing inodilator, have suggested possible beneficial effects on kidney function after major surgery [92] and in septic shock [93]. This effect has some physiological rationale as levosimendan may improve renal perfusion both by augmenting cardiac output and also by venodilation reducing renal congestion and improving microvascular flow. Another multicentre randomized controlled study [94] is nearing completion examining the use of levosimendan in septic shock including detailed reporting of kidney outcomes, but as yet confirmation of benefit in AKI is lacking. Thus, while considerable research is ongoing, currently there is no evidence from high-quality prospective studies that any specific vasoactive drugs are better able to modify the course of AKI than standard care using conventional vasopressors such as noradrenaline.

19.7 Non-dialytic Management of More Severe AKI

While much of the non-dialytic management of AKI relates to the diagnosis and prevention of general clinical deterioration, instances arise when the medical management of the metabolic complications of advanced acute kidney failure is desirable. In the main these approaches are a bridging therapy to the safe initiation of renal replacement therapy rather than definitive treatment. Complications of advanced AKI can be broadly classified according to the functions of the kidney; notably accumulation of nitrogenous end products of metabolism through diminished GFR occurs progressively as kidney function deteriorates so that while common in advanced CKD patients nearing need for dialysis, they are uncommon in acutely unwell AKI patients. Conversely severe electrolyte and acid-base abnormalities occur relatively late in the progression of CKD, but may be prominent in rapidly progressive cases of AKI where kidney function has effectively ceased at the same time as shock, neurohormonal responses, medical therapy and tissue injury are contributing to abnormalities in metabolites normally regulated by the kidney. As a consequence, the most common life-threatening complications of AKI are hyperkalaemia, metabolic acidosis and fluid overload often exacerbated by co-existing conditions such as tissue injury, lactic acidosis and high-volume fluid resuscitation. Conversely conditions like hypertension, uraemia, anorexia, renal bone disease and anaemia that are of key importance in the pre-dialysis management of CKD are rarely clinically important in acute AKI management.

19.7.1 Management of Fluid Overload

Recognition of refractory oligoanuria and the limitation of fluid loading has an essential role in preventing the adverse effects of severe fluid overload in developing AKI. The schema outlined in Fig. 19.4 suggests an active approach to both the prevention and management of fluid overload in AKI patients. Within this approach any role of diuretics is as a method of manipulating fluid balance and not as a treatment of AKI as such [95]. Diuretics are of no proven benefit in altering the course of AKI [96] and may delay definitive treatment [97]; conversely benefit may accrue when diuretics are used to treat fluid overload in patients with AKI diagnoses [55]. Thus any use of diuretics to treat fluid overload must be appropriately indicated for fluid overload and continuously re-evaluated for effectiveness of treatment and need to transit to RRT. Recently it has been suggested that a standardized test dose of loop diuretic (80–120 mg of furosemide) in a so-called *furosemide stress test* might demonstrate renal excretory capacity and thus underlying severity of AKI or need for RRT in AKI patients [98]. Clinically this test has shown better predictive ability for RRT worsening of AKI and death than a number of novel AKI biomarkers [99]. While the *furosemide stress test* is a prognostic test rather than a treatment as patients were kept fluid neutral during the assessment, these findings do at least suggest that if there is an inadequate initial response to diuretic treatment in AKI, continued treatment is likely to be unsuccessful and recourse to RRT should be considered.

19.7.2 Metabolic Acidosis

The function of the kidney in acid-base regulation is to excrete organic acids and ammonium ions thus generating excess bicarbonate allowing the respiratory pH buffer to maintain blood pH around 7.4 rather than at the natural pKa of dissolved carbon dioxide which is 6.1. Thus loss of kidney function leads to depletion of bicarbonate reserves and progressive metabolic acidosis which is partially hypochloraemic (through failure to excrete ammonium chloride) and partially associated with accumulation of unmeasured (renally excreted) strong anions. In addition, during critical illness uremic acidosis is often exacerbated by co-existent lactic or respiratory acidosis. While moderate acidosis may be well tolerated, sustained low pH below 7.25 becomes progressively life-threatening. Non-renal contributions to acidosis should be targeted and treated if possible as renal replacement therapy does not treat any underlying cause of other causes of acidosis. RRT replaces kidney function by donating bicarbonate while removing acid anions including chloride.

However, in extremis sodium bicarbonate can be used to similarly compensate for the lost kidney function allowing clinical stabilization until RRT is available. While formulae for estimation of bicarbonate deficit are available, a better approach is to judiciously titrate bicarbonate dosing to achieve the minimum acceptable pH. Concerns regarding use of bicarbonate include the development of fluid overload and hypernatraemia. In addition, theoretical concerns regarding the development of hypercapnia and cellular acidosis are often raised; in fact the additional carbon dioxide generated in the treatment of metabolic acidosis is a relatively small fraction of the overall CO_2 generation, so as long as some ventilation is occurring, the excess CO_2 generated is extremely rapidly excreted in the lungs [100], so that in physiological conditions significant intracellular acidification does not occur [101].

19.7.3 Hyperkalaemia

Severe hyperkalaemia complicating AKI is often of mixed aetiology resulting from not only marked reduction in potassium excretion by the kidneys but also release of potassium from injured tissues with reperfusion and release from the intracellular compartment with metabolic acidosis particularly ketoacidosis. While there is no standard definition of hyperkalaemia, development of ECG abnormalities and risk of life-threatening arrhythmias increase progressively with serum levels >6.5 mmol/L. There are few if any randomized trials to guide clinicians in the medical management of acute severe hyperkalaemia, and expert consensus continues to drive treatment recommendations [102]. A step-wise approach involving administration of intravenous calcium to aid cardiac membrane stability in patients with ECG changes, followed by strategies to shift potassium into cells, is key to the emergency management—the intention being to allow time to institute definitive treatment by either addressing a reversible cause or providing potassium removal through RRT. Classically attempts to lower serum potassium by cellular uptake use a combination of concentrated dextrose and insulin, possibly aided by high-dose salbutamol nebulizers. Evidence suggests that while salbutamol alone is of limited efficacy, the combination of salbutamol with insulin-glucose is more effective than either treatment alone [103, 104]. Conversely limited evidence available in the chronic haemodialysis population suggests sodium bicarbonate fails to acutely lower potassium in comparison to other potassium-lowering regimens [105, 106]. As an adjunct to treatment, in moderate or chronic hyperkalaemia, enteral potassium-binding resins (sodium polystyrene sulphonate or calcium resonium) are commonly employed; however these are considered to be slow and unreliable to be useful in the emergency treatment of life-threatening hyperkalaemia [102] where emergency medical management is a bridge to definitive treatment with RRT. Recently two novel potassium-binding agents, *patiromer* and *zirconium cyclosilicate*, have been developed that may be effective for the management of mild-moderate hyperkalaemia over a relatively shorter period of time [107]; these may eventually replace current potassium binder in the management of chronic or subacute hyperkalaemia; however it seems unlikely that their introduction will alter the acute management of severe hyperkalaemia complicating AKI where the focus will remain on stabilization prior to RRT.

19.8 Long-Term Follow-Up After AKI

As well as the acute association with risk of death, AKI is now recognized as a major risk factor for the development and progression of CKD [108–110], even if apparent recovery to baseline function occurs [111, 112]. This has significant health implications beyond potential need for long-term renal replacement therapy; AKI and the subsequent development of CKD have been associated with increased risk of death and cardiovascular morbidity [113, 114].

Targeted follow-up for AKI survivors could modify long-term outcomes [115]. A recent UK health economic analysis has suggested that *post-discharge* healthcare costs attributable to

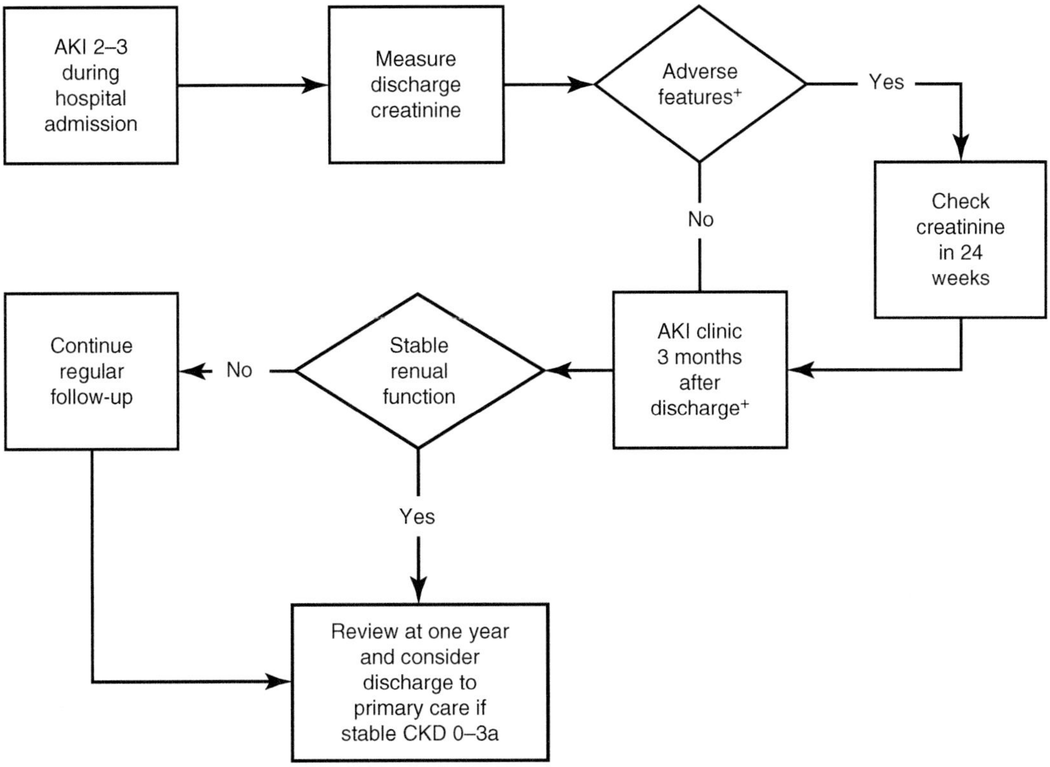

Fig. 19.5 A proposed pathway for follow-up of patients who survive an episode of AKI 2 or 3 (as per KDIGO criteria) while in hospital. Reproduced with permission from: Kirwan CJ et al. Critically Ill Patients Requiring Acute Renal Replacement Therapy Are at an Increased Risk of Long-Term Renal Dysfunction, but Rarely Receive Specialist Nephrology Follow-Up. *Nephron*. 2015 [117]. *Adverse features suggesting need for early follow-up include a significant increase in serum creatinine from premorbid baseline to discharge (new overt CKD or unrecovered AKI) or the presence of significant kidney impairment (suggested as a serum creatinine of >175 µmol/L (2 mg/dL) or eGFR <30 mL/min/1.73 m^2). Consider formal measurement of GFR or creatinine clearance in patients with prolonged critical illness or significant loss of muscle mass. †Patients with specific features including persistent haematuria or proteinuria (urine protein/creatinine ratio >100), proven or suspected glomerulonephritis, refractory hypertension, familial kidney disease, recurrent or extensive nephrolithiasis or likely progression to ESRD within 1 year should be referred directly to the appropriate specialist nephrology clinic

inpatient AKI would be £179 million per year, primarily arising from the development of CKD [1]. Despite potential gains rates of systematic renal follow-up after severe AKI remain very low [116, 117], while it is difficult to predict, at the time of hospital discharge, whether kidney function will subsequently improve, stabilize or worsen. Consequently, some form of systematic approach to follow-up (Fig. 19.5) of patients who experienced significant AKI is a crucial accompaniment to the management of both RRT-requiring and non-RRT-requiring AKI to sustain good outcomes in the longer term.

References

1. Kerr M, Bedford M, Matthews B, O'Donoghue D. The economic impact of acute kidney injury in England. Nephrol Dial Transplant. 2014;29(7):1362–8.
2. Kidney Disease Improving Global Outcomes. KDIGO clinical practice guideline for acute kidney injury; section 2: AKI definition. Kidney Int Suppl (2011). 2012;2(1):19–36.
3. Bellomo R, Ronco C, Kellum JA, Mehta RL, Palevsky P. Acute renal failure—definition, outcome measures, animal models, fluid therapy and information technology needs: the Second International Consensus Conference of the Acute Dialysis Quality Initiative (ADQI) Group. Crit Care. 2004;8(4):R204–12.

4. Mehta RL, Kellum JA, Shah SV, Molitoris BA, Ronco C, Warnock DG, Levin A. Acute Kidney Injury Network: report of an initiative to improve outcomes in acute kidney injury. Crit Care. 2007;11(2):R31.
5. Bywaters EG, Beall D. Crush injuries with impairment of renal function. Br Med J. 1941;1(4185):427–32.
6. Oliver J, Mac DM, Tracy A. The pathogenesis of acute renal failure associated with traumatic and toxic injury; renal ischemia, nephrotoxic damage and the ischemic episode. J Clin Invest. 1951;30(12:1):1307–439.
7. Bull GM, Joekes AM, Lowe KG. Conservative treatment of anuric uraemia. Lancet. 1949;2(6571):229–34.
8. Borst JG. Protein katabolism in uraemia; effects of protein-free diet, infections, and blood-transfusions. Lancet. 1948;1(6509):824–9.
9. Uchino S, Kellum JA, Bellomo R, Doig GS, Morimatsu H, Morgera S, Schetz M, Tan I, Bouman C, Macedo E, et al. Acute renal failure in critically ill patients: a multinational, multicenter study. JAMA. 2005;294(7):813–8.
10. Chawla LS, Eggers PW, Star RA, Kimmel PL. Acute kidney injury and chronic kidney disease as interconnected syndromes. N Engl J Med. 2014;371(1):58–66.
11. Hoste EAJ, Clermont G, Kersten A, Venkataraman R, Angus DC, De Bacquer D, Kellum JA. RIFLE criteria for acute kidney injury are associated with hospital mortality in critically ill patients: a cohort analysis. Crit Care. 2006;10(3):R73.
12. Ostermann M, Chang RW. Acute kidney injury in the intensive care unit according to RIFLE. Crit Care Med. 2007;35(8):1837–43; quiz 1852.
13. Chertow GM, Burdick E, Honour M, Bonventre JV, Bates DW. Acute kidney injury, mortality, length of stay, and costs in hospitalized patients. J Am Soc Nephrol. 2005;16(11):3365–70.
14. Schetz M, Gunst J, Van den Berghe G. The impact of using estimated GFR versus creatinine clearance on the evaluation of recovery from acute kidney injury in the ICU. Intensive Care Med. 2014;40(11):1709–17.
15. Pickering JW, Ralib AM, Endre ZH. Combining creatinine and volume kinetics identifies missed cases of acute kidney injury following cardiac arrest. Crit Care. 2013;17(1):R7.
16. Porter CJ, Juurlink I, Bisset LH, Bavakunji R, Mehta RL, Devonald MA. A real-time electronic alert to improve detection of acute kidney injury in a large teaching hospital. Nephrol Dial Transplant. 2014;29(10):1888–93.
17. Selby NM, Crowley L, Fluck RJ, McIntyre CW, Monaghan J, Lawson N, Kolhe NV. Use of electronic results reporting to diagnose and monitor AKI in hospitalized patients. Clin J Am Soc Nephrol. 2012;7(4):533–40.
18. Wilson FP, Shashaty M, Testani J, Aqeel I, Borovskiy Y, Ellenberg SS, Feldman HI, Fernandez H, Gitelman Y, Lin J, et al. Automated, electronic alerts for acute kidney injury: a single-blind, parallel-group, randomised controlled trial. Lancet. 2015;385(9981):1966–74.
19. Lin J, Fernandez H, Shashaty MG, Negoianu D, Testani JM, Berns JS, Parikh CR, Wilson FP. False-positive rate of AKI using consensus creatinine-based criteria. Clin J Am Soc Nephrol. 2015;10(10):1723–31.
20. Prowle J, Bellomo R. Urine output and the diagnosis of acute kidney injury. In: Annual update in intensive care and emergency medicine 2012; Springer: Berlin/Heidelberg; 2012. p. 628–40.
21. Alge JL, Arthur JM. Biomarkers of AKI: a review of mechanistic relevance and potential therapeutic implications. Clin J Am Soc Nephrol. 2015;10(1):147–55.
22. Cruz DN, Bagshaw SM, Maisel A, Lewington A, Thadhani R, Chakravarthi R, Murray PT, Mehta RL, Chawla LS. Use of biomarkers to assess prognosis and guide management of patients with acute kidney injury. Contrib Nephrol. 2013;182:45–64.
23. AKI Care Bundle. http://www.londonaki.net/clinical/guidelines-pathways.html.
24. Jacobs R, Honore PM, Joannes-Boyau O, Boer W, De Regt J, De Waele E, Collin V, Spapen HD. Septic acute kidney injury: the culprit is inflammatory apoptosis rather than ischemic necrosis. Blood Purif. 2011;32(4):262–5.
25. Prowle JR, Bellomo R. Sepsis-associated acute kidney injury: macrohemodynamic and microhemodynamic alterations in the renal circulation. Semin Nephrol. 2015;35(1):64–74.
26. Lipcsey M, Bellomo R. Septic acute kidney injury: hemodynamic syndrome, inflammatory disorder, or both? Crit Care. 2011;15(6):1008.
27. LeDoux D, Astiz ME, Carpati CM, Rackow EC. Effects of perfusion pressure on tissue perfusion in septic shock. Crit Care Med. 2000;28:2729–32.
28. Marik PE, Baram M, Vahid B. Does central venous pressure predict fluid responsiveness? A systematic review of the literature and the tale of seven mares. Chest. 2008;134:172–8.
29. Michard F, Teboul JL. Predicting fluid responsiveness in ICU patients: a critical analysis of the evidence. Chest. 2002;121:2000–8.
30. Bouhemad B. Isolated and reversible impairment of ventricular relaxation in patients with septic shock. Crit Care Med. 2008;36:766–74.
31. Bouhemad B. Acute left ventricular dilatation and shock-induced myocardial dysfunction. Crit Care Med. 2009;37:441–7.
32. Rudiger A, Singer M. Mechanisms of sepsis-induced cardiac dysfunction. Crit Care Med. 2007;35:1599–608.
33. Di Giantomasso D, May CN, Bellomo R. Vital organ blood flow during hyperdynamic sepsis. Chest. 2003;124:1053–9.
34. Ruokonen E. Regional blood flow and oxygen transport in septic shock. Crit Care Med. 1993;21:1296–303.

35. Fleck A. Increased vascular permeability: a major cause of hypoalbuminaemia in disease and injury. Lancet. 1985;325:781–4.
36. Marik PE, Cavallazzi R. Does the central venous pressure predict fluid responsiveness? An updated meta-analysis and a plea for some common sense. Crit Care Med. 2013;41(7):1774–81.
37. Marik PE, Bellomo R, Demla V. Lactate clearance as a target of therapy in sepsis: a flawed paradigm. OA Critical Care. 2013;1:3.
38. Wan L, Bellomo R, May CN. A comparison of 4% succinylated gelatin solution versus normal saline in stable normovolaemic sheep: global haemodynamic, regional blood flow and oxygen delivery effects. Anaesth Intensive Care. 2007;35(6):924–31.
39. Legrand M, Mik EG, Balestra GM, Lutter R, Pirracchio R, Payen D, Ince C. Fluid resuscitation does not improve renal oxygenation during hemorrhagic shock in rats. Anesthesiology. 2010;112(1):119–27.
40. Wan L, Bellomo R, May CN. The effect of normal saline resuscitation on vital organ blood flow in septic sheep. Intensive Care Med. 2006;32(8):1238–42.
41. Prowle JR, Chua HR, Bagshaw SM, Bellomo R. Clinical review: volume of fluid resuscitation and the incidence of acute kidney injury—a systematic review. Crit Care. 2012;16(4):230.
42. Mouncey PR, Osborn TM, Power GS, Harrison DA, Sadique MZ, Grieve RD, Jahan R, Harvey SE, Bell D, Bion JF, et al. Trial of early, goal-directed resuscitation for septic shock. N Engl J Med. 2015;372(14):1301–11.
43. Investigators A, Group ACT, Peake SL, Delaney A, Bailey M, Bellomo R, Cameron PA, Cooper DJ, Higgins AM, Holdgate A, et al. Goal-directed resuscitation for patients with early septic shock. N Engl J Med. 2014;371(16):1496–506.
44. Pro CI, Yealy DM, Kellum JA, Huang DT, Barnato AE, Weissfeld LA, Pike F, Terndrup T, Wang HE, Hou PC, et al. A randomized trial of protocol-based care for early septic shock. N Engl J Med. 2014;370(18):1683–93.
45. Firth JD, Raine AE, Ledingham JG. Raised venous pressure: a direct cause of renal sodium retention in oedema? Lancet. 1988;1(8593):1033–5.
46. Dalfino L, Tullo L, Donadio I, Malcangi V, Brienza N. Intra-abdominal hypertension and acute renal failure in critically ill patients. Intensive Care Med. 2008;34(4):707–13.
47. Vidal MG, Ruiz Weisser J, Gonzalez F, Toro MA, Loudet C, Balasini C, Canales H, Reina R, Estenssoro E. Incidence and clinical effects of intra-abdominal hypertension in critically ill patients. Crit Care Med. 2008;36(6):1823–31.
48. Malbrain ML. Incidence and prognosis of intraabdominal hypertension in a mixed population of critically ill patients: a multiple-center epidemiological study. Crit Care Med. 2005;33:315–22.
49. Prowle JR, Kirwan CJ, Bellomo R. Fluid management for the prevention and attenuation of acute kidney injury. Nat Rev Nephrol. 2014;10(1):37–47.
50. Payen D, de Pont AC, Sakr Y, Spies C, Reinhart K, Vincent JL, Sepsis Occurrence in Acutely Ill Patients (SOAP) Investigators. A positive fluid balance is associated with a worse outcome in patients with acute renal failure. Crit Care. 2008;12(3):R74.
51. Bouchard J, Soroko SB, Chertow GM, Himmelfarb J, Ikizler TA, Paganini EP, Mehta RL. Fluid accumulation, survival and recovery of kidney function in critically ill patients with acute kidney injury. Kidney Int. 2009;76(4):422–7.
52. Teixeira C, Garzotto F, Piccinni P, Brienza N, Iannuzzi M, Gramaticopolo S, Forfori F, Rocco M, Ronco C, Belluomo Anello C, et al. Fluid balance and urine volume are independent predictors of mortality in acute kidney injury. Crit Care. 2013;17(1):R14.
53. Basu RK, Andrews A, Krawczeski C, Manning P, Wheeler DS, Goldstein SL. Acute kidney injury based on corrected serum creatinine is associated with increased morbidity in children following the arterial switch operation. Pediatr Crit Care Med. 2013;14(5):e218–24.
54. Fulop T, Pathak MB, Schmidt DW, Lengvarszky Z, Juncos JP, Lebrun CJ, Brar H, Juncos LA. Volume-related weight gain and subsequent mortality in acute renal failure patients treated with continuous renal replacement therapy. ASAIO J. 2010;56(4):333–7.
55. Grams ME, Estrella MM, Coresh J, Brower RG, Liu KD, National Heart L, Blood Institute Acute Respiratory Distress Syndrome N. Fluid balance, diuretic use, and mortality in acute kidney injury. Clin J Am Soc Nephrol. 2011;6(5):966–73.
56. Sutherland SM, Zappitelli M, Alexander SR, Chua AN, Brophy PD, Bunchman TE, Hackbarth R, Somers MJ, Baum M, Symons JM, et al. Fluid overload and mortality in children receiving continuous renal replacement therapy: the prospective pediatric continuous renal replacement therapy registry. Am J Kidney Dis. 2010;55(2):316–25.
57. Vaara ST, Korhonen AM, Kaukonen KM, Nisula S, Inkinen O, Hoppu S, Laurila JJ, Mildh L, Reinikainen M, Lund V, et al. Fluid overload is associated with an increased risk for 90-day mortality in critically ill patients with renal replacement therapy: data from the prospective FINNAKI study. Crit Care. 2012;16(5):R197.
58. Dass B, Shimada M, Kambhampati G, Ejaz NI, Arif AA, Ejaz AA. Fluid balance as an early indicator of acute kidney injury in CV surgery. Clin Nephrol. 2012;77(6):438–44.
59. Kambhampati G, Ross EA, Alsabbagh MM, Asmar A, Pakkivenkata U, Ejaz NI, Arif AA, Ejaz AA. Perioperative fluid balance and acute kidney injury. Clin Exp Nephrol. 2012;16(5):730–8.
60. Goldstein SL, Somers MJ, Baum MA, Symons JM, Brophy PD, Blowey D, Bunchman TE, Baker C, Mottes T, McAfee N, et al. Pediatric patients with multi-organ dysfunction syndrome receiving continuous renal replacement therapy. Kidney Int. 2005;67(2):653–8.

61. Prowle JR, Echeverri JE, Ligabo EV, Ronco C, Bellomo R. Fluid balance and acute kidney injury. Nat Rev Nephrol. 2010;6(2):107–15.
62. Jungheinrich C, Neff TA. Pharmacokinetics of hydroxyethyl starch. Clin Pharmacokinet. 2005;44(7):681–99.
63. Finfer S, Bellomo R, Boyce N, French J, Myburgh J, Norton R, Investigators SS. A comparison of albumin and saline for fluid resuscitation in the intensive care unit. N Engl J Med. 2004;350(22):2247–56.
64. Myburgh JA, Finfer S, Bellomo R, Billot L, Cass A, Gattas D, Glass P, Lipman J, Liu B, McArthur C, et al. Hydroxyethyl starch or saline for fluid resuscitation in intensive care. N Engl J Med. 2012;367(20):1901–11.
65. Perner A, Haase N, Guttormsen AB, Tenhunen J, Klemenzson G, Aneman A, Madsen KR, Moller MH, Elkjaer JM, Poulsen LM, et al. Hydroxyethyl starch 130/0.42 versus Ringer's acetate in severe sepsis. N Engl J Med. 2012;367(2):124–34.
66. Guidet B, Martinet O, Boulain T, Philippart F, Poussel JF, Maizel J, Forceville X, Feissel M, Hasselmann M, Heininger A, et al. Assessment of hemodynamic efficacy and safety of 6% hydroxyethylstarch 130/0.4 vs. 0.9% NaCl fluid replacement in patients with severe sepsis: the CRYSTMAS study. Crit Care. 2012;16(3):R94.
67. Bayer O, Reinhart K, Kohl M, Kabisch B, Marshall J, Sakr Y, Bauer M, Hartog C, Schwarzkopf D, Riedemann N. Effects of fluid resuscitation with synthetic colloids or crystalloids alone on shock reversal, fluid balance, and patient outcomes in patients with severe sepsis: a prospective sequential analysis. Crit Care Med. 2012;40(9):2543–51.
68. Haase N, Perner A, Hennings LI, Siegemund M, Lauridsen B, Wetterslev M, Wetterslev J. Hydroxyethyl starch 130/0.38–0.45 versus crystalloid or albumin in patients with sepsis: systematic review with meta-analysis and trial sequential analysis. BMJ. 2013;346:f839.
69. Zarychanski R, Abou-Setta AM, Turgeon AF, Houston BL, McIntyre L, Marshall JC, Fergusson DA. Association of hydroxyethyl starch administration with mortality and acute kidney injury in critically ill patients requiring volume resuscitation: a systematic review and meta-analysis. JAMA. 2013;309(7):678–88.
70. Perel P, Roberts I, Ker K. Colloids versus crystalloids for fluid resuscitation in critically ill patients. Cochrane Database Syst Rev. 2013:2:CD000567.
71. Yunos NM, Kim IB, Bellomo R, Bailey M, Ho L, Story D, Gutteridge GA, Hart GK. The biochemical effects of restricting chloride-rich fluids in intensive care. Crit Care Med. 2011;39(11):2419–24.
72. Shaw AD, Bagshaw SM, Goldstein SL, Scherer LA, Duan M, Schermer CR, Kellum JA. Major complications, mortality, and resource utilization after open abdominal surgery: 0.9% saline compared to Plasma-Lyte. Ann Surg. 2012;255(5):821–9.
73. Yunos NM, Bellomo R, Hegarty C, Story D, Ho L, Bailey M. Association between a chloride-liberal vs chloride-restrictive intravenous fluid administration strategy and kidney injury in critically ill adults. JAMA. 2012;308(15):1566–72.
74. Chowdhury AH, Cox EF, Francis ST, Lobo DN. A randomized, controlled, double-blind crossover study on the effects of 2-L infusions of 0.9% saline and plasma-lyte 148 on renal blood flow velocity and renal cortical tissue perfusion in healthy volunteers. Ann Surg. 2012;256(1):18–24.
75. Bullivant EM, Wilcox CS, Welch WJ. Intrarenal vasoconstriction during hyperchloremia: role of thromboxane. Am J Phys. 1989;256(1 Pt 2):F152–7.
76. Yunos NM, Bellomo R, Story D, Kellum J. Bench-to-bedside review: chloride in critical illness. Crit Care. 2010;14(4):226.
77. Young P, Bailey M, Beasley R, Henderson S, Mackle D, McArthur C, McGuinness S, Mehrtens J, Myburgh J, Psirides A, et al. Effect of a buffered crystalloid solution vs saline on acute kidney injury among patients in the intensive care unit: the SPLIT randomized clinical trial. JAMA. 2015;314(16):1701–10.
78. Bellomo R, Kellum JA, Wisniewski SR, Pinsky MR. Effects of norepinephrine on the renal vasculature in normal and endotoxemic dogs. Am J Respir Crit Care Med. 1999;159(4 Pt 1):1186–92.
79. Anderson WP, Korner PI, Selig SE. Mechanisms involved in the renal responses to intravenous and renal artery infusions of noradrenaline in conscious dogs. J Physiol. 1981;321:21–30.
80. Martin C, Papazian L, Perrin G, Saux P, Gouin F. Norepinephrine or dopamine for the treatment of hyperdynamic septic shock? Chest. 1993;103(6):1826–31.
81. Redfors B, Bragadottir G, Sellgren J, Sward K, Ricksten SE. Effects of norepinephrine on renal perfusion, filtration and oxygenation in vasodilatory shock and acute kidney injury. Intensive Care Med. 2011;37(1):60–7.
82. Badin J, Boulain T, Ehrmann S, Skarzynski M, Bretagnol A, Buret J, Benzekri-Lefevre D, Mercier E, Runge I, Garot D, et al. Relation between mean arterial pressure and renal function in the early phase of shock: a prospective, explorative cohort study. Crit Care. 2011;15(3):R135.
83. Liu YL, Prowle J, Licari E, Uchino S, Bellomo R. Changes in blood pressure before the development of nosocomial acute kidney injury. Nephrol Dial Transplant. 2009;24(2):504–11.
84. Panwar R, Lanyon N, Davies AR, Bailey M, Pilcher D, Bellomo R. Mean perfusion pressure deficit during the initial management of shock—an observational cohort study. J Crit Care. 2013;28(5):816–24.
85. Asfar P, Meziani F, Hamel JF, Grelon F, Megarbane B, Anguel N, Mira JP, Dequin PF, Gergaud S, Weiss N, et al. High versus low blood-pressure target in patients with septic shock. N Engl J Med. 2014;370(17):1583–93.
86. Prowle JR, Bellomo R. Acute kidney injury: specific interventions and drugs. In: Jörres A, et al., editors.

Management of acute kidney problems. Berlin/Heidelberg: Springer; 2010. p. 229–39.
87. Bellomo R, Chapman M, Finfer S, Hickling K, Myburgh J. Low-dose dopamine in patients with early renal dysfunction: a placebo-controlled randomised trial. Australian and New Zealand Intensive Care Society (ANZICS) Clinical Trials Group. Lancet. 2000;356(9248):2139–43.
88. Gillies MA, Kakar V, Parker RJ, Honore PM, Ostermann M. Fenoldopam to prevent acute kidney injury after major surgery-a systematic review and meta-analysis. Crit Care. 2015;19:449.
89. Bove T, Zangrillo A, Guarracino F, Alvaro G, Persi B, Maglioni E, Galdieri N, Comis M, Caramelli F, Pasero DC, et al. Effect of fenoldopam on use of renal replacement therapy among patients with acute kidney injury after cardiac surgery: a randomized clinical trial. JAMA. 2014;312(21):2244–53.
90. Gordon AC, Russell JA, Walley KR, Singer J, Ayers D, Storms MM, Holmes CL, Hebert PC, Cooper DJ, Mehta S, et al. The effects of vasopressin on acute kidney injury in septic shock. Intensive Care Med. 2010;36(1):83–91.
91. Gordon AC, Mason AJ, Perkins GD, Ashby D, Brett SJ. Protocol for a randomised controlled trial of VAsopressin versus Noradrenaline as Initial therapy in Septic sHock (VANISH). BMJ Open. 2014;4(7):e005866.
92. Zhou C, Gong J, Chen D, Wang W, Liu M, Liu B. Levosimendan for prevention of acute kidney injury after cardiac surgery: a meta-analysis of randomized controlled trials. Am J Kidney Dis. 2016;67(3):408–16.
93. Morelli A, De Castro S, Teboul JL, Singer M, Rocco M, Conti G, De Luca L, Di Angelantonio E, Orecchioni A, Pandian NG, et al. Effects of levosimendan on systemic and regional hemodynamics in septic myocardial depression. Intensive Care Med. 2005;31(5):638–44.
94. Orme RM, Perkins GD, McAuley DF, Liu KD, Mason AJ, Morelli A, Singer M, Ashby D, Gordon AC. An efficacy and mechanism evaluation study of Levosimendan for the Prevention of Acute oRgan Dysfunction in Sepsis (LeoPARDS): protocol for a randomized controlled trial. Trials. 2014;15:199.
95. Goldstein S, Bagshaw S, Cecconi M, Okusa M, Wang H, Kellum J, Mythen M, Shaw AD, Group AXI. Pharmacological management of fluid overload. Br J Anaesth. 2014;113(5):756–63.
96. Uchino S, Doig GS, Bellomo R, Morimatsu H, Morgera S, Schetz M, Tan I, Bouman C, Nacedo E, Gibney N, et al. Diuretics and mortality in acute renal failure. Crit Care Med. 2004;32(8):1669–77.
97. Mehta RL, Pascual MT, Soroko S, Chertow GM, Group PS. Diuretics, mortality, and nonrecovery of renal function in acute renal failure. JAMA. 2002;288(20):2547–53.
98. Chawla LS, Davison DL, Brasha-Mitchell E, Koyner JL, Arthur JM, Shaw AD, Tumlin JA, Trevino SA, Kimmel PL, Seneff MG. Development and standardization of a furosemide stress test to predict the severity of acute kidney injury. Crit Care. 2013;17(5):R207.
99. Koyner JL, Davison DL, Brasha-Mitchell E, Chalikonda DM, Arthur JM, Shaw AD, Tumlin JA, Trevino SA, Bennett MR, Kimmel PL, et al. Furosemide stress test and biomarkers for the prediction of AKI severity. J Am Soc Nephrol. 2015;26(8):2023–31.
100. Levraut J, Garcia P, Giunti C, Ichai C, Bouregba M, Ciebiera JP, Payan P, Grimaud D. The increase in CO2 production induced by NaHCO3 depends on blood albumin and hemoglobin concentrations. Intensive Care Med. 2000;26(5):558–64.
101. Goldsmith DJ, Forni LG, Hilton PJ. Bicarbonate therapy and intracellular acidosis. Clin Sci (Lond). 1997;93(6):593–8.
102. Treatment of acute hyperkalaemia in adults. http://www.renal.org/docs/default-source/guidelines-resources/joint-guidelines/treatment-of-acute-hyperkalaemia-in-adults/hyperkalaemia-guideline—march-2014.pdf?sfvrsn=2.
103. Allon M, Copkney C. Albuterol and insulin for treatment of hyperkalemia in hemodialysis patients. Kidney Int. 1990;38(5):869–72.
104. Lens XM, Montoliu J, Cases A, Campistol JM, Revert L. Treatment of hyperkalaemia in renal failure: salbutamol v. insulin. Nephrol Dial Transplant. 1989;4(3):228–32.
105. Allon M, Shanklin N. Effect of bicarbonate administration on plasma potassium in dialysis patients: interactions with insulin and albuterol. Am J Kidney Dis. 1996;28(4):508–14.
106. Blumberg A, Weidmann P, Shaw S, Gnadinger M. Effect of various therapeutic approaches on plasma potassium and major regulating factors in terminal renal failure. Am J Med. 1988;85(4):507–12.
107. Kovesdy CP. Management of hyperkalemia: an update for the internist. Am J Med. 2015;128(12):1281–7.
108. Amdur RL, Chawla LS, Amodeo S, Kimmel PL, Palant CE. Outcomes following diagnosis of acute renal failure in U.S. veterans: focus on acute tubular necrosis. Kidney Int. 2009;76(10):1089–97.
109. Chawla LS, Kimmel PL. Acute kidney injury and chronic kidney disease: an integrated clinical syndrome. Kidney Int. 2012;82(5):516–24.
110. Ishani A, Xue JL, Himmelfarb J, Eggers PW, Kimmel PL, Molitoris BA, Collins AJ. Acute kidney injury increases risk of ESRD among elderly. J Am Soc Nephrol. 2009;20(1):223–8.
111. Bucaloiu ID, Kirchner HL, Norfolk ER, Hartle JE 2nd, Perkins RM. Increased risk of death and de novo chronic kidney disease following reversible acute kidney injury. Kidney Int. 2012;81(5):477–85.
112. Mammen C, Al Abbas A, Skippen P, Nadel H, Levine D, Collet JP, Matsell DG. Long-term risk of CKD in children surviving episodes of acute kidney injury in the intensive care unit: a prospective cohort study. Am J Kidney Dis. 2012;59(4):523–30.

113. Wu VC, Wu CH, Huang TM, Wang CY, Lai CF, Shiao CC, Chang CH, Lin SL, Chen YY, Chen YM, et al. Long-term risk of coronary events after AKI. J Am Soc Nephrol. 2014;25(3):595–605.
114. Chawla LS, Amdur RL, Shaw AD, Faselis C, Palant CE, Kimmel PL. Association between AKI and long-term renal and cardiovascular outcomes in United States veterans. Clin J Am Soc Nephrol. 2014;9(3):448–56.
115. Harel Z, Wald R, Bargman JM, Mamdani M, Etchells E, Garg AX, Ray JG, Luo J, Li P, Quinn RR, et al. Nephrologist follow-up improves all-cause mortality of severe acute kidney injury survivors. Kidney Int. 2013;83(5):901–8.
116. Siew ED, Peterson JF, Eden SK, Hung AM, Speroff T, Ikizler TA, Matheny ME. Outpatient nephrology referral rates after acute kidney injury. J Am Soc Nephrol. 2012;23(2):305–12.
117. Kirwan CJ, Blunden MJ, Dobbie H, James A, Nedungadi A, Prowle JR. Critically ill patients requiring acute renal replacement therapy are at an increased risk of long-term renal dysfunction, but rarely receive specialist nephrology follow-up. Nephron. 2015;129(3):164–70.
118. Kidney Disease. Improving Global Outcomes (KDIGO) Acute Kidney Injury Work Group: KDIGO clinical practice guideline for acute kidney injury. Kidney Int Suppl. 2012;2:1–138.

Diuretics in Acute Kidney Injury

20

Sagar U. Nigwekar and Sushrut S. Waikar

20.1 Introduction

Despite recent advances, the incidence of acute kidney injury (AKI) has continued to increase, and outcomes from AKI remain poor [1, 2]. Oliguria has been one of the most consistently reported risk factors for poor prognosis in AKI, and the presence of oliguria has implications for fluid management in patients with AKI [3]. Thus, it is not at all surprising that diuretic use is a common practice in the setting of AKI especially as clinicians attempt to alter an oligoanuric AKI to a non-oligoanuric AKI [4]. What is surprising is that little evidence is available especially from rigorous randomized controlled trials to support or oppose this common clinical practice [5, 6]. Different diuretic (loop diuretics, thiazide diuretics, and osmotic diuretics) and natriuretic agents have been investigated to prevent and treat AKI. In this chapter, we will review the literature for diuretic and natriuretic agents in AKI management and discuss related mechanisms, experimental evidence, epidemiology, and randomized controlled trials. Implications for clinical practice of AKI management are discussed.

S. U. Nigwekar (✉)
Department of Medicine/Nephrology, Massachusetts General Hospital, Boston, MA, USA
e-mail: snigwekar@mgh.harvard.edu

S. S. Waikar
Division of Renal Medicine, Brigham and Women's Hospital, Harvard Medical School, Boston, MA, USA
e-mail: swaikar@partners.org

20.2 Mechanisms of Action and Experimental Evidence for Diuretic and Natriuretic Agents in AKI

Table 20.1 summarizes the pharmacological characteristics of commonly used diuretics relevant to AKI management.

20.2.1 Loop Diuretics

The principal mechanism of loop diuretic agents involves the Na-K-2Cl transporter blockade on the luminal side of the thick ascending limb of the loop of Henle [7]. Reducing oxygen consumption by interfering with active sodium transport is clearly an appealing therapeutic target in AKI, and experimental evidence has shown that loop diuretics increase renal blood flow, increase renal tissue oxygenation, prevent tubular obstruction by flushing tubular debris, and improve glomerular filtration rate [8]. However, effects of loop diuretics on renal blood flow have been inconsistent in experimental studies [5, 9–11].

Loop diuretics are minimally filtered at the glomerular as they are highly protein bound; however, active secretion facilitated by organic

S. S. Waikar et al. (eds.), *Core Concepts in Acute Kidney Injury*,
https://doi.org/10.1007/978-1-4939-8628-6_20

Table 20.1 Properties of diuretic agents

Diuretic agent	Primary site of action	Onset of action	Duration of action	Protein binding	Elimination half-life	Oral bioavailability
Furosemide	Loop of Henle	Oral, 30–60 min; intravenous, 5 min	Oral, 6–8 h; intravenous, 2 h	>90%	0.5–9 h depending on renal function	~50%
Bumetanide	Loop of Henle	Oral, 30–60 min; intravenous, 2 min	Oral, 4–6 h; intravenous, 2 h	>90%	1–1.5 h	~80%
Torsemide	Loop of Henle	Oral: 30–60 min	Oral: 6–8 h	>90%	3.5 h; prolonged in patients with liver disease	~80%
Ethacrynic acid	Loop of Henle	Oral, 30 min; intravenous, 5 min	Oral, 12 h; intravenous, 2 h	>90%	3–4 h	~100%
Chlorothiazide	Distal tubule	Oral, 120 min; intravenous, 15 min	Oral, 6–12 h; intravenous, 2 h	~40%	1–3 h	<50%
Hydrochlorothiazide	Distal tubule	Oral: 120 min	Oral: 6–12 h	~60%	6–15 h	~65%
Chlorthalidone	Distal tubule	Oral: 120–360 min	Oral: 24–72 h	~75%	40–60 h	~65%
Mannitol	Proximal tubule and loop of Henle	Intravenous: 60–180 min	Intravenous: 2–6 h	None	5 h	NA

acid transporters in proximal renal tubule enables them to reach their sites of action in the loop of Henle. This tubular secretion of loop diuretics is reduced in the setting of hypoalbuminemia and use of other highly protein-bound drugs (e.g., warfarin). Elimination half-life and bioavailability for loop diuretics varies significantly and should be taken into account for dosing decisions (elimination half-life: 1 h for bumetanide, 1.5–2 h for furosemide, and 3–4 h for torsemide; oral bioavailability 50% for furosemide and 80–100% for bumetanide and torsemide) [12, 13]. The dose of loop diuretic needed to achieve an effective diuresis is frequently higher in patients with AKI because of reduced renal blood flow, which slows the delivery of loop diuretics into the loop of Henle [14], and inhibition of tubular secretion by metabolic acidosis and by accumulated organic acids in AKI [12]. Elevated circulating vasopressin levels observed in congestive heart failure augment the expression of the Na-K-2Cl transporter, whereas medications such as nonsteroidal anti-inflammatory agents interfere with prostaglandin synthesis and lead to decreased expression of the Na-K-2Cl transporter [7, 13].

The only way to increase response to a loop diuretic agent once the maximally effective dose and frequency are administered is to concomitantly administer agents that act at other nephron sites such as thiazide diuretics. However, such combination therapy may lead to adverse effects such as hypotension and hypokalemia, and clinical vigilance is needed.

The pharmacological properties of furosemide described above have also been a focus of recent work dedicated to developing a furosemide stress test where a one-time dose of furosemide 1.0 or 1.5 mg/kg has been shown to predict the severity of AKI and may also improve the risk stratification provided by novel biomarkers [15–17]. These findings await further validation in larger studies.

20.2.2 Thiazide Diuretics

Thiazide diuretics interfere with sodium reabsorption by inhibiting sodium–chloride symporter in the distal convoluted tubule [13, 18]. The effectiveness of thiazide diuretics is significantly reduced once the glomerular filtration rate is <30 mL/min; however, these agents can be useful when used in combination with loop diuretics in the setting of AKI.

20.2.3 Mannitol

Mannitol is an osmotic diuretic that exerts its effects at the proximal tubule and loop of Henle [19]. In animal models of ischemic AKI, mannitol has been demonstrated to attenuate the reduction in glomerular filtration rate by acting as a free radical scavenger and inhibiting renin release [20, 21].

20.2.4 Natriuretic Peptides

Agents such as atrial natriuretic peptide, brain natriuretic peptide, and urodilatin have diuretic and natriuretic properties in addition to the potential actions of vasodilatation and angiotensin inhibition [22, 23].

20.3 Clinical Evidence for Diuretic and Natriuretic Agents in AKI Observational Studies

There is abundant data from observational studies and survey studies that highlights the high prevalence of diuretic use in patients with AKI. However, results in terms of efficacy of diuretics in treatment of AKI are disappointing. Summarized below are the key findings from three such studies:

20.3.1 PICARD Study [4]

- A cohort study of severe AKI in critically ill patients ($n = 552$).
- Diuretics used in ~60% of the patients at the time of nephrology consultation.
- Additional 12% patients were prescribed diuretics after nephrology consultation [19].
- Combination diuretics (loop and thiazide diuretics together) used in approximately 1/3 of patients.
- The median (with 10–90% range) doses of furosemide, bumetanide, and metolazone were 80 (20–320), 10 (2–29), and 10 (5–20) mg/day, respectively.
- Older patients and those with presumed nephrotoxic AKI origin, a lower BUN level, acute respiratory failure, and history of congestive heart failure were more likely to receive diuretic therapy.
- A propensity score-adjusted analysis in this population demonstrated that diuretic use was significantly associated with in-hospital mortality or non-recovery of renal function (odds ratio, 1.77; 95% confidence interval, 1.14–2.76).

20.3.2 BEST Kidney Study [24]

- Multicenter, multination (54 centers, 23 countries) cohort of 1713 critically ill patients with AKI.
- Seventy percent received diuretic agents at the time of study enrollment; however, <10% received combination diuretic therapy.
- Diuretic use in a multivariable analysis was not associated with increased mortality (odds ratio, 1.22; 95% confidence interval, 0.92–1.66).

20.3.3 Survey of Intensivists in Australia and New Zealand [25]

- One hundred and forty-six intensivists participated in this study.
- The most likely initial loop diuretic dose reported in this survey was intravenous furosemide 40 mg.
- Key indications for loop diuretic therapy were positive fluid balance, acute pulmonary edema, and acute lung injury (ALI).
- Elevated central venous pressure and AKI were not key indications for loop diuretic therapy.

20.3.4 Mannitol

In a retrospective study of critically ill patients with rhabdomyolysis, mannitol administration was not associated with improvement in clinical outcomes such as the incidence of AKI, need for renal replacement therapy, or mortality [21]. There are also reports that indicate potential harm from mannitol therapy in AKI [26, 27].

20.4 Randomized Controlled Trials

The role of loop diuretics in the prevention and treatment of AKI has been a focus of multiple randomized clinical trials [28–37]. Investigators have focused on a variety of clinical settings including cardiovascular surgery and radiocontrast nephropathy using a wide array of doses of loop diuretics (furosemide infusion rates from 1 to 20 mg/h, bolus dose 1–3 mg/kg in the prevention studies, and daily furosemide 600–3400 mg in the treatment trials). There is no trial to date that has specifically compared combination diuretic therapy (loop and thiazide) to loop diuretic alone in the prevention or treatment of AKI. Overall, these studies show that loop diuretics increase the urine output, as expected, but do not conclusively show any significant improvements in clinical outcomes such as mortality or renal recovery. Most of these studies were inadequately powered, however, to examine clinical outcomes.

Table 20.2 provides a summary of meta-analyses that included randomized clinical trials designed to address the effects of diuretic agents

Table 20.2 Recent meta-analyses of randomized controlled trials examining the efficacy of diuretic and natriuretic agents in the prevention and treatment of AKI

Study	Study objectives	Number of RCTs/patients	Key results
Ho et al. [39]	– To address the potential beneficial and adverse effects of furosemide to prevent or treat AKI in adults	– RCTs: 9 – Patients: 849	– No improvement in in-hospital mortality (relative risk 1.11, 95% confidence interval 0.92–1.33) or risk for requiring renal replacement therapy (relative risk 0.99, 95% confidence interval 0.80–1.22) – Increased risk of temporary deafness and tinnitus in patients treated with high doses of furosemide
Bagshaw et al. [38]	– To address the potential beneficial and adverse effects of loop diuretics to prevent or treat AKI in adults	– RCTs: 5 – Patients: 555	– No improvement in mortality (odds ratio 1.28, 95% confidence interval 0.89–1.84) or renal recovery (odds ratio 0.88, 95% confidence interval 0.59–1.31) – Deafness and tinnitus were the most commonly reported adverse events
Gu et al. [40]	– To address the effect of additional furosemide treatment beyond saline hydration on contrast nephropathy post radiologic procedures	– RCTs: 5 – Patients: 1330	– No reduction in the incidence of contrast-induced nephropathy (relative risk 1.18, 95% confidence interval 0.50–2.78) – No reduction in the incidence of renal replacement therapy (relative risk 1.03, 95% confidence interval 0.41–2.57)
Yang et al. [40]	– To address the potential beneficial and adverse effects of mannitol to prevent AKI in adults	– RCTs: 9 – Patients: 626	– No reduction in AKI or renal replacement therapy requirement in nonrenal transplant population (relative risk 0.29, 95% confidence interval 0.01–6.60) – Possible reduction in AKI or renal replacement therapy requirement in renal transplant population (relative risk 0.34, 95% confidence interval 0.21–0.57)

Table 20.2 (continued)

Study	Study objectives	Number of RCTs/patients	Key results
Nigwekar et al. [45]	– To address the potential beneficial and adverse effects of natriuretic peptides in management of solid transplant organ-associated AKI in adults	– RCTs: 7 – Patients: 238	– Reduction in AKI requiring dialysis (odds ratio 0.50, 95% confidence interval 0.26–0.97) – No adverse events noted
Nigwekar et al. [43, 44]	– To address the potential beneficial and adverse effects of atrial natriuretic peptide to prevent or treat AKI in adults	– RCTs: 19 – Patients: 1861	– Low (but not high) dose atrial natriuretic peptide associated with a reduced need for renal replacement therapy in the prevention studies (relative risk 0.32, 95% confidence interval 0.14–0.71) but no difference in mortality – For established AKI, low (but not high) dose atrial natriuretic peptide was associated with a reduction in the need for renal replacement therapy (relative risk 0.54, 95% confidence interval 0.30–0.98) but no difference in mortality – High dose atrial natriuretic peptide associated with more adverse events (hypotension, arrhythmias)
Nigwekar et al. [42]	– To address the potential beneficial and adverse effects of natriuretic peptides in the management of cardiovascular surgery-associated AKI in adults	– RCTs: 13 – Patients: 934	– Reduction in AKI requiring renal replacement therapy (odds ratio 0.32, 95% confidence interval 0.15–0.66) but no reduction in mortality

in the treatment and prevention of AKI [38–41]. Despite pooling data from multiple small studies, these analyses concluded that there are no beneficial effects of loop diuretics or mannitol in terms of preventing or treating AKI and no improvement in clinical outcomes such as requirement of renal replacement therapy or mortality. This is in contrast to some meta-analyses of randomized trials of natriuretic peptides [42–45].

20.5 Clinical Implications

Loop diuretics should be used for the management of volume overload in AKI, but there is no clear evidence that loop diuretics enhance renal recovery or prevent the development of AKI. However, loop diuretics may be used as a test of likelihood of renal recovery ("furosemide stress test"). Thiazide diuretics augment the efficacy of loop diuretics, but again current available data do not support their specific therapeutic or prevention role in the management of AKI. Similarly, data on mannitol are limited and not convincing. Natriuretic properties may have some role in the prevention and treatment of AKI, but further confirmation is needed in larger clinical trials.

References

1. Wang HE, Muntner P, Chertow GM, Warnock DG. Acute kidney injury and mortality in hospitalized patients. Am J Nephrol. 2012;35:349–55.
2. Okusa MD, Molitoris BA, Palevsky PM, Chinchilli VM, Liu KD, Cheung AK, Weisbord SD, Faubel S, Kellum JA, Wald R, Chertow GM, Levin A, Waikar SS, Murray PT, Parikh CR, Shaw AD, Go AS, Chawla LS, Kaufman JS, Devarajan P, Toto RM, Hsu CY, Greene TH, Mehta RL, Stokes JB, Thompson AM, Thompson BT, Westenfelder CS, Tumlin JA, Warnock DG, Shah SV, Xie Y, Duggan EG, Kimmel PL, Star RA. Design of clinical trials in acute kidney injury: a report from an NIDDK Workshop—prevention trials. Clin J Am Soc Nephrol. 2012;7(5):851.
3. Bagshaw SM, Bellomo R, Kellum JA. Oliguria, volume overload, and loop diuretics. Crit Care Med. 2008;36:S172–8.

4. Mehta RL, Pascual MT, Soroko S, Chertow GM, PICARD Study Group. Diuretics, mortality, and nonrecovery of renal function in acute renal failure. JAMA. 2002;288:2547–53.
5. Nigwekar SU, Waikar SS. Diuretics in acute kidney injury. Semin Nephrol. 2011;31:523–34.
6. Bagshaw SM, Delaney A, Jones D, Ronco C, Bellomo R. Diuretics in the management of acute kidney injury: a multinational survey. Contrib Nephrol. 2007;156:236–49.
7. Shankar SS, Brater DC. Loop diuretics: from the Na-K-2Cl transporter to clinical use. Am J Physiol Renal Physiol. 2003;284:F11–21.
8. Bayati A, Nygren K, Kallskog O, Wolgast M. The effect of loop diuretics on the long-term outcome of post-Ischaemic acute renal failure in the rat. Acta Physiol Scand. 1990;139:271–9.
9. Tenstad O, Williamson HE. Effect of furosemide on local and zonal glomerular filtration rate in the rat kidney. Acta Physiol Scand. 1995;155:99–107.
10. Bak M, Shalmi M, Petersen JS, Poulsen LB, Christensen S. Effects of angiotensin-converting enzyme inhibition on renal adaptations to acute furosemide administration in conscious rats. J Pharmacol Exp Ther. 1993;266:33–40.
11. De Torrente A, Miller PD, Cronin RE, Paulsin PE, Erickson AL, Schrier RW. Effects of furosemide and acetylcholine in norepinephrine-induced acute renal failure. Am J Phys. 1978;235:F131–6.
12. Brater DC. Resistance to diuretics: emphasis on a pharmacological perspective. Drugs. 1981;22:477–94.
13. Brater DC. Diuretic therapy. N Engl J Med. 1998;339:387–95.
14. Wang DJ, Gottlieb SS. Diuretics: still the mainstay of treatment. Crit Care Med. 2008;36:S89–94.
15. Chawla LS, Davison DL, Brasha-Mitchell E, Koyner JL, Arthur JM, Shaw AD, Tumlin JA, Trevino SA, Kimmel PL, Seneff MG. Development and standardization of a furosemide stress test to predict the severity of acute kidney injury. Crit Care. 2013;17:R207.
16. Chawla LS. The furosemide stress test to predict renal function after continuous renal replacement therapy. Authors' response. Crit Care. 2014;18:429.
17. Koyner JL, Davison DL, Brasha-Mitchell E, Chalikonda DM, Arthur JM, Shaw AD, Tumlin JA, Trevino SA, Bennett MR, Kimmel PL, Seneff MG, Chawla LS. Furosemide stress test and biomarkers for the prediction of AKI severity. J Am Soc Nephrol. 2015;26:2023–31.
18. Paton RR, Kane RE. Long-term diuretic therapy with metolazone of renal failure and the nephrotic syndrome. J Clin Pharmacol. 1977;17:243–51.
19. Bosch X, Poch E, Grau JM. Rhabdomyolysis and acute kidney injury. N Engl J Med. 2009;361:62–72.
20. Higa EM, Dib SA, Martins JR, Campos L, Homsi E. Acute renal failure due to rhabdomyolysis in diabetic patients. Ren Fail. 1997;19:289–93.
21. Homsi E, Barreiro MF, Orlando JM, Higa EM. Prophylaxis of acute renal failure in patients with rhabdomyolysis. Ren Fail. 1997;19:283–8.
22. Allgren RL, Marbury TC, Rahman SN, Weisberg LS, Fenves AZ, Lafayette RA, Sweet RM, Genter FC, Kurnik BR, Conger JD, Sayegh MH. Anaritide in acute tubular necrosis. Auriculin Anaritide Acute Renal Failure Study Group. N Engl J Med. 1997;336:828–34.
23. Weisberg LS, Allgren RL, Genter FC, Kurnik BR. Cause of acute tubular necrosis affects its prognosis. The Auriculin Anaritide Acute Renal Failure Study Group. Arch Intern Med. 1997;157:1833–8.
24. Uchino S, Doig GS, Bellomo R, Morimatsu H, Morgera S, Schetz M, Tan I, Bouman C, Nacedo E, Gibney N, Tolwani A, Ronco C, Kellum JA. Beginning, ending supportive therapy for the kidney I: diuretics and mortality in acute renal failure. Crit Care Med. 2004;32:1669–77.
25. Jones SL, Martensson J, Glassford NJ, Eastwood GM, Bellomo R. Loop diuretic therapy in the critically ill: a survey. Crit Care Resusc. 2015;17:223–6.
26. Dorman HR, Sondheimer JH, Cadnapaphornchai P. Mannitol-induced acute renal failure. Medicine (Baltimore). 1990;69:153–9.
27. Fang L, You H, Chen B, Xu Z, Gao L, Liu J, Xie Q, Zhou Y, Gu Y, Lin S, Ding F. Mannitol is an independent risk factor of acute kidney injury after cerebral trauma: a case-control study. Ren Fail. 2010;32:673–9.
28. Solomon R, Werner C, Mann D, D'Elia J, Silva P. Effects of saline, mannitol, and furosemide to prevent acute decreases in renal function induced by radiocontrast agents. N Engl J Med. 1994;331:1416–20.
29. Mahesh B, Yim B, Robson D, Pillai R, Ratnatunga C, Pigott D. Does furosemide prevent renal dysfunction in high-risk cardiac surgical patients? Results of a double-blinded prospective randomised trial. Eur J Cardiothorac Surg. 2008;33:370–6.
30. Majumdar SR, Kjellstrand CM, Tymchak WJ, Hervas-Malo M, Taylor DA, Teo KK. Forced euvolemic diuresis with mannitol and furosemide for prevention of contrast-induced nephropathy in patients with CKD undergoing coronary angiography: a randomized controlled trial. Am J Kidney Dis. 2009;54:602–9.
31. Shilliday IR, Quinn KJ, Allison ME. Loop diuretics in the management of acute renal failure: a prospective, double-blind, placebo-controlled, randomized study. Nephrol Dial Transplant. 1997;12:2592–6.
32. Brown CB, Ogg CS, Cameron JS. High dose frusemide in acute renal failure: a controlled trial. Clin Nephrol. 1981;15:90–6.
33. Cantarovich F, Rangoonwala B, Lorenz H, Verho M, Esnault VL, High-Dose Flurosemide in Acute Renal Failure Study Group. High-dose furosemide for established ARF: A prospective, randomized, double-blind, placebo-controlled, multicenter trial. Am J Kidney Dis. 2004;44:402–9.
34. Cantarovich F, Locatelli A, Fernandez JC, Perez Loredo J, Cristhot J, Debenedetti L. [Treatment of urinary infections with antibiotics and high doses of furosemide]. Rev Clin Esp. 1971;123:59–62.
35. Kleinknecht D, Ganeval D, Gonzalez-Duque LA, Fermanian J. Furosemide in acute oliguric renal failure. A controlled trial. Nephron. 1976;17:51–8.

36. Van Der Voort PH, Boerma EC, Koopmans M, Zandberg M, De Ruiter J, Gerritsen RT, Egbers PH, Kingma WP, Kuiper MA. Furosemide does not improve renal recovery after hemofiltration for acute renal failure in critically ill patients: a double blind randomized controlled trial. Crit Care Med. 2009;37:533–8.
37. Kunt AT, Akgun S, Atalan N, Bitir N, Arsan S. Furosemide infusion prevents the requirement of renal replacement therapy after cardiac surgery. Anadolu Kardiyol Derg. 2009;9:499–504.
38. Bagshaw SM, Delaney A, Haase M, Ghali WA, Bellomo R. Loop diuretics in the management of acute renal failure: a systematic review and meta-analysis. Crit Care Resusc. 2007;9:60–8.
39. Ho KM, Sheridan DJ. Meta-analysis of frusemide to prevent or treat acute renal failure. BMJ. 2006;333:420.
40. Yang B, Xu J, Xu F, Zou Z, Ye C, Mei C, Mao Z. Intravascular administration of mannitol for acute kidney injury prevention: a systematic review and meta-analysis. PLoS One. 2014;9:e85029.
41. Gu G, Zhang Y, Lu R, Cui W. Additional furosemide treatment beyond saline hydration for the prevention of contrast-induced nephropathy: a meta-analysis of randomized controlled trials. Int J Clin Exp Med. 2015;8:387–94.
42. Nigwekar SU, Hix JK. The role of natriuretic peptide administration in cardiovascular surgery-associated renal dysfunction: a systematic review and meta-analysis of randomized controlled trials. J Cardiothorac Vasc Anesth. 2009;23:151–60.
43. Nigwekar SU, Navaneethan SD, Parikh CR, Hix JK. Atrial natriuretic peptide for preventing and treating acute kidney injury. Cochrane Database Syst Rev. 2009;(4):CD006028.
44. Nigwekar SU, Navaneethan SD, Parikh CR, Hix JK. Atrial natriuretic peptide for management of acute kidney injury: a systematic review and meta-analysis. Clin J Am Soc Nephrol. 2009;4:261–72.
45. Nigwekar SU, Kulkarni H, Thakar CV. Natriuretic peptides in the management of solid organ transplantation associated acute kidney injury: a systematic review and meta-analysis. Int J Nephrol. 2013;2013:949357.

21 Emerging Therapies: What's on the Horizon?

Lynn Redahan and Patrick T. Murray

21.1 Introduction

Acute kidney injury (AKI) is a multisystem disease with many potential causes. The mortality and morbidity associated with AKI remain unacceptably high despite advances in critical care and dialysis technologies. There is an expanding body of knowledge of the cellular and molecular mechanisms of AKI, which has led to the discovery of many potential therapeutic targets (see Table 21.1). Despite varied triggers, there are certain common features in the renal response to injury. Here we present the data on emerging therapies, potential drug targets and recent negative trials. We have categorized potential therapies according to their site and mode of action (see Figs. 21.1 and 21.2).

21.2 Mitochondria

The renal tubular cells, particularly those that are highly involved in active solute transport, have a rich concentration of mitochondria. Mitochondrial injury has been found to be a common feature of AKI, regardless of the inciting injury. It is an integral component in the pathogenesis of AKI, but may also play a role in promoting kidney injury. Given this, mitochondria are important potential therapeutic targets (see Fig. 21.2). To date, mitochondria-specific pharmacotherapies have largely been prophylactic rather than therapeutic.

21.2.1 Agents Targeting MPTP Opening

21.2.1.1 Cyclosporine

Mitochondrial permeability transition pore (MPTP) is a cyclosporine-sensitive channel located in the inner mitochondrial membrane. In the setting of ischaemia-reperfusion (IR) injury, MPTP opening mediates cell death. Due to its ability to inhibit MPTP opening, cyclosporine A (CsA) has anti-apoptotic properties and may prevent IR-mediated cell injury. A single dose of CsA has also been shown to reduce inflammatory cell infiltration and tubular cell injury [1]. In animal models of IR, the administration of CsA at the time of resuscitation limited the extent of kidney dysfunction [2]. Lemoine et al. recently proposed that the nephroprotective effect of CsA depends on both the dose and the timing of administration, relative to IR injury [3]. Unfortunately, there are distinct disadvantages

L. Redahan (✉) · P. T. Murray
School of Medicine,
University College Dublin, Dublin, Ireland
e-mail: lynn.redahan@ucd.ie; patrick.murray@ucd.ie

S. S. Waikar et al. (eds.), *Core Concepts in Acute Kidney Injury*,
https://doi.org/10.1007/978-1-4939-8628-6_21

Table 21.1 Summary of potential therapies for the prevention and treatment of AKI

Agent	Site of action	Mechanism of action	Drug development stage	Role in AKI
Cyclosporine	Mitochondria	Inhibition of MPTP opening	Phase 2 underway	Prevention
NIM-811	Mitochondria	Inhibition of MPTP opening	Preclinical	Prevention
Bendavia	Mitochondria	Mitochondrial antioxidant	Phase 2 underway	Prevention and treatment
MitoQ	Mitochondria	Mitochondrial antioxidant	Preclinical	Prevention and treatment
Sildenafil	Mitochondria Vasculature	Induction of mitochondrial biogenesis Local vasodilation	Phase 1 underway	Prevention and treatment
Mdivi-1	Mitochondria	Inhibition of mitochondrial fission	Preclinical	Prevention
4-Phenylbutyrate	Endoplasmic reticulum	Reduction in expression of CHOP/GADD153	Preclinical	Prevention
EET analogues	Endoplasmic reticulum	Reduce ER oxidative stress	Preclinical	Prevention
Fingolimod	Cell membrane	Activation of S1P receptor	Phase 3	Prevention
Nicotine	Nicotinic receptor	Anti-inflammatory effect	Preclinical	Prevention
Endothelin receptor antagonists	Endothelin receptor	Alteration of renal haemodynamics	Preclinical	Prevention and treatment
OPN-305	Toll-like receptor 2	Inhibition of TLR2-induced initiation of innate immune responses following kidney injury	Phase 2 underway	Prevention
Angiopoietin agonists	Endothelium	Anti-inflammatory effects Enhanced endothelial cell survival	Preclinical	Prevention
Endothelial progenitor cells	Endothelium	Endothelial repair and regeneration	Preclinical	Treatment
QPI-1002	Gene silencing	Temporary suppression of p53 expression	Phase 1/2	Prevention
HMGB1 antagonists	Antisepsis	Anti-inflammatory and anti-apoptotic effects	Preclinical	Prevention
Alkaline phosphatase	Antisepsis	Anti-inflammatory effect through generation of adenosine and phosphorylation of endotoxin	Phase 2	Treatment
Caspase inhibitors	Antisepsis	Anti-inflammatory and anti-apoptotic effects	Preclinical	Prevention
Bone morphogenetic protein 7	Antisepsis	Inhibition of TGFβ signalling Anti-inflammatory and anti-fibrotic effects Downregulation of adhesion molecules	Phase 1	Prevention and treatment
EA-230	Antisepsis	Anti-inflammatory effects Improvement in renal blood flow	Preclinical	Treatment

to the use of cyclosporine as a prophylactic agent for AKI. The potent immunosuppressive and renal vasoconstrictor properties of this drug are likely to limit its clinical utility in the prevention of AKI. A phase II trial exploring the ability of cyclosporine to reduce the risk and degree of AKI in the context of cardiac surgery is underway.

21.2.1.2 Other Cyclophilin Inhibitors

N-Methyl-4-isoleucine cyclosporine (NIM-811) is a non-immunosuppressive cyclophilin inhibitor. NIM-811 has been found to improve kidney dysfunction significantly following IR injury in rabbits [2]. It had comparable efficacy to cyclosporine but without the systemic side effects. Preclinical studies suggest that it may have a role

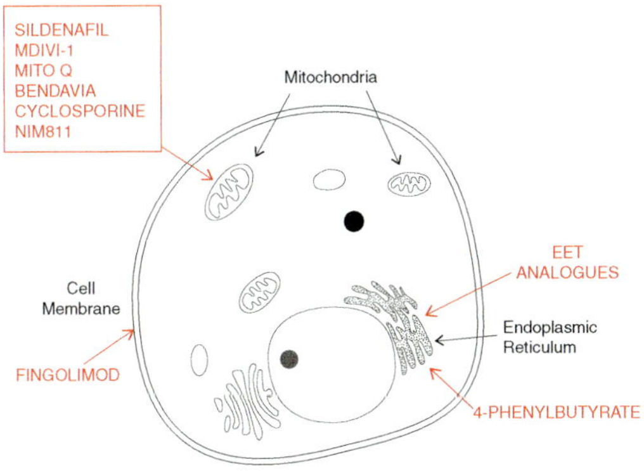

Fig. 21.1 Novel drugs and their target within the renal tubular cell

in preventing irreversible cellular injury. Early clinical trials report a favourable safety profile.

21.2.2 Agents Targeting Mitochondrial Oxidative Damage

21.2.2.1 Mitochondrial-Targeted Antioxidants

Oxidative injury to mitochondria is a prominent feature of IR injury. The inability of damaged mitochondria to recover ATP leads to tubular cell injury and promotes AKI. Most antioxidant

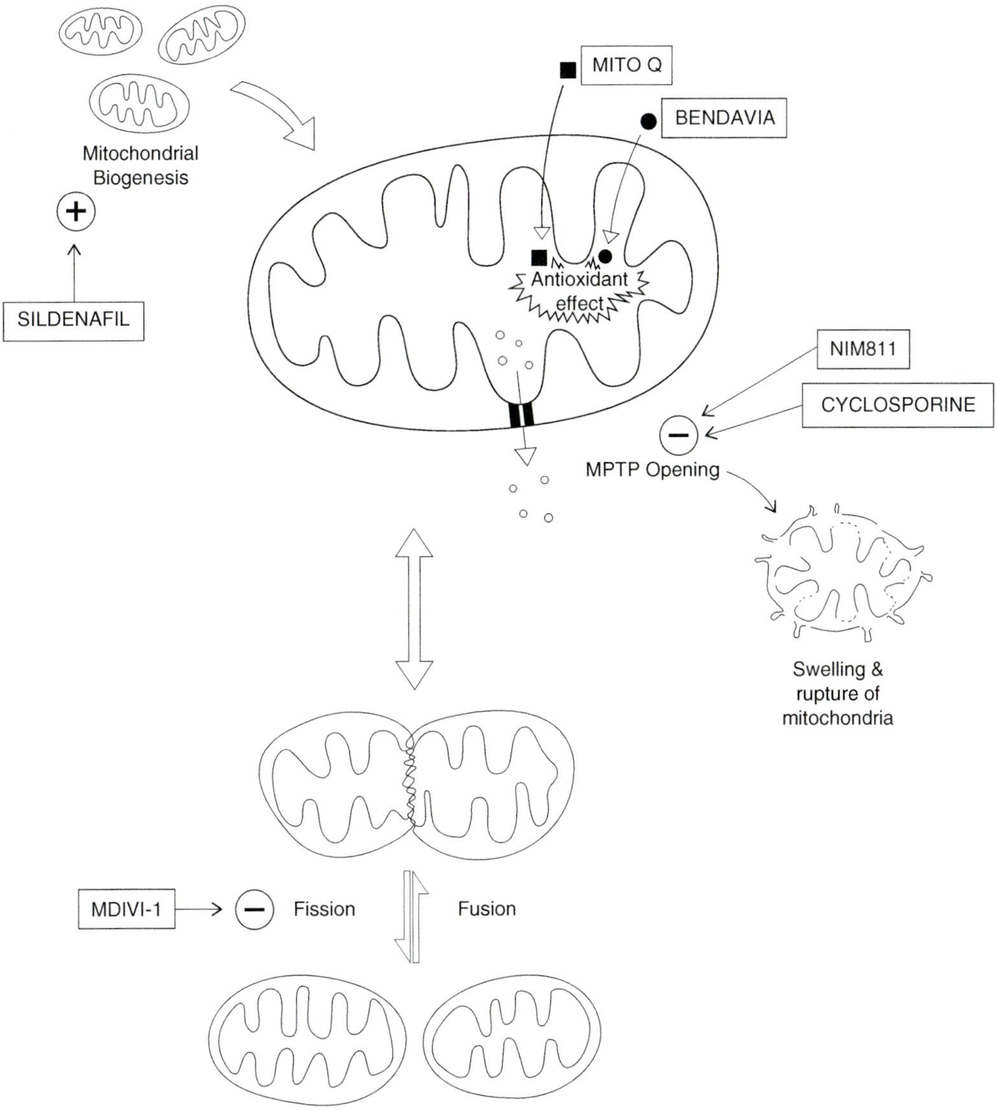

Fig. 21.2 Novel drugs targeting mitochondria and mitochondrial dynamics

agents are clinically ineffective as they are not taken up by mitochondria. Novel mitochondria-specific antioxidants are showing promising results in early clinical trials.

MitoQ is a mitochondria-targeted antioxidant agent that accumulates in mitochondria, localizing within the inner mitochondrial membrane (IMM). Once there, it is continually reduced by the respiratory chain and prevents mitochondrial oxidative damage. It was the first mitochondria-specific antioxidant agent to undergo clinical trials in humans. It has been found to be effective in reducing tubular damage and cell death during cold storage of porcine kidneys [4]. Pretreatment with MitoQ protected mice kidneys from IR-mediated damage and dysfunction [5]. MitoQ has undergone early clinical trials in Parkinson's disease and hepatitis without any serious adverse events [6, 7]. MitoCP, another mitochondria-targeted antioxidant, may have similar protective properties. It has been shown to prevent cisplatin-induced renal dysfunction in mice in a dose-dependent manner [8]. These potent mitochondrial antioxidants hold promise as an effective preventative therapy for AKI.

21.2.2.2 Bendavia

Cardiolipin is a phospholipid, located in the IMM and involved in many essential mitochondrial functions. Ischaemic injury causes peroxidation of cardiolipin through the generation of reactive oxygen species (ROS). Structural and functional defects in the mitochondria occur as a result. The peroxidation of cardiolipin also promotes the dissociation of cytochrome c from the IMM into the cytosol, activating programmed cell death pathways.

Bendavia (SS-31 or MTP-131) is a tetrapeptide that inhibits the peroxidation of cardiolipin [9]. It has been shown to accelerate the recovery of ATP after ischaemic insult and ameliorate kidney injury [10]. Pretreatment of rats with bendavia resulted in improved repair of mitochondrial morphology and reduced tubular apoptosis and necrosis after IR injury. Early studies look promising, and phase 2 trials are underway.

21.2.3 Sildenafil

Sildenafil is a selective inhibitor of cyclic guanosine monophosphate (cGMP)-specific phosphodiesterase type 5 (PDE5), which increases endogenous nitric oxide (NO) activity. The preservation of NO levels has been found to protect the kidney against a range of insults. There is evidence that PDE inhibitors can induce mitochondrial biogenesis, a key step in the recovery of renal function in AKI [11]. Another postulated mechanism for the renoprotective effect of PDE inhibitors is through local vasodilation. In an experimental model of ischaemic kidneys, a more favourable haemodynamic pattern was evident in animals pretreated with sildenafil [12].

Sildenafil may have the potential to accelerate the recovery from AKI in addition to having a prophylactic effect. In animal models, pretreatment with sildenafil has been shown to lessen histological injury, attenuate serum creatinine levels and reduce reactive oxygen species generation [13–15]. Recently, a phase 1 study reported that sildenafil was well-tolerated in cardiac surgery patients [16]. Unfortunately, a randomized placebo controlled trial by Krane et al. did not observe a significant renoprotective effect with a single preoperative dose of sildenafil [17]. The lack of an observed beneficial effect may relate to the dosing regimen used in this study. Sildenafil has a short half-life, and it may be necessary to administer repeated doses for a protective effect. This potential disadvantage of sildenafil could limit its clinical utility.

21.2.4 Mitochondrial Division Inhibitor-1

Mitochondrial dynamics are governed by two key processes: fission and fusion. There is evidence to indicate that proteins involved in mitochondrial fission actively participate in apoptosis. Dynamin-related protein 1 (Drp-1) is an integral mitochondrial fission protein. Inhibition of Drp-1 inhibits mitochondrial fission and delays programmed cell death.

Mitochondrial division inhibitor-1 (mdivi-1) is a selective inhibitor of Drp-1 that partially inhibits apoptosis [18]. Experimental studies have demonstrated that it can prevent mitochondrial fragmentation and tubular cell apoptosis during kidney injury [19]. However, Sumida et al. did not identify a significant renoprotective effect when they administered mdivi-1 to mice with IR injury [20]. In addition to these inconclusive preclinical results, there is concern that permanent inhibition of mitochondrial fission may have detrimental effects on mitochondrial and cellular function.

21.3 Endoplasmic Reticulum

The endoplasmic reticulum (ER) is a network of tubules within the cytoplasm. ER stress contributes to AKI. Tunicamycin is an antibiotic that induces extensive ER stress and has been shown to induce substantial proximal tubular damage. Many researchers have utilized it to induce ER stress and AKI in animal studies. There is evidence to suggest that males may be more vulnerable to ER stress than females [21], which may partly explain gender differences in the response to renal injury.

21.3.1 4-Phenylbutyrate

C/EBP homologous protein (CHOP) is a protein that mediates ER stress-induced apoptosis. Prolonged ER stress in renal cells results in upregulation of CHOP. The chemical chaperone, 4-phenylbutyrate (4-PBA), reduces the expression of CHOP. In mice with tunicamycin-induced AKI, 4-PBA has been shown to protect the kidney and reduce the extent of tubular injury [15, 22]. It appears to protect the kidney through the inhibition of ER stress. Taurodeoxycholic acid is another chemical chaperone, which appears to protect kidney cells through a similar mechanism [23].

4-PBA is approved for use in urea cycle disorders and has undergone clinical trials in non-renal conditions such as neurodegenerative diseases, liver cirrhosis and certain cancers. It has been reported to have an acceptable safety profile in these conditions. At present, its use in renal diseases has not progressed past preclinical testing. It may prove to be an effective prophylactic agent. Those most likely to benefit are patients at high risk of AKI in which ER stress is a prominent pathogenic feature, e.g. cisplatin- and contrast-induced AKI.

21.3.2 Epoxyeicosatrienoic Acid Analogs

Epoxyeicosatrienoic acids (EETs) are metabolites of arachidonic acid, with anti-inflammatory and antioxidant effects. Also, they have potent vasodilatory and antihypertensive properties. Based on the results of experimental models, EET analogues can protect against organ injury in conditions such as diabetes and cardiovascular disease. They have also been found to protect the kidney from cisplatin-induced apoptosis through various mechanisms. Amongst these mechanisms is its ability to reduce ER stress and attenuate renal inflammation secondary to cisplatin [24]. It accomplishes this without attenuating the chemotherapeutic effects of cisplatin. Unfortunately, EETs may promote tumour growth and metastasis [25, 26]. This concerning finding may limit their clinical utility.

21.4 Cell Membrane

The cell membrane is a primary site of damage in AKI. Both necrosis and apoptosis feature alterations in the cell membrane and both forms of cell death can exist in AKI. The plasma membrane is an exciting potential target for therapies to prevent or attenuate AKI.

Fingolimod Sphingolipids are integral components of the cell membrane. The metabolites of sphingolipids, which include sphingosine-1-phosphate (S1P), act as important signalling molecules. S1P is a ligand for a family of five G-protein-coupled receptors. Through its actions on these receptors, it is involved in many cell processes, including cell growth and the suppression of apoptosis. S1P plays a pivotal role in determining cell fate. Activation of the S1P receptors has been shown to protect the proximal tubular cells from IR injury.

Fingolimod (also known as FTY720) is an orally active immunomodulatory agent that activates the S1P receptor. When administered before IR injury, fingolimod was shown to attenuate kidney injury [27–29]. It has been approved for the treatment of multiple sclerosis in many countries. The results of several phase 3 trials of fingolimod in renal transplant patients are awaited.

21.5 Receptors

Many cell surface receptors have been implicated in epithelial injury, and subsequent repair, in AKI. Signalling through certain receptors (e.g. epidermal growth factor receptor and the hepatocyte growth factor receptor) has a protective or regenerative effect. Others, such as TGF-β, can increase apoptosis. There is scope to attenuate or prevent kidney injury by chemically targeting receptors. Here we outline drugs that have successfully manipulated receptor pathways to protect against and treat AKI in experimental models.

21.5.1 Nicotinic Agonists

The cholinergic pathway has been linked with an anti-inflammatory effect, in particular through activation of the α7 nicotinic receptor (α7nAChR). Nicotine is a directly acting cholinergic agonist that mediates its actions through stimulation of the nicotinic acetylcholine receptors. Although chronic nicotine exposure has been linked with adverse renal effects, nicotine has also been found to have a powerful anti-inflammatory effect. Through α7nAChR-dependent regulation of the immune response, nicotine may limit tubular damage and protect renal function after IR injury [30]. Interestingly, although a single pretreatment dose of nicotine prior to IR injury had a protective effect, repeated administration over several days before injury had the opposite effect in a mouse model of IR injury [31].

Nicotinic agonists may prove to be beneficial in the prevention of AKI. However, it has yet to be determined if the protective effects of nicotine are species-specific. GTS-21 is an agent that selectively stimulates the α7nAChR. It has been shown to reduce the infiltration of leucocytes into the kidney [32]. In animal models, GTS-21 has been found to attenuate renal injury in both IR and sepsis-induced AKI. Due to its selective α7nAChR agonist effects, it may have greater potential as a therapeutic agent for the prevention of AKI. Phase 1 studies have commenced.

Exposure to a modified ultrasound regime has been found to attenuate kidney injury in mice that were subject to IR injury. It is postulated to mediate this effect through its actions on the splenic cholinergic anti-inflammatory pathways, particularly via the α7nAChR [33]. At present, data is limited and is insufficient to propose ultrasound as a prophylactic strategy against AKI.

21.5.2 Endothelin Receptor Antagonists

The kidney is extremely sensitive to endothelin and has abundant endothelin receptors. Endothelin plays an integral role in regulating kidney function through its ability to control global and local renal blood flow. During AKI, there is an imbalance between endothelin and nitric oxide, a potent vasodilator. The effect of endothelin dominates and plays an important role in mediating kidney injury. Through the endothelin A receptor (ETA), endothelin mediates vasoconstriction of vascular smooth muscle. Through the endothelin B receptor (ETB), it causes vasodilation. While blockade of ETA receptors has been shown to improve renal blood flow, ETB receptor inhibition has been associated with renal vasoconstriction [34, 35].

The administration of non-selective ET receptor antagonists (such as tezosentan and bosentan) before or after IR injury has been shown to protect and optimize kidney function [36, 37]. They have also been found to protect the kidney from renal damage induced by cisplatin and from cardiopulmonary bypass [38, 39]. Although endothelin has been implicated in the progression of AKI to CKD, selective blockade of the ETA receptor did little to prevent the progression of renal injury in mice exposed to unilateral IR injury [92]. Phase 1 and 2 trials looking at the effects of ETA receptor antagonists in chronic kidney disease are underway. Based on experimental studies, the ETA receptor seems to be a likely target for the prevention and early treatment of AKI.

21.5.3 Toll-Like Receptor 2 Antagonists

Toll-like receptors (TLRs) are a family of transmembrane receptors that play a pivotal role in initiating innate immune responses. TLR2 is widely expressed in the kidney and has been implicated in the pathogenesis of AKI. It has been shown to initiate inflammatory responses after kidney injury and is upregulated in renal tubular cells in IR-induced AKI [40, 41]. Blockade of the TLR2 signalling has been shown to reduce neutrophil infiltration and renal damage in an experimental model of IR injury of the kidney [42]. In murine models, the administration of a mouse anti-TLR2 antibody protected transplanted kidneys from IR injury [43].

A humanized monoclonal antibody (OPN-305) that blocks TLR2 signalling has been developed. A phase 2 trial of its efficacy for the prevention of delayed graft function (DGF) in kidney transplant recipients is underway (NCT01794663). There is optimism that it may also prove to be a novel and effective therapy for the prevention of AKI.

21.6 The Endothelium

Renal endothelial cell dysfunction is prominent in the pathogenesis of AKI. IR injury disrupts endothelial cell integrity which consequently influences vascular tone and inflammatory responses. Endothelial cells play a key role in the initiation, progression and recovery phases of renal IR injury. By targeting endothelial cell damage, kidney injury can be partially prevented.

21.6.1 Angiopoietin-1 and TIE2 Agonists

Angiopoietin-1 (Ang1) is an angiogenic factor that acts on endothelial cells through the tyrosine kinase receptor, TIE2. Through its interaction with TIE2, Ang1 plays a role in inflammation and vascular growth and development. It has anti-inflammatory properties and enhances endothelial cell survival.

Ang1 has beneficial effects in AKI. A stable, potent variant of Ang1, COMP-Ang1, has been shown to have a protective effect in lipopolysaccharide-induced AKI [44]. In a model of cyclosporine-induced renal injury, it was shown to protect peritubular capillaries and reduce inflammation [45]. However, in a model of folic acid-induced AKI, although Ang1 was found to stabilize peritubular capillaries, it also demonstrated pro-fibrotic and pro-inflammatory effects [46]. This contrasts with evidence provided by Jung et al., who observed that COMP-Ang1 reduced interstitial fibrosis 30 days after IR injury [47]. It has been postulated that the effects of Ang1 may depend on the disease model tested. The varying effects may also be explained by differences in the potency of Ang1 and COMP-Ang1. Clinical trials in humans are awaited.

21.6.2 Endothelial Progenitor Cells

Endothelial dysfunction and disruption of the vascular barrier integrity are pivotal steps in the pathogenesis of multiorgan failure in septic shock. Endothelial progenitor cells (EPCs) originate in the bone marrow but migrate to the peripheral circulation, where they play a role in endothelial repair and regeneration. In septic shock, the number of EPCs increases, and there is an inverse relationship between EPC numbers and the extent of organ dysfunction. The number of circulating EPCs correlates with survival. In renal ischaemia, EPCs migrate to the renal parenchyma, where they offer partial protection from injury [48]. EPCs may have an important role in ameliorating the effects of AKI. It has been suggested that the renoprotective effects of ischaemic preconditioning may be partially mediated by enhancing the recruitment of EPCs to the renal parenchyma [49].

Stromal cell-derived factor-1 (SDF-1) is a chemokine with regulatory effects on inflammation and cell migration. Through its interaction with the CXCR4 receptor, SDF-1 plays a major role in the recruitment of EPCs to the injured kidney [50]. Theoretically, agonists of SDF-1-CXCR4 should promote the migration of EPCs to the kidney and repair of endothelial cell damage. A high-affinity CXCR4 agonist has been developed, but its effects on kidney injury have not yet been investigated. EPCs and CXCR4 agonists have the potential to play a role in early renal recovery.

21.7 Gene Silencing Therapy

QPI-1002 Apoptosis triggered by p53 activation has been shown to play an important role in the pathogenesis of AKI [51]. QPI-1002 (also called I5NP) is a synthetic small interfering RNA, designed to temporarily suppress expression of the p53 gene. It inhibits p53-mediated apoptosis after kidney injury, allowing kidney cells to repair and regenerate following injury. After administration, QPI-1002 rapidly accumulates within the kidney, with the main site of uptake being the proximal tubular cell [52]. Once the effect of QPI-1002 has subsided, the irreversibly damaged cells undergo apoptosis. A large phase 1/2 trial in kidney transplant patients suggested it could prevent or attenuate delayed graft function in recipients of deceased donor transplants (NCT00802347). An acceptable safety and toxicity profile was reported. Results of a phase 1 study (NCT00554359) in patients undergoing major cardiovascular surgery are awaited. This novel agent is showing promise as a preventative therapy for AKI and DGF in high-risk patients.

21.8 Antisepsis

21.8.1 HMGB1 Antagonists

High-mobility group box 1 protein (HMGB1) is a nuclear protein that bends DNA and acts as a cofactor for gene transcription. It also acts as an extracellular signalling molecule during inflammation. After release from cells undergoing necrosis, HMGB1 activates and propagates the inflammatory response. It has been implicated as an inflammatory mediator in sepsis and IR injury [53, 54]. Through its high affinity binding to the toll-like receptor 4 (TLR4), HMGB1 is also implicated in the pathogenesis of AKI [54, 55].

The blockade of HMGB1 using a neutralizing antibody has been demonstrated to attenuate neutrophil infiltration, tubular necrosis and renal dysfunction in IR injury [55]. Additionally, preconditioning with recombinant HMGB1 has been shown to downregulate the TLR4 signalling in IR injury and protect the kidney [56]. In mouse models of severe sepsis, monoclonal HMGB1 antibodies improved survival from sepsis and reduced circulating levels of pro-inflammatory cytokines [57]. However, the implications of altering the levels of other important cytokines have not yet been explored.

Ethyl pyruvate (EP), an aliphatic ester, has been found to inhibit HMGB1 release. It has anti-inflammatory and antioxidant effects and has been shown to decrease injury in many organs, including the liver, heart and pancreas. In animal models of sepsis, EP reduced circulating levels of HMGB1, attenuated organ dysfunction and improved survival [58]. In IR injury, EP has been shown to have a nephroprotective effect [59]. Pretreatment of mice with EP resulted in improved short- and long-term kidney function [60]. Phase 1 studies have reported an adequate safety profile. EP and HMGB1 antagonists are potential therapies for sepsis and may have a role in preventing AKI.

21.8.2 Alkaline Phosphatase

Alkaline phosphatase (AP) is showing considerable promise as a treatment for sepsis-associated AKI. There are two proposed mechanisms for this protective effect. AP is an endogenous enzyme that catalyses the conversion of ATP to adenosine, a factor with potent anti-inflammatory and tissue protective effects. It also phosphorylates endotoxins, rendering them non-toxic. When compared with placebo, treatment with bovine AP improved renal function and reduced RRT requirement in patients with severe sepsis [61]. Human recombinant AP (recAP) has been developed, and in animal models of renal IR injury and lipopolysaccharide-induced AKI, it has been shown to exert a renal protective anti-inflammatory effect. A phase 2 trial investigating its efficacy in sepsis-associated AKI has commenced (NCT02182440), and the results will help elucidate if recAP can improve the outcomes of patients with sepsis-associated AKI. This agent may also have protective effects in other forms of AKI.

21.8.3 Caspase Inhibitors

Caspases are a family of intracellular proteases that promote apoptotic cell death and activate pro-inflammatory cytokines. Their ability to trigger, execute and regulate cell death has prompted investigators to explore the potential for caspase inhibition to attenuate organ injury. Caspase inhibitors have been shown to reduce renal damage in animal models of septic, drug-induced and IR-induced AKI [62–65]. The breadth of caspase functionality is being increasingly recognized and so too are the varying roles of individual members of this family. The therapeutic capability of both selective and pancaspase inhibitors is being explored. Pharmacological pancaspase inhibition was well-tolerated by patients with chronic hepatitis C and was shown to reduce markers of hepatocellular injury in a phase 2 trial reported by Shiffman et al. [66]. It seems likely that selective caspase inhibition will yield more predictable clinical effects, compared to pancaspase inhibitors. Human trials of the tolerability and efficacy of selective caspase inhibitors in AKI are awaited. Given the key role these proteases play in programmed cell death, there are grounds for cautious optimism that caspases are novel therapeutic targets for the treatment of AKI.

21.8.4 EA-230

Peptides derived from human chorionic gonadotrophin (hCG) are drawing attention due to the discovery of their potent anti-inflammatory effects. One such peptide is EA-230 (also known as AQGV), a tetrapeptide derived from β[beta] hCG lysates. It has been shown to attenuate multiorgan failure in sepsis and also ameliorates IR-induced kidney injury [67, 68]. In animal models of IR injury, EA-230 was also associated with a substantial survival advantage.

The exact mechanisms of action of EA-230 have not been fully elucidated. It appears to exert an early anti-inflammatory effect on the kidney, thereby preventing organ dysfunction. EA-230 has been shown to reduce neutrophil influx and the release of pro-inflammatory cytokines. It may also improve renal blood flow [69]. Phase 1 trials have been successfully completed and have reported a good safety profile.

21.8.5 Bone Morphogenetic Protein 7 (BMP-7) and THR-184

Bone morphogenetic protein 7, a member of the TGFβ superfamily, plays an important role in nephrogenesis. It may play a role in repair and regeneration in the adult kidney and has been shown to ameliorate kidney damage through its anti-inflammatory and anti-fibrotic properties. In ischaemic injury to the kidney, BMP-7 inhibits neutrophil accumulation by downregulating the expression of intercellular adhesion molecule (ICAM-1) [70]. In animal models of both obstructive and ischaemic AKI, BMP-7 has been shown to reduce kidney injury and inhibit tubular atrophy [70, 71]. It represents a potential target for the treatment of both AKI and chronic kidney disease.

Due to the high doses required and the expense of production of recombinant BMP, BMP-7 agonists may be a more viable clinical option. Small peptide agonists that bind selectively to BMP receptors have been developed. THR-184 is one such agonist, which activates the BMP signalling pathway. It had a good safety profile in early clinical testing, and a phase 2 clinical trial of THR-184 in AKI has commenced.

21.9 Negative Trials

There is currently no specific therapy approved for the treatment of AKI. Despite optimistic preclinical results, only a small number of drugs have progressed to clinical trials. There are several potential reasons for this (see Table 21.2). AKI is a complex and multisystem disease with a multifaceted pathogenesis. The AKI patient is frequently critically ill with multiple comorbidities. Consequently, a multifaceted approach to treatment is often required. It seems likely that there is a narrow therapeutic window for the treatment of AKI, and an early diagnosis is crucial. The ability to demonstrate the success of therapy partly relies on the early detection of kidney injury. If a rise in creatinine is the trigger for treatment initiation, therapy has probably been commenced too late to show a benefit. Biomarkers of AKI are showing promise and are likely to facilitate the earlier diagnosis of AKI and the development of drugs that can be initiated in a timely fashion.

Table 21.2 Barriers to the development of effective therapies for AKI

The disease	Multiple pathogenic factors
	Many and varied aetiologies
	Multisystem disease
	Timing of diagnosis—need for sensitive biomarkers
The patient	Complex patients, often with multiple comorbidities
	Often critically ill
The trial	Definition and selection of endpoints
	Statistical power
	Translation from "bench to bedside"

Trial design has also acted as a limitation to success in this field. Many studies, particularly those of preventative strategies, have been underpowered. To demonstrate the efficacy of preventative therapy, large numbers of patients are required to ensure a sufficient number of AKI cases. The selection and definition of endpoints can also be problematic. The Acute Dialysis Quality Initiative has endeavoured to reach a consensus regarding AKI staging and diagnosis, which has improved trial design. However, other frequently utilized endpoints such as RRT initiation and mortality also present challenges. In practice, there are substantial differences in the utilization of RRT. A consistent approach is lacking. Trials that select mortality as an endpoint may not be powered to detect small alterations in renal function. We have outlined some of the notable agents that showed initial promise but failed to demonstrate a benefit in clinical trials (see Table 21.3).

21.9.1 Fenoldopam

Fenoldopam is a short-acting α1-selective dopamine agonist that increases renal blood flow even at doses that lower systemic blood pressure. A meta-analysis conducted by Gillies et al. reported that perioperative fenoldopam administration may have the potential to prevent AKI after major surgery [72]. However, mortality and the need for RRT were not attenuated. More recently, Bove et al. reported a decisively negative result [73]. Fenoldopam did not reduce the need for RRT or

Table 21.3 Notable negative trials of agents proposed to prevent or treat AKI

Agent	Negative findings	Reference
Fenoldopam	Did not reduce need for RRT or 30-day mortality compared with placebo	Bove et al. [73]
Alpha melanocyte-stimulating hormone	Did not prevent AKI in patients undergoing high-risk surgery	McCullough et al. [78]
Minocycline	Did not prevent AKI in patients undergoing cardiac surgery	Golestaneh et al. [81]
Statins	Did not prevent AKI in patients undergoing cardiac surgery	Lewicki et al. [82]
Insulin-like growth factor 1	Did not accelerate renal recovery in human trials	Hirschberg et al. [86]
Sodium bicarbonate	Did not prevent AKI in patients undergoing cardiac surgery	Haase et al. [87] McGuinness et al. [88] Kristeller et al. [89]
Balanced crystalloid solution	Did not reduce risk of AKI in critically ill patients	Young et al. [91]
Mesenchymal stem cells	Did not accelerate renal recovery or reduce need for RRT in patients undergoing cardiac surgery	Swaminathan et al. [93]

the 30-day mortality when compared with placebo, but those treated with fenoldopam had a higher rate of hypotension. The trial was terminated for futility.

21.9.2 Alpha Melanocyte-Stimulating Hormone (A[Alpha]MSH)

α[Alpha]MSH is an endogenous anti-inflammatory cytokine that may exert a nephroprotective effect by inhibiting apoptotic and inflammatory pathways [74, 75]. Animal studies of the α[alpha]MSH analogue, AP214 acetate (now known as ABT-719), demonstrated a protective effect in AKI induced by IR injury, sepsis and cisplatin [76, 77]. Unfortunately, this benefit has not been substantiated in human trials. McCullough et al. recently reported on the results of their phase 2b clinical trial of ABT-719 [78]. This agent failed to lower the incidence of AKI in high-risk cardiac surgery patients. Furthermore, it did not attenuate increments in novel biomarkers, nor did it improve clinical outcomes at 90 days.

21.9.3 Minocycline

Minocycline is a second-generation tetracycline antibiotic that has anti-inflammatory and anti-apoptotic effects. The mitochondria appear to be an important site for its protective property. In animal models of IR injury, minocycline was shown to reduce renal inflammation and attenuate renal injury [79, 80]. However, in a clinical trial, minocycline did not protect cardiac surgery patients against AKI [81].

21.9.4 Statins

Statins have been found to have many beneficial effects in addition to their lipid-lowering properties. Amongst these was the implication that they may have a role in preventing AKI by inhibiting inflammatory responses. A recent meta-analysis concluded that the data reviewed do not support the ability of statins to prevent AKI in patients undergoing cardiac surgery [82].

21.9.5 Insulin-Like Growth Factor 1

Insulin-like growth factor-1 (IGF-1) is a polypeptide growth factor with a similar molecular structure to insulin. It has been advocated as an important mediator of renal regeneration in models of AKI. Several preclinical studies have indicated that IGF-1 enhances renal recovery in animals with AKI [83–85]. However, the administration of recombinant human IGF-1 to patients with AKI in a multi-centre clinical trial did not accelerate the recovery of renal function [86].

21.9.6 Sodium Bicarbonate

The perioperative administration of sodium bicarbonate initially showed promise as a preventative strategy for AKI post-cardiac surgery. The proposed mechanism of protection was by reducing oxidant damage in the kidney. However, a series of randomized controlled trials have failed to substantiate this [87–89], and in fact, this strategy may increase mortality.

21.9.7 Balanced Crystalloid Solutions

There has been considerable debate regarding the optimal choice of intravenous fluid in critical illness. It has been hypothesized that saline solutions contribute to the development of AKI. Evidence emerged in support of the use of chloride restrictive or "balanced" salt solutions in the prevention of AKI [90]. However, a large randomized trial found that a balanced crystalloid solution did not reduce the risk of AKI when compared with saline [91].

21.9.8 Mesenchymal Stem Cells

Preclinical studies suggested that mesenchymal stem cells (MSCs) had the potential to protect against AKI. Amongst the proposed mechanisms were anti-inflammatory and anti-apoptotic effects. Unfortunately, the beneficial effects of MSC in animal models of AKI have not been replicated in human trials of the disease. A phase 2 trial of mesenchymal stem cell therapy for the prevention of AKI in cardiac surgery patients did not speed up renal recovery or reduce the need for RRT [93].

References

1. Wen X, Peng Z, Li Y, Wang H, Bishop JV, Chedwick LR, et al. One dose of cyclosporine A is protective at initiation of folic acid-induced acute kidney injury in mice. Nephrol Dial Transplant. 2012;27(8):3100–9.
2. Cour M, Abrial M, Jahandiez V, Loufouat J, Belaïdi E, Gharib A, et al. Ubiquitous protective effects of cyclosporine A in preventing cardiac arrest-induced multiple organ failure. J Appl Physiol. 2014;117(8):930–6.
3. Lemoine S, Pillot B, Augeul L, Rabeyrin M, Varennes A, Normand G, et al. Dose and timing of injections for effective cyclosporine A pretreatment before renal ischemia reperfusion in mice. PLoS One. 2017;12(8):e0182358.
4. Parajuli N, Campbell L, Marine A, Brockbank K, MacMillan-Crow L. MitoQ blunts mitochondrial and renal damage during cold preservation of porcine kidneys. PLoS One. 2012;7(11):e48590.
5. Dare A, Bolton E, Pettigrew G, Bradley J, Saeb-Parsy K, Murphy M. Protection against renal ischemia–reperfusion injury in vivo by the mitochondria targeted antioxidant MitoQ. Redox Biol. 2015;5:163–8.
6. Gane E, Weilert F, Orr D, Keogh G, Gibson M, Lockhart M, et al. The mitochondria-targeted antioxidant mitoquinone decreases liver damage in a phase II study of hepatitis C patients. Liver Int. 2010;30(7):1019–26.
7. Snow BJ, Rolfe FL, Lockhart MM, Frampton CM, O'Sullivan JD, Fung V, et al. A double-blind, placebo-controlled study to assess the mitochondria-targeted antioxidant MitoQ as a disease-modifying therapy in Parkinson's disease. Mov Disord. 2010;25(11):1670–4.
8. Mukhopadhyay P, Horváth B, Zsengellér Z, Zielonka J, Tanchian G, Holovac E, et al. Mitochondrial-targeted antioxidants represent a promising approach for prevention of cisplatin-induced nephropathy. Free Radic Biol Med. 2012;52(2):497–506.
9. Birk A, Liu S, Soong Y, Mills W, Singh P, Warren D, et al. The mitochondrial-targeted compound SS-31 re-energizes ischemic mitochondria by interacting with cardiolipin. J Am Soc Nephrol. 2013;24(8):1250–61.
10. Szeto HH, Liu S, Soong Y, Wu D, Darrah SF, Cheng F-YY, et al. Mitochondria-targeted peptide accelerates ATP recovery and reduces ischemic kidney injury. J Am Soc Nephrol. 2011;22(6):1041–52.
11. Whitaker R, Wills L, Stallons J, Schnellmann R. cGMP-selective phosphodiesterase inhibitors stimulate mitochondrial biogenesis and promote recovery from acute kidney injury. J Pharmacol Exp Ther. 2013;347(3):626–34.
12. Lledo-Garcia E, Subira-Rios D, Ogaya-Pinies G, Tejedor-Jorge A, Cañizo-Lopez J, Hernandez-Fernandez C. Intravenous sildenafil as a preconditioning drug against hemodynamic consequences of warm ischemia-reperfusion on the kidney. J Urol. 2011;186(1):331–3.

13. Lauver DA, Carey EG, Bergin IL, Lucchesi BR, Gurm HS. Sildenafil citrate for prophylaxis of nephropathy in an animal model of contrast-induced acute kidney injury. PLoS One. 2014;9(11):e113598.
14. De Almeida LS, Barboza JR, Freitas FP, Porto ML, Vasquez EC, Meyrelles SS, et al. Sildenafil prevents renal dysfunction in contrast media-induced nephropathy in Wistar rats. Hum Exp Toxicol. 2016;35(11):1194–1202.
15. Mohey V, Singh M, Puri N, Kaur T, Pathak D, Singh AP. Sildenafil obviates ischemia-reperfusion injury-induced acute kidney injury through peroxisome proliferator-activated receptor γ agonism in rats. J Surg Res. 2016;201(1):69–75.
16. Ring A, Morris T, Wozniak M, Sullo N, Dott W, Verheyden V, et al. A phase I study to determine the pharmacokinetic profile, safety and tolerability of sildenafil (Revatio®) in cardiac surgery: the REVAKI-1 study. Br J Clin Pharmacol. 2017;83(4):709–20.
17. Krane LS, Peyton CC, Olympio MA, Hemal AK. A randomized double blinded placebo controlled trial of sildenafil for renoprotection prior to hilar clamping in patients undergoing robotic assisted laparoscopic partial nephrectomy. J Surg Oncol. 2016;114(7):785–8.
18. Cassidy-Stone A, Chipuk J, Ingerman E, Song C, Yoo C, Kuwana T, et al. Chemical inhibition of the mitochondrial division dynamin reveals its role in Bax/Bak-dependent mitochondrial outer membrane permeabilization. Dev Cell. 2008;14(2):193–204.
19. Brooks C, Wei Q, Cho S-G, Dong Z. Regulation of mitochondrial dynamics in acute kidney injury in cell culture and rodent models. J Clin Invest. 2009;119(5):1275–85.
20. Sumida M, Doi K, Ogasawara E, Yamashita T, Hamasaki Y, Kariya T, et al. Regulation of mitochondrial dynamics by dynamin-related protein-1 in acute cardiorenal syndrome. J Am Soc Nephrol. 2015;26(10):2378–87.
21. Hodeify R, Megyesi J, Tarcsafalvi A, Mustafa H, Seng N, Price P. Gender differences control the susceptibility to ER stress-induced acute kidney injury. Am J Physiol Renal Physiol. 2013;304(7):F875–82.
22. Carlisle R, Brimble E, Werner K, Cruz G, Ask K, Ingram A, et al. 4-phenylbutyrate inhibits tunicamycin-induced acute kidney injury via CHOP/GADD153 repression. PLoS One. 2014;9(1):e84663.
23. Peng P, Ma Q, Wang L, Zhang O, Han H, Liu X, et al. Preconditioning with tauroursodeoxycholic acid protects against contrast-induced HK-2 cell apoptosis by inhibiting endoplasmic reticulum stress. Angiology. 2015;66(10):941–9.
24. Khan MA, Liu J, Kumar G, Skapek SX, Falck JR, Imig JD. Novel orally active epoxyeicosatrienoic acid (EET) analogs attenuate cisplatin nephrotoxicity. FASEB J. 2013;27(8):2946–56.
25. Jiang J-G, Chen C-L, Card J, Yang S, Chen J-X, Fu X-N, et al. Cytochrome P450 2J2 promotes the neoplastic phenotype of carcinoma cells and is up-regulated in human tumors. Cancer Res. 2005;65(11):4707–15.
26. Jiang J-G, Ning Y-G, Chen C, Ma D, Liu Z-J, Yang S, et al. Cytochrome P450 epoxygenase promotes human cancer metastasis. Cancer Res. 2007;67(14):6665–74.
27. Bajwa A, Jo S-KK, Ye H, Huang L, Dondeti KR, Rosin DL, et al. Activation of sphingosine-1-phosphate 1 receptor in the proximal tubule protects against ischemia-reperfusion injury. J Am Soc Nephrol. 2010;21(6):955–65.
28. Bajwa A, Rosin DL, Chroscicki P, Lee S, Dondeti K, Ye H, et al. Sphingosine 1-phosphate receptor-1 enhances mitochondrial function and reduces cisplatin-induced tubule injury. J Am Soc Nephrol. 2015;26(4):908–25.
29. Park SW, Kim M, Kim M, D'Agati VD, Lee HT. Sphingosine kinase 1 protects against renal ischemia-reperfusion injury in mice by sphingosine-1-phosphate1 receptor activation. Kidney Int. 2011;80(12):1315–27.
30. Yeboah MM, Xue X, Javdan M, Susin M, Metz CN. Nicotinic acetylcholine receptor expression and regulation in the rat kidney after ischemia-reperfusion injury. Am J Physiol Renal Physiol. 2008;295(3):F654–61.
31. Sadis C, Teske G, Stokman G, Kubjak C, Claessen N, Moore F, et al. Nicotine protects kidney from renal ischemia/reperfusion injury through the cholinergic anti-inflammatory pathway. PLoS One. 2007;2(5):e469.
32. Chatterjee PK, Yeboah MM, Dowling O, Xue X, Powell SR, Al-Abed Y, et al. Nicotinic acetylcholine receptor agonists attenuate septic acute kidney injury in mice by suppressing inflammation and proteasome activity. PLoS One. 2012;7(5):e35361.
33. Gigliotti JC, Huang L, Ye H, Bajwa A, Chattrabhuti K, Lee S, et al. Ultrasound prevents renal ischemia-reperfusion injury by stimulating the splenic cholinergic anti-inflammatory pathway. J Am Soc Nephrol. 2013;24(9):1451–60.
34. Matsumura Y, Taira S, Kitano R, Hashimoto N, Kuro T. Selective antagonism of endothelin ET(A) or ET(B) receptor in renal hemodynamics and function of deoxycorticosterone acetate-salt-induced hypertensive rats. Biol Pharm Bull. 1999;22(8):858–62.
35. Chade AR, Krier JD, Textor SC, Lerman A, Lerman LO. Endothelin-a receptor blockade improves renal microvascular architecture and function in experimental hypercholesterolemia. J Am Soc Nephrol. 2006;17(12):3394–403.
36. Herrero I, Torras J, Riera M, Condom E, Coll O, Cruzado JM, et al. Prevention of cold ischaemia-reperfusion injury by an endothelin receptor antagonist in experimental renal transplantation. Nephrol Dial Transplant. 1999;14(4):872–80.
37. Wilhelm SM, Stowe NT, Robinson AV, Schulak JA. The use of the endothelin receptor antagonist, tezosentan, before or after renal ischemia protects renal function. Transplantation. 2001;71(2):211–6.
38. Helmy MM, Helmy MW, Abd Allah DM, Abo Zaid AM, Mohy El-Din MM. Selective ET(A) receptor

blockade protects against cisplatin-induced acute renal failure in male rats. Eur J Pharmacol. 2014;730:133–9.
39. Patel NN, Toth T, Jones C, Lin H, Ray P, George SJ, et al. Prevention of post-cardiopulmonary bypass acute kidney injury by endothelin A receptor blockade. Crit Care Med. 2011;39(4):793–802.
40. Kim B, Lim S, Li C, Kim J, Sun B, Ahn K, et al. Ischemia-reperfusion injury activates innate immunity in rat kidneys. Transplantation. 2005;79(10):1370–7.
41. Wolfs T, Buurman W, van Schadewijk A, de Vries B, Daemen M, Hiemstra P, et al. In vivo expression of toll-like receptor 2 and 4 by renal epithelial cells: IFN-γ and TNF-α mediated up-regulation during inflammation. J Immunol. 2002;168(3):1286–93.
42. Kim H, Park S, Koo S, Cha H, Lee J, Kwon B, et al. Inhibition of kidney ischemia–reperfusion injury through local infusion of a TLR2 blocker. J Immunol Methods. 2014;407:146–50.
43. Farrar C, Keogh B, McCormack W, O'Shaughnessy A, Parker A, Reilly M, et al. Inhibition of TLR2 promotes graft function in a murine model of renal transplant ischemia-reperfusion injury. FASEB J. 2012;26(2):799–807.
44. Kim DH, Jung YJ, Lee AS, Lee S, Kang KP, Lee TH, et al. COMP-angiopoietin-1 decreases lipopolysaccharide-induced acute kidney injury. Kidney Int. 2009;76(11):1180–91.
45. Lee S, Kim W, Kim DH, Moon S-OO, Jung YJ, Lee AS, et al. Protective effect of COMP-angiopoietin-1 on cyclosporine-induced renal injury in mice. Nephrol Dial Transplant. 2008;23(9):2784–94.
46. Long DA, Price KL, Ioffe E, Gannon CM, Gnudi L, White KE, et al. Angiopoietin-1 therapy enhances fibrosis and inflammation following folic acid-induced acute renal injury. Kidney Int. 2008;74(3):300–9.
47. Jung YJ, Kim DH, Lee AS, Lee S, Kang KP, Lee SY, et al. Peritubular capillary preservation with COMP-angiopoietin-1 decreases ischemia-reperfusion-induced acute kidney injury. Am J Physiol Renal Physiol. 2009;297(4):F952–60.
48. Patschan D, Krupincza K, Patschan S, Zhang Z, Hamby C, Goligorsky MS. Dynamics of mobilization and homing of endothelial progenitor cells after acute renal ischemia: modulation by ischemic preconditioning. Am J Physiol Renal Physiol. 2006;291(1):F176–85.
49. Bo C-JJ, Chen B, Jia R-PP, Zhu J-GG, Cao P, Liu H, et al. Effects of ischemic preconditioning in the late phase on homing of endothelial progenitor cells in renal ischemia/reperfusion injury. Transplant Proc. 2013;45(2):511–6.
50. Togel FE, Westenfelder C. Role of SDF-1 as a regulatory chemokine in renal regeneration after acute kidney injury. Kidney Int Suppl (2011). 2011;1(3):87–9.
51. Kelly KJ, Plotkin Z, Vulgamott SL, Dagher PC. P53 mediates the apoptotic response to GTP depletion after renal ischemia-reperfusion: protective role of a p53 inhibitor. J Am Soc Nephrol. 2003;14(1):128–38.
52. Molitoris BA, Dagher PC, Sandoval RM, Campos SB, Ashush H, Fridman E, et al. siRNA targeted to p53 attenuates ischemic and cisplatin-induced acute kidney injury. J Am Soc Nephrol. 2009;20(8):1754–64.
53. Wang H, Bloom O, Zhang M, Vishnubhakat JM, Ombrellino M, Che J, et al. HMG-1 as a late mediator of endotoxin lethality in mice. Science. 1999;285(5425):248–51.
54. Wu H, Ma J, Wang P, Corpuz TM, Panchapakesan U, Wyburn KR, et al. HMGB1 contributes to kidney ischemia reperfusion injury. J Am Soc Nephrol. 2010;21(11):1878–90.
55. Li J, Gong Q, Zhong S, Wang L, Guo H, Xiang Y, et al. Neutralization of the extracellular HMGB1 released by ischaemic damaged renal cells protects against renal ischaemia-reperfusion injury. Nephrol Dial Transplant. 2011;26(2):469–78.
56. Wu H, Steenstra R, de Boer EC, Zhao CY, Ma J, van der Stelt JM, et al. Preconditioning with recombinant high-mobility group box 1 protein protects the kidney against ischemia-reperfusion injury in mice. Kidney Int. 2014;85(4):824–32.
57. Qin S, Wang H, Yuan R, Li H, Ochani M, Ochani K, et al. Role of HMGB1 in apoptosis-mediated sepsis lethality. J Exp Med. 2006;203(7):1637–42.
58. Fink MP. Ethyl pyruvate: a novel treatment for sepsis. Curr Drug Targets. 2007;8(4):515–8.
59. Chung K-YY, Park J-JJ, Kim YS. The role of high-mobility group box 1 in renal ischemia and reperfusion injury and the effect of ethyl pyruvate. Transplant Proc. 2008;40(7):2136–8.
60. Rabadi MM, Ghaly T, Goligorksy MS, Ratliff BB. HMGB1 in renal ischemic injury. Am J Physiol Renal Physiol. 2012;303(6):F873–85.
61. Pickkers P, Heemskerk S, Schouten J, Laterre P-FF, Vincent J-LL, Beishuizen A, et al. Alkaline phosphatase for treatment of sepsis-induced acute kidney injury: a prospective randomized double-blind placebo-controlled trial. Crit Care. 2012;16(1):R14.
62. Servais H, Ortiz A, Devuyst O, Denamur S, Tulkens PM, Mingeot-Leclercq M-PP. Renal cell apoptosis induced by nephrotoxic drugs: cellular and molecular mechanisms and potential approaches to modulation. Apoptosis. 2008;13(1):11–32.
63. Daemen MA, van 't Veer C, Denecker G, Heemskerk VH, Wolfs TG, Clauss M, et al. Inhibition of apoptosis induced by ischemia-reperfusion prevents inflammation. J Clin Invest. 1999;104(5):541–9.
64. Guo R, Wang Y, Minto AW, Quigg RJ, Cunningham PN. Acute renal failure in endotoxemia is dependent on caspase activation. J Am Soc Nephrol. 2004;15(12):3093–102.
65. Homsi E, Janino P, de Faria JB. Role of caspases on cell death, inflammation, and cell cycle in glycerol-induced acute renal failure. Kidney Int. 2006;69(8):1385–92.
66. Shiffman ML, Pockros P, McHutchison JG, Schiff ER, Morris M, Burgess G. Clinical trial: the efficacy and safety of oral PF-03491390, a pancaspase inhibitor—a randomized placebo-controlled study in patients with chronic hepatitis C. Aliment Pharmacol Ther. 2010;31(9):969–78.

67. Khan NA, Khan A, Savelkoul HF, Benner R. Inhibition of septic shock in mice by an oligopeptide from the beta-chain of human chorionic gonadotrophin hormone. Hum Immunol. 2002;63(1):1–7.
68. Khan NA, Susa D, van den Berg JW, Huisman M, Ameling MH, van den Engel S, et al. Amelioration of renal ischaemia-reperfusion injury by synthetic oligopeptides related to human chorionic gonadotropin. Nephrol Dial Transplant. 2009;24(9):2701–8.
69. Gueler F, Shushakova N, Mengel M, Hueper K, Chen R, Liu X, et al. A novel therapy to attenuate acute kidney injury and ischemic allograft damage after allogenic kidney transplantation in mice. PLoS One. 2015;10(1):e0115709.
70. Vukicevic S, Basic V, Rogic D, Basic N, Shih MS, Shepard A, et al. Osteogenic protein-1 (bone morphogenetic protein-7) reduces severity of injury after ischemic acute renal failure in rat. J Clin Invest. 1998;102(1):202–14.
71. Hruska KA, Guo G, Wozniak M, Martin D, Miller S, Liapis H, et al. Osteogenic protein-1 prevents renal fibrogenesis associated with ureteral obstruction. Am J Physiol Renal Physiol. 2000;279(1):F130–43.
72. Gillies MA, Kakar V, Parker RJ, Honoré PM, Ostermann M. Fenoldopam to prevent acute kidney injury after major surgery—a systematic review and meta-analysis. Crit Care. 2015;19(1):449.
73. Bove T, Zangrillo A, Guarracino F, Alvaro G, Persi B, Maglioni E, et al. Effect of fenoldopam on use of renal replacement therapy among patients with acute kidney injury after cardiac surgery: a randomized clinical trial. JAMA. 2014;312(21):2244–53.
74. Chiao H, Kohda Y, McLeroy P, Craig L, Linas S, Star RA. Alpha-melanocyte-stimulating hormone inhibits renal injury in the absence of neutrophils. Kidney Int. 1998;54(3):765–74.
75. Jo SK, Yun SY, Chang KH, Cha DR, Cho WY, Kim HK, et al. alpha-MSH decreases apoptosis in ischaemic acute renal failure in rats: possible mechanism of this beneficial effect. Nephrol Dial Transplant. 2001;16(8):1583–91.
76. Doi K, Hu X, Yuen PS, Leelahavanichkul A, Yasuda H, Kim SM, et al. AP214, an analogue of alpha-melanocyte-stimulating hormone, ameliorates sepsis-induced acute kidney injury and mortality. Kidney Int. 2008;73(11):1266–74.
77. Simmons MN, Subramanian V, Crouzet S, Haber G-PP, Colombo JR, Ukimura O, et al. Alpha-melanocyte stimulating hormone analogue AP214 protects against ischemia induced acute kidney injury in a porcine surgical model. J Urol. 2010;183(4):1625–9.
78. McCullough PA, Bennett-Guerrero E, Chawla LS, Beaver T, Mehta RL, Molitoris BA, et al. ABT-719 for the Prevention of Acute Kidney Injury in Patients Undergoing High-Risk Cardiac Surgery: A Randomized Phase 2b Clinical Trial. Am Heart Assoc. 2016;5(8):e003549.
79. Kelly KJ, Sutton TA, Weathered N, Ray N, Caldwell EJ, Plotkin Z, et al. Minocycline inhibits apoptosis and inflammation in a rat model of ischemic renal injury. Am J Physiol Renal Physiol. 2004;287(4):F760.
80. Wang J, Wei Q, Wang C-Y, Hill W, Hess D, Dong Z. Minocycline up-regulates Bcl-2 and protects against cell death in mitochondria. J Biol Chem. 2004;279(19):19948–54.
81. Golestaneh L, Lindsey K, Malhotra P, Kargoli F, Farkas E, Barner H, et al. Acute kidney injury after cardiac surgery: is minocycline protective? J Nephrol. 2015;28(2):193–9.
82. Lewicki M, Ng I, Schneider AG. HMG CoA reductase inhibitors (statins) for preventing acute kidney injury after surgical procedures requiring cardiac bypass. Cochrane Database Syst Rev 2015;(3):CD010480.
83. Ding H, Kopple JD, Cohen A, Hirschberg R. Recombinant human insulin-like growth factor-I accelerates recovery and reduces catabolism in rats with ischemic acute renal failure. J Clin Invest. 1993;91(5):2281–7.
84. Friedlaender M, Popovtzer MM, Weiss O, Nefesh I, Kopolovic J, Raz I. Insulin-like growth factor-1 (IGF-1) enhances recovery from HgCl2-induced acute renal failure: the effects on renal IGF-1, IGF-1 receptor, and IGF-binding protein-1 mRNA. J Am Soc Nephrol. 1995;5(10):1782–91.
85. Miller SB, Martin DR, Kissane J, Hammerman MR. Insulin-like growth factor I accelerates recovery from ischemic acute tubular necrosis in the rat. Proc Natl Acad Sci U S A. 1992;89(24):11876–80.
86. Hirschberg R, Kopple J, Lipsett P, Benjamin E, Minei J, Albertson T, et al. Multicenter clinical trial of recombinant human insulin-like growth factor I in patients with acute renal failure. Kidney Int. 1999;55(6):2423–32.
87. Haase M, Haase-Fielitz A, Plass M, Kuppe H, Hetzer R, Hannon C, et al. Prophylactic perioperative sodium bicarbonate to prevent acute kidney injury following open heart surgery: a multicenter double-blinded randomized controlled trial. PLoS Med. 2013;10(4):e1001426.
88. McGuinness SP, Parke RL, Bellomo R, Van Haren FM, Bailey M. Sodium bicarbonate infusion to reduce cardiac surgery-associated acute kidney injury: a phase II multicenter double-blind randomized controlled trial. Crit Care Med. 2013;41(7):1599–607.
89. Kristeller JL, Zavorsky GS, Prior JE, Keating DA, Brady MA, Romaldini TA, et al. Lack of effectiveness of sodium bicarbonate in preventing kidney injury in patients undergoing cardiac surgery: a randomized controlled trial. Pharmacotherapy. 2013;33(7):710–7.
90. Yunos N, Bellomo R, Hegarty C, Story D, Ho L, Bailey M. Association between a chloride-liberal vs chloride-restrictive intravenous fluid administration strategy and kidney injury in critically ill adults. JAMA. 2012;308(15):1566–72.
91. Young P, Bailey M, Beasley R, Henderson S, Mackle D, McArthur C, et al. Effect of a buffered crystalloid solution vs saline on acute kidney injury among patients in the Intensive Care Unit: the SPLIT randomized clinical trial. JAMA. 2015;314(16):1701–10.

92. Erika I. Boesen, (2016) Lack of an apparent role for endothelin-1 in the prolonged reduction in renal perfusion following severe unilateral ischemia-reperfusion injury in the mouse. Physiological Reports 4 (21):e13027.
93. Madhav Swaminathan, Mark Stafford-Smith, Glenn M. Chertow, David G. Warnock, Viken Paragamian, Robert M. Brenner, François Lellouche, Alison Fox-Robichaud, Mohamed G. Atta, Spencer Melby, Ravindra L. Mehta, Ron Wald, Subodh Verma, C. David Mazer, Allogeneic Mesenchymal Stem Cells for Treatment of AKI after Cardiac Surgery. Journal of the American Society of Nephrology: ASN.2016101150.

22 Dialytic Therapy of Acute Kidney Injury

Alian A. Al-balas, Keith M. Wille, and Ashita J. Tolwani

22.1 Introduction

Renal replacement therapy (RRT) is used largely for supportive management of patients with severe acute kidney injury (AKI). At present, RRT is initiated for the acute management of life-threatening complications of AKI, including severe hyperkalemia, metabolic acidosis, volume overload, overt uremic manifestations, and dialyzable intoxications. Although several meta-analyses of both randomized controlled trials (RCTs) and cohort studies have suggested that "early" initiation of RRT for AKI (based on a lower urea or creatinine level) is associated with better patient survival, these studies have significant design limitations [1, 2]. Since those earlier studies, two RCTS comparing the timing of RRT initiation in critically ill patients have been published. The Early Versus Late Initiation of Renal Replacement Therapy in Critically Ill Patients with Acute Kidney Injury (ELAIN) trial was a single-center RCT comparing early RRT (starting within <8 h of fulfilling Kidney Disease: Improving Global Outcomes (KDIGO) stage 2 AKI) with delayed RRT (starting within <12 h of developing KDIGO stage 3 AKI or upon an absolute indication) in 231 critically ill patients [3]. Patients were also required to have a plasma neutrophil gelatinase-associated lipocalin (NGAL) level > 150 ng/mL and one other condition from among severe sepsis, use of vasopressors or catecholamines, refractory fluid overload, or development or progression of nonrenal organ dysfunction for enrolment. Mortality at day 90 was significantly lower among patients randomized to the early initiation arm compared with those in the delayed initiation arm (39.3% versus 54.7%; hazard ratio, 0.66; 95% confidence interval [95% CI], 0.45–0.97; $P = 0.03$). Similar benefits were seen with regard to duration of RRT and mechanical ventilation, as well as hospital length of stay, but not RRT dependence at day 90 among survivors or intensive care unit length of stay. The results of this trial are in contrast to the findings of the multicenter Artificial Kidney Initiation in Kidney Injury (AKIKI) trial [4]. In the AKIKI trial, 620 critically ill adults with KDIGO stage 3 AKI who needed mechanical ventilation, vasopressor therapy, or both were randomized to either immediate RRT or the addition of renal support only when medically necessary (severe hyperkalemia, metabolic acidosis, pulmonary edema, or a blood urea nitrogen level greater than 112 mg/dL, or oliguria for more than 72 h). Mortality at 60 days was similar in both groups (48.5% in the early group

A. A. Al-balas · A. J. Tolwani (✉)
Division of Nephrology, University of Alabama at Birmingham, Birmingham, AL, USA
e-mail: aalbalas@uabmc.edu

K. M. Wille
Division of Pulmonary, Allergy, and Critical Care Medicine, University of Alabama at Birmingham, Birmingham, AL, USA
e-mail: wille@uab.edu

S. S. Waikar et al. (eds.), *Core Concepts in Acute Kidney Injury*,
https://doi.org/10.1007/978-1-4939-8628-6_22

and 49.7% in the delayed group). Given the discordant results between the ELAIN and AKIKI trials and fundamental differences in trial design, the results of the ELAIN trial must be interpreted cautiously, especially given the relatively small sample size and limited statistical power. While both trials are important contributions toward informing practice on this issue, additional evidence from large multicenter RCTS is needed. In clinical practice, clinicians characteristically take into account the overall clinical state of the patient, including degree of other organ systems failing and likelihood of rapid renal recovery, and often start RRT prior to the development of overt AKI complications.

Options for RRT for AKI include intermittent hemodialysis (IHD), continuous renal replacement therapy (CRRT), "hybrid" therapies known as prolonged intermittent renal replacement therapy (PIRRT), and peritoneal dialysis (PD) (Table 22.1). IHD, CRRT, and PIRRT, are extracorporeal therapies and require the presence of a vascular access in the form of a large-bore double-lumen central venous catheter; PD requires the placement of an intra-abdominal catheter for dialysis. Selection of renal replacement modality depends on therapy availability, patient hemodynamic status, goals for solute clearance and volume control, need for anticoagulation, and physician preference and expertise.

The various RRTs transport water and solutes across a semipermeable membrane. Solute removal occurs by diffusion, convection, or a combination of both, whereas fluid removal occurs by hydrostatic pressure (in HD and CRRT) or osmotic (in PD) gradients. In diffusion, solute removal across the membrane is driven by the concentration gradient between blood and dialysate. With extracorporeal RRTs, this concentration gradient is maximized along the length of the membrane by running the dialysate countercurrent to the blood flow. Diffusive clearance of solutes depends on the concentration gradient for the solute between the two compartments, the molecular weight of the solute, the membrane properties (surface area, pore size, charge, and water permeability), dialysate flow, and dialyzer blood flow. Some solutes may also be removed by adsorption onto the membrane. Since the diffusivity of a solute is inversely proportional to its molecular weight, dialysis is highly effective in removing small solutes from the circulation, such as urea and creatinine, as compared to larger ("middle-molecular-weight") solutes like β2-microglobulin and vancomycin.

While diffusion is most effective at removing small-molecular-weight solutes (<500 Da), convection provides effective removal of both small- and middle-molecular-weight solutes (500–10,000 Da). In convection, solutes are transported by bulk flow during ultrafiltration. As plasma water is driven across the

Table 22.1 Comparison of different dialysis methods for acute kidney injury

Dialysis modality	IHD	CRRT	PIRRT	PD
Vascular access	Yes	Yes	Yes	No
Anticoagulation	Preferred but not necessary	Preferred but not necessary; regional citrate anticoagulation	Preferred but not necessary	No
Duration (h)	3–5	24	6–12	24
Frequency	3–6 × week	Daily	3–6 × week	Daily
Dialysate flow (mL/min)	500–800	15–60	100–300	––
Severe hyperkalemia	Preferred if hemodynamically stable	––	Preferred if hemodynamically unstable	––
Brain edema	––	Preferred	––	Preferred
Perceived cost	++	++++	+++	+

Abbreviations: *IHD* intermittent hemodialysis, *CRRT* continuous renal replacement therapy, *PIRRT* prolonged intermittent renal replacement therapy, *PD* peritoneal dialysis

semipermeable membrane by either a hydrostatic or osmotic gradient, it "drags" with it both small-molecular-weight solutes and middle-molecular-weight solutes. Convective transport is not size-dependent as long as the molecular weight of the solute is smaller than the membrane pore diameter. Convective solute clearance is generally proportional to the ultrafiltration rate.

22.2 Intermittent Hemodialysis (IHD)

IHD is typically delivered in intermittent sessions of 3–5 h, 3–6 times per week, using a blood flow rate of 300–500 mL/min and a dialysate flow rate of 500–800 mL/min. The duration and frequency of IHD sessions are determined by the patient's specific needs and degree of hemodynamic stability. Solute clearance occurs mainly by diffusion, and volume is removed by ultrafiltration. However, high-flux dialyzers can also provide convective clearance of solutes through increased membrane porosity, enhanced transport capacity, and internal filtration and backfiltration. Given that the advantage of IHD is rapid solute and volume removal, IHD is preferred for correction of electrolyte derangements, such as hyperkalemia, and removal of drug in intoxications. Moreover, when compared to other types of extracorporeal RRTs, IHD can be performed with less or no anticoagulation because of the faster blood flow rate and shorter duration of therapy. The main disadvantage of IHD is hypotension caused by rapid solute and fluid removal, which complicates 20–30% of treatments [5, 6]. Strategies for decreasing dialysis-induced hypotension include sodium modeling, increasing the dialysate calcium concentration, cooling the dialysate, and prolonging the duration of therapy [7]. Despite this, approximately 10% of patients with AKI cannot tolerate IHD because of hemodynamic instability [5, 7–10]. Furthermore, rapid solute removal from the intravascular space can cause cerebral edema and increased intracranial pressure, limiting this therapy in patients with head trauma or hepatic encephalopathy [11].

22.3 Continuous Renal Replacement Therapy (CRRT)

CRRT represents a variety of dialysis modalities developed specifically to manage critically ill patients with AKI who cannot tolerate IHD due to hemodynamic instability. CRRT uses diffusion, convection, or a combination of both for solute clearance and is performed up to 24 h a day with blood flow rates of 100–300 mL/min [12–14]. By providing slower solute and fluid removal per unit of time, CRRT is thought to allow for better hemodynamic tolerance as compared to IHD. Other potential advantages of CRRT over IHD include more efficient solute clearance, better control of volume status, and better clearance of middle-molecular-weight solutes. Disadvantages of CRRT over IHD include decreased patient mobility, increased nursing labor, greater need for anticoagulation, and increased cost. Moreover, since no clear data exists on how to appropriately dose many drugs during CRRT, potential underdosing of drugs, especially antibiotics, can occur.

The CRRT modalities employed for solute removal are continuous venovenous hemofiltration (CVVH), continuous venovenous hemodialysis (CVVHD), and continuous venovenous hemodiafiltration (CVVHDF) [12–14] (Table 22.2). In CVVH, solute removal is solely dependent on convective clearance and is augmented by increas-

Table 22.2 CRRT modalities

CRRT modality	Convection	Diffusion	Replacement fluid	Ultrafiltration rate (mL/min)	Dialysate rate (mL/min)
CVVH	++++	–	Yes	16–50	–
CVVHD	+	++++	No	5–15	16–50
CVVHDF	+++	+++	Yes	16–50	16–50

Abbreviations: *CRRT* continuous renal replacement therapy, *CVVH* continuous venovenous hemofiltration, *CVVHD* continuous venovenous hemodialysis, *CVVHDF* continuous venovenous hemodiafiltration

ing the volume of ultrafiltrate. No dialysate is used. A "replacement" or "substitution" fluid is infused in the blood to replace the excess volume and electrolytes removed through the membrane from the high ultrafiltration rates and to correct acid-base and electrolyte abnormalities. The replacement fluid can be infused prior to the hemofilter (pre-filter or pre-dilution) or after the hemofilter (post-filter or post-dilution) in varying amounts. The use of post-filter replacement fluid is limited by the filtration fraction, which is defined as the ratio of ultrafiltration rate to plasma water flow rate [15]. Clinical practice suggests a filtration fraction >0.30 is associated with increased clotting from hemoconcentration and protein-membrane interactions. Adding some of the replacement fluid pre-filter dilutes the hematocrit, thereby reducing the filtration fraction and likelihood of filter clotting. The downside is that by diluting the concentration of solutes entering the hemofilter, pre-filter replacement fluid decreases solute clearance by 15% with ultrafiltration volumes of 2000 mL/h and up to 34% with volumes of 4500 mL/h [16]. CVVHD removes solutes by diffusion. In contrast to IHD, the dialysate flow rate (typically 1–2 L/h, or 17–34 mL/min) is slower than the blood flow rate (100–300 mL/min), allowing small solutes to equilibrate completely between the blood and dialysate. Ultrafiltration is used only for volume control and, therefore, with rates much lower than required for convective solute clearance. CVVHDF uses a combination of convection and diffusion for solute removal and, as a result, requires both a dialysate and replacement fluid.

Despite increased clearance of middle-molecular-weight molecules with hemofiltration, no study has shown that CVVH improves patient survival when compared to CVVHD. Friedrich et al. published a meta-analysis comparing the outcomes of hemofiltration to hemodialysis for the treatment of AKI [17]. Nineteen RCTs were evaluated, of which 16 used CRRT. The authors found no difference in patient survival or clinical outcomes such as organ dysfunction, vasopressor use, or survivor renal recovery. Hemofiltration was associated with an increased clearance of larger molecules but also a shorter filter life. Although cytokines can be removed by CVVH, most controlled studies have failed to demonstrate a significant and sustained decrease in cytokine plasma concentrations or an improvement in outcome [18–23]. High-volume hemofiltration (HVHF) with ultrafiltration rates >50 mL/kg/h has been attempted to augment the clearance of cytokines in AKI patients with sepsis and septic shock. However, a meta-analysis of four RCTs comparing HVHF to standard-volume CVVH did not show any survival benefit with HVHF [24]. The HEROICS study was a more recent RCT in which patients with severe shock requiring high-dose catecholamines 3–24 h post-cardiac surgery were randomized to early HVHF at 80 mL/kg/h for 48 h followed by standard-volume CVVHDF versus standard care [25]. Standard care involved initiating CVVHDF for conventional indications in the setting of AKI. Early HVHF did not lower 30-day mortality (odds ratio, 1.00; 95% confidence interval, 0.64–1.56; P = 1.00) or improve any other clinical outcomes. Since there is insufficient data to recommend one type of CRRT modality over another, the choice of CRRT modality should be based on clinician preference and expertise.

22.4 Prolonged Intermittent Renal Replacement Therapy (PIRRT)

Hybrid therapies are also known as prolonged intermittent renal replacement therapy (PIRRT), sustained low-efficiency dialysis (SLED), and extended daily dialysis (EDD). These therapies use conventional hemodialysis machines with lower blood-pump speeds (e.g., 200 mL/min) and dialysate flow rates (e.g., 100–300 mL/min) to provide solute and fluid removal slower than IHD but faster than conventional CRRT. The duration of dialysis is extended to 8–16 h daily. PIRRTs combine the advantages of both CRRT and IHD. They allow for improved hemodynamic stability through gradual solute and volume removal while providing the benefits of an intermittent therapy, such as decreased cost, increased patient mobility, and decreased need for anticoagulation. Because they are intermittent, scheduling of required diagnostic and therapeutic procedures can be done without interruption of therapy. Studies have demonstrated that PIRRTs provide comparable hemodynamic control to CRRT [26–29]. As with CRRT, appropriate dosing of drugs is not known and can lead to underdosing of critical medications such as antibiotics.

22.5 Peritoneal Dialysis (PD)

In PD the peritoneum functions as a semipermeable membrane and allows for solute removal through diffusion and volume removal through ultrafiltration. A dialysate solution is instilled into the peritoneal cavity through a catheter, where it dwells for a prescribed period of time allowing solutes to diffuse from blood in the capillaries into the dialysate. The saturated dialysate is then drained and discarded and fresh dialysate reintroduced. High concentrations of dextrose are used in the dialysate to create an osmotic gradient for ultrafiltration. Acute PD can be performed intermittently or continuously and either manually or by an automated cycler. Advantages of PD include wide availability, technical simplicity, hemodynamic stability, lack of need for anticoagulation or vascular access, and lower cost. Disadvantages include complications of PD catheter placement, risk of peritonitis, potential inability to provide sufficient solute clearance in hypercatabolic patients, unpredictable ultrafiltration, albumin loss across the peritoneal membrane, hyperglycemia, and potential respiratory compromise from increased abdominal pressure caused by instilled dialysate [30, 31]. PD is contraindicated in patients with recent abdominal surgery, abdominal drains, or ileus. Acute PD is useful in AKI patients with hemodynamic instability or difficult vascular access issues or in AKI patients located in regions with limited resources.

22.6 Selection of RRT Modality

Evidence for improved outcomes with one specific RRT over another in patients with AKI is lacking. CRRT has been associated with less need for escalation of vasopressors [32] and with greater net negative fluid balance [33]. However, based on RCTs and several meta-analyses, there has been no convincing evidence that CRRT is superior to IHD in terms of survival [32, 34–37]. While observational studies have shown CRRT to be associated with higher rates of renal recovery, the evidence is insufficient [38]. Most studies only evaluated renal recovery in patients who survived, and improved renal recovery with CRRT has not been observed in RCTs.

There are scant data comparing other modalities of RRT in AKI. Although data comparing PIRRT to either IHD or CRRT are limited, similar survival outcomes have been suggested [28, 39, 40]. A recent meta-analysis of studies comparing CRRT and PIRRT shows no difference in mortality, renal recovery, fluid removal, ICU days, or solute control [41]. Several small RCTs have compared PD to other RRT modalities in AKI. In a study from Vietnam comparing CVVH to PD, CVVH was associated with better survival in patients whose predominant etiology of AKI was malaria [31]. The applicability of this study to other causes of AKI is uncertain. A RCT of 120 patients, comparing high-volume PD to daily IHD, demonstrated no difference in survival or renal recovery [42]. Another RCT comparing high-volume PD and PIRRT found no evidence of a survival benefit with PD [43]. A meta-analysis of seven cohort studies and four RCTS comparing PD with extracorporeal therapies in the setting of AKI suggested there were no significant differences in outcomes between patients treated with PD and IHD or hemodiafiltration (HDF) [44].

In the absence of definitive data to support a particular modality, selection of RRT modality should be based on the needs of the patient. Choice of RRT modality is also influenced by availability, expertise, resources, cost, and physician preference. Most clinicians choose IHD for

AKI patients who are hemodynamically stable and CRRT or PIRRT for AKI patients who are hemodynamically unstable and fluid overloaded and/or have sepsis and multi-organ failure. IHD is also favored in patients who need rapid solute removal, such as patients with severe hyperkalemia or drug intoxications. CRRT is preferred in patients with cerebral edema since IHD may worsen neurological status by compromising cerebral perfusion pressure as a result of dialysis-associated hypotension or from rapid intracellular fluid and solute shifts [45–47]. Given the slower rate of volume and solute removal, CRRT is better tolerated by patients with acute brain injury who are at risk for acute herniation [46, 48].

22.7 Anticoagulation

Anticoagulation is frequently required to prevent clotting of the circuit in most types of extracorporeal RRT. Clotting of the filter affects treatment efficacy by decreasing solute and fluid removal and contributes to blood loss in the dialyzer. The most commonly used anticoagulant is unfractionated heparin (UFH). UFH has several significant advantages including its wide availability, low cost, ease of administration and monitoring, and reversibility with protamine. Disadvantages include its unpredictable pharmacokinetics, risk of heparin-induced thrombocytopenia (HIT), heparin resistance due to low patient antithrombin levels, and increased risk of bleeding [49]. Although IHD and PIRRT can be generally performed without anticoagulation given the shorter duration of treatment with higher blood flow rates, CRRT often requires anticoagulation.

The incidence of bleeding episodes with heparin as an anticoagulant for CRRT ranges from 10 to 50%, with mortality from bleeding as high as 15% [50–52]. As a result, regional anticoagulation with citrate has been gaining wider acceptance in CRRT [53–55]. Several methods of regional citrate anticoagulation (RCA) for CRRT are described in the literature [53, 56–66]. Citrate is infused into the blood at the beginning of the extracorporeal circuit where it chelates ionized calcium and inhibits the coagulation cascade [67]. Coagulation is adequately inhibited with an ionized calcium level less than 0.35 mmol/L in the extracorporeal circuit (measured as the post-filter ionized calcium concentration) [67, 68]. Since a portion of the calcium-citrate complex is lost across the hemofilter, calcium has to be infused back to the patient to replace the calcium lost. The remainder of the calcium-citrate complex enters the systemic circulation, where citrate is metabolized to bicarbonate by the liver and ionized calcium is released back to the circulation. By maintaining normal levels of ionized calcium in the systemic circulation, anticoagulation is limited to the extracorporeal circuit.

Advantages of RCA include avoidance of HIT and decreased risk of bleeding since only the CRRT circuit is anticoagulated. The primary disadvantages of RCA are potential electrolyte complications and the complexity of RCA protocols. The electrolyte complications include metabolic alkalosis, metabolic acidosis, hypernatremia when hypertonic citrate solutions are used, and hypocalcemia. Since 1 mole of citrate potentially yields 3 moles of bicarbonate, metabolic alkalosis can occur with excessive citrate administration or use of exogenous bicarbonate. Metabolic acidosis can occur when citrate accumulates in patients who cannot metabolize citrate, such as those with liver failure or severe lactic acidosis. Citrate accumulation and toxicity is characterized by low systemic ionized calcium levels from unmetabolized calcium-citrate complexes, elevated total serum calcium due to the need for higher systemic calcium infusion rates, metabolic acidosis with increased anion gap, and a disproportional rise in total systemic calcium to ionized calcium ratio of greater than 2.5 [69–72]. Frequent monitoring of acid-base status, electrolytes, and ionized calcium in the systemic circulation is necessary to prevent complications. If properly monitored, complications associated with RCA are uncommon.

A recent meta-analysis of 11 RCTs comparing RCA to UFH concluded that RCA significantly increased CRRT circuit lifespan, decreased circuit failure, and lowered bleeding risk [73]. The authors reported the incidence of HIT was higher in the heparin groups, while hypocalcemia was increased in citrate groups. No significant survival difference was observed between the groups. They concluded that RCA should be considered as a better anticoagulant than heparin for CRRT in AKI patients without any contraindication to citrate.

22.8 Dose of Renal Replacement Therapy

It is unclear how to define dose of RRT in patients with AKI. Traditionally, the "dose" or "intensity" of RRT in AKI has been assessed by urea clearance in PD, IHD, and PIRRT and by effluent volume (a surrogate of urea clearance) in CRRT. Urea clearance in IHD is most commonly quantified as the fractional urea clearance per treatment, expressed as Kt/V_{urea}. In CRRT, the effluent is comprised of the ultrafiltrate in CVVH, spent dialysate in CVVHD, and the sum of both in CVVHDF. The ability of a molecule to pass through the membrane is expressed as a ratio of the solute concentration in the effluent to that in plasma and is known as the sieving coefficient (SC) [74–76]. The clearance of a solute during CRRT is equal to the product of the SC and the effluent rate. Under usual conditions, the SC for urea and other low-molecular-weight solutes is close to 1 [76]. Thus, small-solute clearance is approximately equal to effluent flow, and the dose of CRRT is reported as effluent flow in mL/kg body weight per hour (mL/kg/h) [6].

Although several small, single-center trials have suggested that higher doses of IHD and CRRT are associated with improved outcomes, two large multicenter RCTs have not confirmed these findings [77–79]. In the Randomized Evaluation of Normal Versus Augmented Level Renal Replacement Therapy (RENAL) trial, patients were randomized to CVVHDF at 25 or 40 mL/kg/h [80]. In the Veterans Affairs/National Institutes of Health Acute Renal Failure Trial Network (ATN), patients transitioned between modalities as their hemodynamic status varied, receiving IHD with a target Kt/V_{urea} per treatment of 1.2–1.4 either three or six times per week when hemodynamically stable and CVVHDF at 20 or 35 mL/kg/h when hemodynamically unstable [81]. Both studies failed to detect any survival benefit from more intensive CRRT. However, both trials delivered more intense therapy in the "low-dose" arms than what is routinely delivered in clinical practice. In the ATN and RENAL trials, 95% and 88% of the prescribed CVVHDF dose were actually delivered, respectively. In the ATN study, the mean delivered Kt/V_{urea} was 1.3 with IHD. Overall survival rates in both trials were better than what has been reported in previous studies. Based on these results, the best evidence suggests that patients with dialysis-dependent AKI should receive the equivalent of at least three dialysis treatments per week with a delivered Kt/V value of 1.2, or CRRT at 20–25 mL/kg/h, with careful attention to ensuring that the target dose of therapy is actually delivered. More frequent IHD treatments may be needed if the target Kt/V or volume control cannot be achieved with IHD three times a week. In both IHD and CRRT, higher doses of therapy may be needed for hypercatabolic patients or for control of severe hyperkalemia or acidemia. Comparable data are not available to guide dosing of PD or PIRRT.

References

1. Karvellas CJ, Farhat MR, Sajjad I, et al. A comparison of early versus late initiation of renal replacement therapy in critically ill patients with acute kidney injury: a systematic review and meta-analysis. Crit Care. 2011;15:R72.
2. Seabra VF, Balk EM, Liangos O, Sosa MA, Cendoroglo M, Jaber BL. Timing of renal replacement therapy initiation in acute renal failure: a meta-analysis. Am J Kidney Dis. 2008;52:272–84.
3. Zarbock A, Kellum JA, Schmidt C, et al. Effect of early vs delayed initiation of renal replacement therapy on mortality in critically ill patients with acute kidney injury: the ELAIN randomized clinical trial. JAMA. 2016;315:2190–9.
4. Gaudry S, Hajage D, Schortgen F, et al. Initiation strategies for renal-replacement therapy in the intensive care unit. N Engl J Med. 2016;375:122–33.
5. Selby NM, McIntyre CW. A systematic review of the clinical effects of reducing dialysate fluid temperature. Nephrol Dial Transplant. 2006;21:1883–98.
6. Palevsky PM, O'Connor TZ, Chertow GM, et al. Intensity of renal replacement therapy in acute kidney

injury: perspective from within the Acute Renal Failure Trial Network Study. Crit Care. 2009;13:310.
7. Emili S, Black NA, Paul RV, Rexing CJ, Ullian ME. A protocol-based treatment for intradialytic hypotension in hospitalized hemodialysis patients. Am J Kidney Dis. 1999;33:1107–14.
8. Conger J. Dialysis and related therapies. Semin Nephrol. 1998;18:533–40.
9. Briglia A, Paganini EP. Acute renal failure in the intensive care unit. Therapy overview, patient risk stratification, complications of renal replacement, and special circumstances. Clin Chest Med. 1999;20:347–66, viii
10. Paganini EP, Sandy D, Moreno L, Kozlowski L, Sakai K. The effect of sodium and ultrafiltration modelling on plasma volume changes and haemodynamic stability in intensive care patients receiving haemodialysis for acute renal failure: a prospective, stratified, randomized, cross-over study. Nephrol Dial Transplant. 1996;11(Suppl 8):32–7.
11. Davenport A, Finn R, Goldsmith HJ. Management of patients with renal failure complicated by cerebral oedema. Blood Purif. 1989;7:203–9.
12. Cerda J, Ronco C. Modalities of continuous renal replacement therapy: technical and clinical considerations. Semin Dial. 2009;22:114–22.
13. Ronco C, Bellomo R. Basic mechanisms and definitions for continuous renal replacement therapies. Int J Artif Organs. 1996;19:95–9.
14. Ronco C, Ricci Z. Renal replacement therapies: physiological review. Intensive Care Med. 2008;34:2139–46.
15. Clark WR, Turk JE, Kraus MA, Gao D. Dose determinants in continuous renal replacement therapy. Artif Organs. 2003;27:815–20.
16. Brunet S, Leblanc M, Geadah D, Parent D, Courteau S, Cardinal J. Diffusive and convective solute clearances during continuous renal replacement therapy at various dialysate and ultrafiltration flow rates. Am J Kidney Dis. 1999;34:486–92.
17. Friedrich JO, Wald R, Bagshaw SM, Burns KE, Adhikari NK. Hemofiltration compared to hemodialysis for acute kidney injury: systematic review and meta-analysis. Crit Care. 2012;16:R146.
18. De Vriese AS, Colardyn FA, Philippe JJ, Vanholder RC, De Sutter JH, Lameire NH. Cytokine removal during continuous hemofiltration in septic patients. J Am Soc Nephrol. 1999;10:846–53.
19. Farese S, Jakob SM, Kalicki R, Frey FJ, Uehlinger DE. Treatment of acute renal failure in the intensive care unit: lower costs by intermittent dialysis than continuous venovenous hemodiafiltration. Artif Organs. 2009;33:634–40.
20. Heering P, Morgera S, Schmitz FJ, et al. Cytokine removal and cardiovascular hemodynamics in septic patients with continuous venovenous hemofiltration. Intensive Care Med. 1997;23:288–96.
21. Hoffmann JN, Hartl WH, Deppisch R, Faist E, Jochum M, Inthorn D. Effect of hemofiltration on hemodynamics and systemic concentrations of anaphylatoxins and cytokines in human sepsis. Intensive Care Med. 1996;22:1360–7.
22. Morgera S, Slowinski T, Melzer C, et al. Renal replacement therapy with high-cutoff hemofilters: Impact of convection and diffusion on cytokine clearances and protein status. Am J Kidney Dis. 2004;43:444–53.
23. van Deuren M, van der Meer JW. Hemofiltration in septic patients is not able to alter the plasma concentration of cytokines therapeutically. Intensive Care Med. 2000;26:1176–8.
24. Clark E, Molnar AO, Joannes-Boyau O, Honore PM, Sikora L, Bagshaw SM. High-volume hemofiltration for septic acute kidney injury: a systematic review and meta-analysis. Crit Care. 2014;18:R7.
25. Combes A, Brechot N, Amour J, et al. Early high-volume hemofiltration versus standard care for post-cardiac surgery shock. The HEROICS Study. Am J Respir Crit Care Med. 2015;192:1179–90.
26. Fieghen HE, Friedrich JO, Burns KE, et al. The hemodynamic tolerability and feasibility of sustained low efficiency dialysis in the management of critically ill patients with acute kidney injury. BMC Nephrol. 2010;11:32.
27. Kumar VA, Yeun JY, Depner TA, Don BR. Extended daily dialysis vs. continuous hemodialysis for ICU patients with acute renal failure: a two-year single center report. Int J Artif Organs. 2004;27:371–9.
28. Kielstein JT, Kretschmer U, Ernst T, et al. Efficacy and cardiovascular tolerability of extended dialysis in critically ill patients: a randomized controlled study. Am J Kidney Dis. 2004;43:342–9.
29. Wu VC, Wang CH, Wang WJ, et al. Sustained low-efficiency dialysis versus continuous veno-venous hemofiltration for postsurgical acute renal failure. Am J Surg. 2010;199:466–76.
30. Steiner RW. Continuous equilibration peritoneal dialysis in acute renal failure. Perit Dial Int. 1989;9:5–7.
31. Phu NH, Hien TT, Mai NT, et al. Hemofiltration and peritoneal dialysis in infection-associated acute renal failure in Vietnam. N Engl J Med. 2002;347:895–902.
32. Rabindranath K, Adams J, Macleod AM, Muirhead N. Intermittent versus continuous renal replacement therapy for acute renal failure in adults. Cochrane Database Syst Rev. 2007:CD003773.
33. Bouchard J, Soroko SB, Chertow GM, et al. Fluid accumulation, survival and recovery of kidney function in critically ill patients with acute kidney injury. Kidney Int. 2009;76:422–7.
34. Bagshaw SM, Berthiaume LR, Delaney A, Bellomo R. Continuous versus intermittent renal replacement therapy for critically ill patients with acute kidney injury: a meta-analysis. Crit Care Med. 2008;36:610–7.
35. Pannu N, Klarenbach S, Wiebe N, Manns B, Tonelli M. Renal replacement therapy in patients with acute renal failure: a systematic review. JAMA. 2008;299:793–805.
36. Tonelli M, Manns B, Feller-Kopman D. Acute renal failure in the intensive care unit: a systematic review

of the impact of dialytic modality on mortality and renal recovery. Am J Kidney Dis. 2002;40:875–85.
37. Kellum JA, Angus DC, Johnson JP, et al. Continuous versus intermittent renal replacement therapy: a meta-analysis. Intensive Care Med. 2002;28:29–37.
38. Schneider AG, Bellomo R, Bagshaw SM, et al. Choice of renal replacement therapy modality and dialysis dependence after acute kidney injury: a systematic review and meta-analysis. Intensive Care Med. 2013;39:987–97.
39. Baldwin I, Bellomo R, Naka T, Koch B, Fealy N. A pilot randomized controlled comparison of extended daily dialysis with filtration and continuous veno-venous hemofiltration: fluid removal and hemodynamics. Int J Artif Organs. 2007;30:1083–9.
40. Baldwin I, Naka T, Koch B, Fealy N, Bellomo R. A pilot randomised controlled comparison of continuous veno-venous haemofiltration and extended daily dialysis with filtration: effect on small solutes and acid-base balance. Intensive Care Med. 2007;33(5):830.
41. Zhang L, Yang J, Eastwood GM, Zhu G, Tanaka A, Bellomo R. Extended daily dialysis versus continuous renal replacement therapy for acute kidney injury: a meta-analysis. Am J Kidney Dis. 2015;66:322–30.
42. Gabriel DP, Caramori JT, Martim LC, Barretti P, Balbi AL. High volume peritoneal dialysis vs daily hemodialysis: a randomized, controlled trial in patients with acute kidney injury. Kidney Int Suppl. 2008:S87–93.
43. Ponce D, Berbel MN, Abrao JM, Goes CR, Balbi AL. A randomized clinical trial of high volume peritoneal dialysis versus extended daily hemodialysis for acute kidney injury patients. Int Urol Nephrol. 2013;45:869–78.
44. Chionh CY, Soni SS, Finkelstein FO, Ronco C, Cruz DN. Use of peritoneal dialysis in AKI: a systematic review. Clin J Am Soc Nephrol. 2013;8:1649–60.
45. Davenport A. Renal replacement therapy in the patient with acute brain injury. Am J Kidney Dis. 2001;37:457–66.
46. Davenport A. Continuous renal replacement therapies in patients with acute neurological injury. Semin Dial. 2009;22:165–8.
47. Lin CM, Lin JW, Tsai JT, et al. Intracranial pressure fluctuation during hemodialysis in renal failure patients with intracranial hemorrhage. Acta Neurochir Suppl. 2008;101:141–4.
48. Davenport A. Continuous renal replacement therapies in patients with liver disease. Semin Dial. 2009;22:169–72.
49. Hirsh J, Warkentin TE, Shaughnessy SG, et al. Heparin and low-molecular-weight heparin: mechanisms of action, pharmacokinetics, dosing, monitoring, efficacy, and safety. Chest. 2001;119:64S–94S.
50. Davenport A, Will EJ, Davison AM. Comparison of the use of standard heparin and prostacyclin anticoagulation in spontaneous and pump-driven extracorporeal circuits in patients with combined acute renal and hepatic failure. Nephron. 1994;66:431–7.
51. Martin PY, Chevrolet JC, Suter P, Favre H. Anticoagulation in patients treated by continuous venovenous hemofiltration: a retrospective study. Am J Kidney Dis. 1994;24:806–12.
52. van de Wetering J, Westendorp RG, van der Hoeven JG, Stolk B, Feuth JD, Chang PC. Heparin use in continuous renal replacement procedures: the struggle between filter coagulation and patient hemorrhage. J Am Soc Nephrol. 1996;7:145–50.
53. Tolwani AJ, Prendergast MB, Speer RR, Stofan BS, Wille KM. A practical citrate anticoagulation continuous venovenous hemodiafiltration protocol for metabolic control and high solute clearance. Clin J Am Soc Nephrol. 2006;1:79–87.
54. Morgera S. Regional anticoagulation with citrate: expanding its indications. Crit Care Med. 2011;39:399–400.
55. Oudemans-van Straaten HM, Kellum JA, Bellomo R. Clinical review: anticoagulation for continuous renal replacement therapy--heparin or citrate? Crit Care. 2011;15:202.
56. Bagshaw SM, Laupland KB, Boiteau PJ, Godinez-Luna T. Is regional citrate superior to systemic heparin anticoagulation for continuous renal replacement therapy? A prospective observational study in an adult regional critical care system. J Crit Care. 2005;20:155–61.
57. Hofmann RM, Maloney C, Ward DM, Becker BN. A novel method for regional citrate anticoagulation in continuous venovenous hemofiltration (CVVHF). Ren Fail. 2002;24:325–35.
58. Cointault O, Kamar N, Bories P, et al. Regional citrate anticoagulation in continuous venovenous haemodiafiltration using commercial solutions. Nephrol Dial Transplant. 2004;19:171–8.
59. Bihorac A, Ross EA. Continuous venovenous hemofiltration with citrate-based replacement fluid: efficacy, safety, and impact on nutrition. Am J Kidney Dis. 2005;46:908–18.
60. Kutsogiannis DJ, Mayers I, Chin WD, Gibney RT. Regional citrate anticoagulation in continuous venovenous hemodiafiltration. Am J Kidney Dis. 2000;35:802–11.
61. Mehta RL, McDonald BR, Aguilar MM, Ward DM. Regional citrate anticoagulation for continuous arteriovenous hemodialysis in critically ill patients. Kidney Int. 1990;38:976–81.
62. Monchi M, Berghmans D, Ledoux D, Canivet JL, Dubois B, Damas P. Citrate vs. heparin for anticoagulation in continuous venovenous hemofiltration: a prospective randomized study. Intensive Care Med. 2004;30:260–5.
63. Palsson R, Niles JL. Regional citrate anticoagulation in continuous venovenous hemofiltration in critically ill patients with a high risk of bleeding. Kidney Int. 1999;55:1991–7.
64. Swartz R, Pasko D, O'Toole J, Starmann B. Improving the delivery of continuous renal replacement therapy using regional citrate anticoagulation. Clin Nephrol. 2004;61:134–43.
65. Tobe SW, Aujla P, Walele AA, et al. A novel regional citrate anticoagulation protocol for CRRT using

only commercially available solutions. J Crit Care. 2003;18:121–9.
66. Tolwani AJ, Campbell RC, Schenk MB, Allon M, Warnock DG. Simplified citrate anticoagulation for continuous renal replacement therapy. Kidney Int. 2001;60:370–4.
67. Calatzis A, Toepfer M, Schramm W, Spannagl M, Schiffl H. Citrate anticoagulation for extracorporeal circuits: effects on whole blood coagulation activation and clot formation. Nephron. 2001;89:233–6.
68. Pinnick RV, Wiegmann TB, Diederich DA. Regional citrate anticoagulation for hemodialysis in the patient at high risk for bleeding. N Engl J Med. 1983;308:258–61.
69. Apsner R, Schwarzenhofer M, Derfler K, Zauner C, Ratheiser K, Kranz A. Impairment of citrate metabolism in acute hepatic failure. Wien Klin Wochenschr. 1997;109:123–7.
70. Kramer L, Bauer E, Joukhadar C, et al. Citrate pharmacokinetics and metabolism in cirrhotic and noncirrhotic critically ill patients. Crit Care Med. 2003;31:2450–5.
71. Meier-Kriesche HU, Gitomer J, Finkel K, DuBose T. Increased total to ionized calcium ratio during continuous venovenous hemodialysis with regional citrate anticoagulation. Crit Care Med. 2001;29:748–52.
72. Bakker AJ, Boerma EC, Keidel H, Kingma P, van der Voort PH. Detection of citrate overdose in critically ill patients on citrate-anticoagulated venovenous haemofiltration: use of ionised and total/ionised calcium. Clin Chem Lab Med. 2006;44:962–6.
73. Bai M, Zhou M, He L, et al. Citrate versus heparin anticoagulation for continuous renal replacement therapy: an updated meta-analysis of RCTs. Intensive Care Med. 2015;41:2098–110.
74. Clark WR, Ronco C. Renal replacement therapy in acute renal failure: solute removal mechanisms and dose quantification. Kidney Int Suppl. 1998;66:S133–7.
75. Clark WR, Ronco C. CRRT efficiency and efficacy in relation to solute size. Kidney Int Suppl. 1999:S3–7.
76. Troyanov S, Cardinal J, Geadah D, et al. Solute clearances during continuous venovenous haemofiltration at various ultrafiltration flow rates using Multiflow-100 and HF1000 filters. Nephrol Dial Transplant. 2003;18:961–6.
77. Ronco C, Bellomo R, Homel P, et al. Effects of different doses in continuous veno-venous haemofiltration on outcomes of acute renal failure: a prospective randomised trial. Lancet. 2000;356:26–30.
78. Schiffl H, Lang SM, Fischer R. Daily hemodialysis and the outcome of acute renal failure. N Engl J Med. 2002;346:305–10.
79. Saudan P, Niederberger M, De Seigneux S, et al. Adding a dialysis dose to continuous hemofiltration increases survival in patients with acute renal failure. Kidney Int. 2006;70(7):1312.
80. Palevsky PM, Zhang JH, O'Connor TZ, et al. Intensity of renal support in critically ill patients with acute kidney injury. N Engl J Med. 2008;359:7–20.
81. Investigators RRTS, Bellomo R, Cass A, et al. Intensity of continuous renal-replacement therapy in critically ill patients. N Engl J Med. 2009;361:1627–38.

23 Drug Dosing in Acute Kidney Injury

Jeremy R. DeGrado, James F. Gilmore, Benjamin Hohlfelder, Craig A. Stevens, and Steven Gabardi

23.1 Introduction

Acute kidney injury (AKI) has traditionally been defined as the rapid loss of renal function resulting in retention of nitrogenous waste products and impaired regulation of extracellular volume and electrolyte homeostasis. The Acute Kidney Injury Network (AKIN) suggested the use of the broad term, AKI, which represents a complete spectrum of acute renal failure.

The prevalence of AKI in hospitalized patients has sharply increased in recent years. This is alarming as mortality can range from 10% to 80% in this population, depending on the severity of AKI and comorbid disease states [1–5]. To compound matters, many pharmacologic agents act on or are eliminated by the kidneys. The pharmacokinetic and pharmacodynamic properties of these medications may be altered in patients with renal dysfunction. As a result, subtherapeutic or supratherapeutic drug concentrations may be more likely, and poor clinical outcomes can result [6].

Accurate estimation of glomerular filtration rate (GFR) is difficult in patients with AKI. The Cockcroft-Gault equation, the simplified refitted MDRD equation, and the CKD-EPI equation were all shown to be poor predictors of GFR in patients with AKI (Table 23.1) [7, 8]. Total body water changes rapidly in patients with AKI. Therefore, changes in serum creatinine do not always correlate well to improvement or deterioration of kidney function [9].

Historically, the approach to drug dosing in patients with AKI has been the same as in patients with chronic kidney disease (CKD). The majority of dosing recommendations for AKI have been extrapolated from studies performed in patients with stable CKD. Of those patients presenting with AKI, 23–45% will have CKD as a predisposing factor [10–13]. In patients presenting with AKI on CKD, it may be more appropriate to utilize CKD dosing recommendations initially to avoid underdosing therapeutic regimens depending on the nephrotoxic profile of the medication being used, as well as the urgency to achieve steady state (i.e., antibiotics). Close monitoring of medication levels, laboratory values, and

J. R. DeGrado
Pharmacy Department, Brigham and Women's Hospital, Boston, MA, USA
e-mail: jdegrado@partners.org

J. F. Gilmore · B. Hohlfelder · C. A. Stevens
Department of Pharmacy Services, Brigham and Women's Hospital, Boston, MA, USA
e-mail: jgilmore2@partners.org
bhohlfelder@partners.org; castevens@partners.org;

S. Gabardi (✉)
Department of Transplant Surgery, Brigham and Women's Hospital, Boston, MA, USA

Department of Pharmacy Services/Renal Division, Brigham and Women's Hospital, Boston, MA, USA

Harvard Medical School, Boston, MA, USA
e-mail: sgabardi@partners.org

S. S. Waikar et al. (eds.), *Core Concepts in Acute Kidney Injury*,
https://doi.org/10.1007/978-1-4939-8628-6_23

Table 23.1 Common estimations/formulas for renal clearance

Clearance estimation	Equation
Cockcroft-Gault equation	CrCl = [(age − 140) × IBW]/(72 × SCr) × 0.85 (females only)
Modification of Diet in Renal Disease (MDRD)	GFR = 186 × (SCr/88.4) −1.154 × (age) −0.203 × (0.742 if female) × (1.210 if black)
Chronic Kidney Disease Epidemiology Collaboration (CKD-EPI)	GFR = 141 × min (SCr/κ, 1)α × max (SCr/κ, 1) − 1.209 × 0.993 (age) × 1.018 [if female] × 1.159 [if black] κ is 0.7 for females and 0.9 for males α is −0.329 for females and −0.411 for males Min indicates the minimum of S_{cr}/κ or 1, and max indicates the maximum of S_{cr}/κ or 1
Schwartz equation (pediatrics)	GFR = (k × height)/SCr Infant (low body weight, <1 year): k = 0.33 Infant (term <1 year): k = 0.45 Child or adolescent girl: k = 0.55 Adolescent boy: k = 0.7
Counahan-Barratt equation (pediatrics)	GFR = (0.43 × height)/SCr

CrCl creatinine clearance, *IBW* ideal body weight, *SCr* serum creatinine, *GFR* glomerular filtration rate

Table 23.2 Pharmacokinetic alterations in patients with renal injury

Pharmacokinetic parameter	Alteration
Absorption	Increased gastroparesis Delayed gastric emptying Increased gastric pH Reduced intestinal drug metabolism Increased P-glycoprotein-mediated medication transport
Distribution	Decreased medication binding to albumin Increased α1-glycoprotein expression Altered medication ionization, tissue distribution, and clearance Altered volume of distribution due to changes in volume status
Metabolism	Altered nonrenal metabolism of medications (may be preserved early in AKI course, lost later in AKI course) Loss of renal-mediated medication metabolism
Elimination	Decreased tubular secretion and reabsorption Accumulation of endogenous and exogenous acidic and basic compounds that compete for transporters Decreased medication filtration by impaired tubular secretion

hemodynamic parameters can assist in the guiding of clinicians on the renal function of a patient with AKI is often fluctuating and difficult to quantify [14]. Specific medication considerations will be reviewed in this chapter.

Renal drug clearance, comprised of glomerular filtration, tubular secretion, and renal drug metabolism, is affected by renal dysfunction. The type of renal dysfunction may affect several renal and nonrenal parameters of drug handling. Renal injury influences drug disposition through changes in several pharmacokinetic characteristics (Table 23.2). Common pharmacokinetic abnormalities seen in patients with CKD include reduced oral absorption and glomerular filtration, altered tubular secretion and reabsorption, and changes in intestinal and hepatic clearance [15]. The impact of AKI on nonrenal clearance, predominantly hepatic metabolism, is not fully understood [16]. Nonrenal clearance appears to be preserved early in the course of AKI and deteriorates as the course of AKI is prolonged. Thus, dosing strategies extrapolated from patients with CKD may result in subtherapeutic drug concentrations and ineffective treatment. Critically ill patients who present with multi-system organ dysfunction may have alterations in drug pharmacokinetics leading to decreased metabolism and excretion, potentially resulting in supratherapeutic drug concentrations and toxicity. Achieving a balance between under- and overdosing requires rigorous monitoring and individualized dosing.

Several published reviews have discussed in great detail drug dosing strategies in CKD and/or patients with AKI receiving renal replacement therapies (RRT). This review will focus on key concepts surrounding the dosing of medications in patients with AKI not receiving RRT.

23.2 Alterations in Pharmacokinetic Parameters

Understanding pharmacokinetic parameters and how they may fluctuate is critical to effective management of patients with AKI. Pharmacokinetics refers to the movement of a medication throughout the body. Pharmacokinetic parameters are generally grouped into four major categories: absorption, distribution, metabolism, and elimination (Table 23.3) [17]. The few currently available pharmacokinetic analyses have generally been conducted in patients with CKD and rarely in patients actively experiencing AKI. For this reason, clinicians will often need to extrapolate known information about a medication's pharmacokinetic profile to adjust the therapeutic regimen in a patient with AKI.

Table 23.3 Pharmacokinetic parameters and definitions

Pharmacokinetic parameter	Definition
Absorption	The rate and extent to which a medication moves into the systemic circulation after administration
Area under the curve	The area under a drug concentration vs. time graph
Bioavailability	The fraction of a medication that reaches systemic circulation after administration. For intravenous and other direct routes of administration, bioavailability is 100%
Distribution	The movement of medications from the intravascular space to the surrounding tissues and organs
Elimination	Drug handling process by which medications are removed from the body
Half-life	The time needed for the concentration of a medication to be decreased by 50%
Metabolism	The process by which biotransformation of medication takes place in the body
Steady state	The point at which plasma concentrations of a medication remain consistent, as the rate of drug administration is equal to the rate of drug elimination. Steady state is typically achieved after three to five medication half-lives
Volume of distribution	Theoretical volume of plasma that it would take to achieve the observed serum concentration of a medication, in relation to the administered dose. Medications with a large volume of distribution are primarily lipophilic and distribute to peripheral tissues. Medications with a smaller volume of distribution are primarily hydrophilic and are generally contained within the intravascular space

23.3 Absorption

Medication absorption describes the rate and extent to which a medication moves into the systemic circulation after administration. The term bioavailability is used to quantify the fraction of administered drug reaching the systemic circulation. Direct routes of administration, such as the intravenous route, have a bioavailability of 100%. Enteral absorption of a medication will depend on several medication-specific variables such as ionization, lipophilicity, particle size, and solubility [18]. The bioavailability of a medication may also be influenced by numerous physiologic changes in the gastrointestinal (GI) tract, including surface area, regional blood flow, gastric pH, delayed gastric emptying, and intestinal drug metabolism [17, 19, 20].

Depending on the etiology of a patient's AKI, elements of medication absorption may also be impacted. For example, in patients receiving vasoactive agents administered to maintain systemic perfusion may reduce blood flow to the GI tract and SC tissues and cause decreased gastric motility [21]. There is conflicting data on to the degree which vasoactive agents will reduce absorption through the GI tract [22–25].

While there is a lack of data specific to patients with AKI, data examining gastric emptying in patients with CKD have yielded conflicting results regarding clinical relevance [24–28].

Gastric pH is often increased in patients with AKI and will often influence a medication's bioavailability. Although its etiology is likely multifactorial, one proposed mechanism is increased ammonia formation in the gut secondary to conversion of salivary urea by urease enzymes [29]. For some medications, dissolution and ionization are reduced in an environment of increased gastric pH, resulting in reduced bioavailability [17, 30].

Intestinal metabolism is a significant component of drug bioavailability, and CKD-induced reductions in intestinal metabolism and P-glycoprotein-mediated drug transport may result in increased medication bioavailability [31]. We will discuss what is theorized about these changes more in depth in the metabolism section.

23.4 Distribution

Distribution, or volume of distribution (Vd), is a pharmacokinetic variable that can help to quantify the serum concentration achieved after an administered dose. A medication's Vd can also help to classify a medication as lipophilic or hydrophilic. Hydrophilic medications will largely remain in plasma water volume, while lipophilic medications will spread into the body's fat stores. Lipophilic drugs will have a significantly increased Vd [18]. Patients experiencing AKI can experience changes in plasma protein binding and fluid status that can have clinically significant effects on Vd, resulting in changes in a medication's plasma and tissue concentrations, as well as its safety and efficacy.

23.4.1 Plasma Protein Binding

Several medications will bind to plasma proteins in the bloodstream, and AKI brought on by critical illness will commonly lead to alterations in plasma protein concentrations [17]. Plasma proteins are relevant for medications as the unbound concentration of a medication is what will exert its pharmacologic effects. With protein-bound medications, any decrease in plasma proteins or protein binding may influence efficacy and toxicity. The most common plasma proteins described in the literature are alpha-1-acid glycoprotein (AAG) and albumin. Basic medications will generally bind to AAG, and acidic medications (warfarin, phenytoin, valproic acid, and salicylates) will more often bind to albumin [32–34].

The alteration in protein concentration expected in a patient with AKI is dependent on the etiology of the renal injury. Patients with AKI often have low serum albumin levels due to increased vascular permeability, protein catabolism, malnutrition, and/or acute illness. Decreases in serum albumin can lead to an amplified risk for adverse events due to a higher drug free fraction [35]. Although AAG is an acute-phase reactant and would be expected to be increased during trauma, surgery, or acute illness, medication binding this protein tends to be less affected by AKI [36].

Hypoalbuminemia will lead to increased plasma concentrations of highly protein-bound medications, which will often lead to an increased chance for toxic side effects to occur. Antiepileptics, most notably phenytoin and valproate, are frequently cited as having increased concentrations in hypoalbuminemic states. Therapeutic drug monitoring (TDM) of these medications should occur when possible, and adjustment of TDM levels for low albumin should occur to try to mitigate the possibility of toxic effects [37].

Increases in AAG may or may not occur depending on the etiology of patient's AKI. The clinical sequelae of changes in AAG are more difficult to routinely monitor for than changes in serum albumin concentrations. When AAG concentrations rise, clinicians should expect an acute rise in bound medication concentration, decreasing Vd and unbound medication concentration, leading to a prolonged duration of effect due to decreased clearance. Clinicians should be aware of the potential for increased duration of effect in AKI brought on by critical illness while remaining vigilant about the increased potential for adverse effects.

Metabolic acidosis and respiratory alkalosis often accompany AKI. Depending on the pKa of medications, differences in pH between the tissue and plasma compartments may alter drug ionization, tissue distribution, and clearance [38–41].

23.4.2 Fluid Status

Fluid status assessment and resuscitation are common tenants of AKI management. For example, patients with AKI brought on by severe sepsis and septic shock will likely be treated with aggressive goal-directed administration of intravenous fluids. This large volume of fluid administered will increase the total volume of body water, which will ultimately decrease the serum concentration of hydrophilic medications. Accumulation of fluid during other etiologies of AKI may result in lower drug concentrations. Often, if patients with AKI are diuresed, higher drug concentrations may result [35]. Understanding the physiology of the AKI and the patient's intravascular fluid status can help clinicians develop a plan for proper monitoring and dose adjustment. In general, the changes in drug disposition due to fluid status are similar in patients with CKD as they are in AKI; however patients with AKI often will have a fluctuating disease course that can alter Vd rapidly.

23.5 Metabolism

Many medications will undergo biotransformation or metabolism in order to enhance eventual excretion [17]. Traditionally, metabolism is considered to take place primarily in the liver, though metabolism occurs in several other organs including the lung, brain, and kidney. Knowledge of the changes in metabolism can help clinicians plan for variations in effectiveness and risk of side effects of certain medications.

Generally hepatic metabolism consists of two distinct phases. Phase 1 metabolism is largely mediated by chemical reactions of the cytochrome P450 (CYP450) enzyme system to convert the parent compound into metabolites. Metabolites are typically less potent than the parent compound, though some medications have metabolites that are more potent and potentially toxic. Phase 2 metabolism consists of glucuronidation and sulfation reactions.

There is an abundance of clinical evidence demonstrating that CKD significantly influences the nonrenal clearance of several medications [42–50]. Depending on the etiology of AKI, nonrenal clearance appears to be preserved early in the course of illness. Patients with AKI brought on by septic shock in the acute phase may be aggressively fluid resuscitated and may result in increased hepatic blood flow and hepatic metabolism. A limited number of studies have investigated the differences in nonrenal clearance of medications in patients with AKI compared with CKD. Notably, patients with AKI have demonstrated decreased nonrenal clearance of medications such as imipenem, meropenem, and vancomycin [51, 52]. Animal studies have also shown that AKI may alter hepatic metabolism of diltiazem, tacrolimus, and theophylline [53, 54].

Some of these changes in nonrenal medication clearance may be due to the fact that some patients with AKI may present with concomitant conditions that impact drug metabolism and elimination, including hepatic damage (cirrhosis) or dysfunction (shock and decreased hepatic blood flow) and cardiovascular or respiratory failure [55, 56]. Common etiologies of AKI in critically ill patients, including sepsis, pancreatitis, and liver failure, can cause profound vasodilatation and decreases in GFR, renal blood flow, and drug elimination [57]. The use of vasopressors will generally lead to decreased metabolism due to decreased hepatic blood flow, while systemic vasodilators may lead to the opposite effect.

A component of drug biotransformation that cannot be overlooked is the drug-metabolizing capacity of the kidneys. Ordinarily, the kidneys have nearly 15% of the metabolic function of the liver, with the highest amount of metabolic enzymes located in the renal cortex [58].

23.6 Elimination

In patients with AKI, estimates of renal clearance will most likely be unable to accurately predict renal function, as a single laboratory time point is

Table 23.4 Tubular drug secretion by anionic and cationic transport systems

Anion transport		Cation transport	
Acyclovir	Acetazolamide	Amantadine	Amiloride
Ampicillin	Ascorbic acid	Amphetamines	B-blockers
Captopril	Cephalosporins	Cimetidine	Digoxin
Cisplatin	Ethacrynic acid	Dopamine	Epinephrine
Furosemide	Ibuprofen	Ethambutol	Famotidine
Indomethacin	Methotrexate	Metformin	Methadone
Nafcillin	Naproxen	Morphine	Neostigmine
Nitrofurantoin	Penicillin G	Norepinephrine	Procainamide
Phenobarbital	Probenecid	Quinidine	Ranitidine
Quinolones	Salicylates	Trimethoprim	
Sulfonamides	Thiazides		

used in these calculations. Serum creatinine is used as a surrogate marker for renal function and can often lag behind acute changes in GFR. Urine collection and monitoring of hourly urine output may be more up-to-date markers of renal function and elimination activity.

AKI can increase glomerular permeability, resulting in increased clearance rates of highly protein-bound drugs. For example, in patients with nephrotic syndrome, the glomerular basement membrane loses negative charge and allows albumin and other large molecules to leak across the barrier [38]. Tubular secretion is an active process that transports and reabsorbs medications between interstitial fluid and nephron by an anion-cation transport system (Table 23.4). In patients with AKI, this mechanism may be decreased as endogenous and exogenous acids and bases accumulate and compete for transporters [40, 59, 60]. Competition for tubular secretion can alter the pharmacologic effect of the administered medication.

Use of medications without renal clearance mechanisms and appropriate dose adjustments of those with renal clearance mechanisms are required for successful management of a patient with an AKI. Dosing strategies and recommendations regarding specific classes of medications will be discussed in the next section.

23.7 Dosing Theories in Acute Renal Failure

23.7.1 General Considerations

As in patients with normal renal function, the goal in dosing patients with AKI is to achieve goal concentrations of medications in the serum or site of action without underdosing or overdosing. Pharmacodynamic (i.e., antimicrobial agents with time-dependent vs. concentration-dependent killing effects) and pharmacokinetic parameters, potential side effects of drug accumulation, and clinical status of patient (i.e., hemodynamic instability, severe inflammatory state, etc.) must be considered to attain this goal [61]. Specific medication-related factors must also be understood when designing a regimen most likely to achieve these targets. Information regarding notable medication classes will be discussed in a later section.

23.7.2 Loading Dose

The time for a medication to reach steady-state concentration is approximately 3–5 half-lives. Loading doses are considered for drugs with long half-lives that will not achieve therapeutic levels for an extended period of time or in scenarios where a delay in the achievement of therapeutic levels has been associated with worsened patient outcomes. The administration of a loading dose before maintenance dosing allows for more rapid achievement of therapeutic plasma concentrations [17]. Patients with AKI will likely require adjustment of maintenance doses to avoid accumulation of drug. However, the necessity of the loading dose in applicable medications to promptly achieve therapeutic concentrations still remains [43, 45]. The loading dose is dependent on both the volume of distribution and the desired plasma concentration; therefore, patients with excess total body water or increased volumes of distribution may require a higher than normal loading dose to take into account a change in Vd [61, 62]. Conversely, in patients with reduced Vd, a lower loading dose may be appropriate [45, 63].

23.7.3 Maintenance Dose

Maintenance doses are administered to maintain steady-state concentrations of drug in the plasma and at the site of action. These doses may require adjustment depending on the patient's ability to metabolize the drug hepatically or eliminate the drug renally, assuming significant portions of the drug go through these pathways [64]. Medications that require renal dose adjustment can either have their dose decreased, dosing interval extended, or a combination of both [43, 64]. The type of dosing adjustment made will attempt to maximize efficacy while minimizing toxicity resulting from drug accumulation. For example, medications that require higher concentrations to achieve their therapeutic effect should have their interval extended, while those that are likely to accumulate and cause adverse effects may have their dose reduced as well.

23.8 Therapeutic Drug Monitoring

Many medications have laboratory assays that can be utilized to directly measure serum concentrations or the pharmacodynamic effect of the drug. Particularly in patients with AKI, where a patient's drug handling may change rapidly, utilization of these laboratory measures when appropriate is vital to ensure efficacy and safety. Medications with narrow therapeutic indices should undergo close monitoring throughout the course of AKI to maximize patient outcomes. In general, TDM should take place when a medication has reached steady state, although in patients with AKI, TDM may take place earlier in the course of therapy to ensure that medication accumulation has not occurred. A list of medications with commonly measured TDM levels is provided in Table 23.5.

Table 23.5 Medications with commonly utilized therapeutic drug monitoring levels

Medication	Goal TDM levels
Antiepileptic drugs (AEDs)	
Phenytoin	Trough: 10–20 mcg/mL Note: must be adjusted for hypoalbuminemia and renal insufficiency
Carbamazepine	Trough: 4–12 mcg/mL
Valproate	Trough: 50–100 mcg/mL
Phenobarbital	Trough: 10–40 mcg/mL (may choose narrower range, i.e., 20–30 mcg/mL)
Antimicrobials	
Vancomycin	Trough: 10–20 mcg/mL (15–20 mcg/mL for sites of infection with poor vancomycin penetration, i.e., lung, brain)

(continued)

Table 23.5 (continued)

Medication	Goal TDM levels
Aminoglycosides (gentamicin = G; tobramycin = T; amikacin = A)	*Treatment of gram-negative organisms*: HEAT dosing: Peak: generally not required Trough: <1 mcg/mL (G/T); <4 mcg/mL (A) Treatment of patients with cystic fibrosis: Peak: 20–30 mcg/mL (G/T); 40–60 mcg/mL (A) Trough: <1 mcg/mL (G/T); <4 mcg/mL (A) Traditional dosing: Peak: 4–8 mcg/mL (G/T); 20–35 (A) Trough: < 1–2 mcg/mL (G/T); <5–8 mcg/mL (A) *Treatment of gram-positive organisms*: Synergy dosing: Peak: generally not required Trough: <1 mcg/mL (G/T); <4 mcg/mL (A)
Voriconazole	Trough: 2–6 mcg/mL
Posaconazole	Trough: >700 ng/mL
Cardiovascular medications	
Digoxin	*Heart failure*: Trough: 0.5–0.9 ng/mL *Atrial fibrillation*: Trough: <2 ng/mL (digoxin should be titrated to effect in management of atrial fibrillation; trough should be checked when there is concern for toxicity)
Lidocaine	Trough: 1–5 mcg/mL
Warfarin	INR: usual goal 2.0–3.0. Goal based on indication for anticoagulation; may be changed based on patient-specific risk for thrombosis or hemorrhage
Enoxaparin	Anti-Xa monitoring: Peak: 0.6–1.0 units/mL (BID dosing); 1–2 units/mL (daily dosing) Trough: <0.4 units/mL
Dalteparin	Anti-Xa monitoring: Peak: 0.5–1.5 units/mL
Fondaparinux	Anti-Xa monitoring (requires a different assay than LMWHs): Peak, 0.5–1.5 units/mL
Immunosuppressants: goal trough levels will depend on the patient's time in the posttransplant course. Goal levels listed below represent the immediate posttransplant time period	
Tacrolimus	Renal transplant: 8–12 ng/mL Liver transplant: 8–12 ng/mL Lung transplant: 8–12 ng/mL Heart transplant: 8–15 ng/mL HSCT: 5–10 ng/mL
Cyclosporine	Renal transplant: 200–300 ng/mL Liver transplant: 200–300 ng/mL Lung transplant: 250–350 ng/mL Heart transplant: 250–300 ng/mL HSCT: 200–400 ng/mL
Sirolimus	Renal transplant: 3–8 ng/mL Lung transplant: 8–10 ng/mL Heart transplant: 3–10 ng/mL HSCT: 3–12 ng/mL

TDM therapeutic drug monitoring, *HEAT* high-dose extended-interval aminoglycoside therapy, *LMWH* low-molecular-weight heparin, *HSCT* hematopoietic stem cell transplant

23.9 Drugs Requiring Special Attention in Acute Kidney Injury

23.9.1 Nephrotoxins

Medications, in addition to many processes and disease states, are risk factors for the development of AKI. In the ICU setting, medications may contribute to AKI in up to 25% of cases [64]. Patient risk factors for drug-induced nephrotoxicity, such as age, dehydration, hypotension, surgery, and infection, should be recognized and used to help decide on the safest pharmacotherapy regimen. In patients with these risk factors, medications with less risk of nephrotoxicity should be favored. Medication-induced AKI can be broken into three main categories: prerenal, ATN (acute tubular necrosis), and AIN (acute interstitial nephritis) [64]. Also, medication dosing and administration strategies that minimize nephrotoxicity (i.e., once-daily dosing of aminoglycosides, administration of isotonic fluid with nephrotoxins such as foscarnet, etc.) should be employed whenever possible. The first step in AKI is to remove possible offending agent(s) to avoid further insult to the kidneys. Repeated exposure to nephrotoxins, such as contrast dye, aminoglycosides, nonsteroidal anti-inflammatory drugs (NSAIDs), and vasoconstrictive agents may prolong recovery from AKI [65].

23.9.2 Anticoagulants

Anticoagulant-associated adverse drug events are common [66]. Warfarin and unfractionated heparin (UFH) metabolism are not typically significantly altered in patients with renal insufficiency [67]. However, in patients with acute-on-chronic renal failure, uremia may induce platelet dysfunction due to several mechanisms including qualitative von Willebrand factor deficiencies and enhanced nitric oxide and prostaglandin synthesis [68]. These patients have a higher incidence of hemorrhage when utilizing warfarin and UFH, most likely due to platelet dysfunction and interactions with coadministered medications [69, 70].

Low-molecular-weight heparin (LMWH) use has increased following a number of studies demonstrating equal or greater efficacy and their ease of use compared with UFH [71–74]. The clearance of LMWH is primarily through renal excretion, and the risk of hemorrhage is higher when these agents are used in patients with renal insufficiency [75–79]. Dose reductions are recommended for these agents in patients with a creatinine clearance less than 30 mL/min. Additionally, monitoring of LMWH can be achieved using a chromogenic factor Xa assay [77]. Monitoring is typically recommended in obese patients or those with CKD. It may also be employed in patients with AKI to determine if supratherapeutic anticoagulation has occurred. Fondaparinux, a pentasaccharide factor Xa inhibitor, is also cleared by renal excretion and is not recommended for use in patients with a creatinine clearance less than 30 mL/min. Its use has not been extensively studied in AKI. Like the LMWHs, fondaparinux may be monitored using a chromogenic factor Xa assay, but avoidance of its use in AKI may be prudent.

In patients with a contraindication to heparin analogues (i.e., heparin-induced thrombocytopenia), direct thrombin inhibitors, such as argatroban and bivalirudin, and fondaparinux may be used for anticoagulation. All of these medications are cleared by the kidneys and need to be dose reduced or avoided in patients with renal insufficiency [80, 81]. Argatroban may be the preferred alternative anticoagulant in renal disease because it is primarily cleared by the liver and does not need empiric dose adjustment in patients with moderate renal insufficiency [82]. However, contradictory data exists which suggests that acute changes in renal function may impact the pharmacodynamics of argatroban [83, 84]. Additionally, in patients with acute-on-chronic kidney disease, nonrenal clearance of argatroban may be reduced. Use of a nomogram with empiric dose reductions of DTIs in patients with CKD or AKI may improve the likelihood of achieving therapeutic anticoagulation [85].

Table 23.6 Direct oral anticoagulants and dose adjustments in patients with renal dysfunction

Anticoagulant	Mechanism of action	Elimination	Usual half-life	Dosing and dose adjustment
Dabigatran (Pradaxa™)	Direct thrombin inhibitor	80% renal	12–14 h	150 mg PO 2×/day; CrCl <30–75 mg PO 2×/day
Rivaroxaban (Xarelto™)	Direct factor Xa inhibitor	35% renal	6–9 h	VTE: 15 mg PO 2×/day × 3 weeks, then 20 mg PO daily AF: 20 mg PO daily CrCl <30–15 mg daily
Apixaban (Eliquis™)	Direct factor Xa inhibitor	30% renal	8–12 h	VTE: 10 mg PO 2×/day × 1 week, then 5 mg PO 2×/day AF: 5 mg PO 2×/day Dose reduction—2.5 mg 2×/day if 2 or more of the following criteria are present: age > 80, weight < 60 kg, SCr >1.5
Edoxaban (Savaysa™)	Direct factor Xa inhibitor	70% renal	10–14 h	60 mg PO daily CrCl <30–30 mg PO daily

CrCl creatinine clearance, *VTE* venous thromboembolism, *AF* atrial fibrillation

The direct oral anticoagulants (DOACs), dabigatran, rivaroxaban, apixaban, and edoxaban, have emerged as promising oral anticoagulants for the treatment of atrial fibrillation (AF) and venous thromboembolism (VTE) and prevention of VTE after knee and hip replacement. Each of the DOACs is eliminated renally, to varying degrees (Table 23.6). Empiric dose recommendations have been developed for patients with baseline CKD. However, data regarding the use of the DOACs in patients with AKI is limited, and these agents should be used with caution. Serum concentration assays for each of the DOACs are available, but are currently not widely available for use outside of clinical drug trials [86]. Coagulation assays such as the activated partial thromboplastin time (dabigatran) and international normalized ratio (rivaroxaban, apixaban, edoxaban) may be prolonged in patients with AKI who accumulate DOACs [87].

23.9.3 Antihypertensive and Cardiac Medications

23.9.3.1 Angiotensin-Converting Enzyme Inhibitors and Angiotensin Receptor Blockers

Angiotensin-converting enzyme inhibitors (ACEIs) and angiotensin receptor blockers (ARBs) inhibit efferent arteriole vasoconstriction, therefore reducing glomerular filtration rate. In general, ACEIs and ARBs should be held in patients with AKI and reinitiated when renal function has stabilized [88].

23.9.3.2 Diuretics

Oliguria is a poor prognostic factor in patients who develop AKI. Therefore, while diuretics may potentially cause prerenal AKI, they are frequently used to improve urine output and improve oliguria [89–91]. Loop diuretics are the most potent and are most commonly administered as boluses or continuous infusion. Improvements in oxygen consumption and renal blood flow have been seen in smaller experimental settings; however, this has not been demonstrated in larger clinical trials. Loop diuretics, which block sodium and water reabsorption in the loop of Henle, are dependent on renal blood flow for their effect. The efficacy of loop diuretics may be decreased in AKI due to decreased drug delivery, and patients may require doses severalfold higher to achieve adequate diuresis [91].

Despite the administration of higher doses, however, tolerance to loop diuretics and various concomitant disease states, such as liver failure, nephrotic syndrome, and heart failure, may result in diuretic resistance. More frequent dosing, the use of continuous infusions, and the coadministration with thiazide diuretics may be strategies to overcome diuretic resistance [91]. Thiazide diuretics interfere with sodium reabsorption in the distal convoluted tubule. Since loop diuretics increase the amount of sodium available for reabsorption at the distal tubule, using thiazide diuretics results in a synergistic response. Thiazide diuretics may lose their effectiveness in patients with low creatinine clearance due to decreased delivery to the site of action, and there is limited data in patients with AKI. However, metolazone has been shown to retain its efficacy in patients with compromised renal function [92–95]. Intravenous thiazide diuretics, such as chlorothiazide, should be given 30 min before intravenous loop diuretics to maximize synergistic effects. Oral agents, such as chlorthalidone and metolazone, should be given at least 1–2 h before loop diuretic boluses.

23.9.4 Analgesics

23.9.4.1 Nonnarcotic Analgesics

Nonsteroidal anti-inflammatory drugs (NSAIDs) have long been associated with serious adverse effects, such as GI bleeding and AKI [96, 97]. Inhibition of COX-1 results in a decrease in prostaglandin synthesis and therefore a reduction of prostaglandin-mediated afferent arteriole vasodilation and renal blood flow [98]. While traditional NSAIDs such as ibuprofen, ketorolac, and naproxen inhibit COX-1 to a greater degree than COX-2-specific NSAIDs, such as celecoxib, no difference in the risk of AKI development between these types of NSAIDs has been observed [97]. Patients with other risk factors for AKI, such as CHF, hypertension, liver disease, or concomitant use of ACEIs, ARBs, and diuretics, are at higher risk of nephrotoxicity when NSAIDs are administered [99, 100, 101]. In patients with AKI, NSAIDs should be avoided when possible to prevent further nephrotoxicity. Other nonnarcotic agents, such as tramadol, gabapentin, and pregabalin, should be renally adjusted as they may accumulate in AKI.

23.9.4.2 Narcotic Analgesics

Opioid selection and dosing in patients with renal dysfunction, especially AKI, is difficult. As hepatic dysfunction often accompanies AKI, the metabolism of most opioids may be reduced leading to an increase in effect and/or duration. In addition, many of these parent drugs or their active metabolites are cleared renally, leading to accumulation [102, 103]. Meperidine should be avoided in renal insufficiency as its active metabolite, normeperidine, may accumulate and increases the risk of neurotoxicity, including seizures [104, 105].

Morphine may also not be an ideal choice as its primary two metabolites, morphine-3-glucuronide and morphine-6-glucuronide, are eliminated renally and may prolong the effects of sedation and respiratory depression in AKI [102, 106, 107]. Additionally, morphine is associated with the greatest amount of hypotension due to histamine release and may further worsen a patient's overall clinical status. Codeine and propoxyphene are metabolized into active metabolites that accumulate in AKI and should generally be avoided [108–111]. Hydromorphone is passively metabolized by the liver through conjugation and is not significantly cleared by the kidneys [112]. Oxycodone undergoes extensive hepatic metabolism with <20% of the parent drug excreted by the kidneys and may be used in AKI with careful monitoring. Fentanyl and methadone are likely the safest opioids to use in patients with AKI due to their lack of active metabolites and their lack of renal clearance [112].

23.9.5 Antimicrobial Agents

Errors regarding the choice and dosing of antimicrobial agents in patients with renal insufficiency are common [113–115]. There is little data to support reductions of initial dosing of antibiotics in patients with AKI due to changes in protein binding, volume of distribution, extrarenal clearance mechanisms, and hemodynamic state of the patient. As discussed above, a loading dose is often required to achieve an optimal drug concentration within a minimal time period, especially for hydrophilic drugs such as vancomycin [116, 117]. Antibiotics that demonstrate concentration-dependent killing should generally be adjusted to be administered less frequently in order to still maximize the peak to MIC ratio or AUC to MIC ratio [118]. Time-dependent antibiotics can achieve their pharmacodynamic goal of adequate time above the MIC while undergoing dose reductions to minimize adverse reactions [119]. Serum drug concentrations can be drawn for peak or trough assessment or for various pharmacokinetic calculations [120].

23.9.5.1 Aminoglycosides

Aminoglycosides remain an important part of anti-infective therapy in patients with severe gram-negative and some gram-positive bacterial infections [121, 122]. Their use in patients with renal insufficiency is complicated by an increased Vd, decreased clearance, and increased risk of serious adverse reactions, such as ototoxicity and worsening of renal function [123–125]. Aminoglycosides exhibit concentration-dependent bactericidal activity and have a significant postantibiotic effect such that they continue to suppress bacterial growth for a period of time after peak concentrations [126]. The trough serum level is the primary determinant and predictor of aminoglycoside toxicity. For these reasons, the goal in aminoglycoside dosing is to maximize efficacy with a goal peak/MIC ratio of 10–12:1 while allowing for a rapid clearance of drug from the body before dosing again [127]. Extended interval aminoglycoside dosing (7–10 mg/kg once daily of gentamicin and tobramycin or 15–25 mg/kg once daily of amikacin) has been widely used in recent years for the treatment of gram-negative bacterial infections to capitalize on the postantibiotic effect while minimizing nephrotoxicity [125, 128–132]. Currently, the data are lacking regarding the efficacy and toxicity of once-daily aminoglycoside dosing as compared with multiple-daily doses in patients with severely impaired renal function [130]. Moreover, data suggest that errors in dosing are common if extended-interval dosing is used for patients with AKI or CKD [124, 133]. Using a more traditional dose (~1.5–2 mg/kg) may not achieve a peak plasma concentration high enough to optimize bacterial killing and may still increase the risk of worsened nephrotoxicity.

Aminoglycosides have also long been used for synergistic effects against gram-positive organisms in combination with other antibiotics that target bacterial cell wall. Current endocarditis guidelines recommend use of aminoglycosides only for treatment of *Streptococcus* species and in patients with prosthetic heart valves [134, 135]. The recommended use of these agents has decreased, as they may not increase the efficacy of these regimens and may be more toxic than alternatives [136]. Additionally, aminoglycoside resistance has increased among common pathogens of endocarditis [134].

23.9.5.2 Carbapenems

Imipenem is filtered and then metabolized by the renal brush border enzyme, dehydropeptidase [137]. Imipenem is given with cilastatin, an inhibitor of dehydropeptidase, to reduce tubular toxicity and prolong imipenem's half-life [138]. Both medications have a prolonged half-life in patients with renal dysfunction [52], and accumulation of imipenem in renal insufficiency may induce seizures. Patients with severe kidney dysfunction should be monitored closely and have their total daily dose decreased. If there is an especially high concern for seizures, a different carbapenem, such as meropenem, doripenem, or ertapenem, can be initiated at a reduced dose [139, 140]. Meropenem has been shown to be cleared in patients with AKI 1.3 to 2 times faster than in those with ESRD [51, 141, 142]. This is likely due to preserved nonrenal clearance in AKI as compared with ESRD.

23.9.5.3 Penicillins/Cephalosporins

Many of the commonly used penicillins and cephalosporins have prolonged half-lives in patients with renal insufficiency and require a reduction from the normal recommended dosage [118, 139, 143–147]. They have a slow, continuous bactericidal effect that is dependent on the amount of time that tissue levels are above MIC [137, 148]. In most cases, the dose of the cephalosporin should be reduced in order to maintain tissue levels above the MIC for the bacteria being treated while limiting adverse effects [116].

In severe AKI, both the dose and frequency of the cephalosporin may need to be reduced. For critically ill patients, the first dose should not be reduced, allowing for rapid achievement of therapeutic levels [148]. Administration of penicillins and cephalosporins as prolonged or continuous infusions may aid in decreasing overall drug exposure while maximizing pharmacokinetic properties of the medication [149, 150].

23.9.5.4 Fluoroquinolones

The fluoroquinolones have a broad spectrum of activity, including both gram-positive and gram-negative coverage, good tissue penetration, and bioavailability [137, 151]. Most fluoroquinolones are cleared by the kidney and require dosage adjustments in patients with renal insufficiency [152, 153]. Similar to aminoglycosides, fluoroquinolones require high peak concentrations. In order to maximize peak concentrations, the dose of fluoroquinolone is typically not reduced, except in cases of severe AKI. Extending the interval at which fluoroquinolones are administered can be implemented to ensure adequate clearance.

23.9.5.5 Vancomycin

Vancomycin is a glycopeptide antibiotic with a broad gram-positive spectrum of activity. It remains the gold standard to treat methicillin-resistant *Staphylococcus aureus* [137]. Vancomycin is cleared renally and has an increased half-life in patients with AKI. In addition, vancomycin has an increased Vd in patients with sepsis, multiorgan failure, and volume overload [146, 154, 155]. Vancomycin may require a loading dose, typically 25–30 mg/kg, which may need to be increased in critically ill patients. The maintenance dose, however, is generally reduced in patients with renal dysfunction [148, 156]. Proper therapeutic drug monitoring is imperative in patients with AKI receiving vancomycin [120, 157]. Meta-analysis has displayed a measurable risk of AKI with the use of vancomycin; careful assessment should take place to determine the intended site of action of vancomycin and the goal vancomycin trough to maximize the AUC/MIC ratio [158].

23.9.5.6 Antifungals

Amphotericin B is used to treat certain severe systemic fungal infections, including some that may be independent risk factors for AKI [147, 159]. Preexisting renal dysfunction, administration of concomitant nephrotoxic agents, volume depletion, obesity, critical illness, and advanced age may increase the risk of amphotericin B-induced nephrotoxicity [140, 160]. The risk of nephrotoxicity can be reduced by the administration of sodium-containing fluid prior to each dose and with the use of lipid formulations of the drug, which are equivalent to conventional amphotericin B in terms of efficacy [161, 162].

Intravenous voriconazole should be used with caution in patients with moderate to severe renal insufficiency, defined as GFR less than 50 mL/min. While voriconazole itself is not nephrotoxic, there is concern that the vehicle in the IV formulation, sulfobutyl ether beta-cyclodextrin sodium (SBECD), has the potential to accumulate and cause tubular toxicity [163, 164]. However, the combination of newer data showing no increased risk of renal injury along with patient severity of illness may warrant the use of IV voriconazole in moderate to severe renal dysfunction [165]. Itraconazole is highly protein bound and has a high level of extrarenal elimination, including bile elimination [166, 167]. Therefore, itraconazole elimination in AKI is more likely to mirror a patient with normal renal function than that of a patient with CKD.

Isavuconazole, a novel triazole antifungal, is primarily eliminated fecally and unchanged from the kidneys and does not require dose adjustment in patients with renal dysfunction, even ESRD [168]. Additionally, the IV formulation of isavuconazole does not contain SBECD, limiting the risk of drug-induced nephrotoxicity associated with the medication [168]. Finally, because it boasts a more predictable pharmacokinetic profile when compared with voriconazole and posaconazole, isavuconazole typically does not require TDM [169].

23.9.5.7 Nitrofurantoin

A toxic metabolite of nitrofurantoin accumulates in patients with renal insufficiency and can cause peripheral neuritis. For this reason, nitrofurantoin should not be used in patients with moderate to severe renal impairment [103].

Conclusion

Multiple factors need to be considered when dosing medications in patients with AKI, as several pharmacokinetic parameters are impacted by renal dysfunction. The etiologies of AKI are vast, and AKI may be accompanied by underlying renal insufficiency, multiple organ dysfunction, critical illness, and the need for RRT. These parameters should contribute to clinical decision-making and medication dosing formation. Patients presenting with AKI without other organ dysfunction may have preserved nonrenal clearance as compared with those with CKD, and, thus, dosing recommendations established from patients with CKD may be insufficient. While estimation of GFR is often difficult in patients with AKI, it is crucial to routinely assess the degree of renal dysfunction and closely analyze drug-specific pharmacokinetic properties to make the most appropriate dosing recommendations in patients with AKI. A dedicated pharmacist available to the inpatient clinician can be a valuable resource to assist with crafting and monitoring therapeutic regimens in these complex patients.

References

1. Xue JL, Daniels F, Star RA, et al. Incidence and mortality of acute renal failure in Medicare beneficiaries, 1992 to 2001. J Am Soc Nephrol. 2006;17:1135–42.
2. Bagshaw SM, George C, Bellomo R. Changes in the incidence and outcome for early acute kidney injury in a cohort of Australian intensive care units. Crit Care. 2007;11:R68.
3. Uchino S, Kellum JA, Bellomo R, et al. Acute renal failure in critically ill patients: a multinational, multicenter study. JAMA. 2005;294:813–8.
4. Ali T, Khan I, Simpson W, et al. Incidence and outcomes in acute kidney injury: a comprehensive population-based study. J Am Soc Nephrol. 2007;18:1292–8.
5. Yong K, Dogra G, Boudville N, Pinder M, Lim W. Acute kidney injury: controversies revisited. Int J Nephrol. 2011;2011:762634.
6. Udy AA, Roberts JA, Lipman J. Implications of augmented renal clearance in critically ill patients. Nat Rev Nephrol. 2011;7:539–43.
7. Robert S, Zarowitz BJ, Peterson EL, Dumler F. Predictability of creatinine clearance estimates in critically ill patients. Crit Care Med. 1993;21:1487–95.
8. Bragadottir G, Redfors B, Ricksten SE. Assessing glomerular filtration rate (GFR) in critically ill patients with acute kidney injury—true GFR versus urinary creatinine clearance and estimating equations. Crit Care. 2013;17:R108.
9. Moran SM, Myers BD. Course of acute renal failure studied by a model of creatinine kinetics. Kidney Int. 1985;27:928–37.
10. Brivet FG, Kleinknecht DJ, Loirat P, Landais PJ. Acute renal failure in intensive care units—causes, outcome, and prognostic factors of hospital mortality; a prospective, multicenter study. French Study Group on Acute Renal Failure. Crit Care Med. 1996;24:192–8.
11. Mehta RL, Pascual MT, Soroko S, et al. Spectrum of acute renal failure in the intensive care unit: the PICARD experience. Kidney Int. 2004;66:1613–21.
12. Mehta RL, Pascual MT, Gruta CG, Zhuang S, Chertow GM. Refining predictive models in critically ill patients with acute renal failure. J Am Soc Nephrol. 2002;13:1350–7.
13. Mehta RL, McDonald B, Gabbai FB, et al. A randomized clinical trial of continuous versus intermittent dialysis for acute renal failure. Kidney Int. 2001;60:1154–63.
14. Eyler RF, Mueller BA. Antibiotic dosing in critically ill patients with acute kidney injury. Nat Rev Nephrol. 2011;7:226–35.
15. Daemen T, Veninga A, Regts J, Scherphof GL. Maintenance of tumoricidal activity and susceptibility to reactivation of subpopulations of rat liver macrophages. J Immunother. 1991;10:200–6.
16. Macias WL, Mueller BA, Scarim SK. Vancomycin pharmacokinetics in acute renal failure: preservation of nonrenal clearance. Clin Pharmacol Ther. 1991;50:688–94.
17. Winter M. Basic clinical pharmacokinetics. 3rd ed. Philadelphia: Lippincott, Williams and Wilkins; 1994.
18. Wilkinson G. Pharmacokinetics: the dynamics of drug absorption, distribution and elimination. In: Hardman JG, Limbird LE, editors. Goodman and Gilman's: the pharmacological basis of therapeutics. New York: McGraw-Hill; 2001. p. 9–23.
19. Lam YW, Banerji S, Hatfield C, Talbert RL. Principles of drug administration in renal insufficiency. Clin Pharmacokinet. 1997;32:30–57.

20. Etemad B. Gastrointestinal complications of renal failure. Gastroenterol Clin N Am. 1998;27:875–92.
21. Boucher BA, Wood GC, Swanson JM. Pharmacokinetic changes in critical illness. Crit Care Clin. 2006;22:255–71. vi
22. Tarling MM, Toner CC, Withington PS, Baxter MK, Whelpton R, Goodhill DR. A model of gastric emptying using paracetamol absorption in intensive care patients. Intensive Care Med. 1997;23:256–60.
23. Ariano RE, Sitar DS, Zelenitsky SA, et al. Enteric absorption and pharmacokinetics of oseltamivir in critically ill patients with pandemic (H1N1) influenza. CMAJ. 2010;182:357–63.
24. Brown-Cartwright D, Smith HJ, Feldman M. Gastric emptying of an indigestible solid in patients with end-stage renal disease on continuous ambulatory peritoneal dialysis. Gastroenterology. 1988;95:49–51.
25. Wright RA, Clemente R, Wathen R. Gastric emptying in patients with chronic renal failure receiving hemodialysis. Arch Intern Med. 1984;144:495–6.
26. Soffer EE, Geva B, Helman C, Avni Y, Bar-Meir S. Gastric emptying in chronic renal failure patients on hemodialysis. J Clin Gastroenterol. 1987;9:651–3.
27. McNamee PT, Moore GW, McGeown MG, Doherty CC, Collins BJ. Gastric emptying in chronic renal failure. Br Med J (Clin Res Ed). 1985;291:310–1.
28. Freeman JG, Cobden I, Heaton A, Keir M. Gastric emptying in chronic renal failure. Br Med J (Clin Res Ed). 1985;291:1048.
29. St Peter WL, Redic-Kill KA, Halstenson CE. Clinical pharmacokinetics of antibiotics in patients with impaired renal function. Clin Pharmacokinet. 1992;22:169–210.
30. Gugler R, Allgayer H. Effects of antacids on the clinical pharmacokinetics of drugs. An update. Clin Pharmacokinet. 1990;18:210–9.
31. Zhang Y, Benet LZ. The gut as a barrier to drug absorption: combined role of cytochrome P450 3A and P-glycoprotein. Clin Pharmacokinet. 2001;40:159–68.
32. Doucet J, Fresel J, Hue G, Moore N. Protein binding of digitoxin, valproate and phenytoin in sera from diabetics. Eur J Clin Pharmacol. 1993;45:577–9.
33. Gabardi S, Abramson S. Drug dosing in chronic kidney disease. Med Clin North Am. 2005;89:649–87.
34. MacKichan J. Influence of protein binding and the use of unbound (free) drug concentrations. In: Evans W, Schentag JJ, Jusko WJ, editors. Applied pharmacokinetics. 3rd ed. Applied Therapeutics: Vancouver; 1992. p. 1–48.
35. Klotz U. Pathophysiological and disease-induced changes in drug distribution volume: pharmacokinetic implications. Clin Pharmacokinet. 1976;1:204–18.
36. Reidenberg MM. The binding of drugs to plasma proteins and the interpretation of measurements of plasma concentrations of drugs in patients with poor renal function. Am J Med. 1977;62:466–70.
37. Torbic H, Forni A, Anger KE, DeGrado JR, Greenwood BC. Use of antiepileptics for seizure prophylaxis after traumatic brain injury. Am J Health Syst Pharm. 2013;70:759–66.
38. Power BM, Forbes AM, van Heerden PV, Ilett KF. Pharmacokinetics of drugs used in critically ill adults. Clin Pharmacokinet. 1998;34:25–56.
39. Brezis M, Rosen S, Epstein FH. Acute renal failure. In: Brenner B, Rector WG, editors. The kidney. 5th ed. Philadelphia: WB Saunders; 1996. p. 735–79.
40. Reed WE Jr, Sabatini S. The use of drugs in renal failure. Semin Nephrol. 1986;6:259–95.
41. Nissenson AR. Acute renal failure: definition and pathogenesis. Kidney Int Suppl. 1998;66:S7–10.
42. Gibson TP. Renal disease and drug metabolism: an overview. Am J Kidney Dis. 1986;8:7–17.
43. Swan SK, Bennett WM. Drug dosing guidelines in patients with renal failure. West J Med. 1992;156:633–8.
44. Nolin TD, Frye RF, Matzke GR. Hepatic drug metabolism and transport in patients with kidney disease. Am J Kidney Dis. 2003;42:906–25.
45. Aronoff G, Berns J, Brier M. Drug prescribing in renal failure: dosing guidelines for adults. 4th ed. Philadelphia: American College of Physicians; 1999.
46. Wu CY, Benet LZ, Hebert MF, et al. Differentiation of absorption and first-pass gut and hepatic metabolism in humans: studies with cyclosporine. Clin Pharmacol Ther. 1995;58:492–7.
47. Dreisbach AW, Lertora JJ. The effect of chronic renal failure on hepatic drug metabolism and drug disposition. Semin Dial. 2003;16:45–50.
48. Yuan R, Venitz J. Effect of chronic renal failure on the disposition of highly hepatically metabolized drugs. Int J Clin Pharmacol Ther. 2000;38:245–53.
49. Leblond FA, Giroux L, Villeneuve JP, Pichette V. Decreased in vivo metabolism of drugs in chronic renal failure. Drug Metab Dispos. 2000;28:1317–20.
50. Pichette V, Leblond FA. Drug metabolism in chronic renal failure. Curr Drug Metab. 2003;4:91–103.
51. Vilay AM, Churchwell MD, Mueller BA. Clinical review: drug metabolism and nonrenal clearance in acute kidney injury. Crit Care. 2008;12:235.
52. Mueller BA, Scarim SK, Macias WL. Comparison of imipenem pharmacokinetics in patients with acute or chronic renal failure treated with continuous hemofiltration. Am J Kidney Dis. 1993;21:172–9.
53. Lee YH, Lee MH, Shim CK. Decreased systemic clearance of diltiazem with increased hepatic metabolism in rats with uranyl nitrate-induced acute renal failure. Pharm Res. 1992;9:1599–606.
54. Leakey TE, Elias-Jones AC, Coates PE, Smith KJ. Pharmacokinetics of theophylline and its metabolites during acute renal failure. A case report. Clin Pharmacokinet. 1991;21:400–8.
55. Nielson C. Pharmacologic considerations in critical care of the elderly. Clin Geriatr Med. 1994;10:71–89.
56. Westphal JF, Brogard JM. Drug administration in chronic liver disease. Drug Saf. 1997;17:47–73.
57. Horl WH, Druml W, Stevens PE. Pathophysiology of ARF in the ICU. Int J Artif Organs. 1996;19:84–6.

58. Anders MW. Metabolism of drugs by the kidney. Kidney Int. 1980;18:636–47.
59. Somogyi A. Renal transport of drugs: specificity and molecular mechanisms. Clin Exp Pharmacol Physiol. 1996;23:986–9.
60. Schmidt C, Hocherl K, Schweda F, Bucher M. Proinflammatory cytokines cause down-regulation of renal chloride entry pathways during sepsis. Crit Care Med. 2007;35(9):2110.
61. Blot S, Lipman J, Roberts DM, Roberts JA. The influence of acute kidney injury on antimicrobial dosing in critically ill patients: are dose reductions always necessary? Diagn Microbiol Infect Dis. 2014;79:77–84.
62. Himmelfarb J, Evanson J, Hakim RM, Freedman S, Shyr Y, Ikizler TA. Urea volume of distribution exceeds total body water in patients with acute renal failure. Kidney Int. 2002;61:317–23.
63. Gilmore JF, Kim M, LaSalvia MT, Mahoney MV. Treatment of enterococcal peritonitis with intraperitoneal daptomycin in a vancomycin-allergic patient and a review of the literature. Perit Dial Int. 2013;33:353–7.
64. Perazella M. Drug use and nephrotoxicity in the intensive care unit. Kidney Int. 2012;81:1172–8.
65. Kelly KJ, Molitoris BA. Acute renal failure in the new millennium: time to consider combination therapy. Semin Nephrol. 2000;20:4–19.
66. Piazza G, Nguyen TN, Cios D, et al. Anticoagulation-associated adverse drug events. Am J Med. 2011;124:1136–42.
67. Bennett WM, Aronoff GR, Morrison G, et al. Drug prescribing in renal failure: dosing guidelines for adults. Am J Kidney Dis. 1983;3:155–93.
68. Boccardo P, Remuzzi G, Galbusera M. Platelet dysfunction in renal failure. Semin Thromb Hemost. 2004;30:579–89.
69. Levine MN, Raskob G, Landefeld S, Kearon C. Hemorrhagic complications of anticoagulant treatment. Chest. 2001;119:108S–21S.
70. Brinkman WT, Williams WH, Guyton RA, Jones EL, Craver JM. Valve replacement in patients on chronic renal dialysis: implications for valve prosthesis selection. Ann Thorac Surg. 2002;74:37–42; discussion.
71. Howard PA. Low molecular weight heparins in special populations. J Infus Nurs. 2003;26:304–10.
72. Wong GC, Giugliano RP, Antman EM. Use of low-molecular-weight heparins in the management of acute coronary artery syndromes and percutaneous coronary intervention. JAMA. 2003;289:331–42.
73. Hull RD, Pineo GF, Stein PD, et al. Extended out-of-hospital low-molecular-weight heparin prophylaxis against deep venous thrombosis in patients after elective hip arthroplasty: a systematic review. Ann Intern Med. 2001;135:858–69.
74. De Lorenzo F, Noorani A, Kakkar VV. Current trends in the management of thromboembolic events. QJM. 2001;94:179–85.
75. Polkinghorne KR, McMahon LP, Becker GJ. Pharmacokinetic studies of dalteparin (Fragmin), enoxaparin (Clexane), and danaparoid sodium (Orgaran) in stable chronic hemodialysis patients. Am J Kidney Dis. 2002;40(5):990.
76. Sanderink GJ, Guimart CG, Ozoux ML, Jariwala NU, Shukla UA, Boutouyrie BX. Pharmacokinetics and pharmacodynamics of the prophylactic dose of enoxaparin once daily over 4 days in patients with renal impairment. Thromb Res. 2002;105:225–31.
77. Hirsh J, Warkentin TE, Shaughnessy SG, et al. Heparin and low-molecular-weight heparin: mechanisms of action, pharmacokinetics, dosing, monitoring, efficacy, and safety. Chest. 2001;119:64S–94S.
78. Gerlach AT, Pickworth KK, Seth SK, Tanna SB, Barnes JF. Enoxaparin and bleeding complications: a review in patients with and without renal insufficiency. Pharmacotherapy. 2000;20:771–5.
79. Spinler SA, Inverso SM, Cohen M, Goodman SG, Stringer KA, Antman EM. Safety and efficacy of unfractionated heparin versus enoxaparin in patients who are obese and patients with severe renal impairment: analysis from the ESSENCE and TIMI 11B studies. Am Heart J. 2003;146:33–41.
80. Fischer KG. Hirudin in renal insufficiency. Semin Thromb Hemost. 2002;28:467–82.
81. Poschel KA, Bucha E, Esslinger HU, et al. Pharmacodynamics and pharmacokinetics of polyethylene glycol-hirudin in patients with chronic renal failure. Kidney Int. 2000;58:2478–84.
82. Swan SK, Hursting MJ. The pharmacokinetics and pharmacodynamics of argatroban: effects of age, gender, and hepatic or renal dysfunction. Pharmacotherapy. 2000;20:318–29.
83. Arpino PA, Hallisey RK. Effect of renal function on the pharmacodynamics of argatroban. Ann Pharmacother. 2004;38:25–9.
84. Kubiak DW, Szumita PM, Fanikos JR. Extensive prolongation of aPTT with argatroban in an elderly patient with improving renal function, normal hepatic enzymes, and metastatic lung cancer. Ann Pharmacother. 2005;39:1119–23.
85. Gilmore JF, Adams CD, Blum RM, Fanikos J, Hirning BA, Matta L. Evaluation of a multi-target direct thrombin inhibitor dosing and titration guideline for patients with suspected heparin-induced thrombocytopenia. Am J Hematol. 2015;90:E143–5.
86. Harenberg J, Kramer S, Du S, et al. Measurement of rivaroxaban and apixaban in serum samples of patients. Eur J Clin Investig. 2014;44:743–52.
87. Dinkelaar J, Patiwael S, Harenberg J, Leyte A, Brinkman HJM. Global coagulation tests: their applicability for measuring direct factor Xa- and thrombin inhibition and reversal of anticoagulation by prothrombin complex concentrate. Clin Chem Lab Med. 2014;52:1615–23.
88. Wynckel A, Ebikili B, Melin JP, Randoux C, Lavaud S, Chanard J. Long-term follow-up of acute renal failure caused by angiotensin converting enzyme inhibitors. Am J Hypertens. 1998;11:1080–6.
89. Shilliday IR, Quinn KJ, Allison ME. Loop diuretics in the management of acute renal failure: a prospec-

tive, double-blind, placebo-controlled, randomized study. Nephrol Dial Transplant. 1997;12:2592–6.
90. Kellum JA. Use of diuretics in the acute care setting. Kidney Int Suppl. 1998;66:S67–70.
91. Nigwekar S, Walkar S. Diuretics in acute kidney injury. Semin Nephrol. 2011;31:523–34.
92. Agarwal R, Sinha A. Thiazide diuretics in advanced chronic kidney disease. J Am Soc Hypertens. 2012;6:299–308.
93. Segar JL, Chemtob S, Bell EF. Changes in body water compartments with diuretic therapy in infants with chronic lung disease. Early Hum Dev. 1997;48:99–107.
94. Ellison DH. Diuretic resistance: physiology and therapeutics. Semin Nephrol. 1999;19:581–97.
95. Paton RR, Kane RE. Long-term diuretic therapy with metolazone of renal failure and the nephrotic syndrome. J Clin Pharmacol. 1977;17:243–51.
96. Whelton A. Renal aspects of treatment with conventional nonsteroidal anti-inflammatory drugs versus cyclooxygenase-2-specific inhibitors. Am J Med. 2001;110(Suppl 3A):33S–42S.
97. Ungprasert P, Cheungpasitporn W, Crowson C, Matteson E. Individual non-steroidal anti-inflammatory drugs and risk of acute kidney injury: a systematic review and meta-analysis of observational studies. Eur J Intern Med. 2015;26:285–91.
98. DeMaria AN, Weir MR. Coxibs—beyond the GI tract: renal and cardiovascular issues. J Pain Symptom Manag. 2003;25:S41–9.
99. Wen SF. Nephrotoxicities of nonsteroidal anti-inflammatory drugs. J Formos Med Assoc. 1997;96:157–71.
100. Nderitu P, Doos L, Jones PW, Davies SJ, Kadam UT. Non-steroidal anti-inflammatory drugs and chronic kidney disease progression: a systematic review. Fam Pract. 2013;30:247–55.
101. Phan O, Meier P, Burnier M. Are cyclooxygenase-2-selective inhibitors safe for the kidneys? Joint Bone Spine. 2003;70:237–41.
102. Hall LG, Oyen LJ, Murray MJ. Analgesic agents. Pharmacology and application in critical care. Crit Care Clin. 2001;17:899–923. viii
103. Drayer DE. Pharmacologically active metabolites of drugs and other foreign compounds. Clinical, pharmacological, therapeutic and toxicological considerations. Drugs. 1982;24:519–42.
104. Szeto HH, Inturrisi CE, Houde R, Saal S, Cheigh J, Reidenberg MM. Accumulation of normeperidine, an active metabolite of meperidine, in patients with renal failure of cancer. Ann Intern Med. 1977;86:738–41.
105. Hassan H, Bastani B, Gellens M. Successful treatment of normeperidine neurotoxicity by hemodialysis. Am J Kidney Dis. 2000;35:146–9.
106. Osborne R, Joel S, Grebenik K, Trew D, Slevin M. The pharmacokinetics of morphine and morphine glucuronides in kidney failure. Clin Pharmacol Ther. 1993;54:158–67.
107. Chauvin M, Sandouk P, Scherrmann JM, Farinotti R, Strumza P, Duvaldestin P. Morphine pharmacokinetics in renal failure. Anesthesiology. 1987;66:327–31.
108. Morphine. Micromedex Solutions. Truven Health Analytics, Inc. Ann Arbor, MI. Available at: http://www.micromedexsolutions.com. Accessed May 1, 2016.
109. Bailie GR, Johnson CA. Safety of propoxyphene in dialysis patients. Semin Dial. 2002;15:375.
110. Almirall J, Montoliu J, Torras A, Revert L. Propoxyphene-induced hypoglycemia in a patient with chronic renal failure. Nephron. 1989;53:273–5.
111. Roberts SM, Levy G. Pharmacokinetic studies of propoxyphene IV: effect of renal failure on systemic clearance in rats. J Pharm Sci. 1980;69:363–4.
112. Dean M. Opioids in renal failure and dialysis patients. J Pain Symptom Manag. 2004;28:497–504.
113. Salomon L, Levu S, Deray G, Launay-Vacher V, Brucker G, Ravaud P. Assessing residents' prescribing behavior in renal impairment. Int J Qual Health Care. 2003;15:235–40.
114. Pillans PI, Landsberg PG, Fleming AM, Fanning M, Sturtevant JM. Evaluation of dosage adjustment in patients with renal impairment. Intern Med J. 2003;33:10–3.
115. Papaioannou A, Clarke JA, Campbell G, Bedard M. Assessment of adherence to renal dosing guidelines in long-term care facilities. J Am Geriatr Soc. 2000;48:1470–3.
116. Gilbert DN, Bennett WM. Use of antimicrobial agents in renal failure. Infect Dis Clin N Am. 1989;3:517–31.
117. Fissell W. Laboratory assays in renal failure: therapeutic drug monitoring. Semin Dial. 2014;27:614–7.
118. Craig W. Pharmacodynamics of antimicrobial agents as a basis for determining dosage regimens. Eur J Clin Microbiol Infect Dis. 1993;12(Suppl 1):S6–8.
119. Aronoff GR. Antimicrobial therapy in patients with impaired renal function. Am J Kidney Dis. 1983;3:106–10.
120. Hewitt WL, McHenry MC. Blood level determinations of antimicrobial drugs. Some clinical considerations. Med Clin North Am. 1978;62:1119–40.
121. Lacy MK, Nicolau DP, Nightingale CH, Quintiliani R. The pharmacodynamics of aminoglycosides. Clin Infect Dis. 1998;27:23–7.
122. Tulkens PM. Efficacy and safety of aminoglycosides once-a-day: experimental and clinical data. Scand J Infect Dis Suppl. 1990;74:249–57.
123. Humes HD. Insights into ototoxicity. Analogies to nephrotoxicity. Ann N Y Acad Sci. 1999;884:15–8.
124. Kirkpatrick CM, Duffull SB, Begg EJ. Pharmacokinetics of gentamicin in 957 patients with varying renal function dosed once daily. Br J Clin Pharmacol. 1999;47:637–43.
125. Swan SK. Aminoglycoside nephrotoxicity. Semin Nephrol. 1997;17:27–33.
126. Townsend PL, Fink MP, Stein KL, Murphy SG. Aminoglycoside pharmacokinetics: dosage requirements and nephrotoxicity in trauma patients. Crit Care Med. 1989;17:154–7.

127. Duszynska W, Taccone FS, Hurkacz M, Kowalska-Krochmal B, Wiela-Hojenska A, Kubler A. Therapeutic drug monitoring of amikacin in septic patients. Crit Care. 2013;17:R165–R74.
128. Freeman CD, Nicolau DP, Belliveau PP, Nightingale CH. Once-daily dosing of aminoglycosides: review and recommendations for clinical practice. J Antimicrob Chemother. 1997;39:677–86.
129. Anaizi N. Once-daily dosing of aminoglycosides. A consensus document. Int J Clin Pharmacol Ther. 1997;35:223–6.
130. Ali MZ, Goetz MB. A meta-analysis of the relative efficacy and toxicity of single daily dosing versus multiple daily dosing of aminoglycosides. Clin Infect Dis. 1997;24:796–809.
131. Boyer A, Gruson D, Bouchet S, et al. Aminoglycosides in septic shock: an overview, with specific consideration given to their nephrotoxic risk. Drug Saf. 2013;36:217–30.
132. DeGrado JR, Cios D, Greenwood BC, Kubiak DW, Szumita PM. Pharmacodynamic target attainment with high-dose extended-interval tobramycin therapy in patients with cystic fibrosis. J Chemother. 2014;26:101–4.
133. Barclay ML, Kirkpatrick CM, Begg EJ. Once daily aminoglycoside therapy. Is it less toxic than multiple daily doses and how should it be monitored? Clin Pharmacokinet. 1999;36:89–98.
134. Baddour LM, Wilson WR, Bayer AS, On behalf of the American Heart Association Committee on Rheumatic Fever E, and Kawasaki Disease of the Council on Cardiovascular Disease in the Young, Council on Clinical Cardiology, Council on Cardiovascular Surgery and Anesthesia, and Stroke Council. Infective endocarditis in adults: diagnosis, antimicrobial therapy, and management of complications: a scientific statement for healthcare professionals from the American Heart Association. Circulation. 2015;132.
135. Habib G, Lacellotti P, Antunes MJ, et al. 2015 ESC guidelines for the management of infective endocarditis. The Task Force for the Management of Infective Endocarditis of the European Society of Cardiology (ESC). Endorsed by: European Association for Cardio-Thoracic Surgery (EACTS), the European Association of Nuclear Medicine (EANM). Eur Heart J. 36(44):2015, 3075–3128.
136. Fernandez-Hidalgo N, Almirante B, Gavalda J, et al. Ampicillin plus Ceftriaxone is as effective as Ampicillin plus Gentamicin for treating enterococcus faecalis infective endocarditis. CID. 2013;56:1261–8.
137. Bernstein JM, Erk SD. Choice of antibiotics, pharmacokinetics, and dose adjustments in acute and chronic renal failure. Med Clin North Am. 1990;74:1059–76.
138. Verbist L, Verpooten GA, Giuliano RA, et al. Pharmacokinetics and tolerance after repeated doses of imipenem/cilastatin in patients with severe renal failure. J Antimicrob Chemother. 1986;18 Suppl E:115–20.
139. Cunha GM, Moraes RA, Moraes GA, Franca MC Jr, Moraes MO, Viana GS. Nerve growth factor, ganglioside and vitamin E reverse glutamate cytotoxicity in hippocampal cells. Eur J Pharmacol. 1999;367:107–12.
140. Manian FA, Stone WJ, Alford RH. Adverse antibiotic effects associated with renal insufficiency. Rev Infect Dis. 1990;12:236–49.
141. Giles LJ, Jennings AC, Thomson AH, Creed G, Beale RJ, McLuckie A. Pharmacokinetics of meropenem in intensive care unit patients receiving continuous veno-venous hemofiltration or hemodiafiltration. Crit Care Med. 2000;28:632–7.
142. Ververs TF, van Dijk A, Vinks SA, et al. Pharmacokinetics and dosing regimen of meropenem in critically ill patients receiving continuous venovenous hemofiltration. Crit Care Med. 2000;28:3412–6.
143. Kirby WM, De Maine JB, Serrill WS. Pharmacokinetics of the cephalosporins in healthy volunteers and uremic patients. Postgrad Med J. 1971;47(Suppl):41–6.
144. Wright N, Wise R, Hegarty T. Cefotetan elimination in patients with varying degrees of renal dysfunction. J Antimicrob Chemother. 1983;11(Suppl):213 6.
145. Tam VH, McKinnon PS, Akins RL, Drusano GL, Rybak MJ. Pharmacokinetics and pharmacodynamics of cefepime in patients with various degrees of renal function. Antimicrob Agents Chemother. 2003;47:1853–61.
146. Harding I, Sorgel F. Comparative pharmacokinetics of teicoplanin and vancomycin. J Chemother. 2000;12(Suppl 5):15–20.
147. Linden PK. Amphotericin B lipid complex for the treatment of invasive fungal infections. Expert Opin Pharmacother. 2003;4:2099–110.
148. Pinder M, Bellomo R, Lipman J. Pharmacological principles of antibiotic prescription in the critically ill. Anaesth Intensive Care. 2002;30:134–44.
149. Falagas ME, Tansarli GS, Ikawa K, Vardakas KZ. Clinical outcomes with extended or continuous versus short-term intravenous infusion of carbapenems and piperacillin/tazobactam: a systematic review and meta-analysis. Clin Infect Dis. 2013;56:272–82.
150. Hohlfelder B, Kubiak DW, DeGrado JR, Reardon DP, Szumita PM. Implementation of a prolonged infusion guideline for time dependent antimicrobial agents at a tertiary academic medical center. Am J Ther. 2015;Accepted ahead of publication.
151. Nightingale CH. Pharmacokinetic considerations in quinolone therapy. Pharmacotherapy. 1993;13:34S–8S.
152. Rodvold KA, Neuhauser M. Pharmacokinetics and pharmacodynamics of fluoroquinolones. Pharmacotherapy. 2001;21:233S–52S.
153. Boelaert J, Valcke Y, Schurgers M, et al. The pharmacokinetics of ciprofloxacin in patients with

impaired renal function. J Antimicrob Chemother. 1985;16:87–93.
154. Garaud JJ, Regnier B, Inglebert F, Faurisson F, Bauchet J, Vachon F. Vancomycin pharmacokinetics in critically ill patients. J Antimicrob Chemother. 1984;14(Suppl D):53–7.
155. Gonzalez-Martin G, Acuna V, Perez C, Labarca J, Guevara A, Tagle R. Pharmacokinetics of vancomycin in patients with severely impaired renal function. Int J Clin Pharmacol Ther. 1996;34:71–5.
156. Whelton A. Antibiotic pharmacokinetics and clinical application in renal insufficiency. Med Clin North Am. 1982;66:267–81.
157. Marquis KA, DeGrado JR, Labonville S, Kubiak DW, Szumita PM. Evaluation of a pharmacist-directed vancomycin dosing and monitoring pilot program at a tertiary academic medical center. Ann Pharmacother. 2015;49:1009–14.
158. Sinha Ray A, Haikal A, Hammoud KA, Yu AS. Vancomycin and the risk of AKI: a systematic review and meta-analysis. Clin J Am Soc Nephrol. 2016;11:2132–40.
159. Gupta K, Gupta A. Mucormycosis and acute kidney injury. J Nephropathol. 2012;1:155–9.
160. Harbarth S, Pestotnik SL, Lloyd JF, Burke JP, Samore MH. The epidemiology of nephrotoxicity associated with conventional amphotericin B therapy. Am J Med. 2001;111:528–34.
161. Safdar A, Ma J, Saliba F, et al. Drug-induced nephrotoxicity caused by amphotericin B lipid complex and liposomal amphotericin B: a review and meta-analysis. Medicine. 2010;89:236–44.
162. Costa S, Nucci M. Can we decrease amphotericin nephrotoxicity? Curr Opin Crit Care. 2001;7:379–83.
163. Ullmann AJ. Review of the safety, tolerability, and drug interactions of the new antifungal agents caspofungin and voriconazole. Curr Med Res Opin. 2003;19:263–71.
164. Burkhardt O, Thon S, Burhenne J, Welte T, Kielstein J. Sulphobutylether-B-cyclodextrin accumulation in critically ill patients with acute kidney injury treated with intravenous voriconazole under extended daily dialysis. Int J Antimicrob Agents. 2010;36:93–4.
165. Lilly C, Welch V, Mayer T, Ranauro P, Meisner J, Luke D. Evaluation of intravenous voriconazole in patients with compromised renal function. BMC Infect Dis. 2013;13:14–21.
166. Arredondo G, Martinez-Jorda R, Calvo R, Aguirre C, Suarez E. Protein binding of itraconazole and fluconazole in patients with chronic renal failure. Int J Clin Pharmacol Ther. 1994;32:361–4.
167. Grant SM, Clissold SP. Itraconazole. A review of its pharmacodynamic and pharmacokinetic properties, and therapeutic use in superficial and systemic mycoses. Drugs. 1989;37:310–44.
168. Cresemba prescribing information. Astellas, 2015. https://www.astellas.us/docs/cresemba.pdf. Accessed 24 Oct 2015.
169. Cornely OA, Bohme A, Schmitt-Hoffmann A, Ullmann AJ. Safety and pharmacokinetics of isavuconazole as antifungal prophylaxis in acute myeloid leukemia patients with neutropenia: results of a phase 2, dose escalation study. Antimicrob Agents Chemother. 2015;59:2078–85.

Index

S. S. Waikar et al. (eds.), *Core Concepts in Acute Kidney Injury*,
https://doi.org/10.1007/978-1-4939-8628-6

U

V

W

Printed by Printforce, the Netherlands